ADVANCED THERAPEUTIC ENDOSCOPY

SECOND EDITION

Advanced Therapeutic Endoscopy
Second Edition

Editors

Jamie S. Barkin, M.D., F.A.C.P., F.A.C.G.
Professor of Medicine
University of Miami School of Medicine
Chief, Division of Gastroenterology
Mount Sinai Medical Center
Miami Beach, Florida

Cesar A. O'Phelan, M.D.
Associate Professor of Medicine
University of Navarra
Pamplona, Spain
Chief, Section of Gastroenterology
AMI Palmetto General Hospital
Miami, Florida

RAVEN PRESS 〰 NEW YORK

Raven Press, 1185 Avenue of the Americas, New York, New York 10036

Made in the United States of America

Library of Congress Cataloging in Publishing Data

Advanced therapeutic endoscopy / edited by Jamie S. Barkin and Cesar A. O'Phelan.—2nd ed.
  p. cm.
  Includes bibliographical references and index.
  ISBN 0-7817-0155-4
  1. Endoscopic surgery. 2. Endoscopy—Therapeutic use.
I. Barkin, Jamie S. II. O'Phelan, Cesar A.
  [DNLM: 1. Digestive System Diseases—therapy. 2. Digestive System Neoplasms—therapy. 3. Endoscopy, Digestive System—methods. WI 100 A261 1994]
RD33.53.A34 1994
617′.05—dc20
DNLM/DLC
for Library of Congress   94-11968
                                                            CIP

9 8 7 6 5 4 3 2 1

*To our wives, Faith and Mary,
and our children, Jodie, Ryan, and Kristy,
for their love, patience, and support.*

Contents

Contributors

Anthony Albanese, M.D.
Divisions of Gastroenterology and
  Hepatology
University of Miami School of Medicine,
  and Veterans Administration Medical
  Center
Miami, Florida 33101

John Baillie, M.D., M.B., Ch.B., F.R.C.P.
  (Glasgow)
Division of Gastroenterology
Duke University Medical Center
Box 3189
Durham, North Carolina 27710

Jamie S. Barkin, M.D., F.A.C.P.,
  F.A.C.G.
Division of Gastroenterology
Mount Sinai Medical Center
4300 Alton Road
Miami Beach, Florida 33140

Stanley B. Benjamin, M.D.
Department of Medicine
Division of Gastroenterology
Georgetown University Medical Center
Washington, D.C. 20007

David Bernstein, M.D.
Division of Gastroenterology
University of Miami School of Medicine
Jackson Memorial Hospital
Miami, Florida 33101

Kenneth F. Binmoeller, M.D.
Department of Endoscopic Surgery
University Hospital Hamburg-Eppendorf
Martinistrasse 52
2000 Hamburg 20
Germany

Patrick G. Brady, M.D.
Department of Internal Medicine
University of South Florida
College of Medicine
12901 Bruce B. Downs Boulevard
Tampa, Florida 33612; and
Department of Medicine
James A. Haley Veterans Affairs Hospital
Medical Service (111B)
13000 Bruce B. Downs Boulevard
Tampa, Florida 33612

Gustavo A. Calleja, M.D.
Division of Gastroenterology
Mount Sinai Medical Center
4300 Alton Road
Miami Beach, Florida 33140

David L. Carr-Locke, M.D., F.R.C.P.,
  F.A.C.G.
Brigham and Women's Hospital and
  Harvard Medical School
Division of Gastroenterology
75 Francis Street
Boston, Massachusetts 02115

Donald O. Castell, M.D.
Department of Medicine
The Graduate School
1800 Lombard Street
Philadelphia, Pennsylvania 19146

Sidney Chung, M.D.
Chinese University of Hong Kong
Department of Surgery
Prince of Wales Hospital
Shatin, New Territories
Hong Kong

Meinhard Classen, M.D.
Med Klinik Und Poliklinik
Der Technishchen Universitat Munchen
Klinikum Rechts Der Isar
Ismaninger Strasse 22
8000 Munich, Germany

Seth A. Cohen, M.D.
Department of Medicine
Columbia University
60 East End Avenue
St. Luke's-Roosevelt Hospital Center; and
Assistant Attending
Beth Israel Medical Center
New York, New York 10028

John T. Cunningham, M.D.
Department of Medicine
Gastrointestinal Division
Gastroenterology Division
Medical University of South Carolina
College of Medicine
171 Ashley Avenue
Charleston, South Carolina 29425

P. Gregory Foutch, C.O., M.S., F.A.C.P.,
  F.A.C.G.
Department of Medicine
Division of Gastroenterology
University of Arizona
Tucson, Arizona; and
Division of Gastroenterology
Desert Samaritan Hospital
1520 South Dobson Road, Suite 302
Mesa, Arizona 85202

Joseph E. Geenen, M.D.
Department of Gastroenterology
Medical College of Wisconsin
1333 College Avenue
Racine, Wisconsin 53403

Colonel Fred H. Goldner, M.D., F.A.C.P.
Department of Medicine
Department of the Army
Brooke Army Medical Center
HSHE MDG
2450 Stanley Road
Fort Sam Houston, Texas 78234

Markus Goldschmiedt, M.D.
Department of Medicine
Parkland Memorial Hospital
Sixth Floor, South
5201 Harry Hines Boulevard
Dallas, Texas 75235

Pradeep K. Gupta, M.D.
Department of Medicine
Division of Gastroenterology
Georgetown University Medical Center
3800 Reservoir Road N.W.
Washington, D.C. 20007

Gregory B. Haber, M.D., F.R.C.P.(C)
Department of Gastroenterology
University of Toronto
The Wellesley Hospital
160 Wellesley Street, East
Toronto, Ontario M4Y 1J3 Canada

Friedrich Hagenmüller, M.D.
Department of Medicine 1
Allgemeines Krankenhaus
Altona, Paul Erlich-Strasse 1
D-22763 Hamburg, Germany

Robert H. Hawes, M.D.
Department of Medicine
Division of Gastroenterology/Hepatology
Indiana University School of Medicine
Indiana University Hospital and
  Outpatient Center
550 University Boulevard, Room 2300
Indianapolis, Indiana 46202

Stephen K. Heier, M.D., F.A.C.P.,
  F.A.C.G.
Section of Endoscopy
Department of Clinical Medicine
New York Medical College
Valhalla, New York 10595

Ulrich Hildebrandt, M.D.
Department of General Surgery
University of Saarland
6650 Homburg/Saar
Germany

K. Huibregtse, M.D.
Department of Gastroenterology and
  Hepatology
Academic Medical Center
University of Amsterdam
Meibergdreef 9
1105 AZ Amsterdam
The Netherlands

Lennox J. Jeffers, M.D.
Divisions of Gastroenterology and
  Hepatology
University of Miami School of Medicine,
  and
Veterans Administration Medical Center
1201 N.W. 16th Street
Miami, Florida 33101

Dennis M. Jensen, M.D.
Department of Medicine
Division of Gastroenterology
University of California, Los Angeles
Center for the Health Sciences
Center for Ulcer Research and Education
* (CURE)*
10833 Le Conte Avenue
Los Angeles, California 90024; and
West Los Angeles Veterans
*   Administration Medical Center*
Los Angeles, California 90024

Rome Jutabha, M.D.
Department of Medicine
Division of Gastroenterology
University of California, Los Angeles
Center for the Health Sciences,
*   Room 44-138*
Center for Ulcer Research and Education
* (Cure)*
10833 Le Conte Avenue
Los Angeles, California 90024; and
West Los Angeles Veterans
*   Administration Medical Center*
Los Angeles, California 90024-1684

Lieutenant Colonel Shailesh C. Kadakia,
** M.D., F.A.C.P., F.A.C.G., F.C.C.P.**
University of Texas Health Science
*   Center at San Antonio*
San Antonio, Texas; and
Gastroenterology Service
Department of Medicine
Department of the Army
Brooke Army Medical Center
HSHE MDG
2450 Stanley Road
Fort Sam Houston, Texas 78234

Ronald M. Katon, M.D.
Division of Gastroenterology
Oregon Health Sciences University
3181 S.W. Sam Jackson Park Road
Portland, Oregon 97201

A. J. Katz, M.D.
Department of Pediatric Gastroenterology
Newton-Wellesley Hospital; and
Pediatric Gastroenterology Associates PC
319 Longwood Avenue
Boston, Massachusetts 02115

Michael L. Kochman, M.D.
Department of Medicine
Division of Gastroenterology
University of Pennsylvania
3400 Spruce Street
Philadelphia, Pennsylvania 19104

Richard A. Kozarek, M.D.
Gastroenterology Division
Virginia Mason Clinic
1100 9th Avenue
P.O. Box 900 (C3-N)
Seattle, Washington 98101; and
Department of Medicine
University of Washington
Seattle, Washington 98111

Loren Laine, M.D.
Division of Gastrointestinal and Liver
*   Diseases (LAC 12-37)*
Department of Medicine
University of Southern California School
*   of Medicine*
2025 Zonal Avenue, LAC 11-221
Los Angeles, California 90033

John G. Lee, M.D.
Division of Gastroenterology
Duke University Medical Center
Box 3913
Durham, North Carolina 27710

Glen A. Lehman, M.D.
Department of Medicine
Division of Gastroenterology/Hepatology
Indiana University School of Medicine
550 North University Boulevard. #2300
Indianapolis, Indiana 46202

Joseph W. Leung, M.D., F.R.C.P. (Edin),
** F.R.C.P. (Glas)**
Division of Gastroenterology
Duke University Medical Center
Box 3913
Durham, North Carolina 27710

Blair S. Lewis, M.D.
Department of Gastroenterology
Mount Sinai School of Medicine
New York, New York 10028

David Lieberman, M.D.
Department of Medicine
Oregon Health Sciences University
Portland, Oregon 97201; and
Department of Gastroenterology
Veterans Administration Medical Center
3710 S.W. Veteran's Hospital Road
Portland, Oregon 97207

Gustavo A. Machicado, M.D.
Department of Medicine
Division of Gastroenterology
University of California, Los Angeles
Center for the Health Sciences
Center for Ulcer Research and Education
10833 Le Conte Avenue
Los Angeles, California 90024

Howard D. Manten, M.D.
Division of Gastroenterology (D49)
University of Miami School of Medicine
Jackson Memorial Hospital
P.O. Box 016960
Miami, Florida 33101

Norman E. Marcon, M.D.
Division of Gastroenterology
The Wellesley Hospital
121 Jones Building
160 Wellesley Street East
Toronto, Ontario M4Y 1J3
Canada

Lee McHenry, Jr., M.D.
Division of Gastroenterology
Department of Medicine
Medical College of Virginia
Box 711 MCV Station
Richmond, Virginia 23292

John D. Mellinger, M.D.
West Michigan Surgical Specialists
245 Cherry S.E., Suite 102
Grand Rapids, Michigan 49503

Larry S. Miller, M.D.
Department of Medicine
Section of Gastroenterology
Temple University Hospital
3401 North Broad Street
Philadelphia, Pennsylvania 19140

Horst Neuhaus, M.D.
Med Klinik Und Poliklinik
Der Technishchen Universitat Munchen
Klinikum Rechts Der Isar
Ismaninger Strasse 22
8000 Munich, Germany

H. Juergen Nord, M.D., F.A.C.P.
Department of Medicine
Division of Digestive Diseases and
 Nutrition
University of South Florida
College of Medicine
Harbourside Medical Tower, Suite 630
4 Columbia Drive
Tampa, Florida 33606

Cesar A. O'Phelan, M.D.
Department of Medicine
University of Navarra
Pamplona, Spain; and
Section of Gastroenterology
AMI Palmetto General Hospital
2001 West 68th Street
Miami, Florida 33016

V. K. Parasher, M.D.
Departments of Gastroenterology and
 Hepatology
Academic Medical Center
University of Amsterdam
Meibergdreef 9
1105 AZ Amsterdam,
The Netherlands

Haim Pinkas, M.D.
Department of Medicine
James A. Haley Veterans Hospital
13000 Bruce B. Downs Boulevard
Tampa, Florida 33612

Jeffrey L. Ponsky, M.D.
Department of Surgery
Mount Sinai Medical Center
One Mount Sinai Drive
Cleveland, Ohio 44106; and Department
 of Surgery
Case Western Reserve University
Cleveland, Ohio 44106

Marios Pouagare, M.D., Ph.D.
Department of Medicine
James A. Haley Veterans Hospital
13000 Bruce B. Downs Boulevard
Tampa, Florida 33612

Isaac Raijman, M.D.
Gastroenterology & Therapeutic
 Endoscopy
Rosedale Medical Centre, Suite 412
600 Sherbourne Street
Toronto, Ontario M4X 1W4
Canada

Erik A. J. Rauws, M.D., Ph.D.
Department of Gastroenterology and
 Hepatology
Academic Medical Center
University of Amsterdam
Meibergdreef 9
1105 AZ Amsterdam
The Netherlands

Robert A. Sanowski, M.D.
University of Arizona
College of Medicine
Tucson, Arizona; and
Chief of Gastroenterology
Carl T. Hayden Veterans Affairs Medical
  Center
650 E. Indian School Road
Phoenix, Arizona 85012

Richard R. Saxon, M.D.
Dotter Institute of Interventional
  Radiology, L342
Oregon Health Sciences University
3181 Southwest Sam Jackson Park Road
Portland, Oregon 97210

Mark Schiele, M.D.
Fellow, Division of Gastroenterology
Oregon Health Sciences University
3181 S.W. Sam Jackson Park Road
Portland, Oregon 97201

M. N. Schoeman, M.D.
Department of Gastroenterology and
  Hepatology
Academic Medical Center
University of Amsterdam
Meibergdreef 9
1105 AZ Amsterdam
The Netherlands

Henning Schwacha, M.D.
Department of Medicine 1
Allgemeines Krankenhaus
Altona, Paul Erlich-Strasse 1
D-22763 Hamburg
Germany

Jerome H. Siegel, M.D., P.C., F.A.C.P.,
  F.A.C.G.
Department of Endoscopy
Mount Sinai School of Medicine
Beth Israel Medical Center, North
  Division
60 East End Avenue
New York, New York 10028

Stephen E. Silvis, M.D.
Department of Medicine
University of Minnesota School of
  Medicine; and
Gastrointestinal Section (111D)
Department of Veterans Affairs Medical
  Center
One Veterans Drive
Minneapolis, Minnesota 55417

Nib Soehendra, M.D.
Department of Endoscopic Surgery
University Hospital Hamburg-Eppendorf
Martinistrasse 52
2000 Hamburg 20
Germany

Steven J. Squillace, M.D.
Department of Gastroenterology
Carl T. Hayden Veterans Affairs Medical
  Center
650 E. Indian School Road
Phoenix, Arizona 85012

Greg Van Stiegmann, M.D.
Department of Surgery
University of Colorado Health Science
  Center
Box C 313
4200 East 9th Avenue
Denver, Colorado 80262

Thian Lok Tio, M.D., Ph.D.
Division of Gastroenterology
Department of Medicine
Georgetown University Medical Center
Room 2122 Main
Washington, D.C. 20007

Stephen Wise Unger, M.D., F.A.C.S.
Surgical Endoscopy and
  Laparoscopy
Mount Sinai Medical Center
4302 Alton Road
Miami Beach, Florida 33140

Rama P. Venu, M.D.
Department of Medicine
Section of Digestive and Liver Disease
University of Illinois at Chicago
840 S. Wood Street M/C 787
Chicago, Illinois 60612

David T. Walden, M.D.
Division of Gastroenterology
The Wellesley Hospital
121 Jones Building
160 Wellesley Street East
Toronto, Ontario M4Y 1J3, Canada

Jerome D. Waye, M.D.
Department of Medicine
Mount Sinai School of Medicine (City
*   University of New York)*
Gastrointestinal Endoscopy Unit
Mount Sinai Hospital
New York, New York 10028

I. Waxman, M.D.
Department of Gastroenterology and
*   Hepatology*
Academic Medical Center
University of Amsterdam
Meibergdreef 9
1105 AZ Amsterdam
The Netherlands

Maurits J. Wiersema, M.D.
Department of Medicine
Division of Gastroenterology/Hepatology
Indiana University School of Medicine
St. Vincent Hospital and Health Care
*   Center*
Indiana Gastroenterology Inc.
8424 Naab Road
Indianapolis, Indiana 46260

Colonel Roy K. H. Wong, M.D., F.A.C.P.,
**   F.A.C.G.**
Gastroenterology Service
Walter Reed Army Medical Center
Washington, D.C.; and
Department of Medicine
Uniformed Services University of Health
*   Science*
Bethesda, Maryland 20892

William C. Wu, M.D.
Division of Gastroenterology
Department of Medicine
Oregon Health Sciences University
School of Medicine
3181 S.W. Sam Jackson Park Road
Portland, Oregon 97201

Alvin M. Zfass, M.D.
Division of Gastroenterology
Department of Medicine
Medical College of Virginia
Richmond, Virginia 23292

Foreword

What do we expect from therapeutic endoscopy? This procedure should become safer, better, and be used for a wider variety of gastroenterologic and pancreatic disorders. The future of therapeutic endoscopy will be fundamentally influenced by the improvement of the image quality. The standard of high-definition television (HDTV) with excellent resolution and true color reproduction will be reached probably within the next 5 years. Light reflexes and other noise signals such as the "blooming effect" already can be electronically eliminated so that safe operating at very close distances will be achieved. Electronic image enhancement may have a variety of clinical implications such as a detailed diagnosis of mucosal alterations or a differential diagnosis of macroscopically undetermined lesions by a computerized analysis of selected details. Stereoscopic endoscopy already allows a precise three-dimensional (3-D) measurement of circumscript findings. The development of a system that provides therapeutic interventions demonstrated in a 3-D image will probably require the introduction of smaller CCD chips. These devices could also be used for miniscopes, which are today still based on fiber technology with a limited image, quality, and durability.

The improvement of the endoscopic image will be completed by new echoendoscopes and ultrasonic probes that demonstrate the anatomic layers and the infiltration depth of pathological lesions under the mucosal surface of the gastrointestinal, biliary, and pancreatic tract. Therapeutic decisions must be based on these results and endoscopic interventions such as an excision of an early gastric cancer or a transmural drainage procedure should be "tailored" on the basis of the EUS image.

Based on this preoperative staging in the upper and lower gastrointestinal tract, the local management of neoplastic lesions may be improved by modern laser techniques, including photodynamic therapy, and by bipolar electrocoagulation, promising a reduced destruction of the surrounding normal tissue. Sophisticated systems for banding, clipping, and sewing through flexible endoscopes are already available and allow definitive hemostasis of bleeding varices and ulcers, or they could be applied in selected cases of perforation. A combined approach of an endoscopic procedure with a laparoscopic technique seems to be reasonable for removal of larger polyps or perforation of the stomach and the colon.

Miniscopes with an outer diameter of 2 to 4 mm are available for the peroral access to the biliary and pancreatic tree via duodenoscopes. This approach is completed by percutaneous techniques for those patients in whom the peroral route is not possible. The image quality has been considerably improved by the introduction of electronic cameras that are adapted to the thin fiberscopes. Further technical advances require specially designed electronic videoscopes. These methods allow direct visualization of the bile duct system and the main pancreatic duct with a satisfactory image quality. Improvement of our cumbersome biopsy techniques is urgently required to confirm the macroscopic diagnosis by an adequate histological examination. The main purpose of therapeutic endoscopy in the biliopancreatic tract is the safe and effective management of stones and strictures. Laser systems with an automatic cut-out technique upon tissue contact are under experimental and clinical evaluation. This method provides disintegration of bile and pancreatic duct stones into microparticles, with no risk of ductal lesions. Due to the safety of the technique and the use of ultrathin fibers for energy transmission, the procedure can be carried out by conventional duodenoscopes even under fluoroscopic control—or better, under direct vision with miniscopes. Treatment of ductal stones without papillotomy may become possible, at least in selected cases.

The management of malignant or benign stenosis of the gastrointestinal tract and biliopancreatic system will be further improved by endoscopic implantation of self-expandable stents. Many devices are currently under evaluation. The technique offers several advantages over dilatation alone or insertion of conventional plastic prostheses. The implantation procedure is safe and convenient for the patient due to the small diameter of the introducer system. After release, the wide diameter, the macroporous configuration, and the small surface area are associated with lower rates of migration and clogging than are seen with conventional endoprostheses. The risk of tumor infiltration through the wire mesh may be overcome by recently developed plastic covered metal stents. Preliminary experiences indicate that these devices are removable so that they may be useful for benign strictures of the esophagus, the biliary tree, or the main pancreatic duct. The invention of self-absorbing stents may be an appropriate alternative. Recent studies show that initially higher costs of metal stents are equalized by a reduction of reinterventions for complications in the long term.

In conclusion, promising new endoscopic techniques are being currently evaluated *in vitro* and *in vivo*. Previously introduced procedures can be carried out less invasively due to the development of miniscopes with an excellent image quality and appropriate equipment for therapeutic interventions. A prospective futuristic view into the potential of therapeutic endoscopy shows that *carefully designed clinical studies are required to demonstrate clinical advantages in terms of safety, improvement, and new indications.*

Meinhard Classen
Horst Neuhaus

Preface

Advanced Therapeutic Endoscopy Second Edition is a concise text that highlights the most current, advanced techniques and new directions in therapeutic gastrointestinal endoscopy. This book provides a step-by-step guide to the latest and most innovative techniques. The chapters are organized with sections covering individual gastrointestinal organ systems, hemostasis, endoscopic ultrasound, and laparoscopy. Contributions by the world's foremost therapeutic endoscopy experts provide up-to-date, authoritative discussions.

The appropriate use of many therapeutic modalities are presented. These include balloon dilation of gastrointestinal strictures, endoscopic ligation and its effects, selective aspects contrasting pediatric with adult endoscopy, the endoscopic management of problems of the biliary and pancreatic ductal system, advances in the removal of foreign objects from the upper and lower GI tract, and the application of laser technology. In addition, the expanding utility of enteroscopy and the explosion of laparoscopic surgical interventions are addressed. We trust that this new edition will have the same acceptance as the first and that the information imparted will assist in providing better care of our patients.

Jamie S. Barkin
Cesar A. O'Phelan

Acknowledgments

We are grateful to the contributors for their efforts and willingness to share their knowledge with others.

We are indebted to Shirley Vance for coordinating this project. Her dedication and efficiency contributed significantly to the production of this book. We are also grateful to Kathy Lyons and the staff at Raven Press for ensuring that our standards were met.

Advanced Therapeutic Endoscopy, 2nd Ed.,
edited by J. S. Barkin and C. A. O'Phelan.
Raven Press, Ltd., New York © 1994.

CHAPTER 1

Endoscopic Evaluation of the Pharynx and Passage Through the Upper Esophageal Sphincter Made Simple

Robert A. Sanowski and Steven J. Squillace

Every upper gastrointestinal endoscopic procedure should begin with an examination of the pharynx, the laryngeal area, and the vocal cords. Unfortunately, many gastroenterologists ignore this area and consider it simply as the initial hurdle for viewing the tubular esophagus. But in this critical area early carcinoma of the pharynx and vocal cords may be detected and other lesions, such as esophageal webs and diverticula, may be seen. In this region the normal anatomy is tortuous and physiologically constricted, providing a potential site for perforation and endoscopic trauma. Understanding the anatomy and endoscopic landmarks and appreciation of local pathology will permit the endoscopist to pass through this troublesome space with greater ease.

PREPARATION OF THE PATIENT

The technique of endoscopic passage through the upper esophageal sphincter begins with achieving a level of conscious sedation that will relax the patient and afford the examiner the degree of patient cooperation necessary to carry out the endoscopy and required therapy. Topical anesthetic agents such as 20% benzocaine spray are commonly used in conjunction with conscious sedation. While the benefit of a topical agent

is still in question, spraying the pharyngeal area with a local anesthetic prior to endoscopy does appear to ease instrument passage (1). Conscious sedation also greatly facilitates the examination of patients with a hyperactive gag reflex, such as those individuals with substance abuse or chronic alcoholism (2–4). In addition, if therapeutic endoscopy including wire-guided esophageal dilation or laser fulguration of cancer is contemplated, an increased level of sedation will enhance patient cooperation. We have used a combination of intravenous Demerol and benzodiazepines to achieve an acceptable level of conscious sedation and then titrate the amount of these medications to the age and physical condition of each patient.

TECHNIQUE OF ENDOSCOPE PASSAGE

With the excellent videoendoscope systems now available, a panoramic view of the laryngopharynx is gained. The use of a mouth block protects the endoscope and also provides space for constant pharyngeal suction during the procedure. If nasopharyngeal secretions are promptly removed and the patient's head is flexed forward, aspiration may be avoided. The head should be inclined downward so that secretions do not pool in the pharynx, thus further avoiding aspiration into the trachea with attendant coughing and patient discomfort.

When the tip of the endoscope is passed to the base of the tongue an excellent view of the larynx, piriform sinuses, and pharyngeal wall is achieved. The examiner can easily assess the vocal cords and detect paralysis, polyps, and carcinoma. At this point, care must be

R. A. Sanowski: Department of Medicine, University of Arizona College of Medicine, Tucson, Arizona; and Department of Gastroenterology, Carl T. Hayden Veterans Administration Medical Center, Phoenix, Arizona 85012.

S. J. Squillace: Department of Gastroenterology, Carl T. Hayden Veterans Administration Medical Center, Phoenix, Arizona 85012.

taken not to activate the endoscope irrigation button or coughing and aspiration of water may result. When the vocal cords are clearly seen, the examiner avoids passing the scope into the respiratory tree. This may occur in those patients with a poor gag or cough reflex. Such mistaken passage may cause trauma to related structures and induce bronchospasm and compromise respiration.

Figure 1 provides a view of of the anatomical structures that can be identified during endoscopic examination of the pharynx and laryngeal area.

Following a brief examination of these landmarks, the examiner advances the scope with the right hand to the point indicated in Fig. 2. The thumb of the left hand holds the control knob of the scope handle steady and apposes the scope tip to the point shown in Fig. 2. At approximately 18 cm from the incisor teeth the scope tip encounters the cricopharyngeus muscle and resistance is met. The examiner should direct the endoscope centrally between the piriform sinuses to encounter the cricopharyngeus muscle. Now, keeping in view the image on the video monitor and with the scope tip touching point A, the patient is asked to swallow and simultaneously gentle pressure is applied as the swallow occurs. With a swallow, the upper esophageal sphincter relaxes and the instrument enters the tubular esophagus. Often, however, the passage is not this easy, especially in those patients with a hyperactive gag reflex. The tip of the endoscope may slip into the right or left piriform sinus. The endoscopist must withdraw and try again. A slight gentle rolling of the large control knob while applying slight pressure during a

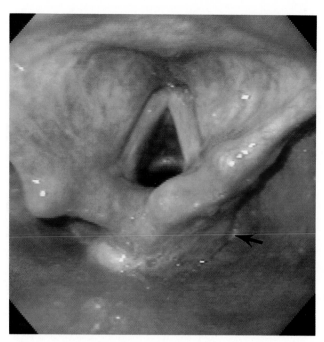

FIG. 2. The point of insertion *(arrow)* of the endoscope tip past the epiglottis into the cervical esophagus.

swallow will also facilitate passage. Timing this maneuver with the patient's swallow is very important.

If there is difficulty in scope passage, patience and care must be exercised to avoid laceration or perforation. A Zenker's diverticulum or carcinoma in this area can certainly impede passage. Symptoms of oropharyngeal dysphagia should alert the examiner to these possibilities. Prior to the endoscopy, any available x-ray studies of this area should be evaluated. In the hyperactive gagger increased sedation may be necessary and on occasion sitting the patient upright and

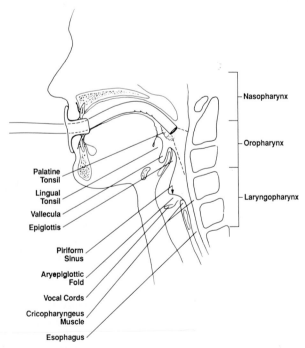

FIG. 1. Anatomical structures identified during endoscopic examination of the pharynx and laryngeal area.

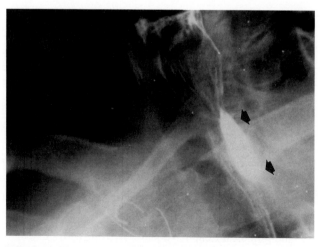

FIG. 3. A Zenker's diverticulum *(arrows)* in a 50-year-old who developed a perforation of this structure following esophagogastroduodenoscopy (EGD).

repeating the above maneuver may facilitate passage of the endoscope.

If a Zenker's diverticulum is suspected on the basis of history or symptoms of oropharyngeal dysphagia, great caution must be exercised to avoid scope impaction in this structure and consequent perforation (Fig. 3). Should there be difficulty in scope passage, a guidewire may be passed with x-ray verification and the endoscope passed over this (5,6).

"Blind" passage of the endoscope using the fingers to depress the tongue while passing the scope through the cricopharyngeal area as the patient swallows is now less commonly used. The direct visualization method described above is easier on the examiner's fingers and allows for a complete examination of the oropharynx.

PATHOLOGY OF THE PHARYNGOESOPHAGEAL AREA

Primary squamous cell carcinoma of the esophagus and secondary involvement of the trachea by primary malignancies of the bronchi are the most common malignancies of this area. Benign tumors are rare.

In 1991, there were approximately 9,400 new cases of pharyngeal cancer with an additional 21,000 cases involving the mouth, lip, and tongue. Unfortunately, the number of cases is on the rise, due to the changes in alcohol and tobacco use among women. The male to female ratio of pharyngeal cancers has changed from 10:1 to 2:1 (7). It is important to note that patients with a history of head and neck cancer are at particularly high risk; up to 14% may develop a second primary tumor (8). Patients with a history of esophageal cancer are also at risk of head and neck tumors, and require surveillance (8). Survival rates depend on the stage of the disease at the time of diagnosis. Careful evaluation of this region with each routine endoscopy may increase the potential for early diagnosis and improved prognosis.

Three intraoral sites are predisposed to develop squamous cell carcinoma. These are the floor of the mouth, the area of the tongue, and the soft palate (9). The most common site for tumor involvement in the hypopharynx is the piriform sinus (9).

Examination of the oral cavity, pharynx, and hypopharynx during routine endoscopy has not received a great deal of attention by gastroenterologists. Kozarek (10) studied the yield of hypopharyngoscopy and nasopharyngoscopy during diagnostic esophagogastroduodenoscopy (EGD). Hypopharyngoscopy involved anterior deflection of the tip of the 8.5 mm endoscope, and the time required was a mean of 30 seconds. A 12% yield for pathologic findings was noted in the 57 patients studied. This simple maneuver may be helpful in detecting pathology in this area such as bleeding telangiectatic lesions.

In addition to discovering cancer, the endoscopist may be called on to remove foreign bodies from the throat. Fish and chicken bones and other foreign materials may lodge in the vallecula, tonsil, pharyngeal wall, hypopharynx, or postcricoid area (11). These may be removed with foreign-body forceps or snares, which the endoscopist has available.

COMPLICATIONS OF PHARYNGOESOPHAGEAL ENDOSCOPY

Traumatic pharyngoesophageal perforation or lacerations may occur during diagnostic and therapeutic procedures. Rigid esophagoscopy for diagnostic and therapeutic management has an incidence of perforation of 0.1% to 1% compared to 0.01% with the flexible endoscope (12). The most common site for perforation is in the cricopharyngeal region (13). The signs and symptoms of pharyngoesophageal injury are subcutaneous emphysema, pain, dysphagia, and sepsis (14). Radiographic studies may confirm the presence of pneumomediastinum and pneumothorax (Fig. 4). An esophagram using water-soluble iodinated radiopaque contrast medium can show the location of a perforation (Fig. 5). Early diagnosis of acute pharyngoesophageal injury is important. If the perforation is small and well contained, medical or conservative management is indicated. Treatment will depend on extent of the perforation and leakage of contrast material. Conservative

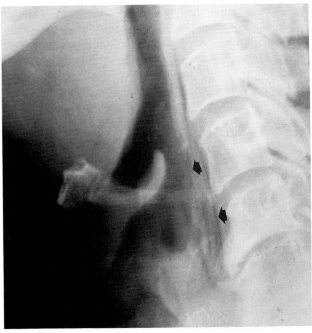

FIG. 4. Air in the soft tissue of the neck *(arrow)* following a perforation of a Zenker's diverticulum.

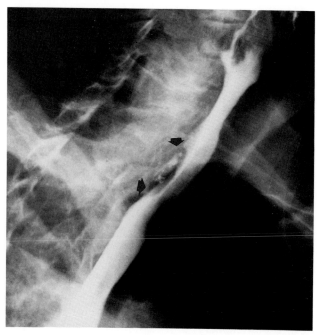

FIG. 5. Esophagram using water-soluble contrast medium in a contained perforation, treated medically with good results.

management of patients with contained perforation includes nothing by mouth, intravenous fluids, and broad spectrum antibiotics with aerobic and anaerobic coverage. Dolgin and colleagues (12) treated ten patients who sustained pharyngoesophageal perforation in this manner, with good results. Surgery is required for large leaks and evidence of sepsis or abscess (15).

Careful examination of the pharyngoesophageal area is an important part of every upper gastrointestinal endoscopic examination. The benefits for the patients include early diagnosis of treatable cancer. The method for maneuvering through this area requires patience and skill, which should characterize all thorough endoscopic examinations. Avoidance of perforation is pos-

sible with careful attention to the local anatomy and by not applying excessive force during instrument passage. Once mastered, the technique of oropharyngoscopy becomes an indispensable part of a complete endoscopic evaluation of the upper gastrointestinal tract.

REFERENCES

1. Lachter J, et al. Topical pharyngeal anesthesia for easing endoscopy: a double-blind, randomized, placebo-controlled study. *Gastrointest Endosc* 1990;36:19–21.
2. Beavis AK, LaBroy S, Misiewicz JJ. Evaluation of one-visit endoscopic clinic for patients with dyspepsia. *Br Med J* 1991;1:1387.
3. Ross WA. Premedication for upper gastrointestinal endoscopy. *Gastrointest Endosc* 1989;35:120–126.
4. Bell GD. Review article: premedication and intravenous sedation for upper gastrointestinal endoscopy. *Aliment Pharmacol Ther* 1990;4:103–122.
5. Catalaro MF, Raijman I. Wire guided endoscope passage (Letter). *Gastrointest Endosc* 1992;38:728.
6. Tsang T, Buto SK. Catheter guided endoscopic intubation: a new technique for intubating a difficult esophagus. *Gastrointest Endosc* 1992;38:49–51.
7. Menck HR, Garfinkel L, Dodd GD. Preliminary report of the National Cancer data base. *CA* 1991;41:7–36.
8. Haughey BH, Arfken CL, Gates GA, Harvey JH. Meta-analysis of second malignant tumors in head and neck cancer: the case for an endoscopic screening protocol. *Ann Otol Rhinol Laryngol* 1992;101:105–112.
9. Harrison DFN. Tumors of the hypopharynx. In: Paparella MM, et al. *Otolaryngology,* 3rd ed. Philadelphia: WB Saunders, 1991.
10. Kozarek RA. Proximal endoscopy: evaluation of the hypo and nasopharynx at time of diagnostic EGD. *Gastrointest Endosc* 1984;191(abst).
11. Jones NS, Lannigan FJ, Salama NY. Foreign bodies in the throat: a prospective study of 388 cases. *J Laryngol Otol* 1991;105:104–108.
12. Dolgin SR, Kumar NR, Wykoff TW, Maniflia AJ. Conservative medical management of traumatic pharyngoesophageal perforations. *Ann Otol Rhinol Laryngol* 1992;101:209–215.
13. Michel L, Grillo HC, Malt RA. Operative and nonoperative management of esophageal perforations. *Ann Surg* 1981;194:56–68.
14. Elleson DA, Rowley SD. Esophageal perforation: its early diagnosis and treatment. *Laryngoscope* 1982;92:678–680.
15. Murphy DW, Roufail WM, Castell DO. Esophageal rupture/perforation: how to select the right treatment. *J Crit Illness* 1992;7:1765–1775.

Advanced Therapeutic Endoscopy, 2nd Ed.,
edited by J. S. Barkin and C. A. O'Phelan.
Raven Press, Ltd., New York © 1994.

CHAPTER 2

Laser Therapy Update: ELT, PDT, LIF, Contact Probes, Low-Power Interstitial Sono-Guided Hyperthermia

Haim Pinkas

Lasers have been used in gastroenterology since 1970 when Youmans et al. (1) treated bleeding gastric erosions with the CO_2 laser via cystoscopy at laparotomy. For the first decade, there was considerable controversy over the selective merits of the argon and neodymium:yttrium-aluminum garnet (Nd:YAG) lasers for control of gastrointestinal hemorrhage. Basic animal studies and clinical trials were carried out with the laser providing a dominant influence on the development of therapeutic endoscopy and turning gastroenterologists into endoscopic surgeons. Some randomized controlled studies and metaanalysis of all the trials using Nd:YAG laser treatment of bleeding ulcers show significant benefit for the treated patients. These studies helped define the predictive value of stigmata of recent hemorrhage and improve patient selection for endoscopic therapy (2). Since cheaper and more portable thermal devices were found to be equal in hemostasis efficacy, the Nd:YAG laser is currently used for the treatment of gastrointestinal tumors.

This chapter is limited to the use of lasers in gastrointestinal oncology.

LASER TUMOR ABLATION (ELT)

The laser's ability to recanalize obstructing esophageal cancer was demonstrated by the innovative work of Fleischer et al. (3). Over the last 10 years, thousands of patients with advanced gastrointestinal (GI) cancers have been treated with Nd:YAG laser, mainly to

H. Pinkas: Department of Medicine, James A. Haley Veterans Administration Hospital; and University of South Florida College of Medicine, Tampa, Florida 33612.

esophageal and low colorectal sites. The results of the enormous clinical experience by multiple investigators are discussed and updated in this section.

Upper Gastrointestinal (UGI) Cancers

The most commonly treated UGI lesions are tumors of the esophagus and the cardia. The main indications for endoscopic laser therapy (ELT) are obstruction and/or bleeding. In general, relief of obstruction does not palliate mediastinal and posterior chest pain, which continue to require analgesic treatment after ELT.

Prognostic factors for the outcome of ELT in UGI tumors were derived from the experience of 26 investigators with 1,098 patients (4–6). Most patients had undergone surgery or radiation therapy before ELT. While recurrence after esophagogastrostomy involved a short segment and quick relief was experienced with ELT (5), recurrence of proximal lesions after radiation therapy, however, presents a frustrating problem for the endoscopist. Radiation-induced pharyngeal muscle dysfunction may be discovered at videoesophagoscopy only after painstaking deobstruction by ELT (6).

The treatment determinants described in Table 1 represent broad guidelines for individualized management of patients with UGI tumors rather than specific indications or contraindications to ELT. In the presence of a tracheoesophageal (TE) fistula, the procedure may be highly beneficial, albeit risky. In this case, carefully performed ELT may establish sufficient esophageal lumen for the placement of a prosthesis, without enlargement of the fistula. Likewise, ELT-induced esophageal patency may permit additional nourish-

TABLE 1. *Prognostic factors of ELT outcome in esophagogastric cancer*

Predictors of good outcome
  Good performance status
  No anorexia
  Mid-esophageal tumor
  Involvement of a straight esophageal segment
  Tumor length <5 cm
  Exophytic lesion
  Mucosal involvement seen at endoscopy
Predictors of poor outcome
  Poor performance status
  Anorexia
  Tumor location in the cervical esophagus
  Fixed horizontal segment at the gastroesophageal junction
  Tumor length >8 cm
  Submucosal involvement at endoscopy/extrinsic compression

TABLE 2. *Results of ELT in UGI tumors*

Indication for the procedure	End point	Occurrence (%)
Obstruction (69)	Luminal patency	97
	Improved dysphagia	83
	Adequate caloric intake	73
	Discharge from hospital	70
Bleeding (34)	Decreased requirement for transfusion	53

ment through a peresophageal percutaneous endoscopic gastrostomy (PEG) placement in patients with persistent anorexia (6).

Technique

The aim of ELT is to vaporize or coagulate the intraluminal tumor. We pass a guidewire through the narrowed lumen and, with the aid of fluoroscopy, perform esophageal polyvinyl bougienage over the guidewire. With the scope inserted through the tumor, we start the treatment distally and advance toward the proximal margin of the tumor. Treatment is applied circumferentially using laser settings of 70 to 90 W for 1 to 2 sec to vaporize the most exophytic intraluminal parts of the tumor, and settings of 40 to 60 W for 0.5 sec to induce coagulative necrosis of the flat tumor areas. In the case of endoscopically impassible stenosis, we use the antegrade technique (3) and some investigators use a laser-resistent guide probe to facilitate the aiming of the laser beam (7).

Repeated sessions are carried out at 48- to 72-hour intervals starting with tapered polyvinyl dilators that push the necrotic debris distally and proceeding with retrograde ELT. Usually two to three treatment sessions in an outpatient setting are required to establish an 11 to 13 mm luminal diameter. To keep the patient dysphagia free, we repeat the laser sessions on a monthly basis or sooner if obstruction recurs. The results of ELT in unselected patients are summarized in Table 2.

ELT is more effective in palliating obstruction than bleeding. We stress the difference between technical and functional success (6).

After relief of obstruction, the performance status of the majority of patients improves. These patients experience a prolongation of survival in comparison to historical controls (8). Karlin et al. (9) and Chatlani et al. (10) found similar impact on survival. The University of South Florida endoscopy team reported the only prospective and randomized study comparing ELT and peroral dilation in the palliation of obstructive esophageal cancer patients undergoing radiation therapy (11). The 1-year survival was 60% for ELT and 20% for peroral dilation (Brady PG, *personal communication*, 1988). The cost-effectiveness of the two treatment modalities expressed as cost per month of survival was comparable. Siegel et al. (12) compared the survival of 36 patients with squamous cell carcinoma of the esophagus treated with ELT and 20 historical controls. The medium survival improved from 5.7 to 9.7 months and the 1-year survival was 38% in ELT patients compared with 20% in controls.

The most frequent complications of ELT are perforation and bacteremia. Perforation rates are usually 5% to 10% (4), while induced bleeding is rarely seen. Kohler et al. (13) reported bacteremia in 33% and sepsis in 10% of patients undergoing ELT. They recommend antibiotic prophylaxis in patients with valvular heart disease or artificial heart valves. Should a fever develop post-ELT, broad-spectrum antibiotics should be administered to prevent sepsis.

Loizou et al. (14) compared ELT with intubation for palliation of malignant dysphagia. Forty-three patients treated with Nd:YAG laser in London were prospectively compared to 30 patients treated with Atkinson endoprosthesis in Nottingham. For thoracic esophageal tumors, the percentage of patients achieving significant improvement in dysphagia grade initially and over the long term was similar (laser, 95% and 77%; intubation, 100% and 86%). For tumors crossing the cardia, intubation was significantly better (laser, 59% and 50%; intubation, 100% and 92%). Thirty-three percent of the ELT patients and 11% of the prosthesis patients were able to eat most or all solid foods. The perforation rate was lower in the laser-treated group (2% vs. 13%). The authors concluded that both forms of therapy need to be used in a complementary fashion tailored to the individual needs of each patient. If the patient was anorectic, endoscopic intubation was preferable with speedy and lasting palliation obviating the need for repeat treatments. If the patient was reasonably healthy with need for near-normal swallowing ability, the laser therapy should be attempted first. If the initial response is good, further treatment sessions should be arranged. If the patient developed only partial or short-term benefit from ELT, endoscopic intubation should be considered early in follow-up. Reed et al. (15) randomized 27 patients with unresectable and obstructing squamous cell carcinoma of the esophagus to one of three treatment groups: (a) insertion of an Atkinson prosthesis alone, (b) insertion of an Atkinson prosthesis followed by radiation therapy, and (c) ELT followed by radiation therapy. Complication rates were 50% in the first group (20% perforations), 38% in the second group, and none in the third group. The quality of palliation was similar in the three small groups and the authors recommend using ELT first, and using stent placement for patients with fistulae on those with extrinsic compression by the tumor.

Sander et al. (16) compared laser alone with laser plus afterloading with iridium-192 for palliation in patients with malignant stenosis of the esophagus. In this prospective randomized study, afterloading prolonged the first dysphagia-free interval (65 vs. 30 days), but overall dysphagia-free time and patient survival were similar. This combination of two local methods of palliation does not offer a significant advantage. Most authors recommend radiation therapy following local palliation. The average period of survival is expected to be twice as long when radiation therapy is combined with a local palliation such as laser or afterloading therapy (17).

The combination of ELT with chemotherapy and radiation therapy promises to increase patient survival in selected cases. In 1985, Pinkas et al. (18) reported a case of squamous cell carcinoma of the esophagus that achieved complete radiologic, endoscopic, and histologic remission after combined treatment by ELT, chemotherapy (5-FU/cisplatin), and radiation therapy. Many other investigators reported similar anecdotal cases (19). Most recently, Lambert (20) reported an overall 5-year survival rate of 9% in 293 patients treated with a multimodality protocol for cancer of the esophagus that involves one ELT session, three radiotherapy courses, and up to 12 chemotherapy courses. He uses ELT at the end of the first chemotherapy course when the tumor sensitivity to thermal injury is the highest. Further dysphagia palliation is achieved by dilation as necessary.

Colorectal Cancers

Surgical resection is the standard treatment for colorectal carcinoma. Endoscopic treatment is usually per-

formed when surgery is contraindicated, for example, when patients are at highest surgical risk, there are metastatic or locally advanced tumors, or when patients refuse surgery. Dittrich et al. (21) used Nd:YAG laser therapy only in 7.1% of 517 patients treated by their surgical department over a period of 5 years. Keifhaber (22) used ELT in surgical candidates with complete colonic obstruction to open the lumen and allow a one-step resection without colostomy. The advantages of preoperative recanalization include adequate large bowel preparation, detection of synchronous neoplasia by full colonoscopy, and performance of an elective colectomy with low mortality versus high morbidity and mortality of multistage surgery involving emergency colostomy.

The accepted goal of ELT in colorectal cancer is palliation of symptoms caused by obstruction, bleeding, rectal discharge, incontinence, and urgency. Pain from extraluminal neoplastic involvement is not an indication for ELT and is alleviated more effectively by radiation therapy.

Technique

Treatment is usually performed on an outpatient basis. A full colonoscopy preparation is usually required before the first ELT session while repeat sessions for rectosigmoid tumors can be done after enema preparation. We use the coaxial CO_2 as the only insufflating gas to avoid thermal ignition and abdominal overdistention. Intermittent suction is needed to remove smoke and necrotic debris. Lesions with a polypoid portion are first debulked with multiple applications of the minisnare electrocautery. Through-the-scope balloon dilation is used to pass the scope above the lesion and apply thermal treatment circumferentially using a power setting of 70 to 90 W over 1 to 2 sec (similar to the retrograde treatment of obstructive esophageal tumors). Repeated sessions are carried out at 48 to 96-hour intervals until palliation is achieved. Maintenance sessions are scheduled at 4- to 8-week intervals.

Initial palliation is achieved in approximately 85% of patients with obstruction and up to 90% of patients with bleeding, diarrhea, mucous discharge, and incontinence (23). The outcome of ELT in colorectal cancer is related to factors listed in Table 3.

Van Cutsem et al. (24) analyzed the long-term results of yttrium-argon garnet (YAG) laser palliation for incurable colorectal carcinoma in 88 patients. Although initial palliation was achieved in 82%, good palliation could only be maintained in 51% and 41% of patients surviving 6 and 12 months, respectively. The selective inefficacy of ELT is due to failure to control extraluminal tumor growth, complications of ELT, and the poor general health condition of the patients.

TABLE 3. *Prognostic factors of ELT outcome in colorectal cancer*

Factors indicating high likelihood of success
  Nonobstructing lesion
  Noncircumferential lesion
  Exophytic lesion
  Rectal location
Factors indicating low likelihood of success
  Obstruction
  Circumferential lesion
  Infiltrative carcinoma
  Location in the sigmoid colon with angulated and narrowed lumen

Mellow (25) compiled the complication rates of ELT for colorectal cancer from surveys of experienced laser endoscopists. Out of 500 patients, 5 patients had free perforation and 15 had a local fistula/abcess formation. Ten patients had a significant hemorrhage requiring transfusion and 15 patients had only minor bleeding. Twenty-one patients developed stenosis while incontinence and pain occurred in five and three patients, respectively. Nineteen patients required surgery, and mortality was 1.2%. Kohler et al. (26) reported bacteremia in 19% of patients undergoing ELT for stenosing colorectal lesions without occurrence of sepsis. They concluded that routine antibiotic prophylaxis is not indicated.

Mellow (27) compared the costs of palliation for adenocarcinomas of the rectum in 35 patients undergoing surgery and 21 patients undergoing ELT. In the surgical patient group complications, length of hospital stay and ICU stay were significantly greater, contributing to mean total cost of surgery of $23,156 compared to $5,333 for inpatient laser treatment and $2,263 for outpatient laser treatment. Lifetime cost calculated in patients with metastasis was $22,900 for surgery and $12,154 for laser therapy.

Complete local destruction of smaller rectosigmoid cancers can be achieved by ELT (28) and is currently used in rare cases of nonsurgical candidates. Endoscopic ultrasonography for accurate tumor staging may facilitate the ELT for cure in selected patients.

Colorectal Adenomas

Laser photocoagulation for colorectal adenomas is indicated in nonsurgical candidates at initial diagnosis or for recurrence after previous treatment. In addition to palliation of mucous secretion/diarrhea (with hypokalemia), bleeding, or obstructive symptoms, we aim at ablation of the lesion.

Technique

Similar to ELT for carcinoma we start with polypectomy snare debulking that provides tissue for histologic diagnosis and improves treatment efficacy. We follow with photocoagulation of the residual polyp using a setting of 50 to 60 W for over 0.5 to 1 sec. Treatment sessions are repeated every 2 to 4 weeks until complete eradication is achieved. Endoscopic surveillance is done at 3- to 6-month intervals and the patients are retreated for recurrence. Multiple biopsies for focal carcinoma are obtained before each thermal treatment.

Symptoms abate in 97% of patients even when the tumor is only reduced in size and not obliterated. Complete oblation is achieved in 82% of adenomas with recurrence rate of 12% to 41%. Only 56% of adenomas bigger than 4 cm can be fully ablated. With current methodology we cannot assume full destruction of neoplastic tissue, and malignant focus remnants are discovered in about 7% to 10%.

The predictors of poor outcome are:

1. Adenoma >4 cm, involving more than two-thirds of the circumference.
2. Proximal location above 10 cm from the anal verge.
3. Predominantly villous histology.

The predictors of good outcome are:

1. Adenomas <1 cm.
2. Located within 10 cm from the anal verge.
3. Tubulovillous histology.

Mathus-Vliegen and Tytgat (28) treated with ELT 241 patients with colorectal adenomas and 30 patients with familial polyposis coli and recurrent polyps in the rectal stump after subtotal colectomy and ileorectal anastomosis. Twenty out of 24 evaluable familial polyposis patients had total polyp elimination and one patient developed malignancy. Complete ablation for at least 12 weeks was achieved in 82% of the colorectal adenomas, but with late recurrences in prolonged follow-up the success rate declined to 77%. ELT for colorectal adenomas is better for small and medium-sized lesions but extensive adenomas require on average nine to ten sessions to achieve 56% eradication. Seven percent of the patients developed major complications of ELT (stenosis, hemorrhage, or perforation) without procedure-related death, and minor complications occurred in 36%. The authors recommend ELT ablation of colorectal adenomas for small and medium-sized polyps (<4 cm; involving less than two-thirds of the circumference) that cannot be removed by polypectomy in inoperable patients *only*. ELT for extensive adenomas seems only appropriate for symptomatic relief.

Brunetaud et al. (29) use the argon laser for the very distal rectum, within 4 cm of the anal verge, when the Nd:YAG laser treatment is painful. The argon laser is used to vaporize superficial tumors, since its green light is readily absorbed by the red pigment, causing mostly superficial tissue ablation with minimal coagulation and "what you see is what you get." This is different than the Nd:YAG laser light, which is poorly absorbed by the tissue components and causes mostly deep coagulation. The newly, rediscovered KTP laser (30) emits green light and can be used like the argon laser. A two-wavelength KTP/YAG laser can be used like a combined electrocautery unit with both "vaporization" and "coagulation" operational modes. Such units are approved by the Food and Drug Administration (FDA) for gastroenterology use.

New wavelength lasers for medical use are already FDA approved or cleared for specific non-GI use while others are still investigational. The mid-infrared range lasers like holmium (gas) or holmium-YAG (2.1 μm; approved for orthopedics) or thulium-holmium-chromium (THC):YAG (2.15 μm, not approved yet) are the future alternatives for endoscopic cutting surgery since they have a much higher absorption coefficient for water than Nd:YAG. Bass et al. (31) compared the tissue effects of the THC:YAG versus the Nd:YAG and found similar ablation rates but much deeper coagulation necrosis by the Nd:YAG with increased risk for delayed perforation of the bowel wall. The mid-infrared lasers may provide safer use in the colon.

Similarly, a highly compact and portable 25-W surgical gallium-aluminum-arsenic (GaAlAs) diode laser has been developed for use through contact and noncontact fibers. With a wavelength of 805 nm the tissue effect is similar to that with Nd:YAG, with predominant coagulation at 2- to 5-mm depth.

PHOTODYNAMIC THERAPY (PDT)

PDT is the destructive action of light irradiation on neoplastic tissue that contains a previously administered photosensitizer. The photosensitizer is initially distributed in all the tissues but is retained for a longer time by the tumor stroma, reaching a larger than 2:1 ratio 40 to 50 hours post administration (32). This difference in photosensitizer concentration enables selective destruction of tumors, since a photodynamic light dose can achieve PDT effect on the tumor while remaining below PDT threshold for the surrounding tissue. The photochemical reaction causes tissue damage by the production of singled oxygen, the cytotoxic agent (33). Tissue studies demonstrate PDT-induced vascular damage with subsequent tumor ischemia and necrosis (34). An important observation was made by Barr et al. (35) about the collagen damage by PDT versus thermal injury. In the normal colon, full-thickness PDT damage spares the submucosal collagen, producing no increase in the risk of perforation. Only transmural invasion by the neoplasm itself can cause PDT-induced perforation.

The photosensitizers used in clinical trials, hemato-

porphyrins, derive from our knowledge about photosensitivity disease processes like porphyria. Lipson et al. (36) isolated a hematoporphyrin derivative (HpD) with tumor localizing and photosensitizing properties that was used in the 1960s for endoscopic detection of carcinomas of the lung, esophagus, and gastric cardia (37). The photodynamically active ingredient of HpD was identified by Dougherty (38) as dihematoporphyrin ether/ester (DHE) and is now produced as Porfimer Sodium (Quadra Logic Technologies, Inc.). It has a major absorption peak (350–450 mm) close to the peak of solar radiation (>400–500 mm) and a minor absorption peak at 630 mm, which is used in clinical PDT.

The light source for PDT at wavelength of 630 mm is usually a dye laser optically pumped by an argon or a copper vapor laser, while a gold vapor laser can emit this wavelength directly.

Technique

We use PDT for cancer of the esophagus as part of a multicenter cooperative study. Eligible patients receive 2 mg/kg Porfimer Sodium by intravenous injection over 3 to 5 min. They become immediately photosensitive to sunlight and follow strict avoidance precautions. Endoscopically delivered red laser light treatment is performed 40 to 50 hours later and can be repeated at a similar time interval, if necessary. The light treatment is performed with a tunable argon-dye laser and is transmitted by a flexible glass fiber that is passed via the endoscope under direct visual control. If the tumor is completely obstructing, the tip of the fiber with a diffuser configuration can be inserted into the tumor central area for interstitial treatment. For small, nonobstructing lesions a microlens is attached to the fiber tip with the light focused on the lesion. The majority of cases are done with a cylindrical diffuser that is placed in the stenotic tumor lumen. The laser power is 400 mW for each centimeter of the diffuser length and the light dose is 300 J/cm, which is translated into treatment time of 12.5 minutes at each treatment level. The diffuser is kept in place under direct fiberoptic endoscopic control and is repositioned after each treatment interval.

The patients are endoscoped for debridement in 2 to 3 days and can be retreated with the laser while still photosensitive. The patients are shielded from sunlight for 1 month and then can carefully expose their skin to sunlight for 5- to 15-min intervals. If no sunburn occurs, sunlight is permitted and the patient is ready for a second cycle of PDT.

Results

Likier et al. (39) followed this protocol and reported on two patients with a completely obstructing cervical esophageal cancer, just below the cricopharyngeus muscle, in whom the guidewire would not pass to permit dilation. In this desperate setting, they were able to establish a lumen with the first cycle of PDT, avoiding potentially more dangerous antegrade Nd:YAG ELT.

Heier et al. (40) reported interim results of a randomized trial of PDT with DHE versus Nd:YAG ELT using the same protocol for obstructing esophageal carcinoma. There was no difference in symptomatic improvement, esophageal patency, or survival. The complication rate was similar for both techniques. The main disadvantage of PDT was difficulty in maintaining the argon-dye laser.

Lightdale et al. (41) reported the initial results of the multicenter randomized trial of PDT versus Nd:YAG ELT for malignant dysphagia, a trial in which we participated. A total of 236 patients were treated and the response rate at 1 week was 44% for PDT and 36% for Nd:YAG (NS). The response rates tend to be better for PDT in the high cervical tumors or the long tumors. Improvement in dysphagia score at 1 week and 1 month was similar for both groups and the median survival was comparable as well (PDT, 127 days versus YAG, 155 days). Treatment-related complications including chest pain, perforation, and bleeding were similar, but photosensitivity reactions were reported in 20% of patients following PDT. Approval of the photosensitizer Porfimer Sodium for this indication by the FDA is pending.

Complications of PDT

Wooten et al. (42) reported cutaneous phototoxicity in 74% of 23 patients treated with HpD. Blisters lasting 5 to 23 weeks occurred in 18% of cases. This high complication rate was ascribed to a lack of compliance with light-avoiding precautions and was deemed a major disadvantage of PDT with HpD. The incidence of cutaneous complications may have been lessened substantially by the use of DHE. Dougherty et al. (43) reviewed the cutaneous phototoxic occurrences in patients receiving DHE. All 180 patients receiving a total of 266 injections of the photosensitizer at doses ranging from 0.5 to 2.0 mg/kg were photosensitive following the injection, but up to 40% of the patients reported some type of phototoxic response presumably due to noncompliance. Some 12% to 14% of the patients reported blistering without apparent relationship to the drug dose. Based on the data, the investigators recommend that patients receiving DHE be cautioned to avoid bright sunlight and other bright lights for at least 6 weeks following injection. Regular UV sunscreen is ineffective and only opaque cream (zinc oxide) provides protection, but it is not cosmetically acceptable. In a pilot study of 12 PDT patients and 12 controls,

treated with oral activated charcoal, Lowdell et al. (44) attempted to reduce the skin photosensitivity but failed to demonstrate a significant pharmacological or clinical difference.

Some patients may experience a burning sensation during treatment and some degree of chest pain and discomfort may persist. Transient dysphagia is common and esophageal strictures may occur later. Sloughing and necrosis of large lesions may cause fever, perforation, and hemorrhage.

Additional Treatment Reports

McCaughan et al. (45) treated 40 patients with advanced cancer of the esophagus including 19 squamous cell carcinomas, 19 adenocarcinomas, and two melanomas. They used a wide range of power settings and added Nd:YAG laser therapy, chemotherapy, and radiation therapy as well as dilation. The average luminal diameter increased from 6 to 9 mm and most patients tolerated soft diet after treatment. Probably part of the tumors treated received a combination of PDT and interstitial hyperthermia when the fiber tip was inserted and the laser power was 1 W. Complications included four perforations, six strictures, nine pleural effusions, and five sunburns.

Thomas et al. (46) treated 15 patients with inoperable esophageal carcinomas, who required a total of 26 treatments with HpD at high light doses. They attempted to increase the treatment area by placing the fiber in the center of a balloon filled with intralipid to scatter the light (similar to urologic PDT in the urinary bladder filled with intralipid). Procedures lasted as long as 70 minutes and general anesthesia was used. All the patients experienced symptomatic improvement, but with the power above 1.5 W the complication rate was high. Complications included fever in seven cases, fistulas in two, mediastinitis in two, and cutaneous photosensitivity in four. The in-hospital mortality was 14%.

Of 120 patients with cancer of the esophagus, stomach, and rectum treated by Jin et al. (47), 73% experienced some type of therapeutic response, which was complete in 10% of cases.

Krasner et al. (48) treated 21 patients with GI neoplasia with PDT. Twelve rectal carcinomas, three esophageal carcinomas, one gastric cancer, and five colorectal sessile villous adenomas were treated with curative/palliative intent. Interstitial PDT of 50 joules at four to seven treatment sites was applied. In some rectal cancers, endoscopic ultrasound was used to assess the depth of tumor invasion and the treatment response. The mean depth of tumor removed was 6 ± 4 mm. Overall, 2 out of the 16 carcinomas and three out of the five adenomas were eradicated. In one case, a major

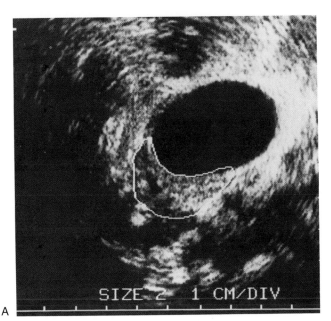
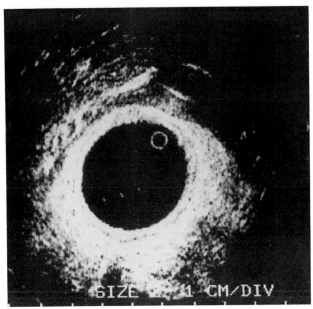

FIG. 1. A: Rectal endoluminal ultrasound of small recurrent rectal carcinoma prior to PDT. Carcinoma outlined in white. **B:** Follow-up rectal endoluminal ultrasound at 1 month after endoscopic PDT. Examination performed at the same site as in A. No tumor was detectable.

hemorrhage complicated the treatment of a large rectal cancer (Fig. 1).

Like many other new cancer treatments, PDT was first tried on patients for whom all else has failed. It is clear that PDT can be used successfully for palliation in desperate cases of complete luminal obstruction but its most promising application should be in the early stage of GI cancer with primary or combined curative intent. In two international surveys of PDT, Spinelli (49) found a worldwide trend toward the treatment of early tumors and preneoplastic lesions.

Sabben et al. (50) treated 43 patients, half of whom were asymptomatic, with superficial esophageal cancer. Complete tumor destruction was obtained in 37 patients, 9 of whom experienced recurrence. Survival was 73% at 1 year and 44% at 2 years.

Lambert (20) achieved complete destruction in 46 of 65 T1,N0 or small T2,N0 esophagogastric tumors treated with PDT, chemotherapy, and radiotherapy. The five-year survival rate was 26% for all cases and 37% for newly diagnosed cases. In 60% of cases, the cause of death was not related to the esophageal cancer.

Patrice et al. (51) used PDT with curative intent in 54 inoperable patients with lesions less than 4 cm in their largest diameter. Twenty-four esophageal squamous cell carcinomas, 14 gastroesophageal adenocarcinomas, and 16 rectosigmoid carcinomas were treated with 33% partial response and 44% complete response. The mean recurrence-free period varied from 13.8 to 17.4 months and 50% of the successfully treated patients were alive at 24 months. This study suggests a

potential efficacy of PDT as curative treatment. Endoscopic ultrasonography staging and better dosimetry could create extension of the PDT indication from palliative to adjuvent or curative.

Karanov et al. (52) used PDT in six patients with early stage cancers of the esophagus, stomach, colon, and rectum. T1,N0,M0 stage was established by computed tomography (CT) scan or endocavitary ultrasound. One to four laser sessions were required to achieve complete response in all the cases. No recurrence was observed over 7 to 16 months of follow-up. Surprisingly, almost all the polyps disappeared from the rectum of a patient with familial polyposis and ileorectal anastomosis.

Overholt (53) treated three patients with early esophageal cancer, achieving complete histologic and endoscopic ultrasonographic response. In one patient with adenocarcinoma in Barrett's esophagus, a reduction in the volume of Barrett's mucosa was noted.

Monnier et al. (54) treated 15 cases of "early" esophageal cancer and achieved complete response in 12. After a long theoretical review of PDT, they concluded that *after 10 years of clinical trials little progress has been achieved in tumor selectivity*. Partial destruction of large tumors is presumed selective because the normal mucosa gets reduced irradiation by red light while we may lose selectivity in small early cancer causing 13% of complications, such as transmural effect with fistulae and stenosis. They developed a transparent light-diffusing cylinder, fixed on a Savary-Gilliard dilatation bougie that permits homogeneous light distribution over the whole length of the cylinder. A similar centering balloon was developed by Panjehpour et al. (55) with uniform light intensities around the lumen. The balloon increases the area illuminated by a 2.5-cm diffuser to 4.0 cm and eliminates the mucosal folds that contribute to uneven light dosimetry. Fleischer et al. (56) developed a similar dilating transparent balloon that is placed over a guidewire and contains a laser fiber for precise dosimetry.

New Photosensitizers

Considerable progress has been made in the search for better sensitizers. Phtalocyanines are porphyrin-like industrial dyes with significant advantages over HpD and DHE, which are an ill-defined mixture of porphyrins with relatively weak tumor selectivity and only a weak absorption peak in the red when tissue penetration by light is the deepest. Phtalocyanines are stable compounds with known structure, easy to synthesize, and with strong absorption peaks at 600 to 750 mm when light penetration in tissue is still good. Their low absorption at wavelengths shorter than 600 mm will potentially reduce the cutaneous photosensitivity. The most promising agent appears to be aluminum chlorosulfonated phtalocyanine (AlSPc) but animal studies (57) demonstrate a similar pattern of uptake by induced colonic and pancreatic cancer with an insubstantial therapeutic ratio to normal tissue that is unlikely to result in significant selective destruction.

When a new photosensitizer, 5-aminolevulinic acid (ALA) was compared to AlS_2Pc by Loh et al. (58), a new promising mechanism of action was discovered. Exogenous ALA leads to accumulation of protoporphyrin IX (PPG), producing photosensitization of the gastric mucosa with very little accumulation in the submucosa and muscularis mucosa (ratio 10:1). PDT with red light resulted in marked mucosal necrosis and sparing of the underlying layers. The mechanism of cell death resulted from direct cellular photodestruction and not from damage to the microvasculature, leading to better healing without scarring. This type of PDT carries application potential for areas with severe mucosal dysplasia such as Barrett's esophagus. ALA causes only short-lived photosensitization, and cutaneous side effects are unlikely after 24 hours (59).

Perspectives

While many other classical photosensitizers (54) are being evaluated (such as naphtalcyanines, purpurins, chlorines, bacteriochlorines, and verdins), selective delivery to tumors is a new way of avoiding PDT side effects. Packaging lipophilic substances in liposome carriers promotes delivery to tumors with enhanced low-density lipoprotein (LDL) receptor activity. Dyes

attached to monoclonal antibodies could combine high tumor selectivity with dye specificity for PDT using more stable and selective compounds.

While gastroenterologists are preoccupied by the application of PDT via endoscopy, laparoscopic surgery is undergoing a mini-revolution. Since initial experimental studies indicated that the liver accumulates porphyrin, PDT for the liver and the pancreas has been studied only to a limited degree (60). With the recent progress in interstitial hyperthermia, possible combination with PDT for solid organs is being reconsidered.

An interesting potential application is in the treatment of malignant ascites. Tochner et al. (61) treated murine ascites tumor by insertion of laser fibers in the abdominal cavity and achieved 85% cure. Is peritoneal carcinomatosis "similar" to carcinoma of the urinary bladder? The urologic application of PDT using porfimer sodium has obtained preliminary approval in Canada.

The future of PDT lies in improved sensitizers, as described earlier, with greater tissue specificity and less cutaneous photosensitivity as well as better, smaller, and cheaper lasers (such as diode lasers) delivering different light wavelengths. While the current clinical applications are relatively crude, the ongoing research efforts by many investigators should rapidly improve PDT over the next few years.

LASER-INDUCED FLUORESCENCE (LIF)

Fluorescence is a physical energy process that occurs when certain compounds absorb electromagnetic radiation, become excited, and then return to an energy level slightly higher than or equal to their original energy level. Since the energy given off is less than that absorbed, the wavelength of the light given off is longer than that absorbed for excitation. A delay time between 10^{-4} and 10^{-8} seconds occurs between the absorption of the energy and the release of part of the energy in the form of light. The spectral distribution of the induced fluorescence can be analyzed by spectroscopic methods and characterizes the physical and chemical properties of tissue.

Low-power laser radiation induces *tissue fluorescence* without tissue damage and may be used for diagnostic fluorescent spectroscopy. The earliest uses of this technique were oriented primarily toward localization of early tumors when using fluorescence from the tumor-seeking substance HpD. The characteristic HpD fluorescence in the red spectral region was used for tumor detection in endoscopic investigation of the lung and the bladder at the Mayo Clinic (62) and in Japan. A krypton laser light (63) was used to stimulate specific HpD fluorescence, which was either "observed" or "translated" into an audible sign or a visible oscilloscopic signal (64). The dose of HpD used was similar to the usual PDT dose with considerable photosensitivity and in most cases the early detection was followed by argon-dye laser PDT for tumor destruction. Further research was conducted on inducing fluorescence of unprepared tissue samples *in vitro* (65) by the use of UV light laser and processing the fluorescence through a spectrograph with a linear diode array capturing the entire UV–visible–near-IR spectral region at a resolution power of 5 nm. The spectra were recorded by accumulating data for 80 pulses then analyzed into specific tissue LIF profiles.

Andersson-Engels et al. (66) evaluated the porphyrin fluorescence of HpD and DHE as well as LIF for localization of tumors in rats. Both an excimer-pumped dye laser and a nitrogen laser were used for different excitation wavelengths and the authors concluded that better tumor demarcation is achieved by LIF induced by an excitation wavelength below 405 nm.

Cardiologists, angiographers, and vascular surgeons faced with a need for a specific targeting device during laser angioplasty started using LIF to discriminate between normal and atherosclerotic parts of the vessels (67). The discrimination is primarily qualitative, based on different peaks seen on pattern analysis. LIF intensity can be variable and does not correlate with histology. Currently their work is oriented toward the building of a "smart" laser angioplasty catheter system incorporating low-power laser radiation for fluorescence spectroscopy to guide delivery of high-power laser radiation for plaque ablation.

Using a similar system Kapadia et al. (68) carried out an *in vitro* study obtaining LIF spectra from normal colonic biopsies as well as resected adenomatous and hyperplastic polyps. They used a helium-cadmium laser at 325 nm UV wavelength and a 5- to 10-mW power, which does not damage the tissue and excites endogenous fluorescence that was analyzed from a 300 to 600 nm wavelength range by an optical multichannel analyzer. A quantitative LIF score was developed to discriminate adenomatous from normal tissue in the fluorescence spectra obtained from the initial 70 tissue specimens with known histology. The LIF scores were obtained prospectively in a validation test including 34 normal mucosal specimens, 16 adenomatous polyps, and 16 hyperplastic polyps. Polyps were classified correctly as adenomatous or hyperplastic with 97% accuracy. One hyperplastic polyp was classified as adenomatous (Fig. 2).

Cothren et al. (69) used an endoscope-compatible optical fiber system to obtain LIF spectra of mucosal abnormalities during colonoscopy *in vivo*. A nitrogen-pumped dye laser was used to deliver excitation light of 370-nm wavelength at 270-mW power delivering 3 nsec pulses at 20 Hz. A diagnostic probe of about 2 mm outside diameter containing one central excitation fiber and nine peripheral collection fibers was placed in direct contact with the tissue surface, and fluorescence emission spectra were collected into an imaging spectrograph coupled to an optical multichannel analyzer. After the fluorescence emission spectra were collected from 350 to 700 nm, a tissue specimen was obtained for histologic examination: 31 adenomas, 4 hyperplastic polyps, and 32 normal mucosal biopsies. Comparison of the average fluorescence intensities at 460 nm and 680 nm shows a significant statistical difference between adenomas and the other specimens. The spectra analysis was used to correctly differentiate adenomas from normal colonic mucosa and hyperplastic polyp in 97% of the specimens with 100% sensitivity, 97% specificity, and positive predictive value of 94%. It is hard to believe that only four hyperplastic polyps were used for this study.

Shomacker et al. (70) used pulsed nitrogen laser at 337 nm wavelength (pulse energy 200 μJ, pulse duration 3 nsec, and repetition rate 20 Hz) for *in vivo* LIF of colonic polyps. Twenty-five hyperplastic polyps and 49 adenomatous polyps were examined and the multivariate regression analysis yielded only 86% positive and 80% negative predictive value. When the histologic diagnosis by the clinical pathology department was compared to the study pathologist's classification, similar 86% to 89% concordance was found; thus, LIF diagnosis accuracy was as good as the clinical pathology. Shomacker et al. carried the experiment further, trying to decipher the observed fluorescence signals. Since the observed tissue fluorescence is produced by a number of molecules in the tissue modified by the absorption by some tissue components, with 337 nm excitation the fluorescence spectra all had peaks at 390 and 460 nm, believed to arise from collagen and reduced nicotinamide adenine dinucleotide (NADH), and a minimum at 425 nm, consistent with absorption by hemoglobin. Normal or hyperplastic histology corresponds to more collagen, while adenomas or adenocarcinomas contain more hemoglobin and less collagen. In fact, since LIF originates within the uppermost 480 μm of tissue, the thickening of the mucosa reduces the collagen signal. The investigators concluded that LIF does not detect changes in fluorophores specific to polyps but senses changes in the polyp morphology.

Once a diagnostic algorithm can be based on one or two emission wavelengths, clinical LIF systems could be greatly simplified using inexpensive narrow-band signal detectors. The potential of LIF in clinical endoscopy includes the following uses:

1. Guide biopsy/polypectomy during endoscopy.
2. Verify eradication site for residual or recurrent neoplasia.
3. Screen for dysplastic epithelium in Barrett's esophagus or chronic ulcerative colitis.

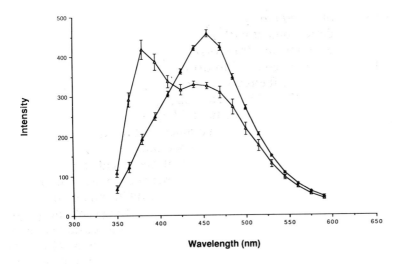

FIG. 2. Mean LIF spectra of normal and adenomatous colonic mucosa. Individual tissue spectra were resampled at 15-nm increments and averaged to derive the mean spectra. The resultant 17 intensity features between 350 and 600 nm are shown ±1 SEM for normal specimens (△) and adenomatous polyps (▲).

4. Differentiate between pseudopolyps and adenomatous polyps in irritable bowel disease (IBD).

CONTACT PROBES

Noncontact ELT is the standard method used by gastroenterologists in the GI tract using high-power bulky and expensive lasers. Since the power density goes up significantly when the fiber is close or in contact to the tissue, less power and a smaller, cheaper laser could be used for ELT. The use of bare fibers gained popularity in France where different investigators use an inexpensive telecommunication quartz fiber (by the running yard). About 30 W is a sufficient power to cause vaporization by this method. Some investigators remove the distal Teflon coating before use while others let the fiber coating burn with the thermal effect at the tissue contact point. Focusing and fiber polishing are irrelevant. Naveau et al. (71) compared the use of noncontact ELT with the contact "in-tissue" bare fiber technique and needed only half the treatment sessions for therapeutic results.

In the mid-1980s sapphire contact probes were introduced and were perceived by gastroenterologists as the laser's industry answer to the coaptive hemostasis instruments like the heater probe. The sapphire tips are attached to the distal end of the laser light guide by a metal connector with two irrigation holes. Irrigation with water is required to avoid overheating of the connector and damage to the tip. Four basic shapes and optical geometry are available:

1. flat tip for coagulation.
2. wedge "chisel" for incision.
3. round tip for vaporization.
4. cone tip for interstitial treatment.

Focusing and defocusing have some role in the distribution of light but surface "frosting" gives diffuse light distribution. With surface carbonization of tissue the high light absorption and heating up turn the sapphire tip into a "hot rod."

The most widely used shape in gastroenterology is the round tip for vaporization. Sahafi (72) measured its thermal behavior with an infrared camera. Light distribution studies showed a focusing effect 2 mm in front of the tip surface. The tip temperature increases with the laser application and adds to the thermal effect of the laser light-tissue interaction. With 15 joules of energy the temperature of the sapphire tip is 80°C; the temperature of focal length is 160°C, and at the tissue contact point 240°C, causing a charred crater. Similarly, when 40 joules of energy is applied the temperature of the sapphire tip is 200°C; the temperature at focal length is 320°C and at the tissue contact point 520°C, causing a clean crater. In addition to the combined thermal effects the sapphire tip can be used for mechanical tumor destruction. The "chisel"-shaped tip has been particularly advocated for such use, but some investigators found it difficult to control.

Metal tips used successfully in laser angioplasty have been adopted for endoscopic use. One metal tip configuration is like a small 2-mm olive attached to the light guide that turns into a "hot rod" by the warming effect of the laser light on the metal. A side "ear" with a hole allows this closed metal tip to pass over a guidewire. Laser power of about 10 W can achieve metal temperature between 300° and 1200°C with red-orange glowing of the tip. It takes 5 sec of 10-W application to turn the metal tip red and cause tissue vaporization. Similar effect with the sapphire tip requires about 18 W and surface charring. Both tips are adherent to the tissue, and while the sapphire tip is irrigated by water, it takes 10 sec for the metal tip to cool and lose its orange glow.

The best adaptation for thermal contact ELT is achieved by a metal tip with a central window that allows combining the thermal effect of the central laser beam on the tissue and the thermal effect of the peripheral laser beam on the metal akin to the thermal behavior of the sapphire tip.

Results

Our initial experience with the sapphire tips was disappointing. The tips were quickly covered with a charred deposit turning them nontransparent and adherent to the necrotic tissue, requiring frequent cleaning during treatment sessions. The chisel tip, more appropriate for "shaving" action, had thermal burnouts of the cutting edge. Considering the cost and the frequent need for cleaning, we reverted to noncontact ELT.

Radford et al. (73) compared contact and noncontact ELT for esophageal tumors and concluded that the contact method offers no advantage with respect to the number of treatment sessions, treatment results, or complications.

Hira (74) used low-power contact ELT for obstructing esophageal and rectal cancer, and found it superior to noncontact ELT because it causes minimal charring and smoke and little surrounding edema, allowing the debulking of the tumor and successfully recanalizing the lumen in one session. The contact method provided less discomfort to the patient since the overdistention of the bowel is eliminated by water cooling of the tip. While contact therapy uses less energy (lower power), more treatment sessions are required to achieve good palliation (75).

Mason (76) used a direct contact sapphire tip (15 W for 5 sec) to traverse a truly obstructed tumor impassible to a guidewire. Whenever the guidewire was able to pass, he proceeded with noncontact ELT for UGI-obstructing tumors.

Faintuch (77) used ELT with contact probes for completely obstructing colorectal carcinoma in ten patients. Tap water enemas were the only preparation. The flexible sigmoidoscope was passed to the level of obstruction and metal contact probe was advanced to the point of maximal obstruction. Power setting of 13 to 15 W over variable pulse durations were used to vaporize the lesion from the midpoint of the colonic lumen circumferentially, gradually increasing the diameter of the lumen. Each treatment session took 20 to 80 minutes, and the therapy was completed in two to three sessions. Initial hospitalization took 3 to 7 days, achieving successful recanalization in all ten patients, all surgically unresectable and subsequently treated as outpatients. This investigator still prefers the noncontact ELT for large localized exophytic tumors, using the "antegrade" approach (78).

Hochberger (79) summarized his center's combined experience of 45 patients treated with the contact tech-

nique and 182 patients with noncontact ELT. The contact laser technique causes less pain and laser edema, less smoke production, and no overdistention of the bowel by gas. It does not cause light guide ignition and is particularly suitable for tumor overgrowth over the esophageal prosthesis or for cases of total stenosis. On the other hand, the therapy requires tissue contact with light guide adhesion and loss of direct vision. The technique is punctiform, slower than the "paint brush" application by noncontact ELT, and requires longer sessions as well as more sessions for large and exophytic tumors.

With the recent advances in interstitial low-power laser therapy, I believe that the contact probes could become more popular in endoscopic use, particularly the long interstitial insertion sapphire tip and the metal tip with a central window.

LOW-POWER INTERSTITIAL LASER THERAPY

Interstitial laser therapy combines the precision of inserted light delivery systems with the tissue effects of deeply penetrating light. It is known as interstitial hyperthermia and its use with the Nd:YAG laser was first reported by Bown in 1983 (80).

The laser fiber is inserted directly into the target organ and the treatment is carried out at very low laser powers, 1 to 2 W, without tip damage or tissue vaporization. Long exposure times are required to allow for heat conduction further into the tissue.

The low absorption and high scattering of Nd:Yag laser light creates an almost spherical distribution pattern at the fiber tip, instead of a wedge or forward-only pattern. The resulting treatment zone is about 16 mm in diameter and the tissue effects depend on the temperature produced (81): temperatures between 40° and 45°C over a few hours can damage tumor cells as well as the tumor microcirculation in a selective fashion, while temperatures above 45°C cause nonselective coagulation necrosis.

This approach is more suitable for tumors of solid organs like the liver and pancreas or for solid lesions in the walls of hollow organs.

Animal Studies

Liver

Matthewson et al. (82) studied the biological effects of low-power Nd:YAG laser photocoagulation in the rat liver model and showed a relationship among the diameter of necrosis, power, and total energy. For a given power setting the necrotic zone diameter increased with the total energy delivered and for a given total energy delivered the necrotic zone diameter increased with power. A plateau effect was observed at 1 W and 800 to 1,000 joules. The necrosis was consistent with a pure thermal, nonspecific, effect.

An increase of the volume of tissue necrosis can be achieved by simultaneous treatment through multiple fibers inserted in juxtaposition under ultrasound control. Steger et al. (83) achieved a 7 × 4 cm necrosis with a four-fiber system.

Van Eyken et al. (84) compared the effects of low-power Nd:YAG laser interstitial hyperthermia to ethanol injection in the dog liver. Interstitial laser hyperthermia by 500 sec exposure of 1 W Nd:YAG laser induced deep, spherical, well-demarcated lesions with a mean diameter of about 1 cm, while the surface of the liver remained normal. In contrast, the dogs treated with alcohol had free intraperitoneal scrosanguineous fluid and the surface of the liver was diffusely abnormal with irregular, pale, depressed areas. The lesions were cylindrical, 1.2 by 0.4 cm, with irregular borders and with necrosis at a distance along the centrilobular veins. The laser method is localized, better controlled, and more reproducible.

Pancreas

Experimental studies on normal canine pancreas using both single or multiple fiber systems have been performed by Steger et al. (85). Hyperamylasemia was seen in all subjects, and lethal pancreatitis occurred in a few, particularly if the pancreatic duct was used for the light guide insertion.

Colon

It takes only 75 to 100 joules to produce full-thickness damage in the rat colon treated endoscopically at 1 W power. When Matthewson et al. (86) treated chemically induced colon cancer in rats, one laser fiber (inserted 2 mm) delivering 1 W of power over 100 to 400 sec caused coagulation necrosis of the tumor as well as full-thickness damage of the colon wall at the base of the tumor. All tumor necrosis resulted in ulceration, but only two perforations and one fistula developed in 52 treated tumors.

Tumor Implants

Karanov et al. (87) compared noncontact, interstitial, and contact Nd:YAG laser treatment of transplanted tumors in mice. Adenocarcinoma was transplanted into 40 mice and on day 15 posttransplant the tumors were treated. Ten mice were treated with noncontact Nd:YAG laser, 90 W over 13 sec, totaling about 1,200 joules. Ten other mice tumors were treated

with contact, water-cooled sapphire tip, 25 W over 48 sec, totaling 1,200 joules. A third group of ten mice tumors were treated by the interstitial method, 1 W over 1,200 sec for total energy of 1,200 joules, while the fourth group of mice served as control. The best treatment results were obtained by the noncontact and interstitial treatment methods with significant tumor weight reduction and both microscopic and histologic necrosis. The contact therapy results were quite similar to the control group, and the authors concluded that the use of the contact sapphire tips does no more than reduce the power output used and raise the cost of a procedure.

Light Delivery Systems

Under sonographic guidance, a thin laser fiber (200 to 600 μm in diameter) is introduced through a 19-gauge needle inserted percutaneously such that 3 to 4 mm of bare fiber tip lies within the lesion. A single fiber can deliver treatment to a small lesion of about 10 to 15 mm in diameter. Larger lesions require the use of a coupling device that can deliver the light simultaneously into four fibers placed in juxtaposition at a distance of 1.5 cm. The position of the fibers is adjusted during the treatment to cover 1 cm of circumferential rim of normal tissue around the lesion.

Real-time sonographic control of interstitial laser hyperthermia (32) is used for:

1. Guidance of organ puncture and laser fiber position.
2. Calculation of the amount of energy required.
3. Assessment of coagulated area by the change of echogenicity.
4. Monitoring for vaporization or gas formation during overheating.

A computer-controlled hyperthermia system was developed by Daikuzono et al. (88) for the use of the interstitial contact sapphire probe. Temperature sensors and thermocouples, placed directly at 6 mm from the probe, can monitor continuously the temperature. Using a computer program interfaced with the laser and the sensors, a controlled temperature can be maintained stable over a prolonged treatment. This thermal control was designed to work for a prototype endoscopic laserthermia system with a two-channel endoscope, one channel for the laser frosted probe and the other for the thermocouple. In clinical use, the thermal control was disrupted by digestive movements and a new single-channel scope method is being developed (89).

Clinical Reports

The first patient application for interstitial laser hyperthermia was reported by Hashimoto et al. (90).

Eight patients with metastatic colon cancer and two patients with hepatocellular carcinomas were treated with a fiber inserted at laparotomy. The Nd:YAG laser power was 5 W, and 1,000 joules were delivered to each cubic centimeter of tumor under intraoperative ultrasound imaging. Illumination was continued until the low echo area was completely replaced by a high echo area. All the patients had transient elevation in liver injury tests and decrease in tumor markers (CEA or α-FP) 2 to 3 months after treatment.

Masters et al. (91) treated ten patients with a total of 18 hepatic metastases from colorectal, stomach, and breast cancers as well as one small bowel carcinoid. The light was delivered by four fibers coupled to a single laser source delivering 1.5 to 2.0 W each over 500 sec. Real-time ultrasonography was used to monitor the treatment and the fibers were repositioned into several sites to incorporate 1 cm of the circumferential rim of normal liver around the metastasis into the treatment space. Ultrasonography demonstrated change in the metastasis from mixed echogenic to bright hyperechoic zones, while contrast CT scans showed change from low enhancement to avascular filling defects. Only 10 out of the 18 metastases showed radiological changes of necrosis, but five out of the ten continued to grow in size, a sign of partial response. Lesions smaller than 2 cm had the best response. None of the patients developed major complications such as bleeding, bile peritonitis, or sepsis, but minor complications included pain at the abdominal needle puncture sites and liver tests elevation (Fig. 3).

Dowlatshahi et al. (92) reported the first case of interstitial laser treatment of recurrent hepatoma in a transplanted liver. The laser fiber was placed into the liver through a 19-gauge needle and the treatment was monitored in real time by sonography. CT and needle biopsy showed no tumor growth for 13 months.

Masters and Bown (93) reported their experience

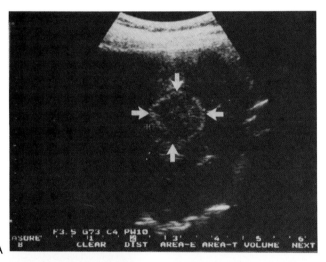
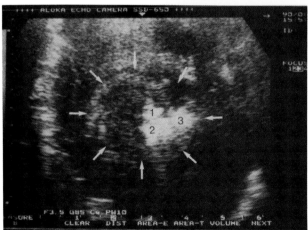
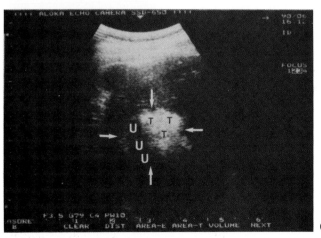

FIG. 3. **A:** Ultrasound appearance of a 4.0 cm diameter mixed echogenic colorectal metastasis *(arrows)* prior to laser treatment. **B:** The appearance of the same lesion *(arrows)* halfway through a 500-sec exposure at a power of 2.0 W per fiber. There are three hyperechogenic foci *(numbered)* each developing around one of the three fibers. **C:** The same metastasis *(arrows)* immediately at the end of treatment. There is a well-defined confluent hyperechogenic area occupying the right half of the lesion. There is clear distinction between the treated (T) and untreated (U) portions.

with three patients with inoperable or recurrent carcinoma of the head of the pancreas. In two patients, partial tumor necrosis was achieved, but more important complications such as acute pancreatitis, bleeding, or perforation were not seen. One patient developed acute common bile duct obstruction and required a biliary stent placement.

Barr and Krasner (94) treated three patients with diffusely bleeding stomach cancers unresponsive to high power Nd:YAG ELT using the interstitial sapphire probe at a power of 1 to 5 W for 200 to 1,000 sec. The treatment achieved lasting hemostasis in all the patients.

Suzuki et al. (89) reported successful treatments of one early and one late gastric cancer with good local control.

Future Trends

Current ELT relies almost exclusively on the immediate visual changes; superficial vaporization or coagulation effects with the Nd:YAG laser also produce deeper coagulation necrosis. The aiming precision of the laser light is underutilized with the constant and practically inevitable changes in the treatment distance; i.e., power density. We are using our knowledge of laser light wavelength effects on the living tissue in a selectively "low-tech" fashion.

The development of the sapphire contact tips brought the laser treatment power to 10 to 20 W. Interstitial laser hyperthermia is bringing it further down to the 1- to 2-W range. A low-power Nd:YAG laser is air-cooled, compact, transportable, and less expensive than our current bulky lasers.

The use of real-time ultrasonographic imaging and computer controlled thermal feedback with multifiber systems is more suitable for tumors of solid organs like the liver and the pancreas. It is probably a better treatment than cryotherapy, microwave hyperthermia, or alcohol injection for complete eradication.

The simpler, one-fiber system without feedback control could become effective in palliative endoscopic use for tumor overgrowth into the prosthesis or for completely obstructing lesions, akin to interstitial PDT, but without the photosensitivity.

For early neoplastic lesion eradication, endoscopic low-power laser hyperthermia requires a precise dosimetry and should become safer with the use of endoscopic sonography and computer-controlled thermal feedback.

In the "high-tech" future, the combination of "on the spot" tissue diagnosis by laser-induced fluorescence and precise staging and sizing by an ultrasound probe, then complete eradication by interstitial laser hyperthermia with computer controlled thermal feedback, followed by posttreatment sonography could become as simple and widely used as today's biopsy and polypectomy. It remains to be seen if interstitial PDT with the advantage of selective damage to neoplasia rather than surrounding normal tissue (but with systemic side effects) could be safer. There is still plenty of work for physicists, engineers, and endoscopists to do.

REFERENCES

1. Youmans CR, Patterson M, McDonald DF, Derrick JR Jr. Cystoscopic control of gastric hemorrhage. *Arch Surg* 1970;100:721–723.
2. Swain CP. Nd:YAG laser for treatment of bleeding peptic ulcers: techniques and results of randomized prospective trials. *Gastrointest Endosc Clin North Am* 1991;1:341–366.
3. Fleischer D, Kessler F, Haye O. Endoscopic Nd:YAG laser therapy for carcinoma of the esophagus: a new palliative approach. *Am J Surg* 1982;143:280–283.
4. Fleischer D. The Washington Symposium on Endoscopic Laser Therapy. *Gastrointest Endosc* 1985;31:397–400.
5. Fleischer D, Sivak MV. Endoscopic Nd:YAG therapy as palliation for esophagogastric cancer. Parameters effecting initial outcome. *Gastroenterology* 1985;89:827–831.
6. Mellow MH, Pinkas H. Endoscopic laser therapy for malignancies affecting the esophagus and the gastroesophageal junction: analysis of technical and functional efficacy. *Arch Intern Med* 1985;145:1443–1446.
7. Ell CH, Reiman JF, Lux G, Demling L. Palliative laser treatment of malignant stenosis in the upper gastrointestinal tract. *Endoscopy* 1986;18(1):21–26.
8. Mellow MH, Pinkas H. Endoscopic therapy for esophageal cancer with Nd:YAG laser: prospective evaluation of efficacy, complications and survival. *Gastrointest Endosc* 1984;30:334–339.
9. Karlin PA, Fisher RS, Krevsky B. Prolonged survival and effective palliation in patients with squamous all cell carcinoma of the esophagus following E.L.T. *Cancer* 1987;59:1969–1972.
10. Chatlani PT, Barr H, Krasner N. Longterm survivors of Nd:YAG laser therapy for upper gastrointestinal carcinoma. *Gut* 1989;30:A1475.
11. Goldschmidt S, Boyce HW, Nord HJ, Brady PG. Nd:YAG laser vaporization versus peroral dilation and or prosthesis in the palliative management of obstructing squamous cell carcinoma. *Gastrointest Endosc* 1988;34:176.
12. Siegel HL, Laskin HJ, Dabezies MA, Fisher RS, Krevsky B. The effect of endoscopic laser therapy on survival in patients with squamous cell carcinoma of the esophagus—further experience. *J Clin Gastroenterol* 1991;13:142–146.
13. Kohler B, Ginsbach CH, Riemann JF. Bacteremia after endoscopic laser therapy of the upper gastrointestinal tract. *Lasers Med Sci* 1988;3:13–15.
14. Loizou LA, Grigg D, Atkinson M, Robertson C, Bown SG. A prospective comparison of laser therapy and intubation in endoscopic palliation for malignant dysphagia. *Gastroenterology* 1991;100:1303–1310.
15. Reed CE, Marsh WH, Carlson LS, et al. Palliation of advanced esophageal cancer: a (laser) light in the end of the tunnel. *Arch Thorac Surg* 1991;51:552–556.
16. Sander R, Hagenmuller F, Sander C, Riess G, Classen M. Laser versus laser plus afterloading with iridium-192 in the palliative treatment of malignant stenosis of the esophagus: a prospective randomized and controlled study. *Gastrointest Endosc* 1991;37:433–445.
17. Bown SG. Palliation of malignant dysphagia: surgery, radiotherapy, laser, intubation alone or in combination? *Gut* 1991;32:841–844.
18. Pinkas H, Cash DK, Neilan BA, Prabhu HR, Shah DE. Endoscopic Nd:YAG laser therapy followed by chemotherapy and

radiation therapy for squamous cell carcinoma of the esopha-gus—case report of complete remission. *Gastrointest Endosc* 1985;31(2):134.

19. Mellow MH. Nd:YAG laser therapy prior to radiation and chemotherapy for the primary "curative" treatment of squam-ous-cell carcinoma of the esophagus. *Lasers Med Sci* 1988;80: 392.

20. Lambert R. Endoscopic therapy of esophago-gastric tumors. *Endoscopy* 1992;24:24–33.

21. Dittrich K, Armbruster C, Hoffer F, Tuchman A, Dinsti K. Nd:YAG laser treatment of colorectal malignancies: an experience of 4½ years. *Lasers Surg Med* 1992;12:199–203.

22. Keifhaber P. Palliative and pre-operative endoscopic Nd:YAG laser treatment of colorectal carcinoma. *Endoscopy* 1987;19: 43–46.

23. Bown SG. Commentary: what role do lasers play in the manage-ment of colorectal disease? *Int J Colorectal Dis* 1989;4:26–29.

24. Van Cutsem E, Boonen A, Geboes G, Coremans G, Hiele M, Vantrappen G, Rutgeerts P. Risk factors which determine the long term outcome of Nd:YAG laser palliation of colorectal car-cinoma. *Int J Colorectal Dis* 1989;4:9–11.

25. Mellow MH. Endoscopic therapy of colorectal neoplasms. *Gas-trointest Endosc Clin North Am* 1992;2(3):543–552.

26. Kohler B, Ginsbach CH, Riemann JF. Incidence of bacteremia following E.L.T. for stenosing colorectal lesions. *Gastrointest Endosc* 1988;34:73–74.

27. Mellow MH. Endoscopic laser therapy as an alternative to pal-liative surgery for adenocarcinoma of the rectum. Comparison of costs and complications. *Gastrointest Endosc* 1989;36(4): 283–287.

28. Mathus Vliegen EMH, Tytgat GHJ. The potential and limita-tions of laser photoablation of colorectal adenomas. *Gastrointest Endosc* 1991;137:9–17.

29. Brunetaud JM, Maunoury V, Ducrotte Cochelard D, Cortot A, Paris JC. Palliative treatment of rectosigmoid carcinoma by laser endoscopic photoablation. *Gastroenterology* 1987;92:663–668.

30. Ginsberg GG, Gupta PK, Newsome JT, Brennecke LH, Fleischer DE. A new laser for therapeutic gastrointestinal endos-copy: initial investigation of the KTP/532 laser in the canine model. *Am J Gastroenterol* 1992;87:1339.

31. Bass LS, Oz MC, Truhel SL, Treat MR. Alternative lasers for endoscopic surgery: comparison of pulsed thulium-holmium-chromium:YAG with continuous-wave neodymium:YAG laser for ablation of colonic mucosa. *Lasers Surg Med* 1991;11: 545–549.

32. Bugelski PJ, Porter CW, Dougherty TJ. Autoradiographic distri-bution in malignant and normal tissue. *Cancer Res* 1979;39: 146–151.

33. Weishaupt KP, Gomer CJ, Dougherty TJ. Identification of sin-glet oxygen as the cytotoxic agent in the photoactivation of a murine tumor. *Cancer Res* 1976;36:2326–2329.

34. Star WM, Marijnissen HPA, Evaunden A. Destruction of rat mammary tumor and normal tissue microcirculation by photora-diation observed in vivo in sandwich observation chambers. *Cancer Res* 1987;46:795–800.

35. Barr H, Tralau CJ, Boulos PB. The contrasting mechanism of colonic collagen damage between photodynamic therapy and thermal injury. *Photochem Photobiol* 1987;46:795–800.

36. Lipson RL, Baldes EJ, Olsen AM. Further evaluation of hema-toporphyrin derivative as a new aid for the endoscopic detection of malignant disease. *Chest* 1964;46:676–679.

37. Lipson RL, Baldes EJ, Olsen AM. Hematoporphyrin-deriva-tive: a new aid for endoscopic detection of malignant disease. *J Thorac Cardiovasc Surg* 1961;42:623–629.

38. Dougherty TJ. PDT: present and future. *Lasers Med Sci* 1988; 3:8.

39. Likier HM, Levine JG, Lightdale CJ. Photodynamic therapy for completely obstructing esophageal carcinoma. *Gastrointest Endosc* 1991;37(1):75–78.

40. Heier SK, Rothnan K, Rosenthal WS, Heier LM. Randomized trial of photodynanic therapy vs. Nd:YAG laser therapy for ob-structing esophageal tumors: interim results. *Gastrointest En-dosc* 1991;37(2):278.

41. Lightdale C, Heier S, Marcon N, McCaughan J, Nava H, Over-holt B, Sobel R, Grose M, Reisman A, Dugan M, and the PDT Esophageal Study Group. A multicenter Phase III trial of photo-dynamic therapy (PDT) vs Nd:YAG laser in the treatment of malignant dysphagia. *Gastrointest Endosc* 1993;39(2):283.

42. Wooten RS, Smith KC, Ahlquist DA, Muller SA, Balm BK. Prospective study of cutaneous phototoxicity after systemic HpD. *Lasers Surg Med* 1988;8:294–300.

43. Dougherty TJ, Cooper MT, Mang TS. Cutaneous phototoxicity occurrences in patients receiving Photofrin. *Lasers Surg Med* 1990;10:485–488.

44. Lowdell CP, Gilson D, Ash DV, Holroyd JA, Vernon D, Brown SB. An attempt to reduce skin photosensitivity in clinical photo-dynamic therapy using oral activated charcoal. *Lasers Med Sci* 1992;7:351–356.

45. McCaughan JS, Nims TA, Guy JT, Hicks WJ, Williams TE, Laufman LR. Photodynamic therapy for esophageal tumors. *Arch Surg* 1989;124:74–80.

46. Thomas RJS, Abbott M, Bhothal PS. High dose photoradiation of esophageal cancer. *Ann Surg* 1987;206:193–199.

47. Jin ML, Yang BQ, Zhang W, Ren P. Photodynamic therapy for the treatment of advanced gastrointestinal tumors. *Lasers Med Sci* 1989;4:183–186.

48. Krasner H, Chatlani PT, Barr H. Photodynamic therapy of tu-mors in gastroenterology—a review. *Lasers Med Sci* 1990;5: 233–239.

49. Spinelli P, Dal Fonte M. PDT—state of the art. In: Waidelich W, ed. *Laser optoelectronics in medicine 1987*. New York: Spring-er-Verlag, 1988;609–618.

50. Sabben G, Souquet JC, Lambert R. PDT in superficial types of esophageal cancer at endoscopy. *Lasers Med Sci* 1988;11.

51. Patrice T, Foultier MT, Yactayo S, Adam F, Galmiche JP, Douet MC, Budic L. Endoscopic photodynamic therapy with hemato-porphyrin derivative for primary treatment of gastrointestinal neoplasms in inoperable patients. *Dig Dis Sci* 1990;35(5): 545–552.

52. Karanov S, Shopova M, Getov H. Photodynamic therapy in gastrointestinal cancer. *Lasers Surg Med* 1991;11:395–398.

53. Overholt BF. Photodynamic therapy and thermal treatment of esophageal cancer. *Gastrointest Endosc Clin North Am* 1992; 2(3):433–455.

54. Monnier PH, Savary M, Fontolliet CH, Wagnieres G, Chatelain A, Cornaz P, Depeursinge CH, Van Den Bergh H. Photodetec-tion and photodynamic therapy in "early" squamous cell carci-noma of the pharynx, oesophagus and tracheo-bronchial tree. *Lasers Med Sci* 1990;5:149–169.

55. Panjehpour M, Overholt BF, DeNovo RC, Sneed RE, Petersen MG. Centering balloon to improve esophageal photodynamic therapy. *Lasers Surg Med* 1992;12:631–638.

56. Fleischer D, Cattau E Jr, Sinofsky E, Newsome J, Lack E, Andreiuk A, Benjamin S. Development of a laser balloon for the treatment of gastrointestinal obstruction. *Endoscopy* 1989; 21:81–85.

57. Barr H. PDT experimental studies. In: Krasner N. ed. *Lasers in gastroenterology*. New York: Wiley-Liss, 1991;233–250.

58. Loh CS, Bedwell J, MacRobert AJ, Krasner H, Phillips D, Bown SG. Photodynamic therapy of normal rat stomach: a compara-tive study between di-sulfonated aluminum phtalocyanine and 5-aminolevulinic acid. *Br J Cancer* 1992;66:452–462.

59. Divaris XG, Kennedy JC, Pottier RH. Phototoxic damage to sebaceous glands and hair follicles of mice after systemic admin-istration of 5-aminolevulinic acid correlates with localized proto-porphyrin IX fluorescence. *Am J Pathol* 1990;136:891–897.

60. Mang TS, Weimann TJ. Photodynamic therapy in the treatment of pancreatic carcinoma: dihematoporphyrin ether uptake and photobleaching kinetics. *Photochem Photobiol* 1987;46: 853–858.

61. Tochner Z, Mitchell JB, Smith P, Harrington F, Glastein E, Russo D, Russo A. Photodynamic therapy of ascites tumors within the peritoneal cavity. *Br J Cancer* 1986;53:733–736.

62. Cortese DA, et al. Clinical applications of a new endoscopic technique for detection of in situ bronchial carcinoma. *Mayo Clin Proc* 1979;34:635–641.

63. Profio AE, et al. Fluorescence bronchoscopy for localization of carcinoma in situ. *Med Phys* 1983;10:35–39.

64. Kato M, et al. Clinical measurement of tumor fluorescence using a new diagnostic system with HpD PRT and a spectroscope. *Lasers Surg Med* 1984;4(1):45–58.
65. Ankerst J. Spectral characteristics in tissue prognostics using L.I.F. *L.I.A. ICALEO* 1984;43:52–60.
66. Andersson-Engels S, Ankerst J, Montan S, Svanberg K, Svanberg S. Aspects of tumor demaraction in rats by means of laser-induced fluorescesce and hematoporphyrin derivatives. *Lasers Med Sci* 1988;3:239–248.
67. Deckelbaum LI, Lam JK, Cabin HS, Clubb, KS, Lors MB. Discrimination of normal and atherosclerotic aorta by L.I.F. *Lasers Surg Med* 1987;7:330–335.
68. Kapadia CR, Citruzzola FW, O'Brien KM, Stetz ML, Enriquez R, Deckelbaum LI. Laser-induced fluorescence spectroscopy of human colonic mucosa. *Gastroenterology* 1990;99:150–157.
69. Cothren RM, Richards-Kortum R, Sivak MV Jr, Fitzmaurice M, Rava RP, Boyce GA, Doxtader M, Blackman R, Ivanc TB, Hayes GB, Feld MS, Petras RE. Gastrointestinal tissue diagnosis by laser induced fluorescence spectroscopy at endoscopy. *Gastrointest Endosc* 1990;36(2):105–111.
70. Shomacker KT, Frisoli JK, Compton CC, Flotte TJ, Richter JM, Deutch TF, Nishioka NS. Ultraviolet laser-induced fluorescence of colonic polyps. *Gastroenterology* 1992;102:1155–1160.
71. Naveau S, Zourabichvilli O, Poynard T, Chaput JC. Comparison of a housed wave guide and a naked wave guide for endoscopic Nd:YAG laser therapy for esophageal and rectal tumors: a randomized clinical trial. *Proceedings of the Congress of the European Laser Association Amsterdam.* 1986.
72. Sahafi F. Light distribution and thermal behavior of a round sapphire tip with Nd:YAG laser. *Am Soc Laser Med Surg* 1988; abst 270.
73. Radford CM, Ahlquist DA, Gostout CJ, Viggiano TR, Balm BK, Zinsmeister AR. Prospective comparison of contact with non-contact Nd:YAG laser therapy for palliation of esophageal carcinoma. *Gastrointest Endosc* 1989;35:394–397.
74. Hira H. The role of contact laser therapy on inoperable rectal cancer. *Am Soc Laser Med Surg* 1988; abst 98.
75. Rutgeerts P, Vantrappen G, D'Heygere F, Geboes K. Endoscopic contact Nd:YAG laser therapy for colorectal cancer: a randomized comparison with non-contact therapy. *Lasers Med Sci* 1987;2:69.
76. Mason RC. The Nd:YAG laser in the relief of malignant gastro-esophageal obstruction. *Lasers Med Sci* 1988;B94.
77. Faintuch JS. Endoscopic contact laser therapy of the totally obstructed colon. *Gastrointest Endosc* 1988;34(2):196.
78. Faintuch JS. Endoscopic laser therapy in colorectal carcinoma. *Hematol Oncol Clin North Am* 1989;3(1):155–170.
79. Hochberger J. Advances in technique: sapphire and metal contact probes. In: Krasner N, ed. *Lasers in gastroenterology.* New York: Wiley-Liss, 1991;261–272.
80. Bown SG. Phototherapy of tumors. *World J Surg* 1983;7:700–707.
81. Matthewson K. Low power laser hyperthermia. In: Krasner N, ed. *Lasers in gastroenterology.* New York: Wiley-Liss 1991;281–299.
82. Matthewson K, Coleridge-Smith P, O'Sullivan JP, Northfield TC, Bown SG. Biological effects of intrahepatic Nd:YAG photocoagulation in rats. *Gastroenterology* 1987;93:550–557.
83. Steger AC, Bown SG, Clark CG. Interstitial laser hyperthermia: studies in normal liver. *Br J Surg* 1988;76:598.
84. Van Eyken P, Hiele M, Fevery J, Geboes K, Vantrappen G, Penninckx F, Desmet VJ, Rutgeerts P. Comparative study of low power neodymium-YAG laser interstitial hyperthermia versus ethanol injection for controlled hepatic tissue destruction. *Lasers Med Sci* 1991;6:35–41.
85. Steger AC, Barr H, Hawes R, Bown SG, Clark CG. Experimental studies on interstitial hyperthermia for treating pancreatic cancer. *Gut* 1987;28:A1382.
86. Matthewson K, Barton T, Lewin MR, O'Sullivan JP, Northfield TC, Bown SG. Low power interstitial laser photocoagulation in normal and neoplastic rat colon. *Gut* 1988;29:27–34.
87. Karanov S, Karaivanova M, Getov H, Karanova S. External beam, sapphire tip contact and interstitial Nd:YAG laser therapy at 1.064 μm on a transplanted adenocarcinoma in mice: a comparative study. *Lasers Med Sci* 1992;7:401–404.
88. Daikuzono H, Suzui S, Tajiri H, Tsunekawa H, Ohyama M, Josse NS. Laserthermia: a new computer-controlled contact Nd:YAG system for interstitial local hyperthermia. *Lasers Surg Med* 1988;8:254–258.
89. Suzuki S, Aoki J, Narumi H, Miwa T. Experimental and clinical studies on laser hyperthermia for gastric cancer. *J Clin Laser Med Surg* 1992;123–125.
90. Hashimoto D, Takami M, Idezuki Y. In-depth radiation therapy by YAG laser for malignant tumors in the liver under ultrasonic imaging. *Gastroenterology* 1985;88(5):1663.
91. Masters A, Steger AC, Lees WR, Walmsley KM, Bown SG. Interstitial laser hyperthermia: a new approach for treating liver metastases. *Br J Cancer* 1992;66:518–522.
92. Dowlatshahi K, Bhattacharye AK, Silver B, Matalon T, Williams JW. Percutaneous interstitial laser therapy of a patient with recurrent hepatoma in a transplanted liver. *Surgery* 1992;112(3):603–606.
93. Masters A, Bown SG. Interstitial laser hyperthermia. *Semin Surg Oncol* 1992;8:242–249.
94. Barr H, Krasner N. Interstitial laser photocoagulation for treating bleeding gastric cancer. *Br Med J* 1989;299:659–660.

Advanced Therapeutic Endoscopy, 2nd Ed.,
edited by J. S. Barkin and C. A. O'Phelan.
Raven Press, Ltd., New York © 1994.

CHAPTER 3

Patient Monitoring During Endoscopy

Pradeep K. Gupta and Stanley B. Benjamin

The role of extracorporeal monitoring equipment during gastrointestinal endoscopic procedures has been a source of debate. Just as the technology of endoscopes has evolved, so too has the complexity and accuracy of monitoring equipment. During the early years of endoscopy, gastroenterologists used rigid scopes, all the while clinically monitoring the patients. Advances in endoscopic equipment now allow the gastrointestinal endoscopist to perform tasks formerly the province of either surgeons or interventional radiologists. Increasingly, these procedures are being performed on an older population of patients. Paralleling the evolution of endoscopic technology, automated extracorporeal monitoring devices recording blood pressure, heart rate, electrocardiogram, respiratory rate, arterial oxygen saturation, and expired carbon dioxide content are currently available. In part due to the paucity of data performed in a randomized, controlled fashion, and partly due to the expense of this equipment [estimated to be in the range of $12,000 to $15,000 (1)], debate has centered on the extent of monitoring required during endoscopic procedures.

This chapter examines the physiologic impact of endoscopy; the potential risks and complications are reviewed by way of clinical trials. The use of specific monitoring devices, most notably pulse oximetry, and the impact on patient safety are also discussed.

ENDOSCOPY: SAFETY

Major complications, i.e., cardiopulmonary in nature, related to gastrointestinal endoscopy are infrequent. However, technological advancements enable the gastrointestinal endoscopist to perform procedures that are arduous and lengthy. These procedures are being carried out on more elderly patients. Coupled with the use of conscious sedation, the combination of all these factors has the potential to be catastrophic.

Cardiopulmonary complications associated with endoscopy were first brought to light in the 1950s with the death of a patient due to ventricular fibrillation during upper endoscopy (2). Since that time, the risk of a fatal complication was found to be 3 in 10,000 in three large studies representing over 250,000 upper endoscopies (3–5). The incidence of death as a complication of colonoscopy ranges from 0% to 0.3% (6–9). A recent survey by the American Society for Gastrointestinal Endoscopy (ASGE) in conjunction with the Food and Drug Administration (FDA) of over 21,000 procedures reported seven deaths, for a mortality rate of 0.3 per thousand procedures (10).

Thus the safety afforded the patient is remarkable. Then why the debate over monitoring? The importance of this issue lies on several fronts. First, although the risk of a complication arising during endoscopy is low, cardiopulmonary complications make up 50% to 60% of these events (11,12). Second, as the population at large trends toward an older age group, the inherent risk of undetected cardiovascular or pulmonary disease increases; further, older patients tend to have less reserve, which would otherwise allow them to physiologically compensate to physiologic stressors such as endoscopy. Third, if we were to utilize selective monitoring, perhaps only on elderly patients or those with known cardiopulmonary disease, how can we justify or defend the absence of monitoring in a younger individual with clinically inapparent cardiomyopathy or other medical illness? Since cardiopulmonary alterations are more readily apparent with extracorporeal monitoring devices, these devices, most notably pulse oximetry, have been the focus of several studies (Table 1).

P. K. Gupta and S. B. Benjamin: Department of Medicine, Division of Gastroenterology, Georgetown University Medical Center, Washington, DC 20007.

TABLE 1. *Summary of studies*

Reference	Sample size	Medications	Age (mean)	Total # or % desaturation (Sqo_2 <90%) or as otherwise noted	# or % desaturation during EGD	# or % desaturation during COL	Findings	Conclusions
O'Connor and Jones (26)	236	Midazolam + meperidine, diazepam + meperidine	55	45%	45%	54%	Medications used, age, type of procedure, or dosages of medications could not reliably predict which patients would desaturate	The authors concluded that pulse oximetry is more sensitive than standard clinical monitoring in detecting desaturation
Bilotta et al. (27)	103	Meperidine + diazepam	61	41%			Sex, obesity, history of heart disease or lung disease did *not* correlate with desaturation; however, age did correlate	No adverse outcomes noted, suggesting that oximetry may not be clinically useful
Steffes et al. (28)	326	Midazolam + meperidine	–		12.9%	17.8%	*EGD group:* Factors associated with desaturation included age, history of cardiac, and/or respiratory disease *Col group:* History of cardiac and/or respiratory disease correlated with desaturation	Pulse oximetry and automated blood pressure was of value during endoscopy, particularly in the elderly and patients with cardiac or pulmonary disease
Dark et al. (29)	115	Midazolam + meperidine	65	70% (74% decrease from baseline saturation) 32% (Sqo_2 <85%)	15% (Sqo_2 <85%)	50% (Sqo_2 <85%)	*EGD group:* Weak correlations between severity of pulmonary disease, age, amount of sedation and desaturation *Col group:* Weak correlation between age and amount of sedation and desaturation	Supported use of continuous exometry as standard procedure for all endoscopic procedures
Lavies et al. (30)	120	Midazolam + diazemuls	58.1 55.1 50.4				The use of i.v. sedation was randomized to three groups, group I—diazemuls, group II—midazolam, group III—normal saline	Operator experience was an important factor affecting desaturation
Hayward et al. (31)	100	Meperidine + midazolam		24%				Authors recommended that continuous oximetry should be routinely performed during endoscopic procedures
Lancaster et al. (32)	63	Midazolam		17% (>8% fall in Sqo_2)			Marked hypotensive episodes (>40% fall in blood pressure) occurred in 17% of all patients No correlation with type of procedure, hypoxia, hypotension Dose of sedation was significantly related to desaturation but not to change in blood pressure	Authors concluded that continuous pulse oximetry and blood pressure monitoring should be performed throughout endoscopic procedure

TABLE 1. *Continued.*

Reference	Sample size	Medications	Age (mean)	Total # or % desaturation (SaO₂ <90%) or as otherwise noted	# or % desaturation during EGD	# or % desaturation during COL	Findings	Conclusions
Murray et al. (33)	20	Pethidine + midazolam					50% of patients developed ectopic foci either supraventricular or ventricular in origin	Authors emphasized the importance of monitoring oxygen saturation, arterial pressure, electrocardiogram and heart rate during endoscopic procedures
DiSario et al. (34)	618	Meperidine and/or diazepam	62				Hemodynamic alterations in 71% 6% of these with severe hypotension (MAP <60) 30% with hypertension, 26% with bradycardia, 32% with tachycardia	Monitoring documents events that are clinically insignificant and that monitoring does not improve outcome
Berg et al. (35)	271	Meperidine, diazepam, midazolam		8.6% (SaO₂ <85%)			There was no difference in desaturation between those undergoing EGD or colonoscopy	The authors concluded this study does not support the use of O₂ monitoring during endoscopic procedures

CLINICAL TRIALS

Arterial oxygen desaturation is now known to be a frequent occurrence during upper and lower endoscopy (13–24). The importance of oxygen desaturation is linked to the physiologic responses associated with decreased oxygen tension. Based on the oxygen-hemoglobin dissociation curve, a saturation of 90% corresponds to an oxygen tension of 60 mm Hg. As oxygen levels decline in the blood, myocardial oxygen levels concomitantly decline, creating a disequilibrium between supply and demand. As a compensatory response, heart rate increases, thereby further raising myocardial oxygen demand. Extraction of oxygen from the coronary arteries provides the main source of myocardial oxygen. An atheroma or noncompliant vessels place the patient at risk for ischemic insult to the myocardium as myocardial oxygen consumption/demands rise in the face of decreased coronary flow (25). Recognizing the significance of hypoxemia, investigators have focused on the role of continuous oximetry during endoscopy.

O'Connor and Jones (26) evaluated 236 consecutive patients scheduled for elective endoscopy. The first 136 patients received midazolam and meperidine; the remaining 100 received diazepam with meperidine. The average age of both groups was approximately 55 years. Baseline oximetry measurements were made and all patients had continuous pulse oximetry during their procedure. Forty-five percent of patients desaturated to less than 90% without manifesting any clinical signs of distress. Of these patients, 45% undergoing upper endoscopy and 54% undergoing lower endoscopy desaturated to <90%. Medications used, age of patient, type of procedure, and dose requirements of medications could not reliably predict which patients would desaturate.

Bilotta and colleagues (27) prospectively monitored 103 consecutive patients undergoing colonoscopy to attempt to ascertain clinical characteristics that may be predictive of oxygen desaturation. Patients requiring medications received meperidine and diazepam as premedication for the procedure. Desaturation of oxygen levels <90% occurred in 41% of patients. The only parameter that correlated with the risk of lowering oxygen tension was age; sex, obesity, history of heart or lung disease, baseline oxygen level, and cardiac medications did not correlate. The authors concluded that since no adverse effects or outcomes were noted, oximetry during colonoscopy may not be necessary. A criticism of this trial may be that monitoring was continued for only 1 minute after the colonoscope was removed, thereby potentially missing periprocedure desaturation. Further, the sample size is far too small to reach validated statistical significance.

Steffes et al. (28) prospectively evaluated continuous oxygen monitoring in 326 patients undergoing esophagogastroduodenoscopy (EGD) and 90 undergoing colonoscopy. Patients were administered titrated doses of midazolam and meperidine. Desaturation was found in 12.9% of patients in the EGD group, and in 17.8% in the colonoscopy group. Continuous blood pressure monitoring, in addition to continuous O_2 saturation monitoring, resulted in 31 therapeutic interventions. Factors associated with desaturation in the EGD group included age, history of cardiac and/or respiratory disease, and a cardiac history alone. Patients in the colonoscopy group were found only to have an association with a history of cardiac and/or respiratory disease. The authors concluded that pulse oximetry and automated blood pressure monitoring proved to be of value, particularly in the elderly and patients with cardiac or pulmonary disease. Their use may guide therapeutic interventions, thereby avoiding cardiopulmonary complications.

Dark and coworkers (29) prospectively studied 115 male patients undergoing endoscopy. The mean age was 62 years in the colonoscopy group and 60 in the EGD group. Patients who had both procedures averaged 65 years. Upper endoscopy was performed with a 9.2 mm diameter scope. All patients underwent pulmonary function tests prior to endoscopy to evaluate the presence of chronic obstructive pulmonary disease. Medications consisted of meperidine and midazolam. Seventy percent of patients exhibited arterial oxygen desaturation (defined by the authors as >4% decrease from baseline oxygen saturation); notably, severe desaturation (SaO_2 <85%, corresponding to a PaO_2 of <50) was found in 32% of all patients. Severe desaturation occurred in 15% of EGD patients, 50% of patients in the colonoscopy group, and 57% of patients requiring both procedures. A weak correlation between severity of pulmonary disease and low arterial saturation was found only in the EGD group. Both groups demonstrated a weak correlation between age and amount of sedation and change in SaO_2. The authors concluded that their data supported the notion of continuous oximetery as standard procedure for all endoscopic procedures.

Lavies et al. (30) compared the risk of desaturation when upper endoscopy was performed by either an experienced endoscopist or an individual in training as well as the influence of i.v. sedation (midazolam and diazemuls) on oxygen tension. They found operator experience an important factor affecting desaturation, whereas the use of i.v. sedation did not significantly affect SaO_2.

Hayward and coworkers (31) studied 100 consecutive patients undergoing endoscopy; of these, 78 underwent EGD and 22 underwent colonoscopy. Pulse oximetry was continued from the time just prior to the endoscopic procedure to 5 minutes after termination of the procedure. Sedation consisted of i.v. meperidine and midazolam. Twenty-four patients exhibited severe hypoxemia (defined by the authors as a SaO_2 <90%, correlating with a PaO_2 of <60), of which 15 had a transient episode without the necessity for intervention. Nine patients required some mode of intervention, i.e., stimulation, supplemental oxygen, i.v. naloxone. Twenty patients developed a tachycardia >120 beats per minute. The authors concluded that continuous oximetry should be routinely performed during endoscopic procedures in order to recognize events that may not be identified clinically, and to initiate corrective measures early.

Lancaster et al. (32) examined the degree of desaturation and change in blood pressure (BP) in 63 patients undergoing either EGD, colonoscopy, or flexible sigmoidoscopy. Intravenous sedation consisted of midazolam. These investigators found that marked hypotensive episodes (defined as a >40% fall in BP) occurred in 13% of the total and that marked hypoxia (defined as >8% fall in SaO_2) occurred in 17% of all patients. There was no significant difference in fall of BP or oxygen saturation based on type of endoscopic procedure. There was no correlation between hypoxia or hypotension and a patient's age or prior medical history. The dose of sedation was significantly related to desaturation but not to change in BP. The authors concluded that hypotension and hypoxia are unpredictable and often not clinically recognizable; thus, continuous pulse oximetry and BP monitoring should be performed throughout endoscopic procedures.

To assess the cardiovascular changes and to determine suitable monitoring techniques, Murray et al. (33) studied 20 consecutive patients undergoing endoscopy. Continuous monitoring of heart rate, electrocardiogram, and arterial oxygen saturation, as well as BP readings at 1-minute intervals, was maintained from prior to the procedure to 1 hour after its completion. Intravenous sedation consisted of pethidine and midazolam. All patients experienced oxygen desaturation to a mean of 82.9% during the procedure and into the recovery stage. Statistically significant changes in arterial pressure were noted. Alterations in heart rate were found in 16 of 20 patients with 10 patients developing ectopic foci that were supraventricular, ventricular, or both, in origin. The authors emphasized the importance of monitoring oxygen saturation, arterial pressure, and the electrocardiogram in addition to the heart rate.

DiSario et al. (34) randomized 618 patients undergoing EGD and/or colonoscopy into two groups: group 1 patients underwent clinical observation throughout the procedure, whereas group 2 patients had automated cardiovascular monitoring during the procedure and 3 minutes after its completion. Meperidine and/or diazepam were the intravenous sedation used. Hemodynamic alterations occurred in 71% of monitored patients with 6% of these evidencing hypotension, defined as mean arterial pressure (MAP) <60. Other alterations noted included hypertension 30%, brady-cardia 26%, and tachycardia 32%. The authors surmised that hemodynamic monitoring documents events that are clinically insignificant and that monitoring does not improve outcome.

Berg and coworkers (35) utilized transcutaneous oxygen saturation monitoring in 271 consecutive patients undergoing EGD and/or colonoscopy. The intravenous sedation consisted of meperidine, diazepam, and midazolam. Significant desaturation, defined as a SaO_2 <85% was observed in 8.6% of patients. There was no difference in desaturation between those undergoing EGD or colonoscopy. The authors concluded that this study does not support the use of O_2 monitoring during endoscopic procedures.

What can one derive from the above data? First, oxygen desaturation is a common event during endoscopy. Second, untoward results from desaturation are uncommon, yet their clinical manifestation is not always readily apparent. None of the studies addressed benefit because of the small sample sizes.

IS SUPPLEMENTAL OXYGEN THE ANSWER?

The predominant factor in desaturation appears to be the use of intravenous sedation. Clearly, some desaturation occurs with intubation, but this is transient (32–35). The combination of benzodiazepines and opiates produces greater desaturation than benzodiazepines alone (36,37). The most reasonable approach is to use intravenous sedation judiciously, with the minimum dosages for the endoscopic examination. The question of use of supplemental oxygen in order to circumvent the issue of continuous monitoring with oximetry has been recently investigated.

Gross and Long (38) prospectively evaluated the effects of supplemental oxygen in patients undergoing colonoscopy. They randomized patients into two groups, those that received supplemental oxygen and those that did not. Patients were medicated with meperidine/midazolam combinations. Patients who received supplemental oxygen were less likely to become hypoxic; however, hypoxemia occurred in this group despite supplemental oxygen. The authors recommended that continuous oxygen monitoring be maintained since desaturation occurs even in the setting of nasal oxygen administration. These finding have been reproduced by Jaffe et al. (39).

Bell and coworkers (40) studied 50 consecutive patients undergoing upper endoscopy. All patients received supplemental oxygen after being sedated with intravenous midazolam. The results were compared to 100 previous patients, none of whom received oxygen.

These investigators found that the use of oxygen via nasal cannula prevented hypoxemia in this group of patients. They suggested that supplemental oxygen be administered to elderly patients, particularly those with cardiovascular disease.

Other investigators have reported similar findings (41–43), that is, that desaturation may occur in those receiving supplemental oxygen. The association of arrhythmias with hypoxemia strengthens the importance in early recognition of desaturation (44–46).

Freeman et al. (47) evaluated the role of carbon dioxide retention during endoscopic retrograde cholangiopancreatography (ERCP), colonoscopy, and upper endoscopy. These investigators prospectively monitored 64 patients, of which 23 underwent ERCP, 20 colonoscopy, and 21 upper endoscopy. Patients were monitored with pulse oximetry for oxygen saturation, transcutaneous carbon dioxide (TCO_2) monitoring, and automated blood pressure and electrocardiogram. Arterial blood gases were obtained to determine the accuracy of TCO_2. Patients received fentanyl and/or midazolam as i.v. sedation. The authors found that TCO_2 correlated well with arterial blood gases. Further, carbon dioxide retention occurred when SaO_2 was less than 90%, and this retention occurred despite supplemental oxygen administration. Supplemental oxygen masked but did not cause CO_2 retention. The authors concluded that CO_2 retention heralded apnea and was associated with hypertension and multifocal PVCs and that pulse oximetry failed to detect significant CO_2 retention. This study puts forth the concept that the administration of supplemental oxygen should be done with caution.

THE DEBATE

Legislative bodies, national organizations, hospitals, and physicians continue to debate the issue of monitoring during endoscopic procedures. As the clinical trials above indicate, there is variance in the conclusions drawn. Furthermore, variability in study design makes direct comparison between trials difficult. Most importantly, the sample size required to create a statistically meaningful study is prohibitively large. The ASGE guidelines (48) do not specifically recommend universal monitoring based on the paucity of scientific data (1). To help delineate the issues, a symposium on sedation and monitoring was convened at the recent World Congress of Gastroenterology meeting in Sydney, Australia. The panel of experts favored universal monitoring, with the incorporation of continuous oximetry into the armamentarium of extracorporeal monitoring devices (49–51). The following sections represent our distillate of the disparities in the literature, and as such, our recommendations.

Role of the Endoscopist

The emergence of the endoscopist as a part-time anesthetist underscores the importance of familiarity with dosages of medications and techniques of administration. An endoscopic nurse/assistant should be present throughout the procedure. A medical history, with specific attention to chronic benzodiazepine use (for the unlikely event that Flumazenil is required), and a physical examination to assess the presence of any contraindications to endoscopy, should be performed prior to endoscopy. Both the endoscopist and endoscopy nurse should clinically observe the patient during the procedure. It is preferable to maintain a log recording the patient's name, age, procedure, indication, duration of procedure, findings, notation of tissue samples, therapeutic interventions, and complication(s) for quality assurance (52).

Resuscitation

Endoscopists and nurse assistants are responsible for ensuring the availability and working order of resuscitation equipment. Essential equipment includes a crash cart with equipment and medications to maintain an airway, breathing, and circulation. It is strongly recommended that members of the endoscopy team be certified in advanced cardiac life support (ACLS). The ASGE survey of endoscopic sedation and monitoring practices (53) revealed that only 30% and 18% of endoscopists and gastrointestinal assistants, respectively, were certified in ACLS.

Sedation

A comprehensive review of sedation is beyond the scope of this chapter; the reader is referred to several recent reviews (54–56). The vast majority of endoscopists in the United States use sedation during endoscopic procedures (53). Meperidine, midazolam, and diazepam are the medications most commonly employed (53). Particular attention to recommended dosing schedules with appropriate adjustments based on age, renal function, etc., should be made. The aim of the gastroenterologist is anxiolysis, analgesia, and amnesia rather than ptosis and hypnosis (57). Protective reflexes should not be abolished. Thus, the minimum dose of sedation to safely complete the endoscopic procedure is sought. A few salient features of these drugs will be discussed.

Benzodiazepines such as midazolam and diazepam, provide anxiolysis, amnesia, sedation, and muscle relaxation. These two drugs differ in onset of action and longevity of effect. Diazepam's onset of action occurs in 1 to 5 minutes with duration of action ranging from 15 to 60 minutes (56). A major characteristic affecting the use of diazepam for gastrointestinal endoscopy is the risk of resedation up to 8 hours after the completion of the procedure due to increased plasma levels of diazepam from gastrointestinal tract absorption of excreted bile (58).

Midazolam has an onset of action of 1 to 5 minutes with a duration of less than 2 hours (56). The FDA received reports of cardiopulmonary complications shortly after midazolam's introduction in 1986. Since that time, it has been determined that several factors contributed to the initial poor outcomes associated with midazolam use. Among these were older age, combination with opioids, doses higher than those recommended by the manufacturer, bolus injection, and lack of adequate monitoring.

Narcotic analgesics provide analgesia and sedation. The recent ASGE survey reported that meperidine is the most commonly administered narcotic for gastrointestinal endoscopy (10).

Dose-dependent respiratory depression is found with both the narcotics and benzodiazepines. The synergistic effects of these drugs enables the endoscopist to reduce the doses of these drugs when used in combination. Bailey et al. (59) recommend that patients receiving a combination of midazolam with fentanyl or other opioid undergo monitoring with pulse oximetry due to the risk of hypoxemia and apnea.

Droperidol, a neuroleptic of the butyrophenone class, has been used in patients who have paradoxical reactions to standard sedation or those in whom standard sedation is inadequate (60). The onset of action is 3 to 10 minutes after intravenous administration with a duration of action of 3 to 6 hours. When combined with a narcotic, a state of analgesia and psychomotor retardation occurs, termed neuroleptanalgesia.

Propofol is the newest medication to be introduced into the armamentarium for conscious sedation. Its use requires the presence of an anesthesiologist for the drug's administration and control of the airway. A continuous intravenous infusion is required to maintain anesthesia. Propofol is a short-acting hypnotic that has the advantage of rapid clearance, enabling the patient's "street readiness" in a shorter time period than with midazolam (61,62).

Barbiturates such as pentobarbital, secobarbital, and thiopental have pharmacokinetics not conducive to use in gastrointestinal endoscopy. These drugs are long-acting with a slow rate of elimination. Most importantly, drugs that have no known antagonists should not be used.

Specific antagonists to opiates and benzodiazepines should be readily available. Once again, dosing schedules, as well as potentially dangerous situations, such as chronic benzodiazepine use and the risk of inducing seizures with flumazenil administration, must be known. The routine use of antagonists to hasten recovery is discouraged, with their utilization limited to medically indicated situations, i.e., cardiopulmonary compromise. The endoscopist must be mindful of the potential complications associated with flumazenil (seizures) and naloxone (arrhythmias, presumably secondary to a generalized sympathetic discharge).

Clinical Monitoring

The use of extracorporeal monitoring devices is not intended to diminish the importance of clinical observation. However, certain factors such as darkened rooms preclude optimum conditions to observe patients. Further, monitoring devices provide early warnings of potentially catastrophic events. The use of automated blood pressure machines, continuous oximetry, and electrocardiographic monitoring is encouraged. Supplemental oxygen should most likely be reserved for prolonged desaturation, with the awareness that CO_2 retention may occur. The majority of endoscopists utilize oximetry and electrocardiographic monitoring, 65% and 55%, respectively (53).

Recovery

Patients should be observed during the recovery period until fully awake. Extracorporeal monitoring should be continued during this period. Written instructions, including significant endoscopic findings, and whom to call in the event of a problem arising, should be given to the patient. Patients who receive sedation should not be permitted to drive for 24 hours. Reversal with antagonists should not sway the endoscopist into allowing the patient to drive home.

SOME FINAL THOUGHTS

As the debate regarding monitoring rages, some would comment on the appearance of a collision between stark reality and lofty philosophical goals. As physicians we strive to provide the best care available, doing what is in our patients' best interests. The lack of large numbers of trials supporting or refuting the use of monitoring devices does not automatically allow us to dismiss it. Rather, it would appear that those opposed to universal, comprehensive monitoring are exhibiting "mural dyslexia" (Dr. Burt Epstein)—that is, they can't read the writing on the wall. The practice of medicine incorporates empiricism in that aspect we call the "art of medicine." Intuitively, we feel that universal, comprehensive monitoring is for the good of our patients, and as such, support its use.

REFERENCES

1. Fleischer DE. Monitoring the patient receiving conscious sedation for gastrointestinal endoscopy: issues and guidelines. *Gastrointest Endosc* 1989;35:262–266.
2. Katz D, Selenick S. *Gastroenterology* 1957;33:650.
3. Mandelstam P, Sugawa C, Silvis SE, et al. *Gastrointest Endosc* 1976;23:16–19.
4. Anderson KE, Clausen N. *Endoscopy* 1978;10:180–183.
5. Schiller KF, Cotton PB, Salmon TR. *Gut* 1972;13:1027.
6. Roger BHG, Silvis SE, Nebel OT, et al. *Gastrointest Endosc* 1975;22:73–77.
7. Smith LF. *Dis Colon Rectum* 1976;19:407–412.
8. Gilbert DA, Hallstrom AP, Shaneyfelt SL, et al. The National ASGE Colonoscopy Survey—complications of colonoscopy. *Gastrointest Endosc* 1984;30:156.
9. Fruhmorgan P, Demling L. *Endoscopy* 1979;11:146–150.
10. Arrowsmith JB, Gerstmann B, Fleischer DE, Benjamin SB. Results from the American Society for Gastrointestinal Endoscopy/U.S. Food and Drug Administration Collaborative Study on Complication Rates and Drug Use during Gastrointestinal Endoscopy. *Gastrointest Endosc* 1991;37:421–427.
11. Silvis SE, Nebel O, Rogers G, Sugawa C, Mandelstam P. *JAMA* 1976;235:928–930.
12. Habr-Gama A, Waye JD. *World J Surg* 1989;13:193–201.
13. Fennerty MB, Earnest DL, Hudson PB, Sampliner RE. Physiologic changes during endoscopy. *Gastrointest Endosc* 1990;36:22–25.
14. Casteel HB, Fiedorek SC, Kiel ER. Effects of upper gastrointestinal endoscopy on blood oxygen saturation and cardiac rhythm in children. *Gastrointest Endosc* 1988;34:214.
15. Hayward SR, Wilson RF, Sugawa C. Cardiopulmonary effects of endoscopy. *Gastrointest Endosc* 1988;34:172.
16. Dark DS, Campbell DR, Wesselius LJ. *Am Rev Respir Dis* 1988;137:163.
17. Bell GD, Reeve PA, Moshiri M, et al. Intravenous midazolam: a study of the degree of oxygen desaturation occurring during upper gastrointestinal endoscopy. *Br J Clin Pharmacol* 1987;23:703–708.
18. Lieberman DA, Wuerker CK, Katon RM. Cardiopulmonary risk of esophagogastroduodenoscopy. *Gastroenterology* 1985;88:468–472.
19. Pecora A, Chiesa JC, Alloy A, et al. The effect of upper gastrointestinal endoscopy on arterial O_2 tension in smokers and nonsmokers with and without medication. *Gastrointest Endosc* 1984;30:284–288.
20. Rozen P, Fireman Z, Gilat T. The causes of hypoxemia in elderly patients during endoscopy. *Gastrointest Endosc* 1982;28:243–246.
21. Rostykes PS, McDonald GB, Albert RK. *Gastroenterology* 1988;78:488–491.
22. Alturi R, Ravry MJR. *Gastrointest Endosc* 1978;24:191.
23. Whorwell PJ, Smith CL, Foster KJ. *Gut* 1976;17:797–800.
24. Bell GD, Spickett GP, Reeve PA, et al. *Br J Clin Pharmacol* 1987;23:709–713.
25. Bell GD. In: Carr-Locke DE, ed. *Balliere's clinical gastroenterology*. London: Balliere Tindall, 1991;5:79–98.
26. O'Connor KW, Jones S. Oxygen desaturation is common and clinically underappreciated during elective endoscopic procedures. *Gastrointest Endosc* 1990;36:S2–S4.
27. Bilotta JJ, Floyd JL, Waye JD. Arterial oxygen desaturation during ambulatory colonoscopy: predictability, incidence, and clinical significance. *Gastrointest Endosc* 1990;36:S5–S8.
28. Steffes CP, Sugawa C, Wilson RF, Hayward SR. *Surg Endosc* 1990;4:175–178.
29. Dark DS, Campbell DR, Wesselius LJ. Arterial oxygen desaturation during gastrointestinal endoscopy. *Am J Gastroenterol* 1990;85:1317–1321.
30. Lavies NG, Creasy T, Harris K, Hanning CD. Arterial oxygen saturation during upper gastrointestinal endoscopy: influence of sedation and operator experience. *Am J Gastroenterol* 1988;83:618–622.
31. Hayward SR, Sugawa C, Wilson RF. Changes in oxygenation and pulse rate during endoscopy. *Am Surg* 1989;55:198–202.

32. Lancaster JF, Gotley D, Bartolo DC, Leaper DJ. Hypoxia and hypotension during endoscopy and colonoscopy. *Aust NZ J Surg* 1990;60:271–273.

33. Murray AW, Morran CG, Kenny NC, Macfarlane P, Anderson JR. Examination of cardiorespiratory changes during upper gastrointestinal endoscopy. *Anaesthesia* 1991;46:181–184.

34. DiSario JA, Waring JP, Talbert G, Sanowski RA. Monitoring of blood pressure and heart rate during routine endoscopy: a prospective, randomized, controlled study. *Am J Gastroenterol* 1991;86:956–960.

35. Berg JC, Miller R, Burkhalter E. Clinical value of pulse oximetry during routine diagnostic and therapeutic endoscopic procedures. *Endoscopy* 1991;23:328–330.

36. Zigsmoid EK, Flynn K, Martinez OA. *J Clin Pharmacol* 1974; 14:377–381.

37. Murray AW, Morran CG, Kenny NC, Anderson JR. Arterial oxygen saturation during upper gastrointestinal endoscopy: the effects of a midazolam/pethidine combination. *Gut* 1990;31: 270–273.

38. Gross JB, Long WB. Nasal oxygen alleviates hypoxemia in colonoscopy patients sedated with midazolem and meperidine. *Gastrointest Endosc* 1990;36:26–29.

39. Jaffe PE, Fennerty MB, Sampliner RE, Hixson LJ. Preventing hypoxia during colonoscopy: a randomized controlled trial of supplemental oxygen. *J Clin Gastroenterol* 1992;14:114–116.

40. Bell GD, Morden A, Bown S, Coady T, Logan RFA. *Lancet* 1987;1:1022–1024.

41. Thompson AM, Park KGM, Kerr F, Munro A. Safety of fibreoptic endoscopy: analysis of cardiorespiratory events. *Br J Surg* 1992;79:1046–1049.

42. McKee CC, Ragland JJ, Myers JO. An evaluation of multiple clinical variables for hypoxia during colonoscopy. *Surg Gynecol Obstet* 1991;173:37–40.

43. Brandl S, Barody TJ, Andrews P, Morgan A, Hyland L, Devine M. *Gastrointest Endosc* 1992;38:415–417.

44. McAlpine JK, Martin BJ, Devine BL. Cardiac arrhythmias associated with upper gastrointestinal endoscopy in elderly subjects. *Scott Med J* 1990;35:102–104.

45. Iber FL, Livak A, Kruss DM. Apnea and cardiopulmonary arrest during and after endoscopy. *J Clin Gastroenterol* 1992;14: 109–113.

46. Danzi JT, Rosado S, Swartz M, et al. The effects of conscious sedation for a variety of endoscopic procedures on patients' vital signs/arterial saturation. *Gastrointest Endosc* 1990;36:186–187.

47. Freeman ML, Hennessy JT, Cass OW. Carbon dioxide retention and oxygen desaturation during conscious sedation for ERCP, colonoscopy, and upper GI endoscopy. *Gastrointest Endosc* 1991;37:233.

48. Standards of Practice Committee American Society for Gastrointestinal Endoscopy. Monitoring of patients undergoing gastrointestinal endoscopic procedures. *Gastrointest Endosc* 1991;37: 120–121.

49. Cousins MJ. Monitoring—the anaesthetist's view. *Scand J Gastroenterol* 1990;25(suppl 179):12–17.

50. Benjamin SB. Overview of monitoring in endoscopy. *Scand J Gastroenterol* 1990;25(suppl 179):28–30.

51. Bell GD. Monitoring—the gastroenterologist's view. *Scand J Gastroenterol* 1990;25(suppl 179):18–23.

52. Fleischer DE, Al-Kawas F, Benjamin SB, Lewis JH, Kidwell J. *Gastrointest Endosc* 1992;38:411–414.

53. Keefe EB, O'Connor KW. 1989 A/S/G/E survey of endoscopic sedation and monitoring practices. *Gastrointest Endosc* 1990; 36:S13–S18.

54. Lauven PM. Pharmacology of drugs for conscious sedation. *Scand J Gastroenterol* 1990;25(suppl 179):1–6.

55. McCloy RF, Pearson RC. Which agent and how to deliver it? *Scand J Gastroenterol* 1990;25(suppl 179):7–11.

56. Ginsberg GG, Nguyen C, Fleischer DE, Al-Kawas FH, Benjamin SB. Medications in endoscopy. In: Lewis JH, ed. In press.

57. McCloy R. Asleep on the job: sedation and monitoring during endoscopy. *Scand J Gastroenterol* 1992;27(suppl 192):97–101.

58. Goodman, Gillman A, eds. *The pharmacological basis of therapeutics.* New York: Pergamon Press, 1990.

59. Bailey PL, Pace NL, Ashburn MA, Moll JW, East KA, Stanley TH. *Anesthesiology* 1990;73:826–830.

60. Wilcox CM, Forsmark CE, Cello JP. Utility of droperidol for conscious sedation in gastrointestinal endoscopic procedures. *Gastrointest Endosc* 1990;36:112–115.

61. Dubois A, Balatoni E, Peters JP, Baudoux M. *Anaesthesia* 1988; 43:S75–S80.

62. Patterson KW, Casey PB, Murray JP, O'Boyle CA, Cunningham AJ. Propofol sedation for outpatients upper gastrointestinal endoscopy: comparison with midazolam. *Br J Anaesth* 1991;67: 108–111.

Advanced Therapeutic Endoscopy, 2nd Ed.,
edited by J. S. Barkin and C. A. O'Phelan.
Raven Press, Ltd., New York © 1994.

CHAPTER 4

Unique Aspects of Pediatric Endoscopy

A. J. Katz

The absence of gastrointestinal (GI) cancer and alcoholic liver disease in the pediatric population radically changes the indications and need for diagnostic and therapeutic endoscopic intervention. Pediatric gastroenterologists still tend to be more diagnostically and less therapeutically oriented, but this is changing. Extensive reviews on pediatric endoscopy are available (1–3). This chapter discusses only selective aspects that distinguish pediatric from adult endoscopy. A consensus of specific indications for pediatric endoscopic procedures is still being evaluated by the North American Society for Pediatric Gastroenterology. Currently, guidelines of the American Society for Gastrointestinal Enterology (ASGE) are modified for pediatric use (Tables 1–4).

ENDOSCOPY SETTING

Pediatric endoscopy is performed in the hospital endoscopy suite or free-standing endoscopy center.

PREPARATION FOR PATIENTS

It is critically important that the parents understand what procedure their child is going to have, and why. Much parent and child anxiety can be allayed simply by ensuring this is done adequately. Parental anxiety, often transmitted to the child, imparts fear and results in lack of cooperation.

At the endoscopy suite, an endoscopy nurse once again explains the procedure and allays any concerns. An IV is placed prior to the procedure. The parents stay in the IV room and are allowed to accompany the child to the endoscopy suite. Some like to stay until

A. J. Katz: Department of Pediatric Gastroenterology, Newton-Wellesley Hospital; and Pediatric Gastroenterology Associates PC, Boston, Massachusetts 02115-5710.

the child is sedated; others prefer to leave earlier. In selective cases, we permit parents to stay and watch the procedure, but one needs to use clinical judgment as to when this is appropriate.

Always evaluate the child for loose teeth prior to the procedure; if a tooth is very loose, remove it prior to the procedure.

Patients under 10 years of age are restrained in a PediWrap. More intensive nursing is needed for pediatric than adult patients. Unlike adult endoscopy, there are at least two assistants in the pediatric endoscopy room, one holding the patient and checking the vital signs, and the other available for biopsy or other assistance. Adequate monitoring includes heart rate, O_2 saturation, and blood pressure.

DOSAGE OF MEDICATIONS

Neonates to 6 Months

In our endoscopy suite we do not always sedate neonates and infants under the age of 6 months for endoscopy. It has been our experience that the procedure is more rapid and effective, and the patients are discharged earlier. Thinner scopes have made this relatively easier. There are, however, differences of opinion. IV Versed 0.5 to 0.7 mg/kg is often used or, very rarely, general anesthesia (1,2).

Six Months to 2 Years

Patients between the ages of 6 months and 2 years are given either p.o. Versed, 0.5 to 0.7 mg/kg 20 minutes prior to procedure, or IV Versed, 0.1 to 0.3 mg/kg, and Demerol, 1 to 2 mg/kg at the time of the procedure.

TABLE 1. *Indications for diagnostic upper endoscopy*

Gastrointestinal bleeding
Dysphagia or odynophagia or persistent refusal to eat
Recurrent abdominal pain
    Signs and symptoms suggesting serious organic disease, such as weight loss, anorexia, or anemia
    Associated significant morbidity: school absenteeism, recurrent hospitalizations, limitation of usual activities, dysfunctional family as a result
    Suspected peptic disease or GE reflux unresponsive to adequate trial of antacid therapy
Reflux esophagitis—evaluation in atypical presentation; failure to respond to treatment; evaluation postfundoplication
Persistent vomiting of unknown cause
Esophageal, gastric, and jejunal tissue or fluid, i.e., for diagnostic purposes, e.g., celiac disease, allergic gastroenteritis, etc.
Clarification or confirmation of x-ray findings of upper GI abnormalities, such as stricture, obstruction, or mass
Ingestion of a caustic material
Unexplained iron deficiency anemia
Surveillance endoscopy, such as in Barrett's esophagus, or following selected ulcer treatment or mucosal abnormality to demonstrate healing if it is likely to alter clinical management

TABLE 2. *Indications for therapeutic upper endoscopy*

Removal of selected polypoid lesions
Sclerotherapy for bleeding esophageal or gastric varices
Dilatation of stenotic lesions
Placement of the feeding tubes, such as percutaneous endoscopic gastrostomy or jejunal tubes, or the placement of catheters for motility studies
Treatment of bleeding, such as ulcers, tumors, or vascular malformations
Removal of foreign bodies
    In the esophagus
    In the stomach

TABLE 3. *Indications for diagnostic colonoscopy*

Unexplained gastrointestinal bleeding
Unexplained iron deficiency anemia
Evaluation of abnormality on barium enema
Chronic intractable diarrhea of unexplained origin
History of familial polyposis
Evaluation of inflammatory bowel disease, diagnosis, extent, results of therapy
Surveillance colonoscopy for cancer screening, e.g., long-standing ulcerative colitis, ureterosigmoidostomy
Intraoperative colonoscopy for identification of specific lesion, e.g., AV malformation, inflammatory bowel disease

TABLE 4. *Indications for therapeutic colonoscopy*

Polypectomy
Dilatation of stenotic lesions
Treatment of bleeding, e.g., AV malformation, postpolypectomy bleeding

Two Years and Older

Two- to five-year-old patients are the most difficult to sedate. They are usually very difficult to placate. IV sedation includes Versed 0.1 to 0.3 mg/kg, Demerol 1 to 3 mg/kg, or fentanyl 1 µg/kg.

SELECTED INDICATIONS FOR UPPER ENDOSCOPY

The indications for upper endoscopy are discussed in the subsections below and include the following:

1. Esophageal disease
   a. esophagitis due to gastroesophageal reflux or allergic disease;
   b. esophageal atresia with or without tracheoesophageal fistula (TEF);
   c. pill esophagitis;
   d. congenital strictures.
2. Stomach
   a. pyloric stenosis;
   b. antral webs;
   c. gastritis secondary to allergy, *Helicobacter pylori*, Crohn's disease, chronic granulomatous disease.
3. Duodenum—duodenal web.

Esophagitis

Gastroesophageal (GE) reflux disease is the commonest cause of esophagitis in infancy, childhood, and adolescents, similar to the adult population. We estimate, however, that 5% to 10% of these infants have allergic esophagitis with no evidence of gastritis, duodenitis, or colitis (Katz et al., *personal observation*).

Simple or uncomplicated GE reflux, i.e., the spitting baby who is thriving, does not need an evaluation, but merely thickening feeds and parental reassurance. GE reflux disease with complications, i.e., reflux associated with failure to thrive, aspiration, choking, gagging, apnea, GI bleeding, and severe irritability, needs therapeutic intervention and further evaluation including endoscopy (1). We always biopsy the esophagus, gastric antrum, and the duodenum of all patients who undergo esophagogastroduodenoscopy (EGD). It has been shown that a normal-looking esophagus at endoscopy may in fact demonstrate actual esophagitis on

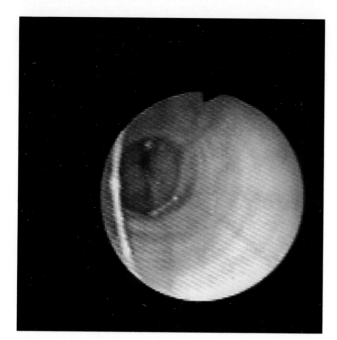

FIG. 1. Esophageal edema.

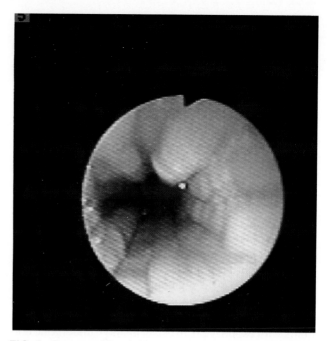

FIG. 2. Same as Fig. 1, but the edema is accentuated by suctioning air.

biopsy and a very erythematous esophagus may be normal (4). Also, for the diagnosis of allergic disease, antral and duodenal inflammation helps differentiate GE reflux from allergic esophagitis (5).

Upper GI series are still usually done prior to endoscopy in young patients with reflux symptoms to rule out congenital abnormalities of the GI tract. These include esophageal stricture, stenosis, TEF, esophageal web, hiatus hernia, pyloric stenosis, antral web, microgastria, and intestinal malrotation.

Endoscopy in most cases reveals edema of the esophagus. This is better appreciated when air is suctioned from the esophagus (Figs. 1 and 2). A ring-like esophagus indicates significant esophagitis (Fig. 3). Ulcerations or erosions may be seen. Allergic disease of the esophagus may look identical. In most cases, however, it is represented by edema, and only occasionally ulceration (5). Biopsies of the esophagus do not differentiate allergy from GE reflux. The degree of eosinophilic infiltration overlaps and pH probe studies may be needed to confirm a diagnosis of reflux esophagitis (5). In conjunction with an endoscopy the pH probe may be passed prior to withdrawal of the endoscope, such that the tip can be visualized in the distal esophagus. The probe is then secured and the endoscope withdrawn. This technique avoids the need for radiographs.

Pill Esophagitis

Pill esophagitis has been reported in adolescents treated on tetracycline for acne (6). They take their tablets prior to sleep with little water, and the tablet usually adheres in the upper esophagus at the level of the aortic arch. These patients present with odynophagia. Treatment includes Carafate slurry and H_2-blockers. It usually takes 5 to 7 days for symptoms to resolve. Physicians and dermatologists should warn their patients to take these medications with meals.

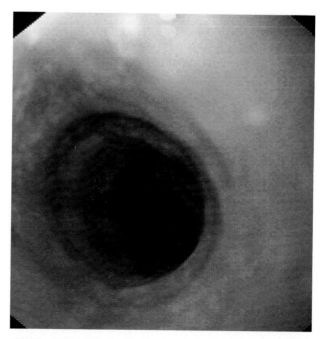

FIG. 3. "Ring-like" esophagus, representing significant esophagitis.

Dysphagia

Dysphagia in pediatrics should always be regarded as pathological. In some patients presenting with dysphagia the upper GI series may miss early strictures (2). Therefore, in any patient with dysphagia, carefully choose which size of scope to start with, since it may lead to a lot of discomfort, and perhaps even perforation if the scope is too large and too much force is used.

Esophageal Atresia, With or Without Tracheoesophageal Fistula

Most patients with esophageal atresia with or without fistula have esophageal motility disorders (1). This is a diffuse process in the distal esophagus and leads to lower esophageal segment (LES) pressure and GE reflux disease. In previous studies, 20% to 30% of these patients underwent fundoplication (7). A number of patients with esophageal atresia who have undergone corrective surgery develop stenosis at the area of anastomosis. The majority, however, are clinically not relevant and do not need to be evaluated or treated. In 30% of patients dilatation is needed (8). Many patients with esophageal atresia with or without TEF will need to be evaluated for chronic GI motility problems and/or esophagitis. Barrett's esophagus has been described in patients with chronic reflux in this group (9).

Congenital Esophageal Stenosis and Web

Congenital stenosis is located in the middle third of the esophagus in 50% of cases, in the distal esophagus in a third of cases, and in the upper third in 15%. These findings may vary from an independent web, usually at the cervical esophagus, a web with inner segmental stenosis, or segmental stenosis on its own (8). Endoscopy is mandatory in these cases to rule out esophagitis.

Pyloric Stenosis

The diagnosis of pyloric stenosis is a clinical one. An "olive" or mass is felt in the area of the pylorus; ultrasound is a reliable tool for diagnosis (10), but in some instances an upper GI series may be needed to confirm the diagnosis. Endoscopy has no role in the straightforward pyloric stenosis.

Patients with pyloric stenosis may present with vomiting and hematemesis (11). Pyloric stenosis is often *not* considered with this presentation. Endoscopy reveals ulcerations or gastritis in the antrum with a closed and edematous pylorus. The new, slim endoscopes (GIF-N30 Olympus) can be passed into the duodenum. Some patients with pyloric stenosis persist with vomiting after adequate pyloromyotomy because of associated GE reflux, not poor surgical results. Whether this is a coincidental or a pathologic finding has not been evaluated. Balloon dilatation of the pylorus instead of surgery has been reported (12), but no extensive study has as yet been done.

Webs are more more common in the antrum than duodenum. Electrocautery has been used to correct these abnormalities.

MANAGEMENT OF FOREIGN BODIES IN THE UPPER GI TRACT

Eighty percent of foreign bodies occur in the pediatric age group, most commonly under the age of 5 years. Coins are the most common, followed by batteries. In contrast, adults tend to have problems with food, such as meat and bone fragments (13).

The management of foreign bodies in children depends on the type of foreign body ingested and whether it is impacted in the esophagus or the stomach.

Long-standing impaction of coins and other foreign objects in the esophagus may lead to perforation, with TEF or rupture into any other thoracic organs. If the coin is impacted in the esophagus and the patient has any respiratory distress, it should be removed endoscopically as an urgent procedure. If the patient is completely asymptomatic, the coin can be removed within 24 hours.

If a coin or a similar soft object remains in the stomach, the patient is observed for 4 to 6 weeks before endoscopical removal. If the patient becomes symptomatic prior to this period, then it should be removed at once. It may be useful to give the patient a 48-hour course of Metacloprimide or cisapride to enhance passage into the small intestine.

If the object is sharp (such as a straight pin or an open safety pin) there is some debate as to what to do. If it is lodged in the esophagus, it should be removed. If it is lodged in the stomach, the problem is that it may pass into the duodenum or the small intestine and lead to perforation or abscess later. Therefore, one would suspect that these probably should be removed if they are seen in the stomach. An overtube is useful to prevent trauma to the esophagus.

Batteries

Litovitz and Schmidtz analyzed 2,382 cases of battery ingestion (14). These cases were accumulated during a 7-year study period. A minimum estimate of 2,100 cases a year of battery ingestion in the United States was derived from their data. Peak incidence was found in 1- to 2-year-olds. Hearing-aid batteries were the most common followed by batteries for watches and toys.

Once the initial x-ray to determine the battery location demonstrates impaction in the esophagus, the battery should be urgently removed. Burns due to esophageal lodging have occurred as early as 4 hours after ingestion and perforation within 6 hours. Removal should be by endoscopy and not Foley catheter. Batteries that have passed into the stomach need not be retrieved unless the patient manifests signs or symptoms of injury to the gastrointestinal tract, such as abdominal pain, tenderness, hematemesis, or if the batteries have a diameter of 15 mm or greater and do not pass within 48 hours.

When mercuric batteries are ingested, blood and urine mercury levels are necessary only if the batteries split in the GI tract or radiopaque droplets are evident in the gut.

If an adolescent or any other pediatric patient presents with a food bolus impaction, one should carefully evaluate those patients for underlying esophagitis or stricture and the patient should undergo a barium swallow and an endoscopy once the obstruction is relieved.

ENDOSCOPIC SCLEROTHERAPY

Endoscopic sclerotherapy in infants and children for varices has been demonstrated to be as effective as with adults. Complications are the same (15).

Percutaneous Endoscopic Gastrostomy

This procedure is performed the same way as in adults (16). The majority of pediatric patients who undergo percutaneous endoscopic gastrostomy are those who are neurologically impaired or have GI motility disturbances. As far as the neurologically impaired children are concerned, there is a controversy as to whether they should have a fundoplication performed at the same time that the G-tube is placed. Data show that those patients who have no reflux prior to the insertion of the G-tube may in fact develop reflux subsequently. It is our policy to recommend fundoplication with G-tube placement in patients with severe neurological impairment who are bedridden (17). If the patient is ambulatory and there has been a negative pH probe prior to the procedure, we do not recommend fundoplication.

Endoscopic Methods of Hemostasis

These methods are the same in pediatric patients as with adults. The heater probe, and injections of adrenaline (1:10,000) or sclerosants appear to be the most effective.

COLONOSCOPY

The indications for colonoscopy are shown in Tables 3 and 4.

Bowel Preparation

1. Clear-liquid diet for 24 hours prior to the procedure.
2. Magnesium citrate, 6 to 10 oz., in the afternoon prior to the procedure at about 4 P.M., 1 to 2 Dulcolax tablets at 6 P.M., Fleet enema at 6 A.M. on the morning of the procedure.
3. NPO after midnight.

Alternative Preparation for Children and Adolescents

1. GoLYTELY, 1 to 4 liters, given at the dose of 1 L/h, perhaps sweetened with Hawaiian punch or Crystal Lite. This is administered orally in most cases. If the patient is unable to tolerate it because of the unpleasant taste, a nasogastric tube may have to be placed and the infusion done via the nasogastric tube as an outpatient the day prior to the procedure.
2. NPO after midnight.

Neonates and Infants

1. Clear liquids for 12 hours prior to the procedure.
2. NPO for 4 to 6 hours.

Sedation Guidelines

These guidelines are the same as for the upper endoscopy, but the doses are usually higher.

Colonoscopic Findings Unique to the Pediatric Patient

Colitis

Allergic colitis is the commonest cause of rectal bleeding in patients under 6 months of age (18). Most infants evaluated as outpatients with this procedure have undergone rigid sigmoidoscopy. The new GIF N-30 (Olympus) scope or other similar-size scopes will probably become the flexible scope of choice. It will permit visualization of the left colon in the office.

The appearance of the colon in allergic colitis looks very similar to any other cause of colitis and cannot be differentiated purely by inspection. It has been reported that about 15% of these infants may have rectal sparing. When complete colonoscopy is performed on these patients, there is usually a pancolitis. Findings include erythema, friability, and ulceration. Biopsies reveal an increased number of eosinophils with eosinophilic cryptitis (18).

Allergic colitis is self-limiting, usually disappearing by 3 to 12 months of age. Occasionally, in the older infant, this may herald the onset of chronic inflammatory bowel disease.

Neonatal Enterocolitis

It is unusual to sigmoidoscope these infants as the diagnosis is made clinically and radiologically. In the rare instance when sigmoidoscopy is performed, extremely severe ulcerations are seen.

Lymphoid Nodular Hyperplasia

At colonoscopy, it should be possible to intubate the ileum in about 70% to 80% of all patients, even in infants. On some occasions, severe lymphoid hyperplasia of ileum may confuse the uninitiated. The lymphoid nodules are usually large and discrete. No bleeding is seen (Fig. 4). Diffuse lymphoid nodular hyperplasia of the small intestine is usually associated with immune deficiency syndromes.

Colonic lymphoid nodular hyperplasia may occur in

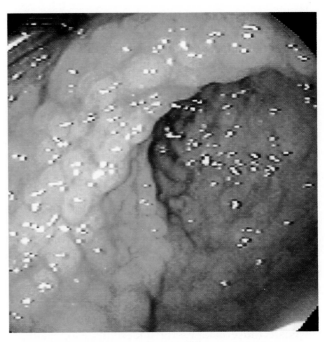

FIG. 5. Lymphoid nodular hyperplasia of the colon.

the left colon or throughout the colon. This finding is not unusual in infants and children and is not associated with immune deficiency (19). There is still no consensus as to whether this is a normal versus a pathological finding. Lymphoid nodular hyperplasia of the colon is found in infants undergoing colonoscopy for rectal bleeding and chronic diarrhea. Significant rectal bleeding may occur with lymphoid nodular hyperplasia. Ulcerations are noted on the surface of these nodules and this probably accounts for the bleeding (Fig. 5). Some of these patients have an associated allergic or infectious colitis, the latter due to *Clostridium difficile*. In the majority of patients the etiology remains idiopathic, and significant bleeding and discomfort may persist. Treatment is empiric, including dietary changes, sulfasalazine, or steroids.

Vasculitis

The hemolytic uremic syndrome (HUS) frequently presents with colitis and moderate-to-severe rectal bleeding as its primary presentation (20). The colitis is usually focal, with ulceration, erythema, friability, and granularity. Specific features cannot be differentiated on rectal biopsy. The main clinical features of hemolytic anemia and renal findings present dramatically on the seventh day after presentation. If this diagnosis is *not* considered, many patients are not adequately followed up or patients with severe colitis undergo needless surgery.

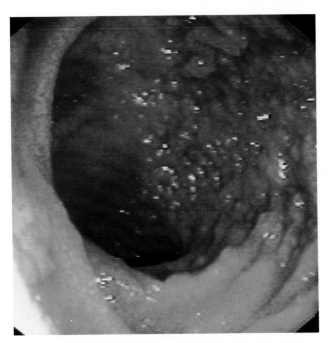

FIG. 4. Lymphoid nodular hyperplasia of the terminal ileum.

Polyps

Juvenile polyps are the most common polyps found in childhood. They are usually not associated with the development of malignancy, although adenomatous transformation has rarely been described. Patients usually present with bleeding and some mucus in the stool. Juvenile polyps may be single or multiple. Fifty percent have more than one polyp and the patient should undergo complete colonoscopy and colon examination (21). The syndrome of multiple juvenile polyposis is different (22) and related to the family of polyp syndromes. Family members may have either juvenile or adenomatous polyposis. These patients are at risk for malignancy later on, as the polyps may undergo adenomatous transformation. These patients are endoscoped frequently for surveillance and electively should have total colectomy with an ileoanal anastomosis at the appropriate time, probably the late teens.

Other types of polyps including adenomatous polyps associated with Gardner's syndrome do occur in children. It is unusual to find polyps before the age of 5. A child may be screened because a family member was found to have polyposis. The child should be observed frequently for the development of polyposis later in life, as this may develop up to the age of 30 years (23). Routine use of genetic markers will identify all patients at risk.

Ureterosigmoidostomy

Ureterosigmoidostomy used to be a common surgical procedure for urinary diversion in children with congenital extrophy of the bladder. Patients with ureterosigmoidostomy have a documented increase in adenocarcinoma of the colon adjacent to the ureteric-sigmoid anastomosis (24). Annual evaluation by sigmoidoscopy is mandatory to rule out dysplasia or early cancer. It is important to note that even if the ureterosigmoidostomy is taken down, the presence of the ureteric stump in the colon still predisposes to cancer, and these patients should undergo annual evaluation (Fig. 6).

Hirschsprung's Disease

Enterocolitis may either be a presenting symptom in patients subsequently diagnosed as having Hirschsprung's disease or present months after surgical correction (25). The etiology is either related to disordered colonic motility or perhaps bacterial overgrowth, or a combination of both.

Motility Studies

Manometric studies of the upper and lower GI tract have enabled us to better evaluate the pathophysiology

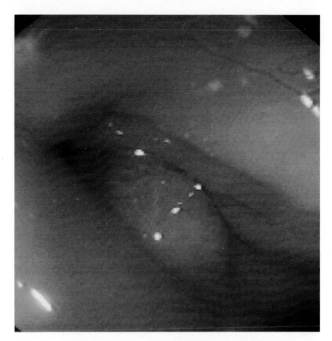

FIG. 6. Ureter in the sigmoid colon.

of many GI disorders (26). The placement of an antro-duodenal motility catheter can be accomplished placing the catheter fluoroscopically. Endoscopic guidance with a biopsy forceps is useful in different cases.

Motility of the colon is accomplished by utilizing the colonoscope to place the catheters, which are advanced by the biopsy forceps and placed into the transverse colon and right colon.

Jejunoscopy

Jejunal feeding tubes have become more common, especially in patients with GI motility disorders who have gastroparesis or severely delayed gastric emptying or severe GE reflux. These patients are not able to eat, cannot tolerate feedings via the stomach, orally, or via the nasogastric tube or G-tube.

Visualization of the jejunum can be easily made using the GIF-N30 endoscope. The gastrostomy tube is removed and the endoscope is placed directly in the jejunum and can be passed either proximally or distally (Fig. 7).

Pediatric Use of Endoscopic Retrograde Cholangiopancreatography (ERCP)

The prototype Olympus 7.5 mm side-view duodenoscope has enabled evaluation of the biliary system in neonates and infants. The indications for pediatric ERCP are shown in Table 5.

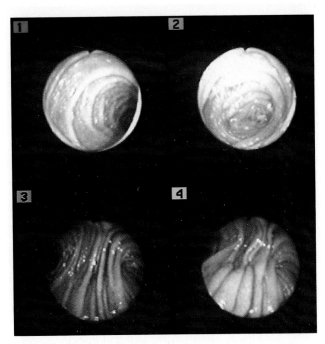

FIG. 7. Jejunoscopy. View of both jejunostomy limbs.

Recurrent Evaluation of Prolonged Neonatal Obstructive Jaundice

Once all secondary causes of obstructive jaundice, such as congenital infection or metabolic disease, have been ruled out, one is faced with the decision of whether this infant has bile duct disease, such as biliary atresia or choledochal cyst, or whether this is cholestasis secondary to hepatitis (Fig. 8). An ultrasound is done first to detect the presence of a choledochal cyst or the absence of a gallbladder. The latter is suggestive but not diagnostic of biliary atresia. Conversely, the presence of a gallbladder does not rule out a distal biliary atresia.

Hepatobiliary scintigraphy is useful only if excretion into the duodenum occurs. If normal, with excretion into the duodenum, biliary atresia is ruled out. However, nonexcretion may be related to severe intrahepatic cholestasis. Once the infant has been demonstrated to have a normal abdominal ultrasound (no

choledochal cyst) and a hepatobiliary scan that shows no excretion, further evaluation depends on the experience of the gastroenterologist. Liver biopsy would be the next step in many centers to differentiate between intrahepatic cholestasis and biliary atresia. Liver biopsy may be able to differentiate 70% to 80% of cases between biliary atresia and hepatitis (27). At this stage, if the diagnosis still remains in doubt, many clinicians would opt for sending the patient for exploratory laparotomy. I believe an ERCP should be performed prior to surgery. The Olympus 7.9 mm side-viewing scope allows access to the biliary tree. Several reports confirm this technique in the diagnosis of biliary atresia or intrahepatic neonatal cholestasis (28,29).

We have adapted Guelrud's technique (29). Infants are sedated with IV Versed 0.5 mg/kg. The presence of bile in the duodenum would obviously favor the diagnosis of a patent biliary tree. Demonstration of a normal biliary system rules out biliary atresia. However, if the biliary tree is not visualized, endoscopists with less experience would have to decide whether this is technical or, in fact, the patient has biliary atresia. The absence of bile in the duodenum during the procedure and demonstration of a normal pancreatic duct but no bile duct visualization make biliary atresia most likely.

We have successfully utilized ERCP to differentiate biliary atresia from neonatal hepatitis in 15 infants. In one patient with Allagile's syndrome, technical difficulty prevented demonstration of the biliary system.

A normal ERCP was found in a neonate presenting with obstructive jaundice, which immediately resolved after the ERCP, suggesting a bile plug that was removed at the time of the procedure (Fig. 9).

Sphincterotomy and Stone Removal

Neonates, infants, and children can develop common duct stones with biliary obstruction. Guelrud has reported successful sphincterotomy in one infant (30). At this stage, the pediatric endoscopist would need assistance from an adult colleague.

Choledochal Cysts

ERCP should be performed preoperatively in patients with choledochal cyst to define exactly the pancreatic biliary anatomy and to determine the type of choledochal cyst and whether there is any intrahepatic involvement.

Recurrent Pancreatitis

Idiopathic pancreatitis is the most common cause of recurrent pancreatitis in childhood. Trauma as a cause

TABLE 5. *Indications for ERCP in infants or children*

Diagnostic	Therapeutic
Neonatal cholestasis; differentiate biliary atresia from neonatal hepatitis	Sphincterotomy with or without stone removal
Choledochal cyst to evaluate anatomy	
Biliary obstruction	
Chronic or relapsing pancreatitis	
Sclerosing cholangitis	

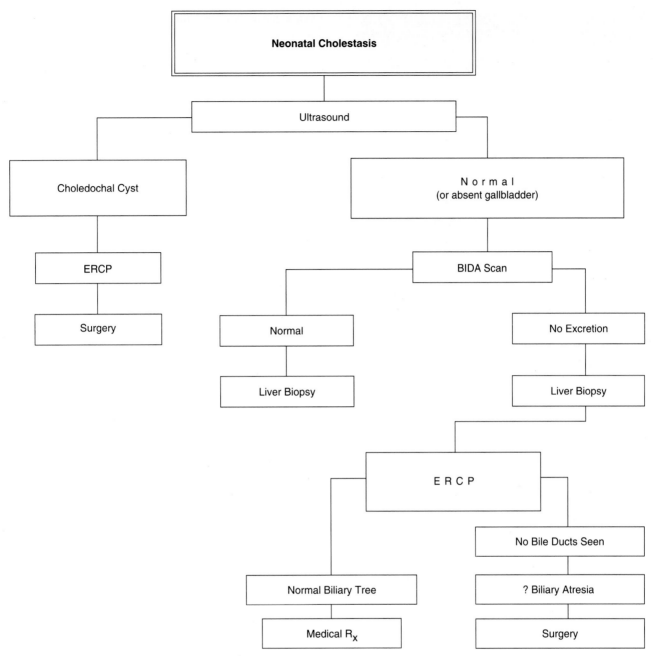

FIG. 8. A decision table for the evaluation of neonatal cholestasis.

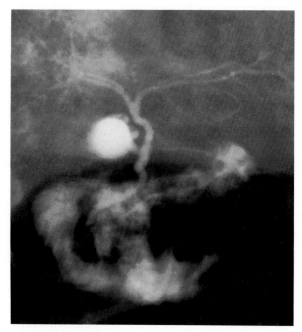

FIG. 9. Normal ERCP in a 4-week-old with obstructive neonatal jaundice.

of pancreatitis is much more common in pediatric patients than in adults. Alcohol and gallstones are not major factors in this age group. ERCP should be performed in pediatric patients with recurrent pancreatitis to determine if there is a remedial anatomical abnormality, such as duodenal duplication, anatomic variations in the pancreatic duct (e.g., pancreas divisum), and the presence of a pancreatic stricture or stone as visualized in Fig. 10.

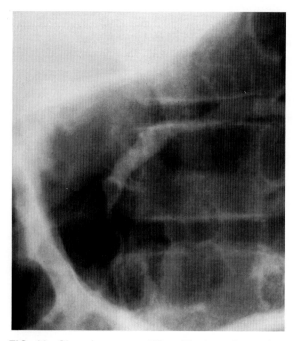

FIG. 10. Chronic pancreatitis with stone formation.

Sphincter of Oddi Motility

The diagnosis of biliary dyskinesia has been established in few pediatric patients. No adequate study has been performed in children with postcholecystectomy syndrome, recurrent pancreatitis, or clinical features suggestive of biliary dyskinesia.

ERCP in the pediatric GI population is still new and in the diagnostic mode. Therapeutic modalities will follow once the pediatric gastroenterologists are comfortable with ERCP. In the meantime an adult colleague will be called upon to assist (31).

REFERENCES

1. Caulfield M, Wylie R, Sivak M, Mitehener W, Steffer R. Upper gastrointestinal endoscopy in the pediatric patient. *J Pediatr* 1989;115:339–345.
2. Ament ME, Berquist WE, Vargas J, Perisic V. Fibreoptic upper intestinal endoscopy in infants and children. *Pediatr Clin North Am* 1988;35:141–155.
3. Rossi T. Endoscopic examination of the colon in infancy and childhood. *Pediatr Clin North Am* 1988;35:331–355.
4. Biller JA, Winter HS, Grand RJ, Allred EN. Are endoscopic changes predictive of histologic esophagitis in children? *J Pediatr* 1983;103:215–218.
5. Katz AJ, Feen D. Allergic esophagitis. (Submitted for publication.)
6. Biller JA, Flores AF, Buie TM, Mazor S, Katz AJ. Tetracycline-induced esophagitis in adolescent patients. *J Pediatr* 1992;120:144–145.
7. Laks H, Wilkinson RH, Schuster SR. Long-term results following correction of esophageal atresia with tracheoesophageal fistula: a clinical and cinefluographic study. *J Pediatr Surg* 1978;7:591–597.
8. Boyle JT. Congenital disorders of the esophagus in diseases of the esophagus. In: Cohen S, Soloway RD, eds. *Contemporary issues in gastroenterology.* 1982;1:97–120.
9. Rothstein FC, Dahms BB. Barrett's esophagus in children. In: Spechler S, Goyal RK, eds. *Barrett's esophagus pathophysiology: diagnosis and management.* New York: Elsevier Science, 1985;129–141.
10. Teele R, Smith EH. Ultrasound in the diagnosis of idiopathic hypertrophic pyloric stenosis. *N Engl J Med* 1977;296:1149–1150.
11. Innon A, Dominguez M, Rivasola A. Congenital pyloric stenosis. An unusual clinical presentation. *J Pediatr Surg* 1982;17:417–419.
12. Hayashi AH, Giacomantorio, Lau Y, Gillis D. Balloon catheter dilatation of hypertrophic pyloric stenosis. *J Pediatr Surg* 1990;25(II):1119–1121.
13. Webb WA. Management of foreign bodies of the upper gastrointestinal tract. *Gastroenterology* 1988;a4:204–216.
14. Litovitz T, Schmidtz BF. Ingestion of cylindrical and button batteries: an analysis of 2382 cases. *Pediatrics* 1992;89:747–757.
15. Hassall E, Ament ME, Berquist WE. Endoscopic sclerotherapy of esophageal varices in childhood. *Gastrointest Endosc* 1988;31:130.
16. Ganderer MWL, Powsky JL, Izant RJ. Gastrostomy without laparotomy: a percutaneous endoscopic technique. *J Pediatr Surg* 1980;15:872–875.
17. Chang J, Coln C, Strickland A, Andersen J. Surgical management of gastroesophageal reflux in severely mentally retarded children. *J Ment Defic Res* 1987;31:1–7.
18. Goldman H, Pronjansky R. Allergic proctitis and gastroenteritis in children. Clinical and mucosal biopsy features in 53 cases. *Am J Surg* 1986;10(2):75–86.
19. Riddlesberger MM, Lebenthal E. Nodular colonic mucosa of

childhood: normal vs. pathologic. *Gastroenterology* 1980;79: 265–270.

20. Berman W. The hemolytic uremic syndrome: initial clinical presentation mimicking ulcerative colitis. *J Pediatr* 1972;81:275.

21. Cymamon HA, Milov DE, Andres J. Diagnosis and management of colonic polyps in children. *J Pediatr* 1989;114(4):593–596.

22. Rozen P, Baratz M. Familial juvenile colonic polyposis with associated colon cancer. *Cancer* 1982;49:1500–1503.

23. Erbe RW. Inherited gastrointestinal polyposis syndromes. *N Engl J Med* 1975;294:1101–1104.

24. Labow SB, Hoexter B, Walrath DC. Colonic adenocarcinomas in patients with uretero-sigmoidostomies. *Dis Colon Rectum* 1979;22(3):157–158.

25. Flores AF, Katz AJ. Enterocolitis following surgery for total colonic aganglionosis. *Pediatr Res* 1984; abstract P.

26. Malagelada JR, Camilleri M, Stanghellini V. Gastric motility disturbances. In: Malagelada JR, Camilleri M, Stanghellini V, eds. *Manometric diagnosis of gastrointestinal motility disorders.* New York: Thieme, 1986;68–69.

27. Watkins JB, Katz AJ, Grand RJ. Neonatal hepatitis. A diagnostic approach. *Adv Pediatr* 1977;24:349–354.

28. Guelrud M, Jaen D, Tones P, et al. Endoscopic cholangiopancreatography in the infant. Evaluation of a new prototype pediatric duodenoscopy. *Gastrointest Endosc* 1987;33:4–8.

29. Guelrud M, Jaen D, Mendoza S, Plaz J, Tones P. Endoscopic retrograde cholangiopancreatography in the diagnosis of extrahepatic biliary atresia. *Gastrointest Endosc* 1991;37:522–526.

30. Guelrud M. Endoscopic retrograde cholangiopancreatography in the infant. In: Barkin J, O'Phelan C, eds. *Advanced therapeutic endoscopy.* New York: Raven Press, 1990;335–356.

31. Brown CW, Werlin SL, Geenen JE, Schualz M. The diagnostic and therapeutic role of endoscopic retrograde cholangiography in children. *J Pediatr Gastroenterol* 1993;17:12–23.

Advanced Therapeutic Endoscopy, 2nd Ed.,
edited by J. S. Barkin and C. A. O'Phelan.
Raven Press, Ltd., New York © 1994.

CHAPTER 5

Injection Therapy for Esophageal Carcinoma

Sydney Chung

For patients with unresectable cancer of the esophagus, the primary therapeutic aim is to restore the ability to swallow. This is most expediently and most rapidly achieved by recanalizing the obstructed esophagus by endoscopic means. The most widely used methods include laser photocoagulation (1) and intubation with a prosthesis (2). These methods are useful in relieving the distressing dysphagia in the remaining life span of the patient. They require, however, expensive equipment or accessories and may not be widely available, especially in developing countries.

Injection sclerotherapy has been widely used for bleeding esophageal varices (3). Esophageal ulceration is a not infrequent complication at the site of injection, especially if a strong sclerosant is used. Of all the sclerosants that have been used, absolute alcohol is probably the most tissue-damaging (4). The tissue-destroying effect of submucosally injected absolute alcohol has been used to destroy small lesions in the stomach (5). More recently, intralesional injection of absolute alcohol has been used to recanalize tumor obstruction of the esophagus (6,7). The initial results are encouraging (Fig. 1).

METHOD

The procedure is performed under intravenous sedation and topical pharyngeal anesthesia. Endoscopy is first performed to survey the tumor. If the stricture is too tight to admit the endoscope, dilatation is performed first. We prefer to use Savary-Gilliard dilators (Wilson-Cook, Winston-Salem, NC) over a guidewire under fluoroscopy.

Alcohol injection is performed with a 23- or 25-gauge

sclerotherapy needle. The needle is inserted into the tumor and 0.5 to 1 ml aliquots are injected intralesionally. Much spillage may occur. Accurate deposition of alcohol into the tumor is indicated by resistance on the syringe and the whitening of the tumor. Care should be taken not to inject into macroscopically normal esophageal wall. Alcohol injection may result in quite marked swelling of the tumor. In patients with long tumors, injection should be started distally so that the edema induced by the injection does not impede the endoscopic view and further injection. We aim to inject all macroscopic tumors at the same session. The total volume injected at any session depends on the extent of the tumor.

After treatment the patients are fasted for 4 hours. If no untoward event occurs they are given a fluid diet the same evening, increasing to soft diet as tolerated the next morning. Low-grade fever and retrosternal discomfort are almost universal after injection treatment. A temporary worsening of the dysphagia because of tumor swelling is also common; this improves when the injected tumor sloughs in a few days. Endoscopy is performed again 3 to 5 days later. Alcohol injections are repeated at twice-weekly intervals until satisfactory relief of dysphagia is achieved.

RESULTS

Payne-James et al. (6) treated 11 patients (9 with adenocarcinoma and 2 with squamous carcinoma). The mean stricture length was 5.27 cm (range 1–10 cm) with six strictures less than 5 cm and five between 5 and 10 cm. The degree of dysphagia was measured using a grading system modified from Bown et al. (1) (Table 1). Two patients had absolute dysphagia, seven patients could swallow fluids only, and two patients could swallow semisolids before treatment. The mean dysphagia score before treatment was 3 ± 0.6.

S. Chung: The Chinese University of Hong Kong; Department of Surgery, Prince of Wales Hospital, Shatin, New Territories, Hong Kong.

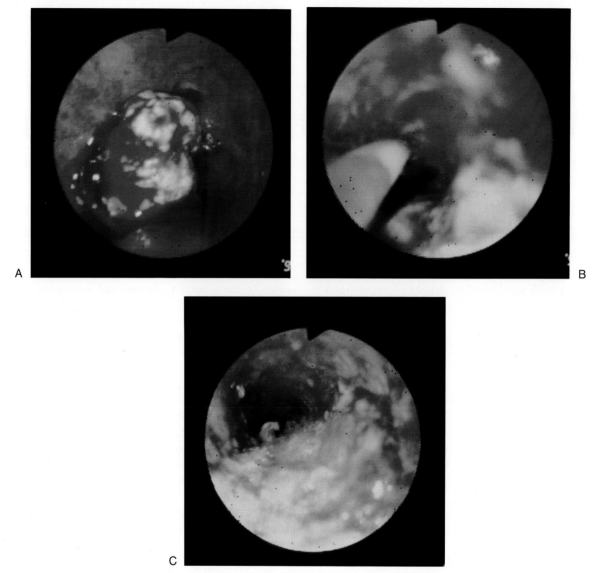

FIG. 1. A: Obstructing carcinoma of the esophagus. **B:** Injection in progress. **C:** Sloughing of the tumor 1 week later.

The patients required a mean of 1.2 ± 1.5 dilatations and 3.3 ± 2.4 sessions of injection. The mean volume of ethanol injected was 9 ± 4.6 ml (1.5 to 22 ml). Ten of the 11 patients improved by at least one grade after one treatment. Dysphagia grades were 1.5 ± 0.8 after one treatment and the best grades attained were 0.9 ± 0.7. The mean survival of this group of patients was 140

days. No complication relating to dilatation or injection was reported.

Chung et al. (7) reported 26 patients with inoperable cancers of the esophagus or the cardia treated by alcohol injection. Since then a total of 36 patients have been treated. Their age ranged from 41 to 92 with a mean of 69 years. Biopsies of the tumor showed squamous cancer in 32 and adenocarcinoma in four. The length of the stricture ranged from 2 to 14 cm.

Before treatment, the dysphagia grades of the patients were as follows: grade 1, 1 patient; grade 2, 16 patients; grade 3, 12 patients; and grade 4, 7 patients. The mean dysphagia grade was 2.7.

The volume of absolute alcohol injected per session ranged from 1.5 to 20.5 ml. The mean volume injected per session was 7.8 ml. Nine patients required one ses-

TABLE 1. *Dysphagia grade*

Grade	Degree of Dysphagia
0	Normal swallowing
1	Occasional difficulty with solids
2	Tolerates semisolids
3	Liquids only
4	Unable to swallow saliva

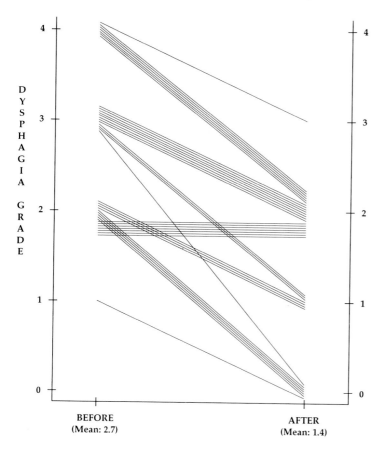

BEFORE
(Mean: 2.7)

AFTER
(Mean: 1.4)

FIG. 2. Dysphagia grades before and after injection.

sion of treatment, 12 patients two sessions, 14 patients three sessions, and 1 patient had four sessions of injection.

The dysphagia grades of the patients before and the best dysphagia grade after treatment are shown in Fig. 2. Twenty-nine of the 36 patients improved at least one grade after treatment. The mean dysphagia grade improved from 2.7 before to 1.4 after treatment ($p < .001$, Wilcoxon's signed rank test).

Three patients in our series developed complications. One patient, who received a total of 36 ml of alcohol 3 days apart, developed high fever, chest pain, and leukocytosis, and blood cultures grew streptococcus and gram-negative rods. He responded to treatment of nothing by mouth, broad-spectrum antibiotics, and nasogastric feeding through a fine-bore tube. Another patient, who had tumors from 25 to 38 cm, had bulging at the carina level on bronchoscopy. Alcohol, 13.5 ml, was injected at one session. He developed a tracheoesophageal fistula 3 days after the procedure that necessitated the insertion of an esophageal prosthesis. A third patient had tumor extending from 32 cm to the esophagogastric junction. The site of obstruction was a shelf-like outgrowth at the proximal end of the tumor. Alcohol, 6 ml, was injected at the top end of the tumor. The patient developed choking with fluid intake 24 hours later. A barium swallow showed fistu-

lation into the right bronchial tree. An esophageal prosthesis was inserted.

Twenty-four patients developed recurrent dysphagia during follow-up. The mean time interval between the end of the alcohol injection and recurrent dysphagia was 35 days. Eleven of these patients were treated by repeat alcohol injection, prosthesis was inserted in four, one had laser treatment, and three had dilatation alone. Five patients were deemed too terminal for further treatment. Thirty of the 36 patients have now died; the median survival was 82 days.

These preliminary results indicate that endoscopic alcohol injection is effective in restoring luminal patency and in relieving dysphagia in patients with inoperable cancers of the esophagus and the cardia. The improvement in swallowing and the duration of palliation obtained compared with those reported after laser therapy.

The obvious advantage of alcohol injection is that, unlike laser therapy, no special equipment or special skills is required. It can be performed easily in any endoscopy unit by endoscopists conversant with esophageal dilatation and variceal sclerotherapy. The technique merits randomized comparative trials with other more established forms of endoscopic recanalization such as laser or bipolar electrocoagulation.

The tissue damage produced by alcohol injection is

not immediately apparent. Sloughing only occurs after a few days. It is therefore difficult to evaluate the extent of tissue damage produced at the time of injection. Overenthusiastic injection at any one site is likely to result in perforation or fistulation into the tracheobronchial tree. We suspect that overaggressive injection into tumor tissue close to the tracheobronchial tree had led to necrosis of the membranous part of the trachea or bronchus in the two patients who developed tracheoesophageal fistula. Similar complications may also occur with laser therapy, as the thermal damage induced by laser photocoagulation also extends beyond the effect visible at the time of endoscopy. Our impression is that the depth of tissue necrosis with alcohol injection is more variable and more difficult to control. We have now adopted the policy of erring on the side of caution, preferring to inject more cautiously during the first session and to repeat the injection a few days later when the injected areas have sloughed.

REFERENCES

1. Bown SG, Hawes R, Matthewson K, Swain CP, Barr H, Boulos PB, Clark CG. Endoscopic laser palliation for advanced malignant dysphagia. *Gut* 1987;28:799–807.
2. Den Hartog Jager FCA, Bartelsman JFWM, Tytgat GNJ. Palliative treatment of obstructing esophagogastric malignancy by endoscopic positioning of a plastic prosthesis. *Gastroenterology* 1979;77:1008–1014.
3. Savin SK, Sachdeva GK, Nanda R, Vij JC, Anand BS. Endoscopic sclerotherapy using absolute alcohol. *Gut* 1985;2:180–182.
4. Rutgeerts P, Gebos K, Vantrappen G. Experimental studies of injection therapy for severe non-variceal bleeding in dogs. *Gastroenterology* 1989;97:610–621.
5. Otani T, Tatsuka T, Kanamaru K, et al. Intramural injection of ethanol under direct vision for the treatment of protuberant lesions of the stomach. *Gastroenterology* 1975;69:123–129.
6. Payne-James JJ, Spiller RC, Misiewicz JJ, Silk DBA. Use of ethanol-induced tumor necrosis to palliate dysphagia in patients with esophagogastric cancer. *Gastrointest Endosc* 1990;36:43–46.
7. Chung SCS, Leong HT, Choi CYC, Leung JWC, Li AKC. Palliation of malignant esophageal obstruction by endoscopic alcohol injection. *Gastrointest Endosc* 1992;38:231(abst).

Advanced Therapeutic Endoscopy, 2nd Ed.,
edited by J. S. Barkin and C. A. O'Phelan.
Raven Press, Ltd., New York © 1994.

CHAPTER 6

Self-Expanding Metallic Stents for Palliation of Malignant Esophageal Obstruction and Esophagorespiratory Fistulae

William C. Wu, Ronald M. Katon, and Richard R. Saxon

Carcinoma of the esophagus frequently presents with progressive, unrelenting dysphagia. When the diagnosis is made, over 60% of patients have tumors that are not amenable to surgical resection. Prognosis is poor, with 1- and 5-year survivals of 18% and 5%, respectively. Although curative resection is occasionally possible, in the majority of patients palliation is the primary therapeutic goal.

Palliative surgery carries an unacceptably high morbidity and mortality rate (1). There are numerous nonsurgical palliative treatments, including radiation therapy (external and intracavitary), chemotherapy, and prosthetic esophageal intubation. Esophageal tumors can be ablated with electrocautery, neodymium:yttrium-aluminum garnet (Nd:YAG) laser, injection of sclerosing agents, and using photodynamic therapy.

The mainstays of endoscopic palliation have been the Nd:YAG laser and the placement of rigid plastic endoprostheses. While both techniques are often effective, they have significant disadvantages. Rigid esophageal stents are of large external bore. Of necessity, placement is traumatic, giving rise to a high perforation rate (5–13%) (2–5). Most commercially available rigid prostheses have a luminal diameter of only 10 to 12 mm, thus limiting intake of solids. Other complications of rigid stents include stent migration, obstruction with food or tumor overgrowth, and late pressure necrosis. Procedure-related mortality is high (4–7%) (2–4).

The Nd:YAG laser is costly to acquire ($80,000–100,000) and thus not widely available. Effective palliation usually requires two to four sessions to obtain esophageal patency (6). Recurrent tumor growth is frequent (30–40%), thereby requiring additional laser sessions in these debilitated patients (7). Laser fulguration is ineffective for submucosal tumor and for those tumors that cause dysphagia by extraluminal compression. Complications of Nd:YAG laser ablation are esophageal perforation, bleeding, and the formation of an esophagorespiratory fistula (8,9).

A dreaded complication in 5% to 15% of patients with esophageal malignancy or its treatment is esophagorespiratory fistula (ERF) (10). Profound morbidity with paroxysms of cough with any oral intake is often debilitating. Surgery is frequently difficult and carries a high mortality rate (11). Esophageal intubation is the treatment of choice in managing ERF. However, rigid endoprotheses are often difficult to place and carry substantial risks already enumerated.

Due to the limitations in current therapy (both endoscopic and radiologic), numerous investigators have sought a more satisfying mode of palliation for malignant esophageal obstruction and esophagorespiratory fistulae. Following successful use within the biliary tree and in the esophagi of experimental animals (12), self-expanding metallic stents (SEMS) have been used in 77 patients in ten published reports (13–22) (Table 1). In 1992 we reported the results in our first six patients (17); to date we have treated a total of 31 patients

W. C. Wu and R. M. Katon: Division of Gastroenterology, Oregon Health Sciences University, Portland, Oregon 97201–3098.

R. R. Saxon: Dotter Institute of Interventional Radiology, Oregon Health Sciences University, Portland, Oregon 97201–3098.

TABLE 1. *Comparison of published reports of the use of self-expanding metallic stents for palliation of malignant esophageal obstruction and esophagorespiratory fistulae*

Reference	Stent type	Diameter (mm)		Number of patients			Mean F/U (wks)[d]	Results	Major complications (n)
		Stent	Del Cath[a]	Dys-phagia	ERF[b]	Both[c]			
Domschke et al., 1990 (13)	Uncovered Wallstent	20	6	1	–	–	16	"Complete relief"	None
Knyrim et al., 1990 (14)	Uncovered Wallstent	14	3	6	–	–	8	6/6 solid food	Tumor ingrowth (2)
Song et al., 1991 (15)	Covered Gianturco	18	12	9	–	–	16	8/9 normal diet 1/9 soft diet	Tumor overgrowth (1)
Song et al., 1992 (16)	"Barbless" covered Gianturco	18 or 22	10 or 12	18	–	3[e]	15	19/21 normal diet 2/21 soft diet 2/2 (ERF) and 1/1 perforation had complete seal	Severe chest pain (4) Migration (1) Food obstruction (2)
Schaer et al., 1992 (17)	Covered Gianturco	15 or 18	10	6	–	–	16	2/6 normal diet 4/6 soft diet	Migration (1) Food obstruction (1) Pressure necrosis/ death (1) Membrane disruption (1)
Neuhaus et al., 1992 (18)	Uncovered Wallstent	20	6	10	–	–	8	3/10 normal diet 7/10 semi-solid diet	Food obstruction (2) Tumor ingrowth (2) Pneumoperitoneum/ death (1)
Kozarek et al., 1992 (19)	Uncovered and covered Gianturco	15	12	3	1	1	N/A[f]	Stents "patent"; no other details available	Migration (1) Tumor overgrowth (1) Pneumothorax/death (1) Erosion into trachea (1) Incomplete stent expansion (1)
Bethge et al., 1992 (20)	Uncovered Wallstent	14	3	8	–	–	11	5/8 normal diet	Tumor overgrowth (1) Tumor ingrowth (1)
Fleischer and Bull-Henry, 1992 (21)	Partially covered Wallstent	20	8	1	–	–	N/A[f]	Failed	Migration requiring conventional stent placement (1)
Sass and Hagenmuller, 1992 (22)	Uncovered Strecker	18	8	10	–	–	N/A[f]	10/10 "successful"	None
Wu et al., 1994 (23)	Covered Gianturco-Rösch Z-stent	18	10	17	1	7	19	14/17 semi-solid diet 6/8 (ERF) complete seal 2/8 (ERF) partial seal	Migration (3) Food obstruction (1) Tumor overgrowth (1) Massive hemorrhage/ death (1)
Totals				89	1	11	17		Complications 32% Deaths 3.9%

[a] Delivery catheter.
[b] Esophagorespiratory fistula.
[c] Both obstruction and ERF.
[d] Mean follow-up.
[e] One of the three patients had obstruction and perforation.
[f] Data not available from published reports.

at our institution using a modified silicone-covered Gianturco-Rösch Z-stent (23).

TYPES OF STENTS AVAILABLE (Table 2)

At the time of this writing there are no self-expanding metallic stents approved for human use by the United States Food and Drug Administration; none are commercially available. However, numerous prototypes are under investigation and have been reported in the world literature.

The Wallstent (Schneider U. S. Stent Division; Minneapolis, MN) was the first self-expanding metallic stent used for the palliation of malignant dysphagia in humans (13,14). This stent is made from surgical-grade stainless steel alloy wires formed into a tubular mesh 14 mm or 20 mm in diameter when fully expanded.

TABLE 2. *Comparison of prototypes of self-expanding metallic esophageal stents currently under investigation*

Stent	Material	Silicone covered?	Diameter (mm)		Shortens on deployment?	Presence of side hooks?
			Stent	Delivery catheter		
Gianturco-Rösch Z-stent (Cook, Inc.)	Stainless steel	Entire stent	18–20	10–12	No	Yes, in some models
Wallstent (Schneider U.S. Stent Division)	Stainless steel	Central portion; flared ends uncovered	18	8	Yes	No
Strecker or Ultraflex (Microvasive)	Nitinol	No	18	8	Yes	No

On elongation, the stent can be loaded into a delivery catheter 9F or 24F in bore (depending upon stent diameter and modifications). The central portion of the Wallstent may be covered with silicone to provide a barrier between the lattices, thereby preventing tumor ingrowth through the stent and allowing the use of the Wallstent in treating ERF (21) (Fig. 1).

An esophageal Strecker stent called the Ultraflex esophageal prosthesis (Microvasive; Watertown, MA) has been fashioned from memory metal filaments made of nitinol into a mesh tube 18 mm in diameter (22) (Fig. 2). Elongation of the stent allows compression into a 24F delivery catheter. No covered Strecker stents have been reported in the literature yet.

The majority of patients treated with SEMS have received the Gianturco-Rösch Z-stent design (Cook, Inc.; Bloomington, IN) (15–17,19,23,24). The basic design consists of individual stent bodies 2 cm in length and 18 or 20 mm in diameter made from 0.018-inch stainless steel wire bent into a cylindrical zigzag con-

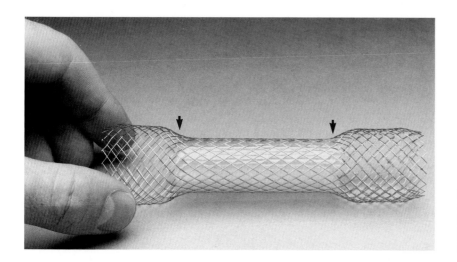

FIG. 1. Prototype of a partially covered esophageal Wallstent (Schneider U.S. Stent Division; Minneapolis, MN) with flared ends. *Arrows* identify margins of the silicone membrane.

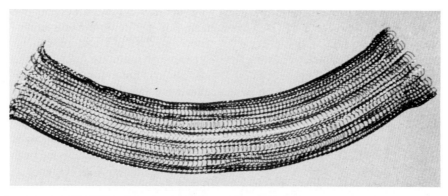

FIG. 2. Prototype of the Ultraflex esophageal prosthesis (Microvasive; Watertown, MA). This stent has no silicone covering.

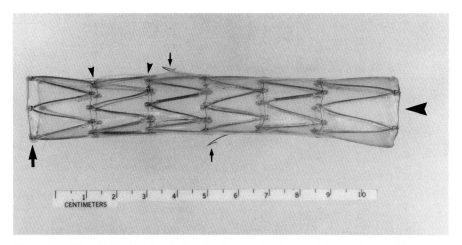

FIG. 3. Gianturco-Rösch Z-stent made by the Dotter Institute of Interventional Radiology (Portland, OR). The stent is comprised of interconnected stent bodies of 2 cm length *(small arrowheads)* and is completely covered with a silicone membrane. The cephalad stent body *(large arrowhead)* is slightly larger (22 mm) than the remainder of the stent (18 mm). Anchoring hooks *(small arrows)* are affixed to the middle stent bodies to prevent migration. The caudad margin of the stent *(large arrow)* has a silicone "bumper," which is difficult to see on this photograph.

figuration of six, eight, or ten bends. Individual stent bodies are interconnected with suture to form stents of any length (usually 8–12 cm) (Fig. 3). The original Gianturco stent has evolved to include numerous modifications: silicone covering, proximal and distal ends with wider diameters, anchoring hooks, and silicone "bumpers" on the leading stent body. A modification by Korean investigators (16) has been dubbed a "barbless" Gianturco stent, which consists of a stent with two wider ends in a dumbbell shape. Stents of Gianturco design are directly compressed and loaded into a delivery catheter 29F or 36F in size. Upon deployment there is no foreshortening of the stent, as seen in the Wallstent or Ultraflex stent.

At our institution each SEMS is custom-designed and handcrafted for each patient by the Dotter Institute of Interventional Radiology. Gianturco-Rösch Z-stents of 18-mm diameter are modified to include a silicone membrane, a proximal flange of 22 mm, six anchoring hooks, and a silicone "bumper" over the caudad margin. The stent is customized to be 4 cm longer than the length of the malignant stricture or ERF. After construction the stent is loaded into a 29F delivery apparatus (also designed by the Dotter Institute) consisting of an outer housing with a side port for injecting intraluminal contrast and a "positioning" tube (Fig. 4).

TECHNIQUE OF STENT PLACEMENT

At our institution the placement of the SEMS is a cooperative effort involving gastroenterology and radiology. The majority of patient care responsibility be-

fore and after stent placement is assumed by the gastroenterologist, while the actual placement of the SEMS is performed by the interventional radiologist. Intimate communication and coordination is paramount for optimum success and enhanced patient outcome.

To begin, the location of the obstruction or ERF is determined by endoscopy and contrast radiography. The length of the lesion is measured to facilitate construction of a SEMS of the correct length. During endoscopy important landmarks are identified, such as the exact location of the cricopharyngeus and squamocolumnar junction relative to the lesion to be stented. In most patients pre-stent dilation is performed to 36 to 45F with American Endoscopy Dilators (Mentor, OH) or 10 to 12-mm angioplasty balloons under fluoroscopic guidance. In most patients premedication consists of conscious sedation using a combination of intravenous meperidine (25–50 mg) and midazolam (2–4 mg). Reversal of sedation at the conclusion of the procedure is not performed routinely.

A 6F angioplasty catheter is manipulated across the lesion over a flexible Bentsen wire guide (Cook, Inc.; Bloomington, IN) and passed beyond the narrowed segment or fistulous tract into the stomach. Next, an exchange is made for a 0.038-inch Amplatz Super Stiff guidewire (Meditech; Watertown, MA). The catheter is removed, and the delivery apparatus with a preloaded stent is advanced over the guidewire and positioned fluoroscopically to allow at least one full stent body (2 cm) to extend beyond both proximal and distal margins of the lesion. If required, radiographic contrast (ionic contrast for patients with obstruction; nonionic contrast for those with ERF) can be injected into the sideport of the delivery apparatus to clearly demon-

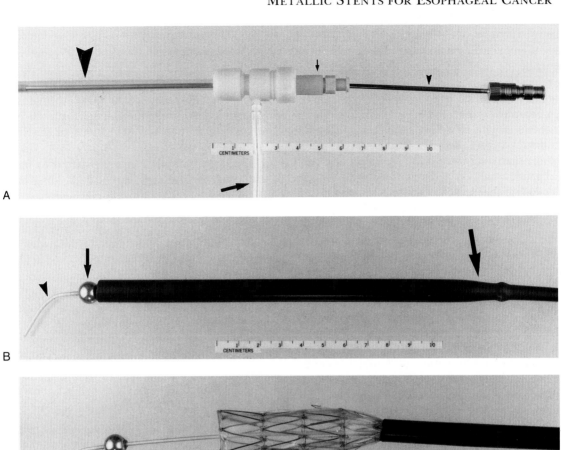

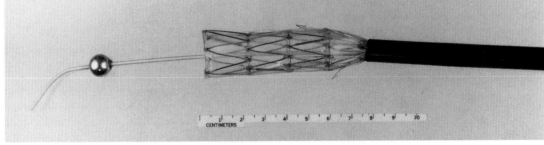

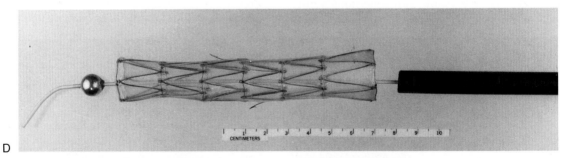

FIG. 4. A: Proximal end of the delivery catheter for the Gianturco-Rösch Z-stent designed by the Dotter Institute of Interventional Radiology (Portland, OR). During stent placement the "positioning" tube *(small arrowhead)* keeps the stent in proper position while the outer housing *(large arrowhead)* is slowly withdrawn. A side port *(large arrow)* is available to inject contrast material to identify the esophageal lesion. A locking device *(small arrow)* is present to prevent inadvertent stent deployment. **B:** Distal end of the Gianturco-Rösch Z-stent delivery apparatus. A guidewire is passed through the positioning tube *(small arrowhead)*. Note the metallic bead *(small arrow)* on the positioning tube covering the end of the apparatus housing the stent, and the tapered portion of the delivery apparatus *(large arrow)*. **C:** Partially deployed covered Gianturco-Rösch Z-stent. **D:** Completely deployed covered Gianturco-Rösch Z-stent. The positioning tube with metallic bead is subsequently removed through the deployed stent.

strate the proximal border of the lesion (Fig. 4). When in correct alignment the positioning tube is held firmly in place while the outer housing is slowly withdrawn, thereby releasing the stent to expand within the esophageal lumen. (Note: the SEMS is not pushed from the delivery apparatus; rather, the outer housing of the delivery catheter is withdrawn over the stent. If the former technique is used, the SEMS may be delivered more distally than intended.) If the stent does not completely expand, a balloon catheter of 12 to 15 mm can be used to dilate the waist to facilitate full expansion. However, it should be anticipated that the stents will gradually expand to their maximal diameter within the first 2 to 3 days. At our institution we have found it necessary to dilate only high-grade residual stenoses seen immediately after SEMS placement.

Endoscopy is performed immediately following SEMS insertion to confirm accurate placement, assess the adequacy of seal between stent and esophagus, and verify the integrity of the stent membrane. When the patient is fully awake, a barium esophagram is performed as further confirmation of luminal patency, stent position, absence of esophagorespiratory communication, perforation, or leakage around the stent. Most patients have the procedure performed while in a short stay or "day surgery" setting, and may be discharged after a 4- to 6-hour period of observation following stent insertion if no untoward symptoms arise.

CARE AFTER SEMS PLACEMENT

Immediately following SEMS placement, patients with obstruction are advised to consume liquids only for the initial 48 hours, followed by a progressively solid diet as tolerated thereafter. Good mastication and avoidance of certain foods (such as meats, raw vegetables, bread, etc.) is suggested. In those patients in whom the lower esophageal sphincter is straddled by the stent, anti-reflux instructions are given and patients are routinely prescribed omeprazole 20 mg a day to minimize anticipated symptoms of gastroesophageal reflux.

Patients with ERF are instructed to begin eating a soft mechanical diet, initially avoiding liquids. If no symptoms of aspiration occur with soft solids, then liquid intake is permitted.

A barium esophagram is routinely obtained at 1 week, 2 months, and 6 months following stent placement. Repeat endoscopy is performed at 6 months. For any symptoms of reobstruction, aspiration, or any complications of stent placement, a routine chest radiograph is initially obtained to confirm the location of the SEMS. Next, esophagoscopy is the diagnostic procedure of choice. For those patients stented for ERF who redevelop symptoms of aspiration, a contrast esophagram is also valuable.

CASE PRESENTATIONS

Case 1

A 57-year-old man with squamous cell carcinoma located in his distal esophagus was referred to the Oregon Health Sciences University for management of dysphagia. Due to the extent of disease, he was considered inoperable and received palliative radiotherapy, which was initially effective. However, his dysphagia

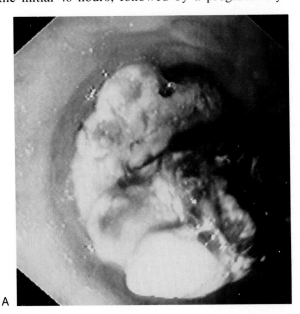 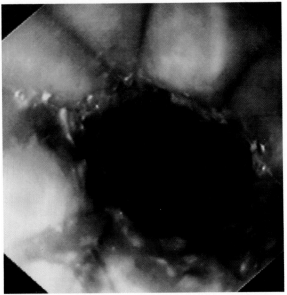

FIG. 5. A: Endoscopic photograph of the proximal margin of malignant esophageal obstruction before stent placement in Case 1. **B:** Endoscopic view within the silicone-covered metallic stent placed for obstruction in Case 1. Note the ability to visualize mucosa through the transparent silicone membrane and the appearance of the metal struts of the stent bodies.

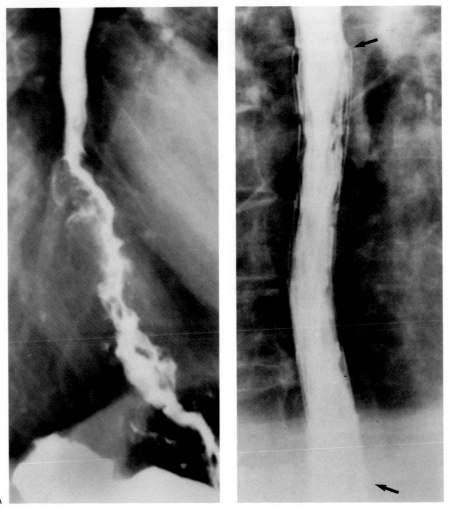

FIG. 6. A: Esophagram of Case 1 demonstrating an 8 cm long malignant stricture before SEMS placement. **B:** Esophagram of Case 1 after stent placement. Note the wide patency through the fully expanded stent. Proximal and distal stent margins are identified *(arrows)*.

returned and was unresponsive to frequent bougie-nage. At the time of referral he was unable to swallow solids or liquids, but could still manage his own secretions.

Esophagoscopy (Fig. 5A) and contrast esophagram (Fig. 6A) confirmed an obstructing malignancy beginning at 37 cm from the incisors and extending for 8 cm to the gastroesophageal junction. Under fluoroscopic guidance, dilation to 45F was accomplished with American Endoscopy dilators. A silicone-covered Gianturco-Rösch Z-stent 18 mm in diameter and 12 cm in length was deployed uneventfully (Figs. 5B and 6B). Following SEMS insertion the patient was able to resume a normal diet until his death 14 weeks later.

Case 2

A 70-year-old man was diagnosed with squamous cell carcinoma of the proximal esophagus 12 months prior to referral to the Oregon Health Sciences University. Since the patient refused surgery he received palliative chemotherapy [*cis*-platinum and 5-fluorouracil (5-FU)] and radiotherapy (4000 cGy) with fair improvement in his dysphagia. However, his course was complicated by radiation esophagitis. His dysphagia recurred 11 months after initial diagnosis; recurrent carcinoma was confirmed endoscopically. A second course of chemotherapy (mitomycin and 5-FU) was undertaken.

The patient subsequently developed paroxysms of cough with food intake. Endoscopy (Fig. 7A) and contrast esophagram (Fig. 8A) revealed the presence of an esophagorespiratory fistula.

A silicone-covered Gianturco-Rösch SEMS was accurately placed straddling the fistulous tract (Fig. 7B). Barium esophagram following SEMS placement confirmed complete sealing of the ERF (Fig. 8B). The patient resumed oral intake of solids and liquids without

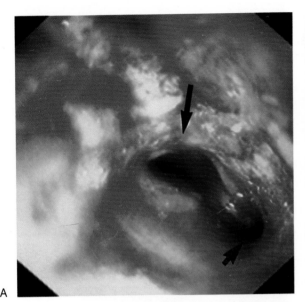 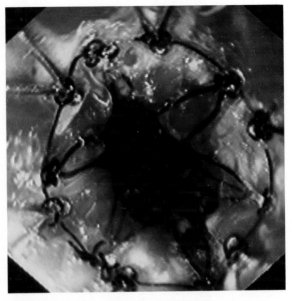

FIG. 7. A: Endoscopic view of the esophagorespiratory fistula *(small arrow)* seen in Case 2. The esophageal lumen is narrowed *(large arrow)*. **B:** Endoscopic view from within the silicone-covered SEMS placed in Case 2. The fistula was completely sealed.

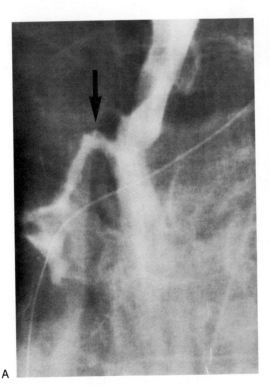 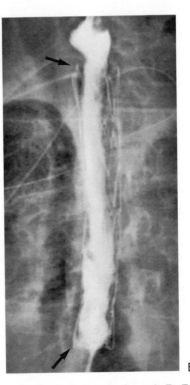

FIG. 8. A: Esophagram showing esophagorespiratory fistula *(arrow)* seen in Case 2. **B:** Esophagram from Case 2 after silicone-covered Gianturco-Rösch Z-stent placement demonstrating complete sealing of the fistulous tract. The proximal and distal margins of the stent are identified *(arrows)*.

symptoms of aspiration. He is still able to consume a normal diet 6 months after stent insertion.

RESULTS

Clinical Response

A review of all published cases reporting SEMS insertion, in addition to our most recent experience in 25 patients (23), reveals a high success rate in palliating malignant obstruction and esophagorespiratory fistula (Table 1). Of 89 patients with malignant dysphagia, 82 (92%) were reported to have resumed a normal or semi-solid diet. Follow-up ranged from 1 week to 12 months, with a composite mean of 17 weeks.

SEMS insertion has been performed in 12 patients (1 with ERF alone, 11 with ERF and obstruction) with 8 patients sustaining a complete seal of the fistulous tract. Two of the 12 patients benefited from a partial seal (able to consume solids orally, but not liquids). The two nonresponders were the only patients who had complications in this group: migration of SEMS into the trachea and tension pneumothorax (19).

In addition to the 12 patients treated for ERF with or without obstruction, Song and colleagues (15) placed a SEMS to occlude a sizable esophageal rupture in one patient with malignant obstruction. The outcome was excellent; the patient required intravenous alimentation and antibiotics over an 8-day hospitalization but surgery was avoided. This is the first reported use of SEMS for this indication.

Major Complications

Major complications consisted of stent migration (7%), food obstruction (6%), tumor ingrowth between struts of uncovered stents (5%), tumor overgrowth around the ends of stents (4%), severe chest pain (4%), migration into trachea (1%), incomplete expansion requiring stent removal (1%), a disrupted stent membrane (1%), and death (4%). Deaths were due to late pressure necrosis with perforation, tension pneumothorax with guidewire insertion through an ERF, pneumoperitoneum likely resulting from esophageal rupture, and massive esophageal hemorrhage. The composite complication rate in 102 patients was 32%. Only two major complications occurred during SEMS insertion, but both resulted in death (pneumoperitoneum and tension pneumothorax).

Many of the complications can be corrected endoscopically without undue morbidity. Food obstructing the SEMS can be removed or pushed into the stomach using the endoscope. Tumor ingrowth, tumor overgrowth, and a torn stent membrane may require the placement of additional overlapping stents. Although

considered permanent, renegade stents that have migrated into the stomach occasionally can be removed endoscopically using various retrieval devices (snare, forceps, basket, or balloon). However, stents modified with anchoring hooks may be very difficult to retrieve and may require laparotomy if the stent is obstructing gastric outflow. Two of our four stent migrations were completely asymptomatic, having been detected on routine follow-up radiographs or endoscopy. In both cases the stents could not be found anywhere within the patients, and neither recalled passing the SEMS rectally.

DISCUSSION

Malignant esophageal obstruction often relentlessly progresses to debilitating dysphagia. The formation of an ERF portends a rapid patient demise with marked morbidity. Effective endoscopic therapy has been limited to laser fulguration or the placement of a rigid endoprosthesis—both of which have significant disadvantages.

The application of self-expanding metallic stents began within the vascular system but has evolved to include the tracheobronchial tree, the biliary system, and now the upper gastrointestinal tract. Experience has been compiled in 102 patients around the world for SEMS use within the esophagus for the management of malignant obstruction and esophagorespiratory fistulae (Table 1). None of these stents are commercially available at this time, but results are promising.

SEMS placement has been effective in relieving malignant dysphagia in over 90% of patients treated thus far. The rate of major complications is approximately 32%, which is comparable to the complication rate for insertion of rigid prostheses. However, many of the complications of SEMS can be managed easily by endoscopy or interventional radiology. Further, our experience in Portland demonstrates the importance of experience in decreasing complications. The rate of complications in our initial eight patients was 63%, while in the latter 23 patients was 26%. This improvement likely reflects enhanced operator experience and/or improved stent design. The mortality rate of 4% is acceptable given the advanced nature of the lesions treated.

In contrast to conventional rigid stents, placement of the SEMS is atraumatic. Large-bore bougienage is not required, thereby decreasing the risk of perforation and death. The diameter of delivery catheters needed to place a SEMS ranges from 18F to 36F. Therefore, the preinsertion dilation requirement is modest. When fully expanded, the luminal diameter of SEMS is 18 to 20 mm compared with 10 to 20 mm for most rigid endoprostheses. A further advantage of SEMS over

TABLE 3. *Comparison of self-expanding metallic stents (SEMS) and rigid esophageal endoprostheses*

Criterion	SEMS	Rigid endo-prosthesis
Pre-insertion dilation requirement (mm)	10–15	18–20
Diameter of delivery apparatus (mm)	8–12	15–18
Traumatic insertion?	No	Yes
Luminal diameter (mm)	18–20	10–12
Ability to overlap stents?	Yes	No

conventional rigid stents is the ability to place one SEMS within another stent already deployed. A second SEMS may be required to extend the length of stenting if tumor overgrowth or stent migration occurs. Covered stents may have membrane disruption necessitating the placement of an overlapping SEMS (Table 3).

Permanent SEMS placement has advantages over Nd:YAG fulguration in managing malignant obstruction (Table 4). First, equipment required to perform SEMS insertion should be inexpensive compared to the sizable investment needed to acquire a Nd:YAG laser. Second, SEMS can manage intraluminal and extraluminal causes of obstruction while laser therapy is limited to the former. Third, only one treatment session is needed to place a permanent SEMS, while Nd:YAG ablation requires repeated visits. Fourth, ERF cannot be managed by laser therapy.

Patients with esophagorespiratory fistulae currently have two palliative options: surgery (which carries a significant mortality rate) and esophageal intubation with a rigid endoprosthesis. Ten of 12 patients with ERF treated to date with SEMS have been able to resume some oral intake without symptoms of aspiration, thereby profoundly improving the quality of life in these debilitated patients. The advantage of SEMS over conventional esophageal intubation in patients with ERF is that palliation can be achieved relatively atraumatically.

While various SEMS designs have been investigated, silicone-covered stents seem to have better effi-

cacy in preventing tumor growth between metal struts (ingrowth). For obvious reasons, only covered stents are acceptable in treating ERF. However, covered stents require a larger delivery catheter; therefore the preplacement dilation requirement is slightly higher. Gianturco-like stents may be easier to accurately deploy within the esophagus compared to the Wallstent or Strecker stent because the Z-stent does not shorten when released from the delivery catheter. Anchoring hooks used by Song and at our institution are intended to prevent SEMS migration. However, these hooks also make it very difficult to safely remove stents nonoperatively once they are inserted. Song's "barbless" Gianturco stent is quite innovative (16). Intended to avoid the trauma of anchoring hooks, the dumbbell shape is designed to funnel food material into the stent and to prevent cephalad or caudad migration. The "barbless" feature theoretically should cause less injury to the esophagus and may make the stent amenable to endoscopic or radiologic removal or relocation if migration does occur. However, 4 of 21 patients treated with the "barbless" Gianturco stent reported severe chest pain requiring analgesia. This complication is unique to this group and may reflect the flared ends (22 or 24 mm in diameter). In spite of the presence of proximal and distal flanges, 1 of 21 patients still had proximal migration of the stent (16). In our experience in 31 patients, stent migration was seen in 4 patients (13%). In all 4 patients the obstruction was located in the distal esophagus and the caudad stent body of the SEMS protruded freely into the stomach. Therefore, if stent placement can be accomplished without extension of the SEMS into the gastric lumen, then the rate of migration likely can be lowered.

SUMMARY

Although worldwide experience using SEMS is limited, early reports suggest that SEMS is highly effective in treating malignant esophageal obstruction and esophagorespiratory fistulae. Stent insertion appears atraumatic and most complications can be easily managed endoscopically. Death occurs in less than 5% of patients. Various designs of esophageal SEMS are in experimental trial, but covered stents have theoretical advantages over uncovered (or partially covered) stents in preventing tumor ingrowth but require a larger delivery vehicle for stent insertion. The Gianturco-Rösch Z-stent design should be easier to precisely place than either the Wallstent or Ultraflex stent because it does not foreshorten on expansion from the delivery apparatus. To optimize patient outcome, we recommend a combined effort between gastroenterology and interventional radiologists in placing expandable stents within the esophagus.

TABLE 4. *Comparison of self-expanding metallic stent (SEMS) and Nd:YAG laser*

Criterion	SEMS	Nd:YAG
Start-up cost	Very low	Extremely high
Treatment sessions needed	1	2–4
Can treat submucosal or extrinsic lesions?	Yes	No
Can treat esophago-respiratory fistulae?	Yes	No

Randomized prospective clinical trials comparing SEMS to conventional rigid stents or laser fulguration are needed. We anticipate that the self-expanding metallic stent will prove to be at least as efficacious as conventional therapy, but with fewer complications, lower cost, and reduced treatment time. Although now only available in selected centers throughout the world on an experimental basis, SEMS offers great hope for effective treatment of malignant esophageal obstruction and esophagorespiratory fistulae. When the self-expanding metallic stent becomes commercially available, it will likely become an integral weapon in our palliative armamentarium.

ACKNOWLEDGMENTS

Special thanks to Josef Rösch, M.D. for his foresight and innovative ideas, which have accelerated the development of a suitable esophageal prosthesis; to Barry T. Uchida, B.S. and Hans A. Timmermans, B.F.A. for their meticulous skill in crafting each stent and for their work in designing the optimal delivery catheter; to Sheri S. Imai, B.S. for producing high quality photographs; and to Schneider U.S. Stent Division and Microvasive for providing photographs of the prototype stents.

REFERENCES

1. Postlethwait RW. Complications and deaths after operations for esophageal carcinoma. *J Thorac Cardiovasc Surg* 1983;85: 827–831.
2. Boyce HW. Palliation of advanced esophageal cancer. *Semin Oncol* 1984;11:186–195.
3. Cavy AL, Rougier PM, Pieddeloup C, Kac J, Laplanche AC, Elias DM, Ducreux MP, Zummer-Rubinstein K, Zimmermann PA, Charbit MA, Crespon BM. Esophageal prosthesis for neoplastic stenosis. *Cancer* 1986;57:1426–1431.
4. Gasparri G, Casalegno A, Camandona M, DeiPoli M, Salizzoni M, Ferrarotti G, Bertero D. Endoscopic insertion of 248 prostheses in inoperable carcinoma of the esophagus and cardia: short-term and long-term results. *Gastrointest Endosc* 1987;33: 354–356.
5. Den Hartog Jager FCA, Bartelsman JFWM, Tytgat GNJ. Palliative treatment of obstructing esophagogastric malignancy by endoscopic positioning of a plastic prosthesis. *Gastroenterology* 1979;77:1108–1014.
6. Mellow MH, Pinkas H. Endoscopic therapy for esophageal carcinoma with Nd:YAG laser: prospective evaluation of efficacy, complications, and survival. *Gastrointest Endosc* 1984;30: 334–339.
7. Ahlquist DA, Gostout CJ, Viggiano TR, Balm RK, Pairolero PC, Hench VS, Zinsmeister AR. Endoscopic laser palliation of malignant dysphagia: a prospective study. *Mayo Clin Proc* 1987; 62:867–874.
8. Lightdale CJ, Zimbalist E, Winawer SJ. Outpatient management of esophageal cancer with endoscopic Nd:YAG laser. *Am J Gastroenterol* 1987;82:46–50.
9. Murray FE, Bower GJ, Birkett DH, Cave DR. Palliative laser therapy of advanced esophageal carcinoma: an alternative perspective. *Am J Gastroenterol* 1988;83:816–819.
10. Duranceau A, Jamieson GG. Malignant tracheoesophageal fistula. *Ann Thorac Surg* 1984;37:346–354.
11. Conlan AA, Nicolaou N, Delikaris PG, Pool R. Pessimism concerning palliative bypass procedures for established malignant esophagorespiratory fistulas: a report of 18 patients. *Ann Thorac Surg* 1984;37:108–110.
12. Binmoeller KF, Maeda M, Lieberman D, Katon RM, Ivancev K, Rösch J. Silicone-covered expandable metallic stents in the esophagus: an experimental study. *Endoscopy* 1992;24:416–420.
13. Domschke W, Foerster EC, Matek W, Rodl W. Self-expanding mesh stent for esophageal cancer stenosis. *Endoscopy* 1990;22: 134–136.
14. Knyrim K, Wagner HJ, Pausch J, Vakil N, Starck E. Expandable metal stents for the palliative treatment of esophageal obstruction. *Gastrointest Endosc* 1990;36:236.
15. Song HY, Choi KC, Cho BH, Ahn DS, Kin KS. Esophagogastric neoplasms: palliation with a modified Gianturco stent. *Radiology* 1991;180:349–354.
16. Song HY, Choi KC, Kwon HC, Yang DH, Cho BH, Lee ST. Esophageal strictures: treatment with a new design of modified Gianturco stent. *Radiology* 1992;184:729–734.
17. Schaer J, Katon RM, Ivancev K, Uchida B, Rösch J, Binmoeller K. Treatment of malignant esophageal obstruction with silicone-coated metallic self-expanding stents. *Gastrointest Endosc* 1992; 38:7–11.
18. Neuhaus H, Hoffmann W, Dittler HJ, Niedermeyer HP, Classen M. Implantation of self-expanding esophageal metal stents for palliation of malignant dysphagia. *Endoscopy* 1992;24:405–410.
19. Kozarek RA, Ball TJ, Patterson DJ. Metallic self-expanding stent application in the upper gastrointestinal tract: caveats and concerns. *Gastrointest Endosc* 1992;38:1–6.
20. Bethge N, Knyrim K, Wagner HJ, Starck E, Pausch J, Kleist DV. Self-expanding metal stents for palliation of malignant esophageal obstruction—a pilot study of eight patients. *Endoscopy* 1992;24:411–415.
21. Fleischer DE, Bull-Henry K. A new coated self-expanding metal stent for malignant esophageal strictures. *Gastrointest Endosc* 1992;38:494–496.
22. Sass NL, Hagenmuller F. First endoscopic implantation of memory metal stents in the esophagus. *Endoscopy* 1992;24:622.
23. Wu WC, Katon RM, Saxon RR, Barton RE, Uchida BT, Keller FS, Rösch J. Silicone-covered self-expanding metallic stents for the palliation of malignant esophageal obstruction and esophagorespiratory fistulas. *Gastrointest Endosc* 1994;40:22–33.

Advanced Therapeutic Endoscopy, 2nd Ed.,
edited by J. S. Barkin and C. A. O'Phelan.
Raven Press, Ltd., New York © 1994.

CHAPTER 7

Photodynamic Therapy for Esophageal Malignancies

Stephen K. Heier

Almost a century after the earliest work with the photo-sensitizers acridine (1) and eosin (2), photodynamic therapy (PDT) is poised to augment our endoscopic armamentarium and emerge from its investigational status. PDT works by injecting a tumor-sensitizing agent intravenously, waiting for the drug to selectively collect in the tumor and clear from normal tissues, and then exposing the tumor to a specific wavelength of light. This activates the drug, which then destroys tumor tissue. The therapy can thus be defined as tumor ablation by photochemical reaction. Technological advances have made the delivery of PDT practicable, and more refinements are anticipated.

Of the many drugs that have been and are being evaluated, dihematoporphyrin ethers (DHE; Photofrin) has taken center stage. Its generic name was recently changed to porfimer sodium, correcting the prior misconception of chemical homogeneity, since the drug consists of oligomers of two to eight porphyrin units connected by ester as well as ether bonds (3). However, the new name has not yet been accepted into current usage or in the literature. DHE is a refined formulation of another mixture called hematoporphyrin derivative (HPD), which is synthesized by acetylation and alkalization of hematoporphyrin (4), an iron-free by-product of hemoglobin breakdown. HPD was used for PDT in hundreds of patients throughout the world from 1966 until the mid-1980s when Dougherty et al. (5) identified its more active components.

During the first 20 hours after intravenous DHE injection, the drug collects in the tumor and is cleared from normal tissue and serum by biliary excretion (6–8). This differential collection of drug in tumor re-

sults partly from large serum aggregates of DHE leaking through the tumor's porous neovasculature (9), partly from transport into the tumor cell of DHE bound to serum low-density lipoprotein (LDL) (10,11), and partly from binding of DHE within tumor cells (12,13). DHE is also concentrated in neovascular stroma, perhaps within cells with phagocytic activity. Few other body sites have affinity for DHE, and almost all are shielded from light, including the liver, kidney, and spleen (9). The exception is skin, which leads to significant photosensitivity of variable duration.

Exposing the DHE-laden tumor to light in the violet range results in the characteristic salmon-colored fluorescence (14). The stimulated fluorescence may be of value for detecting tumors too small to otherwise be visible. Tumor therapy requires red light at 630 nm, a wavelength also absorbed well by DHE. This wavelength was chosen because it has greater tissue penetration and thus greater tumoricidal potential (15). The red photons activate the DHE, which then transfers its unstable energy by generating singlet oxygen, a highly reactive mediator of subsequent cellular damage (16). The tumor's neovasculature is the major target for this photochemical destruction (17,18).

CURRENT STATUS

The era of practicable PDT is due to incremental but only recently coordinated strides in drug refinement, laser technology, and fiberoptic delivery systems. Dye lasers, which generate light at the appropriate wavelength for PDT applications, date their early development to the late 1960s. As recently as several years ago, many hours would be spent before a therapy tweaking the laser's reflective mirrors and making other equally tedious adjustments. An occurrence of

S. K. Heier: Department of Clinical Medicine, Section of Endoscopy, New York Medical College, Valhalla, New York 10595.

minor seismic activity, such as use of a nearby floor-waxing machine, could then throw this delicate balance out of kilter. Present-day laser units allow the gastroenterologist to walk in, throw a switch, and expect automatic alignment for optimum function. Currently available laser fibers, once quite brittle, are sturdy and deliver fairly uniform light with relatively minor care.

PDT can be functionally classified as a laser therapy that, depending upon its intended use, requires skill in gastrointestinal endoscopy, cystoscopy, neurosurgery, etc. However, the Food and Drug Administration (FDA) classifies PDT as a chemotherapy, albeit one with little systemic toxicity, that is delivered by specialists other than oncologists. Because the therapy requires drug administration, it cannot be FDA approved by equivalence to devices, a pathway that has sped many endoscopic advances. Instead, as a drug therapy, it must be proved to have therapeutic benefit by comparison to currently available therapies. Despite many qualitative advantages inherent to PDT (discussed below), at the time of this writing PDT is an investigational therapy pending FDA approval based on multidisciplinary randomized phase III trials.

INSTRUMENTATION

PDT is not a thermal therapy, and the activating 630 nm light need be of only low intensity. Nevertheless, to get sufficient power of this single wavelength to the endoscopic field, a laser is required. The laser of choice is the tunable argon dye laser, a device that is actually two lasers in one. An argon gas laser optically pumps (excites) a circulating dye in the second laser. The dye can emit a spectrum of wavelengths, but by turning a diffraction grating in the second laser, a specific wavelength of light to resonate between mirrors can be selected. Thus, the unit is "tuned" to emit laser light of the appropriate wavelength.

Laser fibers, for carrying the laser light from the laser to the targeted tumor, are available with different types of tips. The two used in gastroenterology are the cylinder diffusing fiber and the microlens fiber. The cylinder diffusing fiber has a cigar-shaped tip, for delivering light circumferentially in luminal cavities such as the esophagus. The fiber is available with tip lengths ranging from 1 to 2.5 cm, in 0.5 cm increments, with a combination of tip lengths selected to sequentially cover the full extent of the tumor targeted. This fiber type can also be inserted directly into a tumor mass, to deliver interstitial laser light. The microlens fiber is used less often, and has a diverging lens on its tip, to deliver a forward uniform beam spot onto a small noncircumferential lesion or protruding tumor region.

A spectrometer is used to determine that the wavelength of light emitted from the fiber tip is 630 ± 2

nm. There are several types of devices available for measuring the power output from different types of fibers, but the only device that will work for cylinder diffusing fibers (and will also work for microlens fibers) is the integrating sphere. The fiber is inserted into the center of the sphere, and the total amount of light emitted is measured. The integrating sphere is precalibrated for the wavelength tested.

DELIVERING THE THERAPY

DHE comes in a lyophilized form, at a concentration of 2.5 mg/ml after reconstitution, and is injected at a dose of 2 mg/kg. The solution should not be exposed to light during injection. We use an opaque-taped syringe and cover the line leading to the injection site with a drape. The volume of solution injected averages 60 ml and should be administered slowly over 5 to 10 minutes, through a line previously established with normal saline. Scrupulous attention is directed to the injection site since extravasation would be clearly undesirable.

The laser is checked for proper functioning before injection, because the laser must be operational at a given time after injection and technical malfunctions can occur. This minimizes the possibility of exposing the patient to potential toxicity of DHE injection (i.e., photosensitivity) and then not being able to perform the therapy. In the event of equipment problems, solutions include emergency technical assistance, a backup laser, or a backup institution that also performs the therapy.

Current recommendations are to wait 40 to 50 hours after injection before therapy to allow DHE clearance out of serum and normal tissue, thereby minimizing normal tissue toxicity during light application. However, waiting this long can be inconvenient for the patient, and may limit in practice which days of the week the therapy can be performed. We have started therapy within 20 hours after injection on many occasions, without adversely affecting the normal tissue response. McCaughan (19) has given therapy to endobronchial obstruction within several hours after injection (i.e., same-day therapy), with efficacy without adverse effects, but he often limits normal tissue exposure by interstitial light delivery.

On the day of the therapy, we prefer to warm up the laser and check its output before the patient is brought into the room, to minimize the appearance of technical wizardry. Safety goggles specifically designed to block the 630-nm wavelength should be worn. Although the amount of light reaching an eye distant from a circumferentially radiating cylinder diffusing fiber is probably not hazardous, if looked at directly it can leave an irritating afterimage in one's visual field. Also, fibers are occasionally interchanged to the fiber connector cable leading from the laser unit, which can unleash a straight and more powerful beam of light with a greater potential for retinal injury. Note that red safety lights and the typical red light-emitting diodes (LEDs) found on many instruments cannot be read through these safety goggles.

Technical preparation for the procedure includes wavelength confirmation by spectrometer, fiber inspection, and power output adjustment. In the case of a microlens fiber, the beam spot should be uniform. In the case of a cylinder diffusing fiber, the fiber tip itself is inspected for any hot spots, with a tip crack often visible only during low-power illumination. A crack will then be identified as a bright transverse line. Next, the power output from the fiber is adjusted, using the integrating sphere. The power readout on the laser unit itself is proportional, but not equivalent, to the power output from the fiber.

If mirrors require minor adjustments to bring the laser's power into therapy range, the output wavelength may change and must be reconfirmed. If the diffraction grating needs readjustment to obtain the right output wavelength, the output power will always be altered. All adjustments are best done after the laser has fully warmed up. Lasers preset to deliver only the 630-nm wavelength are available, with mirrors that automatically adjust to optimize power output; but these accoutrements come at a hefty cost compared to other easily adjustable lasers.

The power for the cylinder diffusing fiber is set to a nonthermal light delivery rate, and no heat will be felt if light from the fiber tip is aimed into one's hand; the rate used is 400 mW/cm fiber tip. Therefore, if the longest tip (2.5 cm) is used, the power would be set at 1,000 mW (400 mW/cm × 2.5 cm). The total energy to be delivered (see Light Dosimetry, below) is 300 joules/cm fiber tip, resulting in a treatment time for each fiber placement of 750 seconds (12 min 30 sec). For example, a 5 cm long tumor may be treated in two segments with a 2.5-cm tipped cylinder diffusing fiber, each segment treated for 750 seconds.

To perform the therapy, the scope is first passed beyond the distal margin of the tumor, and preferably into the stomach. The fiber is then passed through the scope, and the scope withdrawn into the area of the tumor just above the first tumor segment to be treated, so as to treat tumor segments in a retrograde sequence. The scope should not be advanced when the fiber is inside the accessory channel. This is because forward advancement of the scope within tight tumor confines may buckle the scope, cracking the fiber tip within the scope. During the therapy, the fiber is intermittently removed to inspect its tip and its power output. We routinely check the fiber about every 6 minutes (i.e., halfway through the therapy of each tumor segment),

and more frequently if maneuvering is necessary during therapy or if there was any resistance to passing the fiber through the scope.

Overtreatment is minimized by avoiding overlap of light applications to adjacent tumor segments. Conversely, efficacy is maximized when light applications adequately cover all tumor segments. The distal segment is usually best treated by making sure the distal point of the fiber is even with the distal margin of the tumor. The proximal segment can usually be treated by making sure the proximal portion of the fiber tip emitting light is even with the proximal margin of the tumor. The segment treated in between, if any, is often best approached from above the proximal margin of the tumor; fiber placement for the middle segment will be easier if the proximal segment is chosen to be the shortest segment. For example, with a 6-cm tumor, the distal 5 cm would first be treated in two segments each 2.5 cm long, and the proximal segment would then be treated with a 1-cm cylinder-diffusing fiber (Fig. 1). The middle segment of this tumor would therefore have been treated by extending the entire 2.5-cm long fiber tip an estimated 1 cm beyond the proximal margin of the tumor.

If the lower margin of the tumor is not distinct or clearly visible from an intratumor position, it is probably best to err on the side of overextending the therapy field, taking advantage of the selective properties of the therapy. On the other hand, if the upper margin is clearly demarcated and visible, it is best to treat with the endoscope up close to the superior margin, using the tip of the endoscope to block backscatter of light, thus limiting unnecessary exposure of normal tissue.

During treatment, the fiber is centered in the tumor lumen. The fiber tip is kept out of and away from crevices, depressions, and deep ulcerations, thus preventing the concentration of activating light on thin-walled areas. In contrast, an overly prominent and asymmetric tumor bulge may occasionally interfere with adequate distribution of light despite scattering. Furthermore, such a bulge may limit the likelihood of a successful outcome, because luminal recanalization will be dependent upon significant unilateral necrosis of the tumor bulge rather than the additive effects of necrosis of two opposing tumor walls. Such bulges may therefore be best treated by interstitial fiber placement, with the fiber inserted tangentially 3 to 5 mm below the surface. Alternatively, either side of the bulge can be treated separately, perhaps by delivering a lower light dose of 200 joules/cm (treatment time of 500 sec) to both sides.

The endoscopic environment is not static, and the position of the fiber will often change when the patient swallows, coughs, or moves; when the endoscopist changes his position or his torque on the scope; or when the tumor gradually releases its tension around

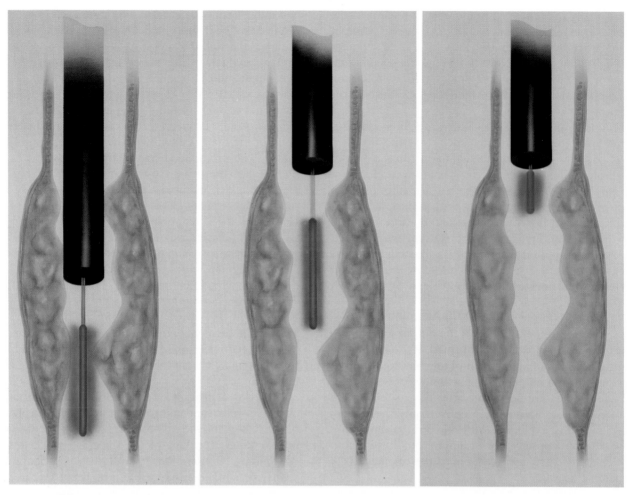

FIG. 1. Treatment of a 6 cm long esophageal cancer using cylinder diffusing fibers in a retrograde sequence. **A:** A 2.5-cm tip with its distal point even with the tumor's distal margin. **B:** A 2.5-cm tip extended an estimated 1 cm beyond the tumor's proximal margin. **C:** A 1.0-cm tip with its proximal point even with the tumor's proximal margin.

the scope. The resulting change in scope tip and fiber tip position may occur despite holding the endoscope shaft a set distance from the patient's mouthpiece. In other words, there may be no change in the length of scope inserted, as indicated by the distance markings along the side of the endoscope. Indeed, the tip of the endoscope can move several centimeters without an overt change in the scope shaft's external position. This paradox can occur due to a release of traction on a tight tumor, which pulled the tumor segment cephalad into the thoracic cavity, or to a release of tension on the endoscope allowing it to attain a freer position within the proximal normal esophageal lumen.

Therefore, once fiber tip position is optimized, it is at least as important, if not more important, to note and maintain tumor landmarks in the visual field as it is to maintain the external station of the endoscope. The briefest puff of air is intermittently used to clear the lens and maintain such visualization; overinsufflation would require advancing the scope beyond the

tumor and lower esophageal segment (LES) for decompression. Suctioning is avoided during therapy, because it can alter the tumor's landmarks. Note that videoendoscopes are best not used for delivering PDT, because when placed on automatic light intensity mode they gray out the picture to compensate for the bright red light, and when on manual intensity mode the light is too bright to distinguish any landmarks. On the other hand, add-on CCD cameras offer the best visualization during therapy.

Blood or secretions covering the tumor field may theoretically limit the penetration of the activating light (20), but in practice have not proved deleterious to the outcome. After initial passage through a very tight and friable tumor, we do, however, use the scope to tamponade the tumor for several minutes. When the scope is then withdrawn into the tumor, minimal water irrigation will usually yield the clearest field that can be achieved.

Despite all the details given above, the majority of

the therapy is performed by remaining still, thereupon developing an appreciation for the activities and distractions of life.

Two to three days after therapy, dead tumor tissue is debrided. Whereas during the actual therapy little response is discernible other than a barely perceptible cyanotic hue, at the time of debridement the tumor surface has coagulated into a curd-like or fibrinous substance that is usually easily sloughed upon passage of the scope. A second light application is not uniformly necessary, and was not required in one-quarter of our patients. In the majority of patients who do require a second light application, retreatment is restricted to those segments that are not fully patent. Whenever a second light application is delivered, debridement is again performed 2 to 4 days later.

Although we did not combine neodymium:yttrium-aluminum garnet (Nd:YAG) laser therapy with PDT, so as to maintain data integrity for unambiguous assessment of each therapy, there may be an advantage to intermingling these therapies if both are available. However, Nd:YAG laser therapy probably should not precede PDT, because the char resulting from thermal carbonization of tissue may interfere with light penetration from PDT. Instead, Nd:YAG laser therapy would probably best follow PDT, and be directed only to those portions of tumor with less than optimum response. In this manner, the advantages of PDT would be preserved as much as possible.

LIGHT DOSIMETRY

One of the first steps in our evaluation of PDT was to analyze its light dosimetry, that is, the effects of various light doses on the degree of tumor necrosis. This testing began with a low light dose (200 joules/cm fiber) (21) that was one-third to one-half those previously used (22) and was intended to have little or no efficacy. Instead, this dose had significant, although not optimum, efficacy.

After testing a variety of light doses, we found a correlation between the tissue dose of light (joules/cm²) and the resulting depth of tumor necrosis (23). The tissue dose of light varies inversely with the luminal diameter of a tumor segment (when the light dose delivered from the fiber tip is held constant), and was calculated by figuring the surface area of an open cylinder. By using this type of analysis and then working backward from tissue doses, the light dose of 300 joules/cm fiber was determined to give a safe yet effective range of tumor necrosis. This light dose was still lower than those that had been previously used. Furthermore, it was independently reported that the higher light doses previously used were associated with untoward com-

plications (e.g., pleural effusions, mediastinitis, fistulas) (24).

The dose of 300 joules/cm for the palliative therapy of malignant esophageal obstruction signifies a standardization of light dosing for PDT. Most studies to date have used a range of light doses, with individual doses selected based upon tumor bulk or clinical severity. Light dose standardization, however, both simplifies therapy delivery and exploits a safety feature of PDT. When the light dose is held constant, the tissue dose decreases as the luminal radius increases. Thus, those portions of tumor segments with more patent lumens will be spared from significant necrosis at the low light dose now selected. As a result, the risk of fistula formation should be minimized.

CLINICAL RESPONSE

We have now analyzed 44 PDT treatment courses delivered to 32 patients, who required a total of 77 light applications.

Dysphagia was relieved in almost all patients, with a concordant and statistically significant increase at 1 month in Karnofsky performance status and esophageal grades (23). However, patients did not gain weight, although their rate of progressive weight loss was certainly ameliorated. Some modest weight loss did occur initially, at the time of the therapy and debridement endoscopies. Subsequent weight gain did not occur despite functional improvement, probably because dietary advancement was tempered by tumor-induced anorexia.

Patients who may not respond as well to therapy include those with the most prolonged and severe obstruction (perhaps due to external tumor compression or anoxic tumor areas), those with marked inflammatory components complicating their tumor (perhaps because PDT intensifies the inflammatory response), and those with long tumors [due to difficulty clearing food through the channel despite an adequate lumen, similar to the outcome noted after Nd:YAG laser therapy (25,26)]. Submucosal lesions, however, do respond to PDT because the wavelength used adequately penetrates beyond the mucosa.

Adenocarcinomas and squamous cell carcinomas responded similarly in terms of clinical parameters, concordant with their similar response by our light dosimetry analysis (27).

By comparison to the extent of tumor necrosis, damage to adjacent normal tissue exposed to activating light during therapy was minimal. However, limited edema, discoloration, and surface erosions of normal tissue did occur.

PDT CONTRASTED WITH Nd:YAG LASER THERAPY

We became interested in PDT because of its possible qualitative advantages compared to Nd:YAG laser therapy, and its potential for the fluorescence detection and therapy of early tumors. We anticipated few quantitative differences if both therapies were capable of achieving luminal patency in the palliative relief of malignant esophageal obstruction. However, in our randomized comparison of the two therapies involving 42 patients (20 PDT and 22 Nd:YAG laser therapy), the duration of response before symptom progression required repeat therapy was longer after PDT (median 66 vs. 45 days, $p < .01$ by Kaplan-Meier techniques). With PDT, at 1 month there was an associated increase in Karnofsky performance status, and a statistically greater improvement in esophageal grade compared to Nd:YAG laser therapy.

The longer duration of response and greater improvement in associated parameters may relate to an hypothesized immunological effect of PDT (28) leading to suppression of the tumor's growth rate. There are some limited clinical and animal data suggesting immunological mechanisms do play a role in the response to PDT (29,30). Furthermore, in our studies two patients who each received three courses of therapy (three DHE injections) developed strictures that were characterized by confluent inflammatory exudates; one of these patients had a complete tumor response (although autopsy showed residual nests of tumor cells). An alternative explanation for PDT's prolonged duration of response relative to Nd:YAG laser therapy is that the extensive thermal injury after Nd:YAG laser ablation may shorten the duration of its effective palliation. Because Nd:YAG laser thermal ablation may injure normal muscle both transmurally through the tumor and at the proximal margin of the tumor, propulsive forces for food boluses may be adversely affected. Therefore, with tumor progression after either PDT or Nd:YAG laser therapy, a similar reduction in luminal patency may lead to an earlier relapse of symptoms after Nd:YAG laser therapy.

The qualitative differences between the therapies are predictable, and relate to the differences in their mechanisms of action. Because PDT is a nonthermal therapy, there is less pain during therapy, as high intrathoracic temperatures are not generated. Furthermore, there is no thermal damage to endoscopes and no smoke generation. The smoke generation associated with Nd:YAG laser therapy obscures operator vision, causes gaseous distension in the patient, and is noxious to endoscopy personnel when eructated by the patient. With PDT each tumor segment is treated circumferentially with little endoscopic maneuvering, whereas with Nd:YAG laser therapy multiple and precisely aimed

pulses to address different sites call for frequent endoscopic maneuvering. PDT may also be less likely to cause normal tissue injury resulting from either operator error or heat transmission.

A disadvantage of PDT is skin photosensitivity (see below).

As previously noted, if both therapies are available to the endoscopist, it may be advantageous in some circumstances to deliver some limited Nd:YAG laser therapy after a course of PDT.

TOXICITY

The actual intravenous administration of DHE was not associated with any toxicity, but we did take special precautions in the one instance of limited drug extravasation at the injection site. As it was reasonable to speculate that there would be enhanced photosensitivity at the site of extravasation, this area was covered with an opaque dressing until swelling subsided.

The only known systemic toxicity associated with PDT is skin photosensitivity (Fig. 2). This usually lasts about a month, but we did have one patient who developed a photoreaction 72 days after DHE injection. Perhaps because patients follow precautions against sun exposure, photoreactions have been few (affecting seven patients), and most are mild, consisting of the equivalent of a first-degree sunburn with erythema. However, one patient did develop blistering (second-degree reaction). Our patients did not require any sig-

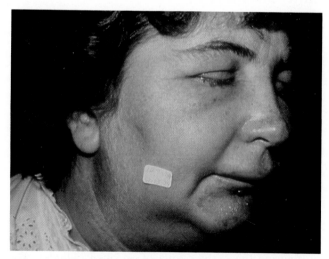

FIG. 2. An unusually severe photoreaction in a patient to receive PDT for skin metastases of breast cancer. Her face was inadvertently exposed to direct sunlight for several hours within one day of HPD (an early formulation of DHE) injection. She had fallen asleep on a sofa behind her front door, later left open by a visiting friend. The photoreaction cleared after several days without treatment. (Courtesy of T. J. Dougherty, Roswell Park Cancer Institute.)

nificant change in their life-styles when adhering to photosensitivity precautions, perhaps partly because of their advanced age and medical difficulties.

As for complications at the site of therapy, one patient developed a fistula and two patients developed strictures requiring dilatation, one of whom also required Nd:YAG laser recanalization. As noted, both patients who developed strictures had undergone three PDT therapy courses. Finally, a few patients have developed transient low-grade fever during therapy not related to evident infection, and a few patients required additional endoscopy to clear necrotic debris blocking the tumor lumen.

Hemorrhage has been reported as a complication of PDT for endobronchial carcinoma (as with Nd:YAG laser therapy for these tumors) (31), and has been cited by some as a difficulty that might be generally associated with PDT of large tumors (32,33). However, none of our patients with malignant esophageal obstruction treated with PDT suffered this complication. There have also been no complications due to normal tissue reactions, when areas adjacent to tumors were exposed to the activating light.

In the randomized trial, there were no significant differences in toxicity between the two therapies, other than the skin photosensitivity reactions that were unique to PDT. Toxicity in the randomized trial (PDT: YAG) included fistula (1:2), stricture (0:2), and skin photoreactions (4:0).

PATIENT INSTRUCTIONS

Patients are instructed to avoid exposure to sunlight for a period of about 1 month. Typical room lighting, including fluorescent lighting, poses no hazard. However, very bright light, as from a dentist's operating lamp, should be avoided. If a patient must go outdoors, precautions should include wearing a wide brimmed hat and covering all exposed areas (e.g., by wearing gloves). Some clothes, such as knitted apparel, may permit sun penetration. Typical sunscreens are ineffective, as they guard against ultraviolet light and not against the activating visible wavelengths. Some preparations are effective (e.g., zinc oxide), but they are not generally acceptable cosmetically.

At the end of the month, the patient may gradually increase his exposure to sunlight as tolerated, usually starting with a 10-minute exposure of an uncovered hand. While patients may possibly decrease their duration of photosensitivity through drug photobleaching, achieved by gradual exposure to sunlight (34), we do not recommend this practice.

Because of DHE retention in the reticuloendothelial cells of the liver, kidney, and spleen, we also warn patients that we must be notified if they require any emergency abdominal surgery. We would then notify the operating surgeon that these organs must be draped during surgery; alternatively, filters on the operating room lights may be used.

Other instructions are similar to those relayed to patients after Nd:YAG laser therapy. For example, solid food should be well chewed and followed by liquid, and all food should be eaten in an upright position.

INDICATIONS FOR PDT

The indications for PDT for the palliative relief of malignant esophageal obstruction can be easily summarized by stating that PDT can be considered as an alternative to Nd:YAG laser therapy. However, if a patient is being considered for surgical intervention in the near future, yet needs immediate establishment of luminal patency, I would opt for Nd:YAG laser therapy to avoid having to drape abdominal organs intraoperatively.

PDT has also been used as a curative therapy to ablate early esophageal and gastric cancers, with complete response rates ranging from 52% to 100% (35–39). Furthermore, successful ablation of early cancer and carcinoma in situ in the setting of Barrett's esophagus has been reported (40–42). The reports of successful therapy have mostly originated from France, Switzerland, Japan, and China. Many studies have either used multimodal therapy or had limited follow-up. Nevertheless, these studies are forging another niche for PDT, as the therapy may ablate microscopic areas of cancer extension that are not visible. PDT for early cancer would probably benefit from endoscopic ultrasound definition of the extent of tumor involvement combined with the careful application of light dosimetry.

PDT has also been successfully performed in the duodenum (43) and the colon (44), although data are insufficient to delineate the indications for such therapy.

CONTRAINDICATIONS TO PDT

Patients with outdoor occupations or recreational activities may be best treated with alternative therapies, to avoid the skin photosensitivity. Patients with a severe inflammatory component to their tumors, as a residual effect of recent radiation therapy or severe reflux, may not respond as well to PDT. Patients with fistulas should not be treated with PDT, and would be best served by an endoscopically placed prosthesis.

Bulky tumors are not a contraindication to therapy, but may require interstitial therapy (see above). Bleeding tumors are not a contraindication to therapy, although blood covering the tumor may theoretically limit light penetration. Most bleeding tumors have actually become less friable after therapy.

FUTURE DIRECTIONS

Certain technical improvements would further enhance PDT. A balloon containing, centering, and fixing the cylinder-diffusing fiber in the tumor lumen would make the therapy even easier to deliver. Solid state lasers would probably decrease the cost of therapy, and would do away with certain maintenance considerations, such as the need to reload dye because of gradual degradation. Drugs associated with less skin photosensitivity would broaden PDT's application. Such drugs are being explored. For example, benzoporphyrin derivative effectively clears from skin within days (45,46).

Gastrointestinal indications other than the palliative relief of malignant esophageal obstruction require further evaluation. These include use of the therapy for other sites in the gastrointestinal tract, and for curative potential in adenomas, dysplasia, and early cancer. The combination of PDT with other modalities, such as Nd:YAG laser therapy, chemotherapy, radiation therapy, and surgery, also requires in-depth evaluation.

Finally, technological advances enabling the exploration of DHE's tumor-localizing and fluorescent properties may lead to even more important clinical benefits.

CONCLUSIONS

Although PDT is still investigational, available studies indicate it to be both effective and safe. Its full potential, perhaps impacting on the curative therapy of early cancer and dysplasia, and the localization of early tumors, should be fully explored.

REFERENCES

1. Raab O. Uber die wirkung fluorescirender stoffe auf infusorien. *Z Biol* 1900;39:524–546.
2. Von Tappeiner H, Jesionek A. Therapeutische versuche mit fluoreszierenden stoffen. *Munchen Med Wochenschr* 1903;47: 2042–2044.
3. Dougherty TJ. Studies on the structure of porphyrins contained in Photofrin II. *Photochem Photobiol* 1987;46:569–573.
4. Lipson RL, Baldes EJ. The photodynamic properties of a particular hematoporphyrin derivative. *Arch Dermatol* 1960;82: 508–516.
5. Dougherty TJ, Boyle DG, Weishaupt KR, Henderson BA, Potter WR, Bellnier DA, Wityk KE. Photoradiation therapy—clinical and drug advances. In: Kessel D, Dougherty TJ, eds. *Porphyrin photosensitization.* New York: Plenum Press.
6. Gomer CJ, Dougherty TJ. Determination of [³H]- and [¹⁴C]hematoporphyrin derivative distribution in malignant and normal tissue. *Cancer Res* 1979;39:146–151.
7. Bellnier DA, Ho YK, Pandey RK, Missert JR, Dougherty TJ. Distribution and elimination of Photofrin II in mice. *Photochem Photobiol* 1989;50:221–228.
8. Profio AE. Dosimetry for photoradiation therapy. *Laser Inst Am* 1983;37:10–15.
9. Bugelski PJ, Porter CW, Dougherty TJ. Autoradiographic distribution of hematoporphyrin derivative in normal and tumor tissue of the mouse. *Cancer Res* 1981;41(11 Pt 1):4606–4612.
10. Kessel D. Porphyrin-lipoprotein association as a factor in porphyrin localization. *Cancer Lett* 1986;33:183–188.
11. Maziere J, Morliere P, Santus R. The role of low density lipoprotein receptor pathway in the delivery of lipophilic photosensitizers in the photodynamic therapy of tumors. *J Photochem Photobiol B: Biol* 1991;8:351–360.
12. Christensen T, Sandquist T, Feren K, Waksvik H, Moan J. Retention and photodynamic effects of haematoporphyrin derivative in cells after prolonged cultivation in the presence of porphyrin. *Br J Cancer* 1983;48(1):35–43.
13. Gibson SL, Hilf R. Photosensitization of mitochondrial cytochrome *c* oxidase by hematoporphyrin derivative and related porphyrins in vitro and in vivo. *Cancer Res* 1983;43:4191–4197.
14. Lipson RL, Baldes EJ, Olsen AM. A further evaluation of the use of hematoporphyrin derivative as a new aid for the endoscopic detection of malignant disease. *Dis Chest* 1964;46: 676–679.
15. Moan J, Sommer S. Action spectra for hematoporphyrin derivative and Photofrin II with respect to sensitization of human cells in vitro to photoinactivation. *Photochem Photobiol* 1984;40: 631–634.
16. Weishaupt KR, Gomer CJ, Dougherty TJ. Identification of singlet oxygen as the cytotoxic agent in photoinactivation of two murine tumors. *Cancer Res* 1976;36:2326–2329.
17. Henderson B, Waldow S, Mang T, Potter W, Malone P, Dougherty T. Tumor destruction and kinetics of tumor cell death in two experimental mouse tumors following photodynamic therapy. *Cancer Res* 1985;45:572–576.
18. Star WM, Marijnissen HPA, van den Berg-Blok AE, Versteeg JA, Franken KAP, Reinhold HS. Destruction of rat mammary tumor and normal tissue microcirculation by hematoporphyrin derivative photosensitization observed in vitro in sandwich observation chambers. *Cancer Res* 1986;46:2532–2540.
19. McCaughan JS. Effect of photodynamic therapy on same day of injection of dihematoporphyrin ether on endobronchial tumors. *Laser Surg Med* 1992;12(suppl 4):212(abst).
20. Vincent GM, Fox J, Charlton G, Hill JS, McClane R, Spikes JD. Presence of blood significantly decreases transmission of 630 nm laser light. *Laser Surg Med* 1991;11:399–403.
21. Heier SK, Lebovics E, Rothman K, Rosenthal WS. Photodynamic therapy (PDT) of esophageal malignancy (EM) using dihematoporphyrin ethers (DHE): a comparison to Nd:YAG endoscopic laser therapy (ELT). *Am J Gastroenterol* 1987;82: 980(abst).
22. McCaughan JS, Williams TE, Bethel BH. Palliation of esophageal malignancy with photodynamic therapy. *Ann Thorac Surg* 1985;40:113–119.
23. Heier SK, Rothman K, Heier LM, Rosenthal WS. Randomized trial and light dosimetry of palliative photodynamic therapy. *Gastrointest Endosc* 1992;38(2):279(abst).
24. Thomas RJ, Abbott M, Bhathal PS, St John DJB, Morstyn G. High-dose photoirradiation of esophageal cancer. *Ann Surg* 1987;206:193–199.
25. Spinelli P, Dal Fante M, Mancini A. Endoscopic palliation of malignancies of the upper gastrointestinal tract using Nd:YAG laser: results and survival in 308 treated patients. *Laser Surg Med* 1991;11:550–555.
26. Bown SG, Hawes R, Matthewson K, et al. Endoscopic laser palliation for advanced malignant dysphagia. *Gut* 1987;28: 799–807.
27. Heier SK, Rothman K, Heier LM, Rosenthal WS. Adenocarcinoma vs. squamous cell carcinoma of the esophagus: the response to palliative photodynamic therapy. *Gastrointest Endosc* 1992;38(2):279(abst).
28. Logan PM, Newton J, Richter A, Yip S, Levy JG. Immunological effects of photodynamic therapy. *SPIE* 1990;1203:153–158.

29. Evans S, Matthews W, Perry R, Fraker D, Norton J, Pass HI. Effect of photodynamic therapy on tumor necrosis factor production by murine macrophages. *J Natl Cancer Inst* 1990;82: 34–39.
30. Nseyo UO, Whalen RK, Duncan MR, Berman B, Lundahl S. Urinary cytokines following photodynamic therapy for bladder cancer. A preliminary report. *Urology* 1990;36:167–171.
31. McCaughan JS, Barabash R, Hawley P. Stage III endobronchial squamous cell cancer: survival after Nd:YAG laser combined with photodynamic therapy vs. Nd:YAG laser or photodynamic therapy alone. *SPIE* 1991;1426:279–286.
32. Bown SG. Laser-tissue interactions. In: Krasner N, ed. *Lasers in gastroenterology.* London: Chapman & Hall, 1991;37–50.
33. Horton R. Oseophageal cancer: laser palliation of malignant dysphagia. *Lancet* 1993;341:348.
34. Boyle DG, Potter WR. Photobleaching of Photofrin II as a means of eliminating skin photosensitivity. *Photochem Photobiol* 1987; 46:997–1001.
35. Tian M, Qui S, Qing J. Preliminary results of hematoporphyrin derivative-laser treatment for 13 cases of early esophageal carcinoma. In: Kessel D, ed. *Methods in porphyrin photosensitization.* New York: Plenum Press.
36. Fujimaki M, Nakayama K. Endoscopic laser treatment of superficial esophageal cancer. *Semin Surg Oncol* 1986;2:248–256.
37. Wagnieres G, Monnier P, Savary M, Cornaz P, Chatelain A, Bergh H. Photodynamic therapy of early cancer in the upper aerodigestive tract and bronchi: instrumentation and clinical results. *SPIE* 1990;IS6:249–271.
38. Tajiri H, Oguro Y. Laser endoscopic treatment for upper gastrointestinal cancers. *J Laparendosc Surg* 1991;1:71–78.
39. Lambert R, Sabben G, Souquet JC, Valette PJ, Bonvoisin S. Clinical experiences. In: Riemann JF, Ell C, eds. *Lasers in gastroenterology.* New York: Thieme, 1989;93–99.
40. Nava HR, Zera R, Douglass HO, Mang T, Cooper M, Dougherty T. Photodynamic therapy in carcinoma in situ in Barrett's esophagus. In: *Proceedings of the 3rd Biennial Meeting of the International Photodynamic Assoc,* 1990;32(abst).
41. Heier SK, Rothman K, Heier LM, Rosenthal WS. Complete responses of esophageal adenocarcinoma to photodynamic therapy. *Gastrointest Endosc* 1992;38(2):279(abst).
42. Overholt B, Panjehpour M, Teftellar E, Rose M. Photodynamic therapy for treatment of early adenocarcinoma in Barrett's esophagus. *Gastrointest Endosc* 1993;39:73–76.
43. Swain CP, Allardyce JT, Dean R, et al. Photodynamic therapy for malignant tumors of the ampulla of Vater. *Gastrointest Endosc* 1992;38:263(abst).
44. Barr H, Krasner N, Boulos PB, Chatlani P, Bown SG. Photodynamic therapy for colorectal cancer: a quantitative pilot study. *Br J Surg* 1990;77:93–96.
45. Richter AM, Kelly B, Chow J, et al. Preliminary studies on a more effective phototoxic agent than hematoporphyrin. *J Natl Cancer Inst* 1987;79:1327–1332.
46. Richter AM, Yip S, Waterfield E, Logan PM, Slonecker CM, Levy JG. Mouse skin photosensitization with benzoporphyrin derivatives and Photofrin: macroscopic and microscopic evaluation. *Photochem Photobiol* 1991;53:281–286.

Advanced Therapeutic Endoscopy, 2nd Ed.,
edited by J. S. Barkin and C. A. O'Phelan.
Raven Press, Ltd., New York © 1994.

CHAPTER 8

Pneumatic Dilatation in Treatment of Achalasia

Larry S. Miller and Donald O. Castell

Achalasia is a motility disorder of the esophagus that is characterized by the failure of the lower esophageal sphincter (LES) to relax and loss of esophageal peristalsis. Dilatation of the LES is a time honored and effective therapy.

In this chapter we discuss various types of dilators, techniques of dilatation, complications of dilatation and treatment of these complications, and ways of assessing the efficacy of dilatation including radiographic and manometric studies. We discuss comparison of surgery versus dilatation, comparison of various dilators, and comparison of various sizes of the same type of dilator, predictors of outcome, and factors that may affect the outcome of pneumatic dilatation including premedication, size of the dilator bag, graduated versus single-sized dilatation, dilatation pressure, duration of dilatation, and the effect of repeat dilatation.

TYPES OF MECHANICAL AND PNEUMATIC DILATORS

There are four types of dilators used to dilate the LES in achalasia: mechanical, hydrostatic, pneumatic, and endoscopic (Table 1). Mechanical dilators were developed in the 1920s for dilatation of the lower esophageal sphincter in achalasia. The principle on which the device works is expanding metal arms with the dilating diameter determined by manual force. Starck (1) reported on the uses of such dilators in 1924. The device was the first commercially available dilator. It was sup-

planted by the use of hydrostatic and pneumatic balloon dilatation. In general, the rigidity of the instrument made it difficult to pass through a sigmoid-shaped esophagus. A fascinating account of the use of the Starck dilator was reported by Schindler (2) in 1956 in which he successfully dilated 80 of 84 patients (95%) with achalasia. Four patients (5%) did not obtain symptomatic relief and five patients (6%) had complications. However, his fatality rate in this series was zero. All of these dilatations were done under fluoroscopic guidance. Schindler reports:

> The instrument is then carefully introduced into the stomach. The position of its dilating portion exactly at the point of narrowing is verified fluoroscopically. At this moment it is a good policy to excite the patient by telling him that he will feel an atrocious pain but that under no conditions must he move. Then, when the patient is as tense as possible, the instrument is opened forcefully, often against a marked resistance. In fact, the operator's hand often has the most disagreeable feeling of hard tissue being broken. If that happens, success can be predicted, although sometimes cures are obtained if this frightening sensation is not experienced.

Another type of dilator that has been replaced by modern pneumatic dilators is the hydrostatic dilator. Hydrostatic dilators consisted of single bags of fixed diameter that were distended with water under various degrees of pressure. Use of the Plummer hydrostatic dilator was reported in 1908. This instrument was usually passed over a previously swallowed string and positioned by a measurement of the distance from the incisors. The inflated diameter of the Plummer hydrostatic dilator was 3.6 cm. However, there was difficulty passing this dilator through a sigmoid-shaped esophagus (3). The use of the Negus dilator was reported in 1955 by Thomas et al. (4). This hydrostatic dilator was

L. S. Miller: Department of Medicine, Section of Gastroenterology, Temple University Hospital, Philadelphia, Pennsylvania 19140.

D. O. Castell: Department of Medicine, The Graduate School, Philadelphia, Pennsylvania 19146.

TABLE 1. *Studies evaluating the use of*

	Premedication	Dilator diameter	Pressure[a]	Duration
Mechanical				
Stark dilator				
Schindler (2)	–	Instrument opened by hand grip	–	Continued squeeze until resistance disappears
Hydrostatic				
Negus				
Lawrence and Shoesmith (34)	–	–	–	–
Plummer				
Olsen et al. (35)	–	–	9.5–10.3 psi (490–533 mm Hg)	Several seconds
Sanderson et al. (36)	–	–	9.5–10.3 psi (490–533 mm Hg)	Several seconds
Pneumatic				
Mosher				
Nanson (6)	Opium alkaloids (Pantopon), meperidine, scopolamine	3.6	15 psi (780 mm Hg)	15 sec
Heimlich et al. (7)	Scopolamine, meperidine	–	1.38 kg/cm (1,013 mm Hg)	5 min
Csendes et al. (8)	Atropine 0.5 mg	5.0	12–15 psi (620–790 mm Hg)	3–5 sec
Sippy				
Kurlander et al. (10)	–	2.38–4.78[b]	5.8 psi (300 mm Hg)	3 min
Van Goidsenhovern et al. (11)	–	3–5[c]	First at 200 mm Hg/1 min	Second at 300 mm Hg/1 min
Vantrappen et al. (12)	–	See Van Goidsenhoven	See Van Goidsenhoven	–
Hurst-Tucker				
Bennett and Hendrix (13)	Atropine, opiate	3.0	9–15 psi (465–533 mm Hg)	30–60 sec
Wong and Maydonovitch (14)	Meperidine	3.0[d]	9–15 psi (460–780 mm Hg)	60 sec
Brown-McHardy				
Stark et al. (17)	–	3.5	>9 psi (>465 mm Hg)	60 sec
Lishman and Dellipiani (15)	Omnopon, chlorpromazine, atropine	–	15 psi (780 mm Hg)	15 sec
Dellipiani and Hewetson (16)	Diazepam	3.0	15 psi (780 mm Hg)	15–20 sec
Rider-Moeller				
Fellows et al. (19)	General anesthesia	–	5.4–5.8 psi (280–300 mm Hg)	3 min
Jacobs et al. (37)	Diazepam	–	12–15 psi (620–780 mm Hg)	–
Adams et al. (20)	Diazepam	–	5.8 psi (300 mm Hg)	3 min
Rigiflex				
Witzel (27)	Light sedation	4.0	5.8 psi (300 mm Hg)	2 min
Endoscopic balloon dilatation				
Cox et al. (21)	Diazepam	3.0	2–15 psi (105–780 mm Hg)	60 sec
Levine et al. (22)	–	3.0	15 psi (780 mm Hg)	60 sec
Gelfond and Kozarek (23)	None	3.0 3.5	5–12 psi (X = 7.16 psi) (258–620 mm Hg)	30 sec
Stark et al. (17)	–	3.5	>9 psi (>465 mm Hg)	60 sec

X = mean of population.

[a] 1 psi = 51.7 mm Hg; 1 kg/cm = 14.2 psi.

[b] Diameter increased by 0.4 cm.

[c] Diameter increased by 3.5, 3.8, 4.0, 4.3, and 4.5 cm.

[d] If poor clinical response at 1 month or greater, the next dilator size was employed (3.3, 3.7, 4.1 cm). No more than one dilation per hospitalization.

[e] One dilatation.

various dilators used to treat achalasia

No. of dilatations during hospitalization	No. of patients	Response (%)			No. of perforations	Surgery for complications
		Excellent	Fair	Poor		
–	84	95	–	5	5	2
–	100	59	–	41	1	1
X = 1.67	452: 332 (73%),[e] 94 (21%),[f] 26 (6%)[g]	61,[e] 39,[f] 19[g]	–	39,[e] 61,[g] 81[g]	10[e]	2[e]
–	408	81	–	19	14	10
3 times in 1 session	13	84	–	15	–	–
–	25	84	–	16	–	–
2	18: 12 (67%),[e] 3 (17%),[f] 3 (17%),[j] 1 (7%)[k]	60		40	0	0
Several	62	32	56	8	10	–
2–4	57	98	–	2	1	–
3.16–3.26	133	77	17	6	3	1
1–2 total, not more than 2 per session	48	70	11	19	3	1
1	30: 12 (40%),[e] 8 (27%),[f] 3 (10%),[g] 2 (7%),[h] 5 (17)[j]	.... 83		17	0	0
1	10 (3.5 cm)	100			0	0
2	18: 2 (11%)[k]	55.5	33.3	11.2	0	0
1	45: 38 (84%),[e] 2 (4%),[f] 2 (4%),[g] 4 (9%)[k]	53	31	16	4	1
1	63: 37 (59%),[e] 9 (14%),[f] 5 (7.9%),[g] 5 (7.9%),[h] 2 (3.2%),[i] 5 (7.9%)[j]	.... 61		39	–	1 (1.6%)
1	30: 25 (83%),[e] 5 (17%),[f] 2 (7%)[j]	.... 83		17	1	0
1	44: 32 (73%),[e] 10 (23%),[f] 2 (5%)[g]	.... 70		30	0	0
Several prior to 2 minute dilation	39: 9 (23%),[f] 30 (77%)[g]	.... 90		10	0	0
1	8: 7 (87.5%),[e] 1 (12.5%)[f]	.... 88		13	0	0
3–5	17	.... 100			2(?)	
1	10 (3.0 cm): 7 (70%),[e] 2 (20%)[f]	.... 93		7		
	14 (3.5 cm): 13 (93%),[e] 1 (7%)[e,j]					
1	10 polyurethane (3.5 cm)	70		30	0	

[f] Two dilations.
[g] Three dilations.
[h] Four dilations.
[i] More than four dilations.
[j] Failed; underwent myotomy.
[k] Developed gastroesophageal reflux.

positioned through a large endoscope under direct visual placement. It was usually used under general anesthesia.

Currently, the most commonly used dilators are pneumatic dilators of various sizes, shapes, and materials. However, the concept of their use is basically the same. These are bag dilators that distend under various degrees of pressure with air. The various maximum diameters of distention are fixed so that the balloon is not overdistended leading to perforation of the esophagus. Use of the Mosher dilator was reported in 1923 (5). The dilating apparatus consisted of a cylindrical bag with six stripes of radiopaque material set into the wall of the bag. Nanson (6) used the Mosher dilator under opium alkaloids, meperidine, and scopolamine premedication. The dilator diameter was 3.6 and the pressure 15 psi. Time duration was 15 seconds with three dilatations during the session. In 1978, Heimlich et al. (7) reported on the use of the Mosher dilator under scopolamine and meperidine presedation with a pressure of 1.38 kg/cm or 1,013 mm Hg. They sustained the dilatation for a duration of 5 minutes. Twenty-five patients were treated in this manner with 84% excellent results. There was minimal morbidity and no mortality. Csendes et al. (8) reported the use of the Mosher dilator in 1981. This was used under premedication of atropine 0.5 mg with a dilator diameter of 5 cm under 12 to 15 psi (620 to 780 mm Hg). The duration of balloon inflation was 3 to 5 seconds and there were two dilations during the hospitalization. Eighteen patients were dilated using this technique. These investigators obtained good or excellent results in 60% of the patients and failure in 40%. In a follow-up study Csendes et al. (9) evaluated 39 patients using a Mosher dilator. Patients were premedicated with 0.5 mg of atropine and light pharyngeal anesthesia. The Mosher bag was rapidly inflated to 5.4 lb/inch² for 10 to 20 seconds and this procedure was repeated twice. Maximum diameter of the Mosher bag at the gastroesophageal junction when completely inflated was 4 cm. It was not possible for the bag to remain inflated for more than 20 seconds each time, because all patients experienced intense pain and discomfort. Two patients (5.17%) experienced perforation of the abdominal esophagus. There were good results in only 64% of the patients (follow-up median 58 months).

The Sippy dilator consists of a series of bags from 3 to 5 cm in diameter that can be placed sequentially on a metal bougie. The bags are hourglass-shaped. The bougie can be passed over a guidewire. Kurlander et al. (10) reported on the use of the Sippy pneumatic dilator in 1963. In this report the dilator diameter was 2.38 to 4.78 cm with the pressure of 5.8 psi (300 mm Hg). Duration of dilatation was 3 minutes and several dilatations were done during the hospitalization. The procedures were done under fluoroscopic positioning.

Pneumatic dilatation was attempted in 92 patients. Of these 92, results in 62 were available for analysis and 39 were observed for more than 10 years. Fifty-two of the 62 patients (84%) received satisfactory benefit from the pneumatic dilatation. Twenty-two patients received ten or more dilatations. Van Goidsenhoven et al. (11) reported their experience with the Sippy dilator in 1963. The dilator diameter was 3 to 5 cm and was increased by 3.5, 3.8, 4.0, 4.2, and 4.5 cm. The initial pressure used was 200 mm Hg for 1 minute. The second and subsequent dilatations were done at a pressure of 300 mm Hg for 1 minute and two to four dilatations were done during the hospitalization. Fifty-seven patients were evaluated. Excellent results were obtained after one (95% of the cases) or two (4% of the cases) series of pneumatic dilatations. There was no mortality. However, one patient sustained an accidental perforation of the esophagus and recovered without surgery. Vantrappen et al. (12) evaluated 264 selected patients with achalasia over a period of 13 years who were dilated with a Sippy dilator. His report gave the late results in 133 patients who had been treated more than 3 years prior to the report. The late results were classified as excellent in 45%, good in 32%, moderate in 17%, and poor in 6%. The best results were obtained in patients with a history of achalasia for 5 to 20 years and a moderately dilated esophagus. By the end of the treatment all patients were able to eat without distress and regurgitation had disappeared completely. Mortality rate was zero. A septic pleural effusion occurred in three patients and a pericardial effusion in one with prompt recovery of all patients. Hemorrhage was seen in two patients and a febrile reaction without any demonstrable lesion in four patients. The procedure was carried out in the same manner as that described by Van Goidsenhoven et al. with the number of dilatations per hospitalization being approximately three.

The Hurst-Tucker and Brown-McHardy pneumatic dilators are virtually identical dilators with cylindrical radiopaque balloons. These dilators consist of a mercury-filled rubber tube surrounded by the radiopaque dilator balloon. These dilators are heavy and semi-pliable and were used without the assistance of a guidewire. Thus, they were often difficult to pass through a sigmoid-shaped esophagus. Bennett and Hendrix (13) published their experience with the use of the Hurst-Tucker dilator in achalasia in 1970. They used atropine and opiate premedication, a dilator diameter of 3 cm, 9 to 15 psi (465 to 533 mm Hg), a duration of 30 to 60 seconds, and one to two dilatations per hospitalization with not more than two dilatations per session. Sixty-one dilatations were studied in 51 patients. Successful dilatation with good immediate results were achieved in 54 of the procedures (88.5%). The dilator failed to enter the cardia in three procedures (4.9%). There was failure to erase constriction in one procedure (1.6%)

and perforation of the esophagus in three procedures (4.9%). Wong and Maydonovitch (14) reported on the use of the Hurst-Tucker dilator in 1989. They used meperidine as premedication with a dilator diameter of 3 cm. The dilator was increased by 0.4 cm increments. Pressure used was 9 to 15 psi (460 to 780 mm Hg) and the duration of dilatation was 60 seconds with only one dilatation per hospitalization. Thirty untreated achalasia patients were evaluated. All patients initially received a 2.7-cm dilator and subsequently larger dilators (3.3, 3.7, 4.1 cm) spaced at least 1 month apart depending on success. Sixty-seven percent of patients were successfully dilated by the second dilatation (3.3 cm) and 87% by the fourth dilatation (4.1 cm). Thirteen percent of the patients in this series ultimately required surgical myotomy.

Lishman and Dellipiani (15) also utilized a modified Brown-McHardy dilator system. The patients were premedicated with chlorpromazine and atropine. Balloon pressure was 15 psi (780 mm Hg) and the duration of balloon dilatation was 15 seconds. There were two dilatations per hospitalization. Eighteen patients were subjected to pneumatic dilatation with a satisfactory result obtained in 16 patients (89%). Ten patients remained asymptomatic, while six patients had mild symptoms on follow-up of a period up to 10 years. Dellipiani and Hewetson (16) used a modified Brown-McHardy hourglass balloon dilatation system in their 1986 report analyzing balloon dilatation in 45 patients. Premedication was given with diazepam and the dilator diameter was 3 cm with a psi of 15 cm (780 mm Hg). The duration of balloon dilatation was 15 to 20 seconds and one dilatation was given during the hospitalization. Eighty-seven percent of the 45 patients had either no symptoms or only minor symptoms following the procedure. Perforation occurred in four patients (8.9%) and one of these patients required surgical intervention. All of the others were managed conservatively. Four patients (8.9%) developed reflux. One patient died of myocardial infarction. Eighty-four percent of the patients needed one dilatation only and no patients required cardiomyotomy. The modified Brown-McHardy esophageal dilator consisted of a mercury-filled bougie with a radiopaque hourglass balloon at the distal end that was inserted under fluoroscopic control until the waist of the balloon was seen at the gastroesophageal junction.

Stark et al. (17) reported their experiences with the Brown-McHardy dilator in 1990. The dilator diameter was 3.5 cm with >9 psi of pressure (>465 mm Hg), duration of dilatation was 60 seconds, and one dilatation was used during the hospitalization. The success rate at 1 month follow-up was 100% (ten of ten patients) and there were no complications. Parkman et al. (18) retrospectively analyzed the results of 123 patients undergoing an initial pneumatic dilatation for achalasia

from 1976 to 1986. These patients underwent pneumatic dilatation with the Brown-McHardy dilator. Each patient received Cetacaine spray applied to the pharynx and were medicated with either diazepam or midazolam. In addition, many patients received meperidine and Vistaril. Dilatation was performed by several different gastroenterologists with an inflation pressure in the range of 7.5 to 17 psi (median = 9.5), and inflation duration ranging from 10 to 75 seconds (median = 30 seconds), using one to three inflations (median of one). Of the 123 patients undergoing an initial pneumatic dilatation for achalasia, 71 (58%) have not needed a subsequent procedure, whereas 52 (42%) have undergone subsequent treatment with pneumatic dilatation and/or esophagomyotomy. Of the 47 patients undergoing a second pneumatic dilatation, follow-up information was available in 45 patients over 3.6 ± 2.5 years. Of these 45 patients, 26 (58%) required subsequent treatments, in contrast to the 42% needing additional treatments after the initial dilatation. There were 24 patients undergoing a third pneumatic dilatation (0.7 ± 0.6 years after the second dilatation), with follow-up information available in 22 patients over 3.5 ± 2.2 years. Sixteen of the 22 patients (73%) have required subsequent treatments. Only 15 of the 123 patients (12%) eventually underwent surgical esophagomyotomy (2 for perforation during pneumatic dilatation, 13 for persistent or recurrent symptoms).

The Rider-Moeller balloon dilator is an hourglass-shaped bag of variable size. The bag is not radiopaque and the dilator is passed over a guidewire. Fellows et al. (19) reported on the use of the Rider-Moeller balloon dilatation system in 1983. General anesthesia was used instead of conscious sedation. The pressure given was 5.4 to 5.8 psi (280 to 300 mm Hg) and the duration of balloon dilatation was 3 minutes with one dilatation given during the hospitalization. Sixty-three patients underwent a total of 107 Rider-Moeller dilatations. There was a marked improvement in swallowing immediately after dilatation in all but two patients. There were no deaths attributable to the procedure and only 1.6% of the patients had serious complications. In the patients who were followed long-term (9 to 73 months), 59% did not require further dilatation. Thirty-eight percent required between one and three further dilatations and 5% required four or more dilatations. It was found that there was a significantly greater continuing need for further dilatation in those patients aged 45 years or older. Cardiomyotomy was necessary in five patients (8%) because of poor response to pneumatic dilatation. Adams et al. (20) reported on their use of the Rider-Moeller dilatation system in 1989. Premedication was given with diazepam. The maximum pressure was 5.8 psi (300 mm Hg) with a duration of 3 minutes and one dilatation per hospitalization. Forty-four patients were evaluated. Balloon dilatation was performed once in

32 patients, twice in 10 patients, and three times in 2 patients during the course of the study. Complications included seven esophageal tears and two complete esophageal ruptures. Patients developed classical features of perforation including abdominal pain, tenderness, and pyrexia. All patients were successfully managed conservatively with no patient requiring surgery.

The Rigiflex dilator is of similar design to the Grunsick angioplasty catheter. The cylindrical balloon is made of nonradiopaque polyethylene and mounted on a flexible bougie. The dilator can be passed over a guidewire. The balloon is inelastic so that when inflated it maintains its size and shape despite high inflation pressures. Increasing the pressure when the balloon is fully inflated makes the balloon harder and not larger, and therefore a net placed over the balloon is not necessary to control the balloon diameter. Should the balloon rupture, the design ensures that it does so through a safe longitudinal tear rather than a damaging transverse blowout. The burst pressure is 20 psi or 1,050 mm Hg. The 10 cm long balloon comes in three sizes and inflates to a maximum diameter of 30, 35, and 40 mm (90 French). The catheter on which the balloon is mounted has a soft tapered radiopaque tip. Radiopaque tantalum markers identify the proximal and distal end of the balloon to help in positioning of the uninflated balloon during fluoroscopy. The balloon can be inflated with air or with contrast media. Cox et al. (21) reported their use of the Rigiflex polyurethane balloon dilator in 1986. In their series they used diazepam as premedication with balloon inflation diameter of 3 cm. The balloon was dilated at 105 to 708 mm Hg for 60 seconds, with one dilatation per hospitalization. Seven patients were dilated using this procedure. All patients reported improved symptoms at 4 weeks without dysphagia or heartburn. Six of the seven patients remained well, while one patient had recurrence of symptoms at 8 months and was referred to surgery.

Since this initial report a number of other investigators have reported on the use of the polyurethane balloon dilators. Levine et al. (22) published on the use of a polyurethane dilator with a diameter of 3 cm using 15 psi (780 mm Hg) for a length of 60 seconds and three to five dilatations during the hospitalization. These dilators were positioned endoscopically and not fluoroscopically. All patients showed prompt relief of symptoms with the use of this polyurethane dilator. One patient developed pain for 6 hours after the dilatation. A second patient had fever and discomfort for 24 hours after dilatation and then made an uneventful recovery.

Gelfond and Kozarek (23) reported on the use of Rigiflex polyurethane achalasia dilators in 1988. The dilatation was done without any premedication. The dilator diameter was 3 cm to 3.5 cm with 5 to 12 psi (256 to 620 mm Hg pressure). The duration of dilatation was 30 seconds with one dilatation per hospitalization.

Twenty-four consecutive patients were treated with 70% satisfactory result using a 30-mm balloon. A 35-mm balloon was used with a 94% satisfactory result including two patients who did not achieve a good response with the smaller balloon. No complications of the procedure occurred.

Stark et al. (17) utilized the 3.5-cm polyurethane Rigiflex-type dilator in their study reported in 1990. All studies were performed under fluoroscopic guidance. The dilator was passed until the balloon straddled the area of the gastroesophageal junction and rapid inflation was performed to a maximum diameter with sufficient pressure (>9 psi) until the waist was obliterated. Ten patients were evaluated using this system. Seven of the ten patients (70%) had satisfactory results. There were no complications of the procedure.

Kadakia and Wong (24) utilized the polyethylene balloon Rigiflex dilators in a total of 47 dilatations in 29 consecutive patients with achalasia. Using a standard technique of balloon inflation to the point of waist obliteration and maintenance of balloon inflation for 1 minute, a 3-cm balloon was used. If there was no symptomatic response, a 3.5-cm balloon was used after 4 to 8 weeks. If there was still no symptomatic response, a 4-cm dilator was again used after 4 to 8 weeks. In this manner 18 (62%) of the patients were successfully dilated with a 3-cm balloon only. Of 11 patients not responding to a 3-cm balloon, 5 were dilated successfully with a 3.5-cm balloon. Of 6 patients not responding to a 3.5-cm balloon, 4 were successfully dilated with a 4.0-cm balloon dilator. Two patients eventually required surgery. The overall success with Rigiflex balloon dilators was achieved in 27 of 29 (93%) patients. In these cases the Rigiflex balloon dilator was passed over a guidewire that was placed endoscopically and positioned fluoroscopically so that half the dilator was above the diaphragmatic hiatus and half below the diaphragmatic hiatus.

Barkin et al. (25) evaluated the efficacy of the Microvasive Rigiflex balloon dilator in 50 patients at two centers. The diameters of the three balloon dilators used were 30, 35, and 40 mm. Local anesthesia of the oral pharynx with Cetacaine was used in both centers. Sedation was induced with an intravenously administered combination of diazepam and meperidine at one center, while few of the patients were sedated at the other center and then only diazepam was used. To obliterate the waist of the balloon dilator, the balloon was inflated to pressures ranging from 15 to 20 psi for a mean time of 67.8 seconds at center A, whereas at center B all balloons were inflated to 15 psi for 15 seconds. Sixty-one procedures were performed on 50 patients at the two centers and an overall treatment success rate of 94% (47 of 50 patients) was achieved. Two patients had elective surgical treatment and a third underwent surgery for perforation secondary to dilatation. A total of three patients complained of postprocedure chest pain within 4 hours and were hospitalized. Two had perforations; one required surgical repair. One hundred percent of patients available for long-term follow-up had relief of symptoms.

A new method of esophageal dilatation described by Tytgat and Derltartogjager (26) and Witzel (27) also uses pneumatic dilatation. However, the dilator is mounted on a forward viewing endoscope making it possible to position the dilator under direct visual guidance. The Witzel dilator is made of a nonradiopaque polyethylene material and is used after light sedation. The dilator diameter is 4 cm and is inflated with 5.8 psi (300 mm Hg). The duration of dilatation is 2 minutes, with several dilatations prior to the final 2-minute dilatation.

TECHNIQUES OF DILATATION

The esophageal dilatation technique described below is the one performed by the authors at Thomas Jeffer-

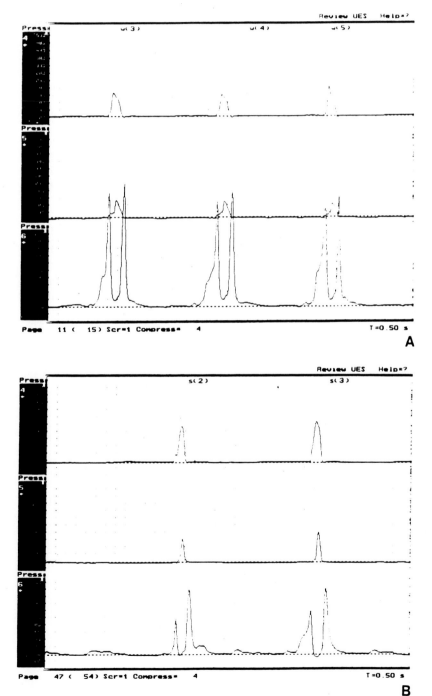

FIG. 1. A: Pressure changes during three swallows in a patient with achalasia. The bottom tracing records the output of the sphincter transducer. The top two tracings record the output of transducers located in the pharynx, 3 and 6 cm above the sphincter transducer. Here the nadir of the upper esophageal sphincter (UES) relaxation is above the baseline, representing a positive UES residual pressure. **B:** Pressure changes during two swallows in a healthy volunteer, with transducers located as in A. Note the nadir of the UES relaxation below the baseline; this represents a negative UES residual pressure. Time is along the *x* axis and pressure along the *y* axis.

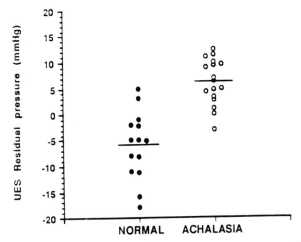

FIG. 2. Distribution of the UES residual pressures in achalasia patients and controls.

son University Hospital and Graduate Hospital in Philadelphia, Pennsylvania, using the Rigiflex achalasia dilator system (Figs. 1 and 2). The patient is given a liquid diet for 3 days and is fasted overnight and taken to the fluoroscopy suite where the entire procedure is performed. If required, an Ewald tube is used to empty and irrigate the esophagus. Premedication is given with a local anesthetic spray to the mouth and throat; 50 to 75 mg of IV Demerol and 2 to 10 mg of IV diazepam is given as necessary to produce mild sedation and subsequent anesthesia. The patient is placed in the left lateral decubitus position for fluoroscopic monitoring. The esophagogastric junction is carefully evaluated endoscopically to exclude any evidence of malignancy. A guidewire is placed through the biopsy channel of the endoscope after the endoscope is positioned in the antrum of the stomach. The guidewire is then left in the antrum of the stomach and the endoscope withdrawn as the guidewire is placed forward. The Rigiflex balloon dilator is placed over the guidewire until the balloon has straddled the area of the gastroesophageal junction. The balloon is slowly inflated to its maximum diameter with sufficient pressure >9 psi until the waist has been obliterated. The balloon is then left inflated for 1 minute. After deflation the Rigiflex dilator is removed and a nasogastric tube is inserted into the midesophagus. With the patient sitting a water-soluble contrast material (60 ml) is injected through the nasogastric tube to evaluate the esophagus for possible perforation. If there is no obvious perforation seen, this material is aspirated and the examination is repeated with 60 ml of barium sulfate suspension. Films of the esophagogastric junction are obtained and compared with predilatation esophagrams. This examination is to identify complications and not to assess the adequacy of dilatation or predict the clinical response of the patient.

If recovery proceeds normally, the patient is allowed to drink 4 to 6 hours after the procedure. The patient remains in the hospital overnight and receives a normal breakfast in the morning, or can be totally managed in an outpatient short procedure unit and released later on the day of the procedure. If a small confined perforation is seen then the patient is usually treated conservatively (see Treatment of Esophageal Perforation, below).

COMPARISON OF VARIOUS DILATORS

As discussed above, there have been many reports of successful treatment of patients with achalasia using different kinds of balloon dilators and numerous types of dilators that have been available in the past. There have been, however, no direct prospective comparisons of various types of dilators except for one study evaluating the Brown-McHardy dilator against the Microvasive Rigiflex polyurethane dilator by Stark et al. (17). The questions asked in this study were: Should the new polyurethane dilator replace the old, more established dilator? Is the new polyurethane dilator as effective and safe as existing technology or even superior to existing technology? In this study 20 achalasia patients were randomly assigned to be treated with either the older Brown-McHardy dilator or the new Microvasive Rigiflex dilator. Overall success occurred with 10 of 10 patients who underwent dilatation with a Brown-McHardy dilator and only 7 of 10 patients who underwent dilatation with the Microvasive Rigiflex dilator. One patient not improved with the Rigiflex dilator underwent myotomy. The other two patients who were not successfully treated with the Microvasive Rigiflex dilator were successfully treated with the Brown-McHardy dilator. No complications occurred with either type of dilator. In this study both types of balloon dilator had a diameter of 3.5 cm and pressure used was >9 psi (>465 mm Hg). The duration of dilatation was 60 seconds with one dilatation during the hospitalization. The investigators felt that the Microvasive Rigiflex dilator was effective and their results were similar to those reported by Gelfond and Kozarek (23) in that 70% of both groups were successfully dilated. The Microvasive Rigiflex dilator also appeared to be safe in that there were no complications. This was also shown by Gelfond and Kozarek, who had 24 consecutive patients dilated without complications. Ten of these dilatations were done with a 30 mm diameter dilator balloon and 14 dilatations with a 35-mm balloon. However, the Microvasive Rigiflex dilator did not appear as good as the Brown-McHardy dilator since only 70% of the dilatations were successful with the Microvasive Rigiflex dilator compared with 100% of the Brown-McHardy dilatations.

COMPARISON OF SURGERY VERSUS DILATATION

There is only one prospective randomized study comparing forceful dilatation using the Mosher dilator with esophagomyotomy in patients with achalasia of the esophagus (8). In this study 18 patients dilated with the Mosher dilator were compared to 20 operated patients. All of these patients were studied before and after treatment except for one patient who was lost to follow-up. Clinical, radiologic, and manometric evaluations were performed before and after the treatment and an acid reflux test was performed in the late follow-up period. Immediately after treatment a significant improvement was seen clinically, by radiologic studies and manometric evaluation. However, in the late follow-up period all the operated patients showed a permanent improvement but dilated patients remained asymptomatic in only 50% of the cases. The rest of these patients had to be redilated or reoperated due to failure of primary dilatation, leading to final good or excellent results in 60% and failure in 40% of patients. In summary, this study showed that significantly better long-term results were obtained using surgical esophagomyotomy rather than after forceful dilatation using a Mosher dilator. However, the work of Csendes et al. (8) has been subjected to criticism because of the technique used in dilatation, in that partial or absent improvement in the dilatation group may have been related to technical difficulties. In this study maximal dilatations with the Mosher bag lasted only 2 to 5 seconds. This was because of severe pain experienced by the patients. Patients refused subsequent dilatations because of the pain intensity. Most other studies were done with the Mosher bag dilated for a period of 15 seconds to 3 minutes. The other complicating factor in this study is that atropine was used as a premedication, which might have relaxed the sphincter and rendered stretching less effective.

In a follow-up study Csendes et al. (9) evaluated the late results in 81 patients with achalasia treated in a prospective randomized study comparing forceful pneumatic dilatation with the Mosher bag and surgical anterior esophagomyotomy. Two patients (2.5%) had a perforation of the abdominal esophagus after pneumatic dilatation and were excluded from late follow-up. One patient in both the surgical group and the pneumatic dilatation group was lost to follow-up and one patient in both the surgical group and pneumatic dilatation group died of esophageal carcinoma. The results of this study showed that 95% of the patients in the surgical group had excellent results at late follow-up (a median of 62 months), while only 65% of the patients in the pneumatic dilatation group had good results (with follow-up of a median of 58 months). There were

30% failures in the pneumatic dilatation group. The authors found that measurement of the resting gastroesophageal sphincter pressure after dilatation was highly predictive of outcome and felt that surgical treatment offered a better final clinical result than pneumatic dilatation with the Mosher bag.

Two large studies that are not related but have been compared because of the number of patients and the duration of follow-up morbidity and mortality and late complications are a surgical report from the Mayo Clinic (28,29) and the Belgian Progressive Dilatation study (30,31). Early morbidity (1% vs. 2.6%) and mortality (0.2% vs. 0.2%) were similar. However, the number of successful procedures was higher in the myotomy series (85% vs. 77%).

Parkman et al. (18) undertook a retrospective study to determine the long-term clinical outcome and cost of treating achalasia initially with pneumatic dilatation as compared to esophagomyotomy; 123 patients underwent an initial pneumatic dilatation for achalasia with the Brown-McHardy dilator. Of the 123 initial patients 71 (58%) required no further treatment for achalasia during a mean follow-up of 4.7 ± 2.8 years. Fifty-two (42%) patients underwent subsequent treatment with pneumatic dilatation and/or esophagomyotomy. Two patients (1.6% of patients, 1.0% of dilatations) had an esophageal perforation during pneumatic dilatation and underwent emergent surgery for esophageal repair with Heller esophagomyotomy and partial fundoplication. An additional 13 patients (11%) underwent elective esophagomyotomy for persistent or recurrent symptoms. Thus, 15 patients (12%) initially treated with pneumatic dilatation ultimately underwent esophagomyotomy. Of the 47 patients undergoing a second pneumatic dilatation, follow-up information was available for 45. Of these 45 patients 26 (58%) required subsequent treatment, in contrast to the 42% needing additional treatments after the initial dilatation. There were 24 patients undergoing a third pneumatic dilatation with follow-up information available in 22 patients. Sixteen of the 22 patients (73%) required subsequent treatments.

During the same period of time, 26 patients underwent Heller esophagomyotomy for achalasia. However, this was the initial treatment for only six patients. The authors concluded that subsequent pneumatic dilatations to treat persistent or recurrent symptoms were less beneficial then an initial pneumatic dilatation. The cost of esophagomyotomy was five times greater than the cost of pneumatic dilatation. When costs were analyzed to include subsequent treatments of symptomatic patients, the total expectant cost of treating with an initial esophagomyotomy remained 2.4 times greater than treating with an initial pneumatic dilatation. This study suggests that an initial pneumatic dilatation will be the only treatment needed for the majority of patients with achalasia. A treatment regimen starting with pneumatic dilatation has less overall cost than starting with esophagomyotomy. For each subsequent pneumatic dilatation, however, the clinical benefits lean toward surgery.

COMPARISONS OF BALLOON SIZE

It is difficult to directly compare patient outcome as a variable dependent on balloon diameter since various studies use different techniques for dilatation. However, in a study by Gelfond and Kozarek (23) two sizes of Rigiflex dilators (30 mm and 35 mm) were used utilizing the same technique of dilatation. Dilation pressure, which averaged only 7 psi, was determined by insufflating 1 to 2 psi more than needed for complete gastroesophageal waist expansion at fluoroscopy. The 30-mm balloon was used in ten patients. Seven (70%) had a satisfactory result. Two patients elected to have a repeat dilation, one performed 8 and the other 9 months after the first dilatation, with the 35-mm balloon producing an excellent response in both. The 35-mm balloon was used initially in 14 patients and yielded satisfactory results in 13. One continued to be symptomatic, but rather than return for follow-up testing and consideration of dilation with a 40-mm balloon, underwent a Heller myotomy. The satisfactory response rate to dilation with the 35-mm balloon was 94% (15 of 16 patients) (21).

USE OF MERCURY BOUGIENAGE FOLLOWED BY PNEUMATIC DILATATION

In 1991, McJunkin et al. (32) evaluated the treatment of 33 achalasia patients with dilatation therapy using either large diameter mercury bougienage or pneumatic balloon dilatation. Maloney bougies (range 52 to 60 F, mean 56 F) were used. Patients received 0.4 mg of atropine intramuscularly, oral Cetacaine, and intravenous diazepam. Twenty of the 33 patients underwent large diameter bougienage as initial therapy. Bougienage was successful in 10 patients (50%) with 8 excellent and 2 good outcomes over a mean period of 34 months (range 6 to 117). One patient required two dilatations to achieve response. Three of the 10 successful bougie dilatation patients required repeat dilatation. Twenty-three patients underwent pneumatic dilatation, 10 of whom had failed bougienage. Pneumatic dilatation was successful in 19 patients (83%) using a Mosher dilator or Rigiflex achalasia balloon (30- or 35-mm balloon), with 15 excellent and 4 good outcomes over a mean follow-up period of 37 months (range 6 to 113). More than one dilatation was required in two patients to acquire an adequate response. Six of the 19

patients (32%) eventually developed recurrent symptoms requiring repeat dilatation. There was a total of 31 pneumatic dilatations with a 3.2% complication rate (1 perforation requiring surgery). Three other pneumatic dilatation failures, all relating to persistent symptoms, required surgical myotomy. The combined efficacy of both forms of dilatation was 88% with a complication rate of 1.4%. The authors felt that these data indicate that mercury bougienage should be considered initial therapy for achalasia in view of its simplicity, safety, and acceptable efficacy, followed by pneumatic dilatation if bougienage is unsuccessful.

ENDOSCOPIC MYOTOMY

Endoscopic myotomy has been reported in which an anteriorly placed incision was made above the Z-line with a sheathed wire. Eighty-eight percent of patients treated had good to excellent relief of dysphagia (33). However, this technique is still considered investigational and should be used only in clinical trials.

EFFICACY OF DILATATION

Mechanical Dilators

In 1956 Schindler (2) published a series of 84 patients with achalasia who he dilated with the Stark mechanical dilator with expanding arms. He found that 95% of these patients had an excellent response.

Hydrostatic Dilators

In 1959, Lawrence and Shoesmith (34) evaluated the response of 100 patients with achalasia to the Negus hydrostatic dilator. They found that 59% of the patients had an excellent response. In 1951 Olsen et al. (35) evaluated 452 patients with achalasia using the Plummer hydrostatic dilator. Of these patients, 332 (73%) underwent one dilatation, 94 patients (21%) underwent two dilatations, and 26 patients (6%) underwent three dilatations. Of the patients undergoing one dilatation, 61% had an excellent response. Of the patients undergoing two dilatations, 39% had an excellent response. Of the patients undergoing three dilatations, 19% had an excellent response. Sanderson et al. (36) also reported their experience in 1970 with hydrostatic dilatation using Plummer dilatation in 408 patients with achalasia. Of these patients, 81% had an excellent response.

Pneumatic Dilators

Mosher

In 1962, Nanson (6) published his series dilating 13 achalasia patients with the Mosher pneumatic dilator.

Eighty-five percent of these patients had an excellent response. Heimlich et al. (7) also published on the series of achalasia patients dilated with the Mosher dilator in 1978. In the evaluation of 25 patients, 84% had an excellent response. Csendes et al. (8) evaluated 18 achalasia patients using the Mosher pneumatic dilator at the lower esophageal sphincter. In this report published in 1981, 12 patients (67%) underwent one dilatation, 3 patients (17%) underwent two dilatations, and 3 patients (17%) failed dilatation and underwent myotomy. Of the patients undergoing dilatation, 66% had an excellent response. In a follow-up study Csendes et al. (9) evaluated 39 patients using a Mosher dilator. There were good results in 65% of patients (follow-up median 58 months).

Sippy

Using the Sippy dilator, Kurlander et al. (10) published on a series of 62 achalasia patients in 1963. Of the 62 patients, 32% had an excellent response to dilatation, 56% had a fair response, and 8% had a poor response. Van Goidsenhoven et al. (11) also published on a series of 57 pateints in 1963 using the Sippy pneumatic dilator. Of the 57 patients undergoing dilatation, 98% had an excellent response. In 1971, Vantrappen et al. (12) published on a series of 133 patients using the Sippy dilator. Of these patients undergoing dilatation, 77% had an excellent response, 17% a fair response, and 6% a poor response.

Hurst-Tucker Dilator

In 1970, Bennett and Hendrix (13) reported on the use of the Hurst-Tucker dilator in 48 achalasia patients. Of the 48 patients undergoing dilatation, 70% had an excellent response, 11% a fair response, and 19% a poor response. In 1989, Wong and Maydonovitch (14) evaluated 30 patients undergoing dilatation with the Hurst-Tucker dilator. Of these patients 12 (40%) underwent one dilatation, 8 (27%) underwent two dilatations, 3 (10%) underwent three dilatations, and 2 (7%) underwent four dilatations. Five (17%) failed dilatation and underwent myotomy. Of the patients undergoing dilatation, 83% had an excellent or fair response.

Rider-Moeller Dilator

In 1983, Fellows (19) evaluated 63 patients using the Rider-Moeller pneumatic dilator. Of these 63 patients, 37 (59%) underwent one dilatation, 9 (14%) underwent two dilatations, 5 (8%) underwent three dilatations, 5 (8%) underwent four dilatations, 2 (3%) underwent more than four dilatations, and 5 (8%) failed dilatation

and underwent myotomy. Of the patients undergoing dilatation, 61% had an excellent to fair response. Jacobs et al. (37) also evaluated patients undergoing dilatation with the modified Rider-Moeller dilator in 1983. Thirty patients underwent dilatation. Of these 30 patients, 25 (83%) underwent one dilatation, 5 (17%) underwent two dilatations, and 2 (7%) failed dilatation and underwent myotomy. Of the patients undergoing dilatation, 83% had an excellent to fair response. Adams et al. (20) in 1989 evaluated 44 patients undergoing dilatation with the Rider-Moeller dilator. Of these patients, 32 (73%) underwent one dilatation, 10 (23%) underwent two dilatations, and 2 (5%) underwent three dilatations. This paper did not evaluate the efficacy of dilatation but was centered more on complications and radiographic diagnosis of the complications in patients undergoing dilatation with the Rider-Moeller dilator.

Brown-McHardy Dilator

Lishman and Dellipiani (15) evaluated a modified Brown-McHardy dilator in 1982. Eighteen patients underwent balloon dilatation. Of these 18 patients, 56% had an excellent response, 33% had a fair response, and 11% had a poor response. Dellipiani and Hewetson (16) evaluated 45 patients undergoing dilatation with a modified Brown-McHardy dilator in 1986. Of these 45 patients, 38 (84%) underwent one dilatation, 2 (4%) underwent two dilatations, and 2 (4%) underwent three dilatations. Of these patients, 53% had an excellent response, 31% had a fair response, and 16% had a poor response. Stark et al. (17) evaluated 10 patients undergoing dilatation with a Brown-McHardy dilator in 1990. Of these 10 patients, 100% had an excellent response to dilatation. Parkman et al. (18) in a retrospective study evaluated 123 patients undergoing pneumatic dilatation. Seventy-one (58%) had a satisfactory result and received no further treatment for achalasia, whereas 52 (42%) required subsequent treatment with pneumatic dilatation and/or esophagomyotomy. Of the 47 patients undergoing a second dilatation, follow-up information was available for 45 patients. Of these 45, 26 required subsequent treatments, in contrast to 42% needing additional treatments after the initial dilatation. Ten of 45 patients (22%) required an esophagomyotomy (one for perforation). There were 24 patients undergoing a third pneumatic dilatation. Sixteen of these 22 patients (73%) required subsequent treatments. Eight of the 22 patients (36%) required an esophagomyotomy. Thus, it appeared that subsequent pneumatic dilatations, although beneficial, were less successful for treatment of symptoms than the initial pneumatic dilatation.

Rigiflex Dilators

In 1986, Cox (21) evaluated eight achalasia patients undergoing dilatation with the Rigiflex dilator. Of these patients, 7 (87.5%) underwent one dilatation and 1 (12.5%) underwent two dilatations. Eighty-eight percent of these patients had an excellent to fair response. Levine et al. (22) evaluated 17 patients in 1987 using the Rigiflex dilator. Of these 17 patients, 100% had either an excellent or fair response to dilatation. Stark et al. (17) evaluated ten patients undergoing dilatation with the polyurethane Rigiflex dilator. Of these ten patients, 70% had an excellent response.

Kadakia and Wong (24) evaluated the efficacy of the use of increasing balloon size in 29 consecutive patients. A total of 47 dilatations were performed. The response of balloon dilatation was considered excellent if there were no or rare dysphagia, good if there was intermittent dysphagia, or poor if there was persistent daily mealtime dysphagia. Twelve patients had an excellent response and six patients had a good response to 3 cm balloon dilatation (total, 18 of 29, 62%). Eleven patients with poor response to a 3-cm balloon were dilated with 3.5 cm at a mean interval of 5.7 weeks. Two patients had an excellent response and three patients had a good response (total, 5 of 11 patients). Six patients with poor response to a 3.5-cm balloon were dilated with a 4-cm balloon at the mean interval of 6.2 weeks. Two patients had an excellent response and two patients had a good response. Overall, 27 patients (93%) had either excellent ($n = 16$) or good ($n = 11$) response to balloon dilatation performed in the graded manner. Two patients who failed to respond to the 4 cm balloon dilatation had modified Heller's esophagomyotomy with excellent response. Barkin et al. (25) performed 61 procedures on 50 patients at two centers using the Microvasive Rigiflex balloon dilator. These authors found an overall treatment success rate of 94% (47 of 50 patients).

PREDICTORS OF OUTCOME IN PATIENTS WITH ACHALASIA TREATED BY PNEUMATIC DILATATION

Although a great many studies have shown that forceful dilatation of the gastric cardia is effective treatment for patients with achalasia, the criteria for improvement have not been defined in most of these reports and patient satisfaction is taken as the determinant of treatment success. Unfortunately, it is difficult to use subjective impressions of patient satisfaction as a guide for treatment success and for further treatment since severely symptomatic patients may be satisfied with minimal improvements and others may not. Various factors may affect the outcome of pneumatic dilatation: (a) The premedication may have an effect on the lower esophageal sphincter and dilatation outcome. These include anticholinergics (atropine), which may cause relaxation of the lower esophageal sphincter and thereby decrease the effectiveness of dilatation, analgesics (meperidine, morphine), and muscle relaxants (diazepam), which may also cause muscle relaxation. (b) The size of the dilator bag. (c) Graduated versus single-sized dilatation. (d) The rate of inflation of the dilator bag. (e) The dilatation pressure. (f) Duration of dilatation, in other words, the time the dilator remains inflated. (g) The number of repeat dilatations in a single session (how many repeats are considered safe in a single session) (38).

Various pre- and post-balloon dilatation indicators have been proposed as predictors of outcome including patient characteristics, relief of symptoms, radiographic and manometric improvement, balloon characteristics, balloon size, manometric pressure during dilatation, and the need for repeat dilatation or the number of dilatations during the procedure. In an attempt to address the predictors of long-term outcome, Eckardt et al. (39) undertook a prospective long-term investigation designed to answer the following questions: (a) Do patients' characteristics at the time of the initial presentation determine the response to pneumatic dilatation? (b) Does the response to therapy depend on the vigor with which dilatation is performed? (c) Can long-term prognosis be predicted on the basis of the results of post-dilatation investigation? (d) Are repeated dilatations followed by progressively longer clinical remissions, or should surgery be recommended if the initial treatment does not succeed (38)? In their study 54 consecutive patients with newly diagnosed achalasia underwent standard pre-balloon dilatation and post-balloon dilatation investigation including evaluation of symptoms by a symptom score, manometric studies of the lower esophageal sphincter, radiographic studies using a barium meal, and 13 patients underwent radionucleotide studies.

Pneumatic dilatation was performed using a Brown-McHardy pneumatic dilator. The results of the study after a mean follow-up period of 45.7 months were that 26 of the 54 patients underwent a single dilatation, 17 a second, and 11 a third. Repeated dilatations increased the likelihood of progressively longer remissions. Among the patient characteristics evaluated at the time of initial presentation (age, sex, duration of symptoms, and radiographic and manometric findings) only young age adversely affected outcome after a single dilatation. Patients younger than 40 years of age had a significantly poorer response to dilatation and the least satisfactory treatment results occurred in adolescents (less than 18 years of age). Evaluation of treatment characteristics revealed that the maximum diameter of the waist of the balloon predicted long-term outcome after a single dilatation. Those patients in whom the diameter of the balloon exceeded 3.6 cm had a significantly better chance of remaining symptom-free for 1 and 2 years than those in whom the balloon was inflated to a lesser degree. Although the pressure applied during the procedure was less predictive, it did indicate that patients with the lowest balloon pressures (<7 psi) had a poor treatment result. Evaluation of post-dilatation investigations revealed that radiographic findings post-dilatation did not predict the long-term clinical course. In addition, the esophageal emptying of barium as evaluated by 1-minute retention and 20-minute retention did not correlate with outcome. Post-dilatation esophageal sphincter pressure was highly predictive of the long-term clinical course ($p < .001$). All patients in whom an LES pressure of <10 was attained remained in remission for at least 2 years.

Evaluation of the duration of clinical remission using Kaplin-Meyier plots showed that a single dilatation resulted in a 1-year remission rate of 59% and a 5-year remission rate of only 26%. The data from this study suggest that additional balloon dilatation treatments are followed by progressively longer durations of remission. In this study, a repeat dilatation was safe and effective. In summary, this study showed that the only treatment variable that predicted successful long-term outcome was the diameter of the waist of the bag. The only inherent patient factor that affected long-term outcome unfavorably was young age and the only post-dilatation investigation that predicted a positive long-term outcome was a lower esophageal sphincter pressure of <10 mmHg post-dilatation.

In a study by Parkman et al. (18), a retrospective analysis of pneumatic dilatation using the Brown-McHardy dilator in 123 patients found that older patients (≥45 years) needed fewer subsequent treatments and had a greater improvement in dysphagia at follow-up. In this study, duration of symptoms, esophageal dilatation or tortuosity, or LES pressure did not influence the benefit from pneumatic dilatation.

In a study by Csendes et al. (9) in which the authors looked at the late results in 81 patients with achalasia treated in a prospective randomized study comparing forceful pneumatic dilatation with Mosher bag and surgical anterior esophagomyotomy by the abdominal route, there was a significant decrease in resting gastroesophageal sphincter pressure after both treatments. The bahavior of the sphincter in the dilated patients showed three distinct patterns recorded among 32 patients in whom it was possible to do manometric studies. Patients who were well and asymptomatic at late follow-up had significantly decreased sphincter pressure (median 54 months with a range of 26 to 149 months), which remained at a similar level 5 years after treatment. In patients who needed further dilatation,

this decrease in resting pressure was less, although significant compared with values before treatment. After redilatation, resting sphincter pressure remained at a similar level to the previous values after first dilatation. In the patients who needed surgery, the decrease in resting sphincter pressure was not significant compared with pressure before treatment. Sphincter pressures after dilatation correlated closely with clinical results and were predictive of the late outcome of the procedure.

OTHER FACTORS THAT MAY AFFECT THE SUCCESS OF DILATATION

Repeat Dilatation in the Same Session

The effect of repeat dilatation using the same-size dilator was studied by Cox and coworkers (21) in 1986 using the Rigiflex type dilator. In this study dilatation was repeated with a 3-cm dilator to 15 psi (780 mm Hg) for 1 minute three to five times during a single session. Good short-term results were reported suggesting that submaximal stretch repeated several times may weaken the esophageal circular smooth muscle.

Progressive Increase in Dilator Size Over Time

Vantrappen et al. (40) and Van Goidsenhoven et al. (11) used an interesting technique of increasing the dilator size from 3 to 5 cm over a number of days. The Sippy dilator was used in both of these studies. Vantrappen et al. had an excellent response in 77% of patients, a fair response in 17% of patients, and a poor response in only 6% of patients. They did have three perforations. Similarly, Van Goidsenhoven et al. had an excellent response in 98% of patients and a poor response in only 2% of patients, but also had one patient with perforation that occurred as a result of defective nylon bag when the dilator exploded. Van Goidsenhoven et al. used a maximum diameter of the dilator of 3 cm in 4 patients, 3.5 cm in 20 patients, 4 cm in 23 patients, and 4.5 cm in 7 patients. Two patients had a recurrence of symptoms after dilatation up to 3.5 and 4.5 cm, respectively. They obtained complete symptomatic relief after repeat dilatation up to 4 and 5 cm, respectively. However, relief was only temporary in the patient dilated to 5 cm. Vantrappen et al. determined the number of dilatations with the maximal diameter of the dilating balloon according to clinical, radiological, and manometric criteria. They noted that the maximum diameter of the dilating balloon was not significantly different in patients with satisfactory and in those with unsatisfactory results. Similarly, the maximal diameter of the dilator used was not significantly different in patients who did and those who did not develop a recurrence. Wong and Maydonovitch (14) also used increasing sizes of dilators. However, instead of using them in a single hospitalization, these investigators used progressively larger dilators over several months to years depending on the clinical response. They noted no perforations in 30 patients with 64 dilatations. Wong and Maydonovitch feel that these data suggest that gradually increasing the dilator size is an effective form of therapy, but perforations may occur if large sizes are repeated too soon or prior to testing longer-term clinical efficacy (34).

Kadakia and Wong (24) performed a total of 47 dilatations in 29 consecutive patients with achalasia using the Rigiflex dilator. These dilatations were done in a standardized manner with inflation of the Rigiflex dilator until the waist was obliterated and maintenance of that pressure for 1 minute then reinflation until no waist was seen and maintenance of that pressure once again for 1 minute. If the patients had an excellent or good response then the dilatation was not repeated. However, if the patient had a poor response (persistent daily mealtime dysphagia) then another dilatation was repeated in 4 to 8 weeks with a 3.5-cm balloon using the same technique. Finally, if the patient had a poor response to a second dilatation a third dilatation was again repeated in 4 to 8 weeks using a 4-cm balloon. Using this technique of progressive increase in dilator size over time a success rate of 93% was achieved with no complications.

Maximum Dilator Pressure

Theoretically, using the polyethylene Rigiflex balloons the maximum dilator pressure should not affect the efficacy of dilatation, since the Rigiflex balloons are designed to expand only to a specific size. However, as noted by Wong and Maydonovitch (38), many authors such as Kurlander et al. (10), Vantrappen et al. (12), Van Goidsenhoven et al. (11), Witzel (27), and Frimberger et al. (41) employed large Sippy or Mosher dilators but inflated with pressures (200–400 mm) insufficient to expand the dilator fully. Hence, the maximum dilatation size obtained during these procedures is unknown, but probably less than full expansion.

Patient Factors That May Affect the Efficacy of Dilatation

Vantrappen et al. (12) and Fellows et al. (19) noted that older patients responded best to pneumatic dilatation. Similarly, Eckardt et al. (39) noted that the only inherent patient factor that affected long-term outcome unfavorably was young age. Vantrappen et al. reported better results in patients with a long history of dysphagia (mean duration 8.2 years) compared to patients with a shorter history of dysphagia (2.5 years).

COMPLICATIONS

There are a number of complications that can occur with balloon dilatation in achalasia. One is the potential development of gastroesophageal reflux due to incompetence of the lower esophageal sphincter after dilatation, although reflux does not appear to be a major problem. The incidence of this complication varies from 0% to 17%. No evidence was found for gastroesophageal reflux in the study by Vantrappen and coworkers (12). Csendes et al. (8) reported a single case of gastroesophageal reflux in 18 patients. Reflux was noted in 4 of 45 (9%) dilated patients in the study by Dellipiani and Hewetson (16). However, Bennett and Hendrix (13) found an incidence of gastroesophageal reflux of 17%. Another potential complication is the development of peptic stricture secondary to gastroesophageal reflux. However, this complication has only been noted in the study by Dellipiani and Hewetson in which one peptic stricture developed.

The complication most feared is perforation of the esophagus. Wong and Maydonovitch (38) state, "There have been 70 reports of perforation in the literature. Sixty-four percent of the patients did well with conservative management whereas 26% underwent surgery with a 4% mortality. It should be noted that the reported incidence of esophageal perforation has decreased over the last 10 years which may be related to the fixed size of the polyurethane dilators."

In a retrospective review undertaken by Fried et al. (42) patients who had undergone balloon dilatation for achalasia at Beth Israel Hospital in Boston were evaluated over a 6-year period. A total of 94 dilatations in 72 patients were identified. Of these, 58 were performed with the Brown-McHardy dilator, 22 with the Rigiflex, and 12 with the Mosher bag. In the 94 dilatations, 5 perforations occurred (5.3%) (defined as extravasation of contrast on Gastrografin swallow after the procedure). It was found that four of the five perforations occurred after dilatation with the Rigiflex balloon, two of which required thoracotomy. There were no procedure-related deaths. Only one perforation occurred after dilatation with the Brown-McHardy or Mosher bag. No other factor could be identified as an independent variable, including number of dilatations, size of dilator, duration of inflation, or other factors such as Candida esophagitis, paraesophageal diverticula, or hiatal hernia. The authors speculate that the rigidity of the polyethylene balloon of the Rigiflex dilator compared with that of the rubber balloon of the Brown-McHardy may somehow play a role in the observed complication rate.

Rate of Perforation According to Dilator

Stark Dilator

Schindler (2), using the Stark dilator, had five perforations in 84 patients. Two patients required surgery for complications.

Hydrostatic Dilator

Lawrence and Shoesmith (34), using the Negus dilator, had one perforation out of 100 patients, with that patient requiring surgery.

Plummer Dilator

Olsen et al. (35), using the Plummer dilator, had 10 perforations in 452 patients. Two of these patients required surgery. Sanderson et al. (36), using the Plummer dilator, had 14 perforations in 408 patients. Ten of these patients required surgery.

Pneumatic Dilators

Mosher Dilator

Csendes et al. (8) had no perforations in 18 patients dilated with the Mosher dilator.

Sippy Dilator

Kurlander et al. (10), using the Sippy dilator, reported 10 perforations in 62 patients. Van Goidsenhoven et al. (11) reported seven perforations in 57 patients using the Sippy dilator. Vantrappen et al. (12) reported three perforations in 133 patients using the Sippy dilator. One patient required surgery.

Hurst-Tucker Dilator

Bennett and Hendrix (13) reported three perforations in 48 patients dilated with the Hurst-Tucker dilator. One patient required surgery. Wong and Maydonovitch (14) reported no esophageal perforation in 30 patients dilated using the Hurst-Tucker dilator. Lishman and Dellipiani (15) reported no perforations and no surgery in 18 patients dilated with a modified Brown-McHardy dilator. Dellipiani and Hewetson (16) had four perforations in 45 patients who were dilated with a modified Brown-McHardy dilator. One patient required surgery. Stark et al. (17) had no perforations and no patients requiring surgery in 10 patients who were dilated with the Brown-McHardy dilator. Parkman et al. (18) in a retrospective study found that 2 of 123 patients undergoing pneumatic dilatation with a Brown-McHardy dilator (1.6% of patients, 1.0% of dilatations) had an esophageal perforation during pneumatic dilatation. These patients underwent emergent surgery for esophageal repair with a Heller esophagomyotomy and partial fundoplication. Seventy percent of the patients had excellent results, 11% had fair results, and 19% had poor results.

Rider-Moeller Dilator

Fellows et al. (19) reported 1 patient out of 63 requiring surgery for complications due to dilatation using the Rider-Moeller dilator. Jacobs et al. (37) noted one perforation in 30 patients dilated with a modified Rider-Moeller dilator. No patients required surgery for complications. Adams et al. (20) reported seven esophageal tears and two complete esophageal ruptures in 44 patients undergoing dilatation with the Rider-Moeller dilator.

Rigiflex Dilator

Cox et al. (21) had no perforations and no patients required surgery in eight patients dilated with the Rigiflex dilator. Levine et al. (22) reported an incidence of 2 perforations in 17 patients dilated with the Rigiflex dilator. Gelfond and Kozarek (23) reported no perforations in 24 patients undergoing dilatation with Rigiflex dilator and Stark et al. (17) reported no perforations in 10 patients undergoing dilatation with the Rigiflex dilator. Kadakia and Wong (24) had no perforations in 29 patients dilated at a total of 47 times using the Rigiflex dilator. Barkin et al. (25) in a study evaluating 50 patients treated with balloon dilatation found that 2 of the 50 patients required elective surgical treatment and a third surgery for perforation secondary to a dilatation. In addition, two other patients had post-procedure chest pain and were found to have perforations. One required surgical repair.

Endoscopic Dilator

Witzel (27) reported no perforation in 39 patients undergoing dilatation with the Witzel dilator.

TREATMENT OF ESOPHAGEAL PERFORATION

Esophageal perforation is the most feared complication of balloon dilatation in achalasia. However, most patients do well using conservative medical treatment and it is the minority of patients that require surgery to close the perforated esophagus (38). Post-dilatation radiographic studies should be performed to determine whether or not a perforation has occurred. Contained perforations can be treated with intravenous antibiotics, making the patient NPO, and parenteral nutrition. Free perforations usually require immediate thoracic surgery and drainage. However, medical treatment with intravenous antibiotics and hyperalimentation has been used successfully (43–45). It appears that the LES muscle itself is relatively resistant to complete tears and that the musculature proximal and distal to the LES are more frequently the sites of perforation. In a study by Lendrum (46) anatomic features of the cardiac orifice of the stomach were looked at with special reference to cardiospasm. It was found that sites of esophageal perforation originate 5 to 10 mm proximal to or 5 mm distal to the squamocolumnar junction. Most perforations occur in the distal left lateral aspect of the esophagus and are noted on anterior radiographic projections. However, lateral projections are required to exclude posterior perforation (38). Immediately after dilatation a Gastrographin swallow is performed. If no perforation is noted, the patient is asked to drink barium to generate a barium column and fully distend the distal esophagus.

PRE- AND POST-DILATATION EVALUATION

Radiographic

Barium study radiographs are characteristic for the diagnosis of achalasia. Early on in the disease, the esophagus is not dilated and there may be evidence of a spasm or tertiary contractions. However, as the disease progresses the body of the esophagus becomes widened and dilated. The esophagus may become tortuous with a smooth tapering "bird beak" as a characteristic finding at the lower esophageal sphincter. In addition, there is often an air fluid level in the chest. Absence of the gastric air bubble is noted in at least 50% of patients (12,47). Post-dilatation there is often an increase in the mean diameter of the esophagogastric junction. Ott et al. (48) noted an increase in mean diameter at the gastroesophageal junction from 4.2 mm before dilatation to 7.5 mm immediately following dilatation. Vantrappen and Hellemans (30) noted a mean increase in diameter from 2 mm before to 9 mm many months after the pneumatic dilatation. They also noted that the gastric bubble was absent in 85% of the patients before treatment and in only 10% many months later.

Manometric Studies

Esophageal manometry is the definitive test to differentiate between achalasia and other esophageal motility disorders. Characteristic manometric findings in achalasia include normal to elevated resting LES pressures, incomplete relaxation on deglutition, and lack of esophageal peristalsis. Manometric studies post-dilatation show decreases in gastroesophageal sphincter pressure and intraesophageal pressure immediately after dilatation. However, sphincter pressure tends to rise after dilatation (49,50). Although relaxation of the sphincter with swallowing does not return, the residual pressure tends to be lower after dilatation. The traditional view has been that the esophageal peristalsis does not return after pneumatic dilatation (49). However, a number of case reports (49,51,52) have questioned this traditional view. Lamet et al. (52) have demonstrated the return of distal progressive peristaltic contraction in 7 of 34 (21%) of patients with achalasia successfully treated with pneumatic dilatation. Kadakia and Wong (24) performed repeat esophageal manometry in 13 patients pre- and post-dilatation. After balloon dilatation, the mean LES pressure was 11 ± 4 mm Hg, compared with 37 ± 9 mm Hg ($p < .001$) in 13 patients in whom repeat esophageal manometry was done. The fall in LES pressure from pre- to post-dilatation in those with excellent (5 patients), good (5 patients), and poor (3 patients) results was not significantly different (24 ± 7 vs. 27 ± 9 vs. 22 ± 7 mm Hg).

Nuclear Scintigraphy

Nuclear scintigraphy esophageal emptying studies have also been used to evaluate the achalasia esophagus before and after balloon dilatation. Gross and colleagues (53) noted differences in esophageal emptying between treated and untreated patients using scintigraphy to monitor clearance of a meal consisting of 250 ml of milk and corn flakes radiolabeled with 99m technetium–diethylenetriamine penta-acetic acid (^{99m}Tc-DPTA). Berger and McCallum devised a similar study utilizing a radiolabeled egg salad sandwich meal to quantitate esophageal emptying following dilatation, surgery, and nifedipine administration. Kadakia and Wong (24) performed radionucleotide esophageal emptying before dilatation and within 4 to 7 days after dilatation, with the patient ingesting an egg salad sandwich containing technetium-labeled sulfur colloid followed by a small glass of milk in 25 of 29 patients dilated. The esophageal retention was measured with the patient in the sitting position at 300 seconds and was expressed as a percentage of ingested isotope retained. The esophageal retention measured by scintigraphy improved from $78 \pm 47\%$ to $44 \pm 34\%$ in 25 of 29 ($p < .001$) patients in whom it was measured before and after balloon dilatation. The esophageal emptying improved in $37 \pm 15\%$ in excellent responders ($n = 14$), compared with 32 ± 14% (not significant) in good responders (*n* = 10).

DILATION AS AN OUTPATIENT PROCEDURE

In 1990, Barkin et al. (25) evaluated the safety and efficacy of pneumatic dilatation as an outpatient procedure. Sixty-one procedures were performed in 50 patients at two centers. An overall treatment success rate of 94% (47 of 50 patients) was achieved. Two patients had elective surgical treatment and a third underwent surgery for perforation secondary to dilatation. A total of three patients complained of post-procedure chest pain within 4 hours and were hospitalized. Two had perforations; one required surgical repair. The third patient had resolution of symptoms. These authors concluded that performing balloon dilatation with the Microvasive Rigiflex balloon dilator as an outpatient procedure was safe, efficacious, and cost-effective. A post-procedure esophagram was done in each patient and revealed intact mucosa in 60 of 61 procedures with one patient exhibiting a mucosal tear. Patients in 8 of 61 procedures (13%) complained of post-dilatation chest pain. Five of the 8 had resolution of their pain within 1 hour of the procedure, whereas chest pain persisted for more than 4 hours post-procedure for 3 patients who were hospitalized at one of the centers. One of these patients, whose post-procedure esophagram showed a mucosal tear, was treated with antibiotics and discharged after 2 days of hospitalization. A second patient continued to have chest pain. The initial barium swallow did not reveal a perforation. However, because of persistent pain a repeat swallow was performed that revealed a delayed perforation. Forty-seven percent of the 15 patients in the study were discharged from the outpatient facility within 4 hours of recovery from sedation. These authors recommend that for outpatient achalasia dilatation patients be evaluated post-procedure for a minimum of 4 hours, especially for pain, nausea and/or vomiting and hypotension. In addition, the authors recommend following patients by direct contact for a period of 2 days. The authors note that in the past they had hospitalized all patients for achalasia dilatation for a minimum of 2 days with the average hospital cost of $1,000 per day. Outpatient dilatation can reduce the cost of treatment for achalasia considerably.

REFERENCES

1. Starck H. *Munch Med Wochenschr* 1924;71:334–336.
2. Schindler R. *Ann Intern Med* 1956;45:207.
3. Plummer HS. *JAMA* 1908;51:549–554.
4. Thomas S, Negus VE, Bateman GH. *A textbook for students and practitioners*, 6th ed. London: Cassel, 1955;776.
5. Mosher HP. *Post Med J* 1923;26:240–246.
6. Nanson EM. *Can Med Assoc J* 1962;86:1107.
7. Heimlich JJ, O'Connor TW, Flores DC. *Ann Otol* 1978;87:519.
8. Csendes A, et al. *Gastroenterology* 1981;80:789.
9. Csendes A, Braghetto I, Henríquez A, Cortés C. *Gut* 1989;30:299–304.
10. Kurlander DJ, et al. *Gastroenterology* 1963;45:326.
11. Van Goidsenhoven GE et al. *Gastroenterology* 1963;45:326.
12. Vantrappen G, et al. *Gut* 1971;12:268.
13. Bennett JR, Hendrix TR. *Mod Treat* 1970;7:1217.
14. Wong RKH, Maydonovitch CL. *Am J Gastroenterol* 1989;84(9):1153.
15. Lishman AH, Dellipiani AW. *Gut* 1982;23:541.
16. Dellipiani AW, Hewetson KA. *Q J Med* 1986;58:253.
17. Stark GA, et al. *Am J Gastroenterol* 1990;85(pt 10):1322.
18. Parkman HP, Reynolds JC, Ouyang A, et al. *Dig Dis Sci* 1993;38:75–85.
19. Fellows IW, Ogilvie AL, Atkinson M. *Gut* 1983;24:1020.
20. Adams H, Roberts GM, Smith PM. *Clin Radiol* 1989;40:53.
21. Cox J, Buckton GK, Bennett JR. *Gut* 1986;27:986.
22. Levine ML, et al. *Am J Gastroenterol* 1987;82(4):311.
23. Gelfond MD, Kozarek RA. *Am J Gastroenterol* 1988;84:924.
24. Kadakia S, Wong KH. *Am J Gastroenterol* 1993;88:34–38.
25. Barkin JS, Guelrud M, Reiner DK, Goldberg RI, Phillips RS. *Gastrointest Endosc* 1990;36:123–126.
26. Tytgat GN, Derltartogjager FL. *Endoscopy* 1977;9:211–215.
27. Witzel L. *Endoscopy* 1981;13:176–177.
28. Richter JE, Castell DO. In: Bennett JR, Hunt RH, eds. *Therapeutic endoscopy and radiology of the gut*. London: Chapman and Hall Medical, 1990;82–90.
29. Ohike N, Payne WS, Neufeld DM, et al. *Ann Thorac Surg* 1979;28:119–125.
30. Vantrappen G, Hellemans J. *Gastroenterology* 1980;79:144–154.
31. Vantrappen G, Janssens J. *Gut* 1983;24:1013–1019.
32. McJunkin B, McMillan WO, Duncan HE, Harman KM, White JJ, McJunkin JE. *Gastrointest Endosc* 1991;37:18–21.
33. Ortega JA, Madwieri V, Perez L. *Gastrointest Endosc* 1980;26:8.
34. Lawrence K, Shoesmith JH. *Thorax* 1959;14:211.
35. Olsen AM, et al. *J Thorac Cardiovasc Surg* 1951;22:164.
36. Sanderson DR, Ellis FH Jr, Olsen AM. *Chest* 1970;58:116.
37. Jacobs JB, Cohen NL, Mattel S. *Ann Otol Rhinol Laryngol* 1983;92:353.
38. Wong RKH, Maydonovitch CL. In: Castell DO, ed. *The esophagus*. Boston: Little, Brown, 1991;233–260.
39. Eckardt VF, Krause J, Bolle D. *Dig Dis Sci* 1989;34(5):655.
40. Vantrappen G, et al. *Gastroenterology* 1963;45:317.
41. Frimberger E, et al. *Endoscopy* 1981;13:173.
42. Fried RL, Rosenberg S, Goyal R. *Gastrointest Endosc* 1991;37:405.
43. Cameron JL, et al. *Ann Thorac Surg* 1978;27:404–408.
44. Michel L, Grillo HC, Malt RA. *Ann Surg* 1981;194:57.
45. Swedlund A, et al. *Dig Dis Sci* 1989;34(3):379.
46. Lendrum FC. *Arch Intern Med* 1937;59:474.
47. Orlando RC, Call DL, Bream CA. *Ann Intern Med* 1978;88:60.
48. Ott DJ, Richter JE, Wu WC, et al. *Dig Dis Sci* 1989;32:962–967.
49. Mellow MH. *Gastroenterology* 1976;70:1148–1151.
50. Holloway RH, Krosin G, Lange RC, et al. *Gastroenterology* 1983;84:771–776.
51. Vantrappen G, Janssens J, Hellemans J, Coremans G. *Gastroenterology* 1979;75:450–451.
52. Lamet M, Fleshler B, Achkar E. *Am J Gastroenterol* 1985;80:602–604.
53. Gross R, Johnson LF, Kaminski RJ. *Dig Dis Sci* 1979;24:945.

Advanced Therapeutic Endoscopy, 2nd Ed.,
edited by J. S. Barkin and C. A. O'Phelan.
Raven Press, Ltd., New York © 1994.

CHAPTER 9

Transendoscopic Balloon Therapy: What Is Its Role for Esophageal Strictures and with Which Balloon?

Shailesh C. Kadakia and Roy K. H. Wong

Esophageal dilatation is a commonly performed procedure to relieve dysphagia in patients with esophageal stenoses (1–5). It is a safe and effective method of treating most esophageal strictures. The mercury-filled rubber bougies (e.g., Maloney) are the most frequently used dilators because they are easy to use and, in most cases, do not require fluoroscopic monitoring, although monitoring has been recommended by some authors (6). A small number of patients requiring very frequent dilatations can even manage self-dilatations at home using mercury-filled rubber bougies (7,8). While most esophageal strictures can be easily and safely dilated with mercury-filled bougies, very tight, tortuous, and/or complex strictures require either a guidewire dilatation system or balloon dilatation. This is because the soft mercury-filled bougies can easily curl up in the esophagus above the stricture resulting in failure of effective dilatation. In 1955, Puestow (9) described a technique of esophageal dilatation that utilized a system of metal olives passed over an "accident proof" steel guidewire. Although it proved to be too dangerous, it was a significant improvement over the semi-rigid flexible guidewire inserted by gastrostomy and leaded guidewire used in the 1880s. The Eder-Puestow system has now been largely replaced by the Savary

and the American Endoscopy dilator systems consisting of polyvinyl bougies passed over a guidewire that are easier to use, possibly safer, and more effective (10,11). We and others have found dilatation of esophageal strictures with American Endoscopy dilators using a marked guidewire without fluoroscopy to be quite effective and safe (12,13). A modified system consisting of only two solid, stepped, radiopaque dilators passed over a guidewire has been described by Celestin and Campbell (14) and compared with the Eder-Puestow technique by them and other investigators (15).

Recently, balloons have been widely used in the treatment of a variety of gastrointestinal strictures. It is a relatively new technique, but one that shows a great deal of promise. Transendoscopic technique, as well as over the guidewire technique with fluoroscopy, has been used widely during the last decade to dilate esophageal strictures in adults (16–29) and children (30–34). Balloon dilators have been used for the treatment of a variety of gastrointestinal stenosis including esophageal (16–34), gastric (18,35–41), small intestinal (42,43), colonic (44,45), and anastomotic strictures (33,46–51). The major indication for balloon dilatation of esophageal strictures is to provide symptomatic relief of dysphagia due to anatomic and functional narrowing of the esophagus (5). Established indications for such treatment include peptic, neoplastic, corrosive, postsclerotherapy, postradiation, postinfectious, postsurgical, pill-induced strictures, and achalasia (1–5,13,52). Other conditions causing esophageal stenosis such as rings and webs can be effectively dilated by other modalities such as Maloney or over the guidewire dilators and do not require balloon dilatation in most instances. Balloon dilatation is primarily used in

S. C. Kadakia: Department of Medicine, University of Texas Health Science Center; and Gastroenterology Service, GI Endoscopy, Department of Medicine, Department of the Army, Brooke Army Medical Center, San Antonio, Texas 78234-6265

R. K. H. Wong: Gastroenterology Service, Walter Reed Army Medical Center, Washington, DC 20307; and Department of Medicine, Uniformed Services University of Health Science, Bethesda, Maryland 20892.

instances in which conventional techniques have been initially unsuccessful (53). It may be the procedure of choice when the strictures are severe, lengthy, irregular, and complex in nature.

Certain basic principles apply to any method of esophageal dilatation including balloon dilatation. Before starting dilatation of any esophageal stricture, complete evaluation of the stricture is necessary. This may be accomplished by barium radiographic studies or during the initial endoscopy. Appropriate biopsies and/or brushing should also be obtained to evaluate for malignancy. If this is not possible during initial endoscopy, repeat endoscopy should be done after the stricture has been dilated. Complete evaluation of the stricture and accessible upper gastrointestinal tract with biopsy and brushing of the stricture should be done. There are certain absolute and relative contraindications to esophageal dilatation that also apply to transendoscopic balloon dilatation of esophageal strictures. Acute or incompletely healed esophageal perforation is an absolute contraindication for esophageal dilatation including balloon dilatation (5). The American Society for Gastrointestinal Endoscopy (ASGE) considers bleeding disorders, severe pulmonary disease, recent myocardial infarction, recent esophageal perforation or surgery, recent laparotomy, and large thoracic aneurysm as relative contraindications, but states that dilatation can be performed if the clinical situation warrants (5). Concomitant chest radiation therapy is not considered to be a contraindication (5). We routinely perform esophageal dilatations in patients with esophageal or nonesophageal malignancy who are receiving concomitant chest radiation therapy and have not had any complications.

TECHNICAL ASPECTS OF TRANSENDOSCOPIC BALLOON DILATATION

Most endoscopists perform transendoscopic balloon dilatation of the esophageal strictures without using a guidewire; therefore, only this particular technique will be described. The technique of balloon dilatation of esophageal strictures (23–29,31,32) and primary esophageal achalasia (52) using guidewire and fluoroscopy has been described in great detail in the literature.

Equipment

Currently, there are three companies that manufacture balloon dilators for esophageal strictures. Balloon dilators manufactured by Wilson-Cook (Wilson-Cook Medical, Inc., Winston-Salem, NC) are available in only two sizes of 8 mm and 15 mm inflated balloon diameter. The balloons are 8 cm long with a 2-cm long tip and cost $135 per balloon. The dilators are passed

over a 0.89-mm (0.035-inch) guidewire. The large shaft sizes of 9 French for the 8-mm balloon and 14 French for the 15-mm balloon make them too large for transendoscopic placement, although the 8-mm balloon can be passed through the large channel (3.8 mm or 4.2 mm) of a therapeutic endoscope.

The Eliminator balloon dilators manufactured by Bard (C. R. Bard, Inc., Tewksbury, MA) have balloon length of 8 cm, catheter outer diameter of 1.9 mm, catheter length of 180 cm, and are available in balloon diameter sizes of 6, 8, 10, 12, 15, and 18 mm. Unfortunately, these balloons are disposable and are designed for one-time use only. The dilator kit, which includes all size balloons, an inflator, and disposable manometer, costs $650 with the price per balloon ranging from $115 to $155. A single use of the balloon at this price makes it quite cost-ineffective.

The Rigiflex TTS (Through The Scope) balloons manufactured by Microvasive (Boston Scientific Corporation, Watertown, MA) have balloon length of 8 cm, catheter outer diameter of 1.7 mm, catheter length of 180 cm, and are available in balloon diameter sizes of 6, 8, 10, 12, 15, and 18 mm. The system with balloons inflated to their maximum diameter is shown in Fig. 1. Each balloon costs $175 and the entire kit, which includes all six balloon dilators, an inflator, and a pressure monitor costs $1,780. The major advantage of these balloons is that they are not designed for one-time use only, which makes them quite cost-effective. We have been able to use each of these balloons several times.

Technique

As mentioned previously, an endoscopy is performed for complete evaluation of the esophageal stricture with biopsies and/or brushing before actual dilatation is started. Once the decision to dilate the stricture by using the transendoscopic technique is made, the balloon system is set up as shown in the Fig. 2. An appropriate-size balloon is selected depending upon the size of the esophageal stricture. We select the next larger balloon for the estimated stricture size. For example, if the esophageal stricture is estimated to be 9 mm, we start with a 10-mm balloon. The selected balloon(s) is tested to ensure absence of air leak by immersing it in water while it is inflated. The system is then set up by attaching the plastic dome to the manometer and connecting the supplied tubing to each arm of the dome (Fig. 2). An inflator is connected to the tubing with a two-way stopcock between the inflator and the tubing. The second tubing connected to the other arm of the dome is connected to the dilator with a two-way stopcock between the two. The entire system is filled with water or contrast such that there is

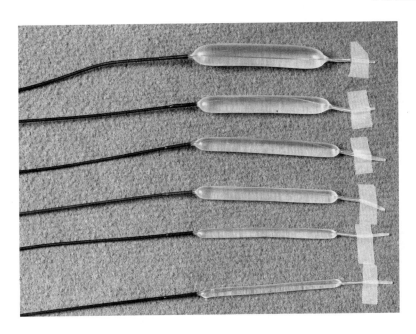

FIG. 1. Completely inflated Rigiflex TTS balloons of 6, 8, 10, 12, 15, and 18 mm sizes.

complete absence of air in the system. The two-way stopcocks are extremely important to maintain the air-free system since they allow the inflator and the dilator to be disconnected from the tubing at any time without risking entrance of air in the system. While the dilatation can be done using air, water, or contrast (4), most endoscopists prefer to use water or contrast (hydrostatic dilatation) rather than air (pneumatic dilatation), which is used primarily during balloon dilatation of esophageal achalasia (52). We use water for most transendoscopic balloon dilatations in our patients. Use of contrast is reserved for the dilatation performed under fluoroscopic guidance.

When an esophageal stricture is encountered during endoscopy, the stricture may be wide enough for the endoscope to pass through it or it may be too tight for the endoscope to pass through (Fig. 3). Once the endoscope passes through the esophageal stricture, the balloon is advanced through the biopsy channel of the endoscope until it emerges through the tip of the endoscope. It must be emphasized that the balloon should be well lubricated by silicone to facilitate its passage through the endoscope (3). While small balloons (6 and 8 mm) can be passed relatively easily through the standard-size endoscope (channel size 2.8 mm), larger balloons (10 mm and larger) should preferably be passed through therapeutic endoscope with large biopsy channel (e.g., Olympus GIF-2T10, GIF-1T10 or its equivalent). In our experience, one of the many reasons for balloon rupture is the use of a small biopsy channel

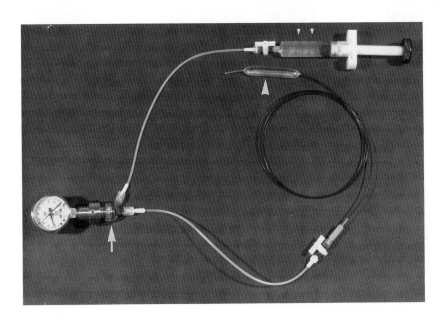

FIG. 2. Standard setup of transendoscopic balloon dilatation. The transducer dome *(arrow)* is tightly screwed onto the pressure monitor. The balloon *(large arrowhead)* and an inflator *(small arrowheads)* are connected to the dome by appropriate tubing and two-way stopcocks.

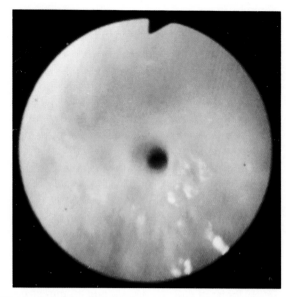

FIG. 3. A tight peptic stricture of the lower esophagus. The endoscope could not be negotiated through the stricture.

(2.8 mm) endoscopes for large (10 mm and greater) balloons. Once the balloon exits through the tip of the endoscope, the endoscope is withdrawn until the balloon is placed across the stricture. Since most esophageal strictures are less than 8 cm in length, and all esophageal balloons are 8 cm in length, the entire balloon can be positioned across the stricture. If the stricture is longer than 8 cm it may be dilated in segments. If the endoscope fails to pass the markedly narrowed esophageal stricture, it may be slowly and carefully advanced through the stricture as shown in Fig. 4. Pre-

vious knowledge of the stricture anatomy is essential and very helpful in this situation to ensure absence of marked angulations that may make this "blind" advancement risky. Absence of resistance is also mandatory during this "blind" advancement. If the advancement of the balloon is considered risky for whatever reason(s), alternative techniques such as polyvinyl bougie dilatation over a guidewire using fluoroscopy or marked guidewire must be utilized (3–5,12,13,28,29).

Once the balloon is placed properly across the stricture, it is inflated until the pressure is just below that recommended by the manufacturer for that particular balloon. The pressure within the balloon is monitored by the pressure manometer as shown in Fig. 2. We routinely use the inflator during our dilatation since it significantly facilitates the rise and maintenance of desired pressure within the balloon. Extreme care is exercised not to exceed the pressure recommended by the manufacture. We believe that this is another common reason for balloon rupture, which is totally and easily avoidable. During this phase of dilatation, the stricture can actually be seen dilating by the inflating balloon through the transparent balloon wall as shown in Fig. 5. In most instances, dilatation is achieved long before the manufacturer's recommended pressure is reached (4). In some instances, the strictures may be too fibrotic and the waist of the balloon is never obliterated, as can be seen when fluoroscopy combined with the use of contrast for balloon dilatation is used. Some authors have suggested that a sudden fall in pressure signifies that the stricture has dilated (4). However, this does not seem to be our own experience and we rely on the maximal dilatation using pressure monitor-

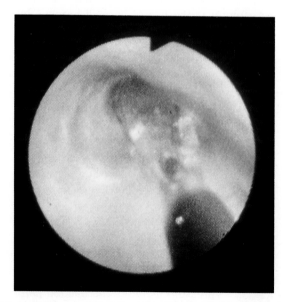

FIG. 4. The balloon is placed across the tight esophageal stricture. The black shaft can be seen emerging through the endoscope.

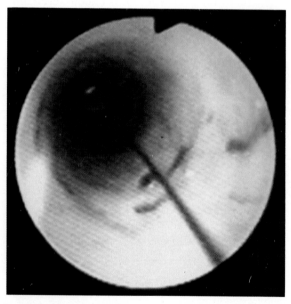

FIG. 5. The inflated balloon across the stricture. The wall of the stricture being dilated is easily visible through the transparent balloon wall.

ing. Since these balloons are made of highly non-compliant material, they will inflate to their designated maximal diameter with maximal pressure. Further increase in pressure beyond that recommended by the manufacturer will result in rupture of the balloon without further increase in the size of the balloon. This "noncompliant" nature is one of the greatest advantages of all modern balloon dilators in contrast to compliant balloons, which increase further (beyond their designated balloon diameter) in diameter with increasing pressure, thereby increasing the chances of esophageal perforation.

The balloon is maintained in inflated position for 60 seconds. The technique varies to some extent from institution to institution. For example, the duration for which the inflation should be maintained is not standardized. While we maintain the inflation for 60 seconds, others have done so for 30 to 45 seconds (4), or for 2 to 5 minutes (53), and still others have not mentioned the duration of inflation at all (3,19,20). The rate of inflation of the balloon is also unknown. We inflate the balloon as rapidly as possible. It is also unknown if there is any advantage to inflating the same-size balloon more than once. Once the stricture is dilated with the balloon as shown in Fig. 6, it is withdrawn through the endoscope after it is emptied of water or contrast. Attempts to withdraw the balloon before it is completely empty of any fluid is yet another reason for the rupture of the balloon. We have found that disconnecting the balloon catheter from the two-way stopcock and aspiration of water is much quicker than aspiration via the inflator. In addition, it also allows one to keep the system (pressure monitor, dome, and tubing) closed at all times. Dilatation is accomplished by dilat-

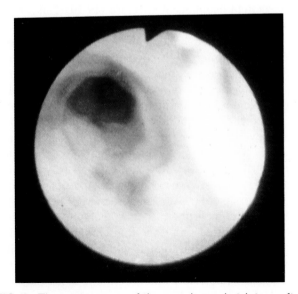

FIG. 6. The appearance of the esophageal stricture after the balloon dilatation is completed.

ing the stricture using sequentially larger balloons until the desired diameter of the stricture is achieved.

EFFICACY OF BALLOON DILATATION OF ESOPHAGEAL STRICTURES

Use of hydrostatic balloon dilatation of the esophageal stricture has increased dramatically over the last 12 to 13 years. Most of the reports in the literature are in the form of a single case or a series of case reports. Only a handful of studies involving more than a few cases are available and even then the number of patients is still small. A national survey of 1,093 ASGE members in 1987 showed that 22% of the respondents used balloon for dilatation of a variety of gastrointestinal strictures and 61% of them had used it for esophageal stenosis (39). Endoscopists found balloon dilatation of reflux strictures easier than dilatation of malignant strictures with a technical success of 88% and 75%, respectively. The immediate symptomatic relief in reflux disease was 89% compared to 68% in cancer, with 65% and 20% symptomatic relief at greater than 3 months, respectively. Unfortunately, this survey did not address the types of dilators or the final size of the balloon used by the endoscopists. However, the success was only 30% when the balloon size was ≤20 French compared to 95% with balloon sizes of ≥51 French.

Graham and Smith (19) used 15 mm or larger (20 mm) Rigiflex TTS balloons in 22 patients at the initial dilatation attempt. While the balloon dilatation was technically successful in all patients, the issue of its clinical efficacy in terms of symptomatic relief of dysphagia as well as the selection of patients was not addressed. In another study, Graham et al. (20), evaluated the effectiveness of Rigiflex TTS balloons in 37 patients with benign and malignant esophageal strictures. Final balloon diameter was 10 mm in 3 patients, 12 mm in 2, 15 mm in 31, and 18 mm in 1. Despite significant increase in final luminal diameter after balloon dilatation, the efficacy in relieving the symptoms was not addressed.

A recent study by Joyce et al. (22), showed that Rigiflex TTS balloon dilatation in 70 outpatients relieved dysphagia in 91% of the patients. Forty-seven (67%) patients required a single dilatation, 8 (11%) patients required two dilatations, and 15 patients (21%) required more than three dilatations to relieve symptoms. Interestingly, the starting size and the final size of the balloon were not mentioned. It appears from these and other studies that benign and malignant esophageal strictures can be successfully dilated with high technical as well as high immediate, but only moderate, clinical success (defined as relief of dysphagia).

Despite this insurgence of transendoscopic balloon

dilatation and great enthusiasm among endoscopists to use the technique, there is very little information in the literature concerning its comparison with other techniques. Cox et al. (54) compared Rigiflex TTS balloon (n = 35) with Celestin bougie (n = 30) dilatation of benign esophageal strictures. Both groups had dilatation to 20 mm, although patients randomized to bougie were dilated with Eder-Puestow after 54 French Celestin bougie dilatation was done in all cases. The mean difference in the baseline dysphagia score was significantly better in the bougie group compared to the balloon group. The strictures remained wider in the bougie group compared to the balloon group. This study suggests that bougie dilatation is more effective than balloon dilatation in reducing dysphagia and maintaining stricture patency.

Shemesh and Czerniak (55) compared the Savary-Gilliard and balloon dilatation of benign esophageal strictures in 64 patients. Savary-Gilliard dilators ranging from 6 to 17 mm were passed through the stricture in 30 patients with significant subjective resistance on the part of the endoscopist being the end point. Rigiflex TTS balloon dilatations were done in 30 patients using 6- to 18-mm sizes with easy passage of an 18-mm balloon through the stricture being the end point. Immediate relief of dysphagia occurred in all patients in both groups. Recurrence of dysphagia within 12 months occurred in 11 patients (37%) in the Savary group compared to 17 (57%) patients in the balloon group. The Savary-Gilliard dilators were slightly more effective and simpler to use than the balloon dilator in achieving both an increase in luminal diameter and in duration of symptomatic improvement. Balloon dilators were more helpful in long, tortuous strictures and in multiple closely placed strictures mainly in the cervical esophagus. Another recent study compared balloon with Eder-Puestow dilators in the treatment of benign esophageal strictures and found similar outcomes in both randomized and nonrandomized groups with a slightly higher complication rates with Eder-Puestow dilators. However, the importance of this study is not quite obvious since Eder-Puestow dilatation has been largely abandoned by most endoscopists. We have used Savary-Gilliard or American Endoscopy dilators over the guidewire exclusively instead of Eder-Puestow dilators since 1986.

Despite significant technological advancement as well as widespread use of transendoscopic balloon dilatation of esophageal strictures, several issues remain unaddressed, unanswered, and/or controversial: Why use balloon dilatation? When and how to use balloon? Which balloon to use? Is it safe to use balloon?

Why Use Balloon?

The bougies such as Maloney, Savary, American Endoscopy, and Celestin dilators dilate the strictures by exerting both longitudinal and radial forces on the stricture causing a "shearing" effect or in the case of metal olives of Eder-Puestow a "splitting" effect (56). In contrast, balloons dilate the strictures by exerting the radial force causing only the "stretching" effect (21). It has been suggested that these differences in the mechanisms of dilatation may reduce the incidence of esophageal perforation with balloon; but studies have failed to show that there is an increased perforation rate with balloons (19,20,22,54,55). Whether these differences are really important clinically in terms of relieving dysphagia, achieving higher technical success, performing dilatation easily, and/or reducing the incidence of complications (especially esophageal perforation) is not obvious. Balloons are clearly more fragile than bougies and therefore more expensive in the long run. Although a balloon can be used several times before it ruptures and sometimes up to 90 uses of a single balloon can be achieved (54), a Savary or American Endoscopy bougie can be used hundreds of times. (We are still using our American Endoscopy dilators bought in 1987.) Another distinct disadvantage of the balloon is that the "tactile sensation" and the "feel for resistance" used by most endoscopists as an end point for dilatation is lost during balloon dilatation. Once again, we do not know the real significance and importance of this "feel" in managing esophageal strictures. A theoretical advantage of balloon dilatation is that it dilates only the stricture instead of the entire esophagus but even the clinical significance of this is unknown (21).

When to Use Balloon?

Most investigators have used a balloon for dilatation of the benign esophageal stricture (19,20,22,39,54,55) with good technical but variable long-term clinical success. The use of a balloon in malignant esophageal strictures is limited with good technical success but poor long-term symptomatic relief (19,39). In all studies, the criteria of selection of patients for balloon dilatation have not been defined. The strictures are generally not considered dilatable by rubber bougies because of the severity of strictures such that rubber bougies are likely to curl up in the esophagus above the stricture. But the question still remains as to why balloon dilatation is preferred over Savary or American Endoscopy dilators passed over the guidewire. The randomized studies comparing these two techniques have led one to believe that strictures that can be dilated with a balloon can also be dilated with polyvinyl bougies over a guidewire. In fact, the bougie and balloon dilatation appear equally safe and acceptable to the patients (54,55). The bougie dilatation can probably be done with more ease, have better long-term success, have lower restenosis rate, and be less expensive due to longer durability (54,55).

In most studies using balloon dilatation, the esophageal strictures are less than 10 mm in diameter (22,54,55). This is interesting because a review article by Webb (3) recommends that balloons be used only when the esophageal stricture diameter is more than 12 mm. Others have recommended that balloons be used for particularly narrow or tortuous strictures and in patients who fear bougie dilatation (54). One situation where balloons may be preferred over bougies is in patients with previous gastrectomy where bougie dilatation may be difficult to accomplish due to their length. At our institution, polyvinyl bougies are used ten times more frequently than balloon dilatation for similar indications and similar stricture characteristics with physician preference and experience being the major determining factors. We believe that the use of balloon or polyvinyl bougies most likely depends upon the endoscopist's preference, level of comfort, and experience in using a particular technique and ready availability of the equipment. Based on the published literature and our own experience, we believe that most esophageal strictures that can be dilated with balloon can be also dilated with polyvinyl bougies, and that polyvinyl bougies are less expensive and more effective in relieving dysphagia for longer duration compared to balloons.

How to Use Balloons?

Although, the general principles of balloon dilatation technique are well defined in the literature (3,17, 19,20,22,54,55), the technique varies from one institution to another in terms of specific details. In general, we use the technique as described above (Technical Aspects section) in most patients who undergo balloon dilatation. The technical issues that remain ill-defined and controversial are as follows:

1. *What should be the size of the starting balloon?* Most authors consider the baseline diameter of the stricture as the major determining factor. Since most strictures treated with balloons are less than 8 to 10 mm in size, the initial balloon used is 8 to 10 mm (19,20,22,54,55). We recommend the 8- or 10-mm balloon as the starting point for all strictures less than 10 mm.

2. *How many balloons should be used during one session and what should be the size of the final balloon?* Most endoscopists have recommended that when bougies are used, the rule of three or four dilators be applied (5,57,58). This rule states that no more than three or four dilators be passed during any one session. Since most bougies are only two or three French apart, the difference between

the first bougie and the last bougie may be only 6 or 9 French (2 or 3 mm), at the most. In all case reports, case series, and randomized trials published to this date, the authors have routinely dilated esophageal strictures using three or more balloon dilators during a single session. If one uses an 8-, 10-, and a 12-mm balloon sequentially during a single session, the difference between the first dilator and the last dilator is 7 mm or 21 French. This would translate into at least ten Maloney dilators that are 2 French apart and seven Savary dilators that are 3 French apart. This is clearly what we would consider a major violation of the well-known rule of three or four that we are so religiously supposed to follow, and teach our fellows at all times. Interestingly, this issue has never been addressed in any study utilizing balloons and is also not emphasized by ASGE in their guidelines for esophageal dilatation (5). Is it all right to dilate the stricture by 21 French total increment with balloons instead of 6 to 8 French when using Maloney or Savary? Unfortunately, we do not know the answer to this question but it seems reasonable to rapidly dilate very tight strictures to 10, 12, 15, or 18 mm as long as the experience and common sense of the treating physician are all that stands between success and perforation (21). Is this safety present because of different physical principles involved in dilatation with bougies compared to balloons? The answer to this question is speculative but unknown.

3. *Is sizing of the stricture after balloon dilatation important?* The strictures can be sized to assess technical success after dilatation using either balloon or bougies (19,20). This can be accomplished by withdrawing the inflated balloon through the stricture and assessing the ease with which it can be withdrawn or by inflating the balloon within the stricture and moving it to and fro within the strictured area. It can also be assessed by passing mercury or polyvinyl dilator to assure that the balloon's diameter has been approximated. However, these maneuvers are not so reliable (21). We and others do not find it unusual to inflate the balloon within or beyond a stricture and to be able to pull that balloon through a stenosis without undue force, and the waist(s) can be seen at various levels of the balloon under fluoroscopy (21). Therefore, we consider symptomatic and objective improvement as the ultimate success and not the technical ability to dilate a stricture to a defined diameter. In our opinion, the stricture is technically dilated when the fluoroscopy shows complete absence of the waist. Since our ability to pass bougies or inflated balloon through a stricture does not necessarily mean that the stricture has been dilated to

that diameter, we do not size stricture diameters using these techniques.

4. *How long should the balloon be kept inflated in the stricture*? The duration for which the inflated balloon is maintained within the stricture varies from 10 seconds (22), to 30 to 45 seconds (18), to up to 1 minute (55). In fact, most authors do not address this issue in their techniques at all (3,4,19,20,39,54). We do not know the exact duration for which the inflation be maintained. Our practice is to maintain inflation (once the balloon is inflated to its maximal diameter or maximal psi designated for that particular balloon) for 1 minute. Based on the literature, it is not known if repeat dilatation of the stricture with the same size balloon is necessary or advantageous.

5. *Which balloon to use*? Most authors have used Rigiflex balloons for transendoscopic balloon dilatation (19,20,22,39,54,55). We use Rigiflex balloon dilators in our practice. One of the distinct advantage of Rigiflex and other similar types of dilators is their noncompliant characteristic. This means that the balloon will inflate maximally to its designated diameter only. Further inflation of the balloon will result in an increase in psi within the lumen of the balloon without resultant increase in the diameter of the balloon. Once the designated maximum psi for any given balloon is exceeded, it will simply rupture without ever increasing the diameter. This noncompliant character may not be present in other balloons that are not made of polyethylene and may result in esophageal perforation due to their high compliance (59). We prefer Rigiflex TTS balloons because they are more durable than the Eliminator by Bard, in our experience. Also, Rigiflex TTS balloons are more cost-effective since they can be used repeatedly in contrast to Eliminator balloons, which are single use only. The Wilson-Cook balloons are not ideal because of their larger shaft diameter, only two sizes of 8 and 15 mm, and the need for a guidewire.

Is it Safe to Use Balloon Dilators?

The most dreaded complication of esophageal dilatation is perforation. The overall rate of esophageal perforation related to dilatation appears to be about 0.1% to 0.3% (3–5,58). The experience with balloon dilatation is less extensive at present. Graham et al. (19,20) dilated 55 patients with benign and malignant esophageal strictures without any complications. Most patients were dilated to the 15 mm Rigiflex TTS balloon. Maynar et al. (25) performed 170 dilatations in 35 patients with three perforations (8.6%). However, the dilatations were done over a guidewire using fluoroscopy

without endoscopy and the perforations occurred when the strictures were dilated with 22- to 25-mm balloons (26). Cox et al. (54) in their randomized trial comparing balloon with bougie dilatation reported no perforations in 35 patients dilated to 20 mm using Rigiflex TTS balloons. Yamamoto et al. (60) reported one incidence of bleeding requiring no blood transfusion among 74 patients treated by Medi-Tech (Medi-Tech, Inc., Watertown, MA) balloons over the guidewire balloons. All strictures were dilated to 20 mm. Lindor et al. (18) using the Medi-Tech balloons had 3% complication (two chest pain, one minor mucosal tear) among 77 benign esophageal and 11 malignant esophageal strictures. The strictures were dilated with 12- through 22-mm balloons. Shemesh and Czerniak (55), in a randomized trial comparing Savary with balloon dilatation, performed 84 balloon dilatations using Rigiflex TTS balloons in 30 patients and reported no perforations. All strictures were dilated to 18 mm balloon diameter. Joyce et al. (22) reported respiratory depression as the only complication in 1 of 70 patients who underwent 100 dilatations using Rigiflex TTS balloons. Finally, the national survey of hydrostatic balloon dilatation of 617 patients with esophageal strictures reported an overall complication rate of 2.1% (39). Of 486 patients with reflux strictures, two had perforation and ten had hemorrhage for an overall complication rate of 2.5%. Of 95 patients with malignant esophageal strictures, none had perforation and one had hemorrhage for an overall complication rate of 1%.

From current data, it appears that the complications from balloon dilatation are uncommon and range from 0% to 2%, but the experience is still limited. As Graham has pointed out, no complications in more than 100 dilatations does not mean that the procedure is as safe as previous techniques (20,61). For example, there is a 43% probability of observing no complications in a consecutive series of 167 procedures when the real complication rate is 5/1,000 (20,62). The perforation rate may be minimized by using gradual dilatation for very tight strictures. It may not be wise to dilate all strictures to a fixed balloon diameter but common sense should be used. Parameters such as chest pain during dilatation, overlying mucosal changes, amount of blood present on the dilator, and the type of dilator are not sensitive enough to define when balloon dilatation should be terminated to minimize the risk of perforation. Other complications such as bleeding and chest pain/discomfort are more common than perforation but are not of significant consequences.

CONCLUSIONS AND RECOMMENDATIONS

Transendoscopic balloon dilatation of esophageal strictures is a significant technical advancement. While it has a definite role in dilatation of other gastrointestinal strictures such as pyloric stenosis, anastomotic stenosis, biliary strictures, and colorectal strictures, the exact role in esophageal strictures remains undefined. It may be the procedure of choice when the strictures are severe, lengthy, irregular, and complex in nature. More specifically, its choice over other devices such as over the guidewire dilators (Savary or American Endoscopy) in the management of esophageal strictures is ill defined. We and other endoscopists use balloon dilators (mostly Rigiflex TTS) on the basis of preference, experience, and availability. Immediate improvement of dysphagia occurs in most patients. Long-term efficacy remains undefined and in randomized trials appears to be significantly inferior to polyvinyl bougie dilatation. The technique is simple but many fine aspects of the technique such as balloon type, initial and final balloon size, need for assessing the technical success, and duration of balloon inflation within the stricture remain unknown. The most important thing is to use a noncompliant balloon. The goal of therapy is to provide symptomatic and objective improvement despite the final diameter of the stricture. The complication rates, including bleeding and esophageal perforation, are low but the number of patients described in the literature is small. Available data and our own experience indicate that polyvinyl bougies are easier to use, more effective in relieving dysphagia (long-term), and more cost-effective than balloon dilators. More prospective, well-controlled, randomized trials are necessary to define the exact place of balloon dilatation and its safety in the management of esophageal strictures.

ACKNOWLEDGMENT

The opinions and assertions herein are the private views of the authors and are not to be construed as reflecting the views of the Department of the Army or the Department of Defense.

REFERENCES

1. Lanza FL, Graham DY. Bougienage is effective therapy for most benign esophageal strictures. *JAMA* 1978;240:844–847.
2. Wesdorp ICE, Bartelsman JFWM, Den Hartog Jager FCA, Huibregtse K, Tytgat GN. Results of conservative treatment of benign esophageal strictures: a follow-up study in 100 patients. *Gastroenterology* 1982;82:487–493.
3. Webb WA. Esophageal dilatation: personal experience with current instruments and techniques. *Am J Gastroenterol* 1988;83:471–475.
4. Tytgat GNJ. Dilation therapy of benign esophageal stenosis. *World J Surg* 1989;13:142–148.
5. Anonymous. Esophageal dilation: guidelines for clinical application. *Gastrointest Endosc* 1991;37:122–123.
6. McClave SA, Wright RA, Brady PG. Prospective randomized study of Maloney esophageal dilation—blinded versus fluoroscopic guidance. *Gastrointest Endosc* 1990;36:272–275.
7. Grobe JL, Kozarek RA, Sanowski RA. Self-bougineage in the treatment of benign esophageal stricture. *J Clin Gastroenterol* 1984;6:109–112.
8. Kim CH, Groskreutz JL, Gehrking SJ. Recurrent benign esophageal strictures treated with self-bougienage: report of seven cases. *Mayo Clin Proc* 1990;65:799–803.
9. Puestow KL. Conservative treatment of stenosing diseases of the esophagus. *Postgrad Med* 1955;18:6–14.
10. Monnier PH, Hsieh V, Savary M. Endoscopic treatment of esophageal stenosis using Savary-Gilliard bougies: technical innovations. *Acta Endoscopica* 1985;15:1–5.
11. Dumon JF, Meric B, Sivak MV, Fleischer D. A new method of esophageal dilatation using Savary-Gilliard bougies. *Gastrointest Endosc* 1985;31:379–382.
12. Fleischer DE, Benjamin SB, Cattau EL, et al. A marked guidewire facilitates esophageal dilatation. *Am J Gastroenterol* 1989;84:359–361.
13. Kadakia SC, Cohan CF, Starnes EC. Esophageal dilation with polyvinyl bougies using a guidewire with markings without the aid of fluoroscopy. *Gastrointest Endosc* 1991;37:183–187.
14. Celestin LR, Campbell WB. A new and safe system for oesophageal dilatation. *Lancet* 1981;1:74–75.
15. Hine KR, Hawkey CJ, Atkinson M, Holmes GKT. Comparison of the Eder-Puestow and Celestin technique for dilating benign oesophageal strictures. *Gut* 1984;25:1100–1102.
16. Siegel JH, Yatto RP. Hydrostatic balloon catheters: a new dimension of therapeutic endoscopy. *Endoscopy* 1984;16:231–236.
17. Kozarek RA. Endoscopic Gruntzig balloon dilatation of gastrointestinal stenosis. *J Clin Gastroenterol* 1984;6:401–407.
18. Lindor KD, Ott BJ, Hughes RW. Balloon dilatation of upper digestive tract strictures. *Gastroenterology* 1985;89:545–548.
19. Graham DY, Smith JL. Balloon dilatation of benign and malignant esophageal strictures: blind retrograde balloon dilatation. *Gastrointest Endosc* 1985;31:171–174.
20. Graham DY, Tabibian N, Schwartz JT, Smith JL. Evaluation of the effectiveness of through-the-scope balloons as dilators of benign and malignant gastrointestinal strictures. *Gastrointest Endosc* 1987;33:432–435.
21. Kozarek RA. To stretch or to shear: a perspective on balloon dilators. *Gastrointest Endosc* 1987;33:459–461.
22. Joyce WP, Walker AJ, Rees M. Trans-endoscopic balloon dilatation of benign oesophageal strictures: a prospective study as an out-patient procedure. *J R Nav Med Serv* 1991;77:103–105.
23. Song HY, Han YM, Kim HN, Kim CS, Choi KC. Corrosive esophageal stricture: safety and effectiveness of balloon dilation. *Radiology* 1992;184:373–378.
24. Starck E, Paolucci V, Herzer M, Crummy AB. Esophageal stenosis: treatment with balloon catheters. *Radiology* 1984;153:637–640.
25. Maynar M, Guerra C, Reyes R, Mayor J, Garcia J, Facal P, Castaneda-Zuniga WR, Letourneau JG. Esophageal strictures: balloon dilation. *Radiology* 1988;167:703–706.
26. Cohen ME, Goldberg RI, Barkin JS. Esophageal strictures: balloon dilation. *Radiology* 1989;171:285–286.
27. Dawson SL, Mueller PR, Ferrucci JT, Richter JM, Schapiro RH, Butch RJ, Simeone JF. Severe esophageal strictures: indications for balloon catheter dilatation. *Radiology* 1984;153:631–635.
28. McLean GK, Cooper GS, Hartz WH, Burke DR, Meranze SG. Radiologically guided balloon dilation of gastrointestinal strictures part II: results of long-term follow-up. *Radiology* 1987;165:41–43.
29. McLean GK, Cooper GS, Hartz WH, Burke DR, Meranze SG. Radiologically guided balloon dilation of gastrointestinal strictures part I: technique and factors influencing procedural success. *Radiology* 1987;165:35–40.
30. Myer CM, Ball WS, Bisset GS. Balloon dilatation of esophageal strictures in children. *Arch Otolaryngol Head Neck Surg* 1991;117:529–532.
31. Sato Y, Frey ED, Smith WL, Pringle KC, Soper RT, Franken EA. Balloon dilatation of esophageal stenosis in children. *AJR* 1988;150:639–642.

32. Dux AEW, Hall CM, Spitz L. Balloon catheter dilatation of oesophageal strictures in children. *Br J Radiology* 1984;57:251–254.
33. Tam PKH, Sprigg A, Cudmore RE, Cook RCM, Carty H. Endoscopy-guided balloon dilatation of esophageal strictures and anastomotic strictures after esophageal replacement children. *J Pediatr Surg* 1991;26:1101–1103.
34. Goldthorn JF, Ball WS, Wilkinson LG, Seigel RS, Kosloske AM. Esophageal strictures in children: treatment by serial balloon catheter dilatation. *Radiology* 1984;153:655–658.
35. Benjamin SB, Glass RL, Cattau EL, Miller WB. Preliminary experience with balloon dilatation of pyloric stenosis. *Gastrointest Endosc* 1984;30:93–94.
36. Benjamin SB, Cattau EL, Glass RL. Balloon dilatation of the pylorus: therapy for gastric outlet obstruction. *Gastrointest Endosc* 1982;28:253–254.
37. Solt J, Rauth J, Papp Z, Bohensczky G. Balloon dilation of postoperative gastric outlet stenosis. *Gastrointest Endosc* 1984;30:359–361.
38. Hogstrom H, Haflund U. Technique of endoscopic balloon dilatation of pyloric stenosis. *Endoscopy* 1985;17:224–225.
39. Kozarek RA. Hydrostatic balloon dilation of gastrointestinal stenosis: a national survey. *Gastrointest Endosc* 1987;31:15–19.
40. Eckhauser FE, Knol JA, Strodel WE, Cho K. Hydrostatic balloon dilatation for stomal stenosis after gastric partitioning. *Surg Gastroenterol* 1984;3:43–50.
41. Bemelman WA, Brummelkamp WH, Bartelsman JFWM. Endoscopic balloon dilation of the pylorus after esophagogastrostomy without a drainage procedure. *Surgery* 1990;170:424–426.
42. Nealon WH, Beauchamp RD, Halpert R, Thompson JC. Combined endoscopic and fluoroscopic balloon dilatation of a complex proximal jejunal stricture. *Surgery* 1989;105:113–116.
43. Brower RA. Hydrostatic balloon dilatation of a terminal ileal stricture secondary to Crohn's disease. *Gastrointest Endosc* 1986;32:38–40.
44. Brower RA, Freeman LD. Balloon catheter dilation of a rectal stricture. *Gastrointest Endosc* 1984;30:95–97.
45. Ball WS Jr, Siegel RS, Goldthorn JF, Kosloske AM. Colonic strictures in infants following intestinal ischemia. Treatment by balloon catheter dilation. *Radiology* 1983;149:469–472.
46. Fregonese D, Di Falco G, Di Toma F. Balloon dilatation of anastomotic intestinal stenoses: long-term results. *Endoscopy* 1990;22:249–253.
47. Musher DR, Boyd A. Esophagocolonic stricture with proximal fistulae treated by balloon dilation. *Am J Gastroenterol* 1988;83:445–447.
48. Neufeld DM, Shemesh EL, Kodner IJ, Shatz BA. Endoscopic management of anastomotic colon strictures with electrocautery and balloon dilation. *Gastroenterol Endosc* 1987;33:24–26.
49. Bedogni G, Ricci E, Pedrazzoli C, Conigliaro R, Barbieri L, Bertoni G, Contini S, Serafini G. Endoscopic dilation of anastomotic colonic stenosis by different techniques: an alternative to surgery? *Gastroenterol Endosc* 1987;33:21–24.
50. Whitworth PW, Richardson RL, Larson GM. Balloon dilatation of anastomotic strictures. *Arch Surg* 1988;123:759–762.
51. Hoffer FA, Winter HS, Fellows KE, Folkman J. The treatment of post-operative and peptic esophageal strictures after esophageal atresia repair. *Pediatr Radiol* 1987;17:454–458.
52. Kadakia SC, Wong RKH. Graded pneumatic dilatation using Rigiflex achalasia dilators in patients with primary esophageal achalasia. *Am J Gastroenterol* 1993;88:34–38.
53. Taub S, Rodan BA, Bean W, et al. Balloon dilatation of esophageal strictures. *Am J Gastroenterol* 1986;81:14–18.
54. Cox JGC, Winter RK, Maslin SC, Jones R, Buckton GK, Hoare RC, Sutton DR, Bennett JR. Balloon or bougie for dilatation of benign oesophageal stricture? An interim report of a randomized controlled trial. *Gut* 1988;29:1741–1747.
55. Shemesh E, Czerniak A. Comparison between Savary-Gilliard and balloon dilatation of benign esophageal strictures. *World J Surg* 1990;14:518–522.
56. Aste H, Munizzi F, Saccomanno S, Pugliese V. "Splitting" and stretching dilation of esophageal strictures. *Endoscopy* 1983;15:41–43.
57. Boyce HW, Palmer ED. *Techniques of clinical gastroenterology*, section III. Springfield, IL: Charles C. Thomas, 1975.
58. Tulman AB, Boyce HW. Complications of esophageal dilation and guidelines for their prevention. *Gastrointest Endosc* 1981;27:229–234.
59. Rabinovici R, Katz E, Goldin E, et al. The danger of high compliance balloons for esophageal dilatation in achalasia. *Endoscopy* 1990;22:63–64.
60. Yamamoto H, Hughes RW, Schroeder KW, Viggiano TR, DiMagno EP. Treatment of benign esophageal stricture by Eder-Puestow or balloon dilators: a comparison between randomized and prospective nonrandomized trials. *Mayo Clin Proc* 1992;67:228–236.
61. Graham DY. Treatment of benign and malignant strictures of the esophagus. In: Silvis SE, ed. *Therapeutic gastrointestinal endoscopy*. New York: Igaku-Shoin, 1985;1–30.
62. Hanley JA, Lippman-Hand A. If nothing goes wrong, is everything all right? *JAMA* 1983;249:1743–1745.

Advanced Therapeutic Endoscopy, 2nd Ed.,
edited by J. S. Barkin and C. A. O'Phelan.
Raven Press, Ltd., New York © 1994.

CHAPTER 10

Elastic Band Ligation of Esophageal and Gastric Varices

Greg Van Stiegmann

Elastic band ligation of internal hemorrhoids was introduced by Blaisdell (1) in 1958 and refined by Barron (2) in 1963. Prior to the introduction of this technique, sclerotherapy was the most commonly employed treatment method. In North America, elastic band ligation has replaced sclerotherapy as the treatment of choice for patients with symptomatic internal hemorrhoids who fail medical treatment. Complications of elastic band ligation for internal hemorrhoids are uncommon and include delayed bleeding, ulceration, and pain (3). Several deaths have resulted from pelvic cellulitis secondary to infection at the treated site (4). Two of three prospective trials that compared elastic band ligation with sclerotherapy for treatment of hemorrhoids concluded that elastic band ligation was superior with regard to prevention of recurrent symptoms and bleeding (3,5,6). Patients treated with elastic band ligation also needed fewer treatments to achieve these goals.

In the mid-1980s our group postulated that elastic band ligation could be used to treat esophageal and gastric varices if a device to effect ligation were designed to attach to a flexible gastroscope (7). We also hypothesized, based on results of the controlled trials that compared sclerotherapy with elastic band ligation for hemorrhoids, that this new treatment could be safer and perhaps more effective than sclerotherapy when used to treat esophagogastric varices. Subsequent experimental and clinical investigation supports this thesis. This chapter presents the technique of endoscopic ligation, details the effects of this treatment, and highlights the results of clinical studies.

ENDOSCOPIC LIGATING DEVICE

The endoscopic ligating device (C. R. Bard, Tewksberry, MA) consists of an outer cylinder, an inner cylinder, a trip wire, and a latex "O" ring. The outer cylinder attaches to the end of a standard gastroscope by a friction mount. The inner cylinder is a smaller cylinder fitted with a clasp that allows insertion of the trip wire. It is constructed to fit snugly, yet slide smoothly, inside the outer cylinder. The trip wire is a monofilament strand to which a flange has been created at the distal end. Small latex "O" rings are stretched open and mounted on the inner cylinder.

The device is assembled with the endoscope by attaching the outer cylinder to the end of the instrument (Fig. 1). The trip wire is passed through the vacuum lock of the biopsy channel entry port and advanced until it exits at the distal end of the endoscope. The trip wire is secured to the clasp in the inner cylinder and the inner cylinder is then backed into the outer cylinder. The elastic band is positioned such that from 1 to 2 mm of the inner cylinder protrudes beyond the "O" ring. The "O" ring is seated against the end of the outer cylinder. The trip wire, which protrudes from the operator's end of the biopsy channel, is held on slight tension by a handle, which also serves as an extraction tool to facilitate removal of a spent inner cylinder from the outer cylinder after firing.

The endoscopic ligating device is used via an endoscopic overtube, which facilitates passage of the endoscope through the hypopharynx and allows the endoscopist to remove, reload, and reinsert the device for multiple applications. After passing the endoscope to the treatment area and identification of a target varix, the endoscope is advanced under direct vision until the inner cylinder is in contact with the target. Once full

G. Van Stiegmann: Department of Surgery, University of Colorado Health Science Center, Denver, Colorado 80262.

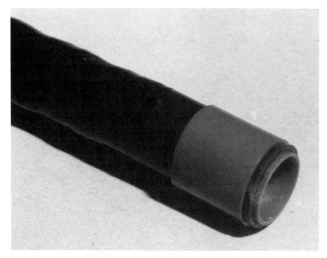

FIG. 1. The endoscopic ligating device consists of an outer cylinder that is mounted on the endoscope. An elastic "O" ring is stretched over an inner cylinder which has been backed into the outer cylinder. The trip wire (not visible) is connected to a clasp in the inner cylinder and runs via the working channel of the endoscope to the operator. The operator pulls the trip wire to move the inner cylinder toward the endoscope and eject the elastic band around the varix (see Fig. 2).

but gentle contact is made, the endoscopic suction is activated. Negative pressure draws the varix inside the inner cylinder (Fig. 2). When the target has filled the chamber the trip wire is pulled and the latex "O" ring is ejected and constricts around the base of the entrapped tissue bolus. The entrapped tissue is held inside the inner cylinder by sustained application of suction for a few moments after firing to allow the elastic band to maximally contract around the varix, after which insufflation is used to eject the varix from the inner cylinder. The ligated tissue is briefly inspected, after which the endoscope is removed and the device reloaded and reinserted to complete as many ligations as needed.

EFFECTS OF ELASTIC BAND LIGATION

Assessment of the tissue effects resulting from elastic band ligation was first done in a portal hypertensive canine model (8). Treatments were confined to the distal esophagus. Ligated varices initially blanched and become cyanotic within 3 to 7 minutes. Repeat endoscopy at 24 hours showed little change in appearance of ligated tissue boluses and all elastic "O" rings remained in place. Animals sacrificed at 24 hours posttreatment had neither bleeding nor evidence of damage to the esophageal wall. Microscopic examination of treatment sites showed ischemic necrosis of mucosa and submucosa with intact muscularis propria (Fig. 3). By days 3 to 7 there was slough at all treatment sites

with shallow (1–2 mm) ulcerations from 8 to 12 mm in length. All elastic "O" rings had been displaced at this time. Microscopic examination showed granulation tissue, sloughing necrotic tissue, and intense inflammatory reaction in the ulcer base with early scar tissue formation (Fig. 4). At 14 to 21 days there were minimal residual varices. Sites previously occupied by shallow ulcers had healed, resulting in slight depressions in the esophageal mucosa measuring from 6 to 10 mm in diameter. Microscopy showed full-thickness replacement of vascular structures in the submucosa with maturing scar tissue. Continued inflammatory response was present at this time. At 50 to 60 days treated sites maintained the appearance of shallow, smooth depressions in the esophageal mucosa. Reepithelialization was complete and the entire submucosa at treated sites was replaced by dense mature scar tissue (Fig. 5). The underlying muscular wall was consistently intact and no animals suffered clinically apparent ill effects.

Jensen and his colleagues (9–11) reported additional experimental studies comparing endoscopic ligation with sclerotherapy in a portal hypertensive canine model. Active bleeding was induced by puncture of an esophageal or gastric varix after administration of intravenous heparin. Test animals received one form of endoscopic treatment and control animals had no therapy. Active bleeding from both esophageal and gastric varices was effectively controlled with either ligation or sclerotherapy. The majority of control animals continued to bleed for periods of greater than 15 minutes. Ulceration occurred at all treatment sites in the stomach with either ligation or sclerotherapy while 90% of ligated esophageal sites ulcerated in contrast to only 10% of sites treated with sclerotherapy. Treatment-induced ulcers at the site of ligation of gastric varices were larger and deeper than those induced by sclerotherapy, but healed rapidly and resulted in diminution in size or eradication of varices.

Young et al. (12), in a controlled clinical trial, compared ulcers caused by sclerotherapy with those caused by ligation and found sclerotherapy ulcers were consistently deeper. Ligation-induced ulcers were larger in surface area and circular in shape compared to the linear lesions resulting from sclerotherapy. One hundred percent of ligation treatment sites had ulcerated at 7 days in contrast to a 90% incidence of ulceration at the sites of sclerosant injection. Ligation-induced ulcers healed in a mean of 14 days compared with a mean of 21 days for those resulting from sclerotherapy. Two of the 13 sclerotherapy treated patients developed esophageal stricture compared with none of the 10 in the ligation-treated group. Bleeding from ulcers was not observed in either cohort. These findings confirm other clinical observations that the majority of ligated sites slough and ulcerate at from 3 to 7 days

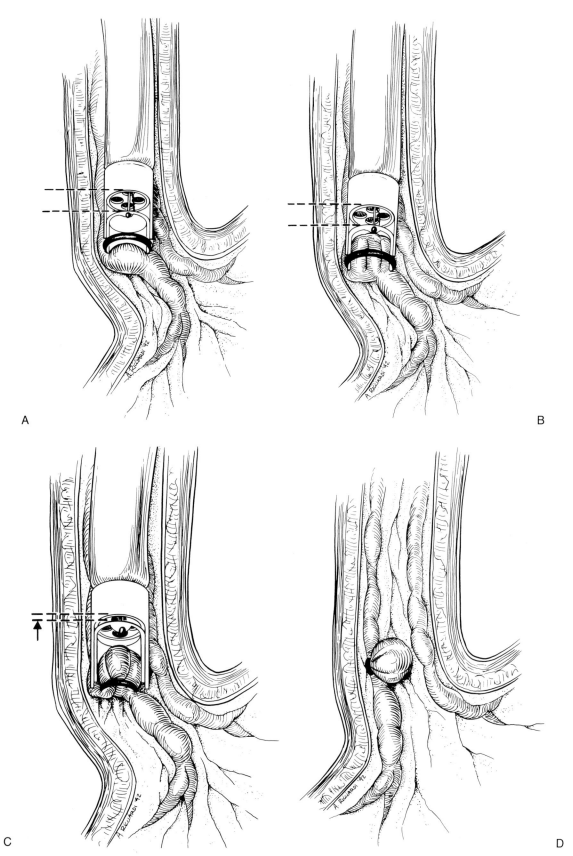

FIG. 2. A: The endoscopist makes contact between the end of the inner cylinder and the varix. **B:** Endoscopic suction is activated and draws the varix inside the inner cylinder. **C:** The trip is pulled, resulting in movement of the inner cylinder toward the endoscope and ejection of the "O" ring around the base of the target. **D:** The ligated varix. (From ref. 28, with permission.)

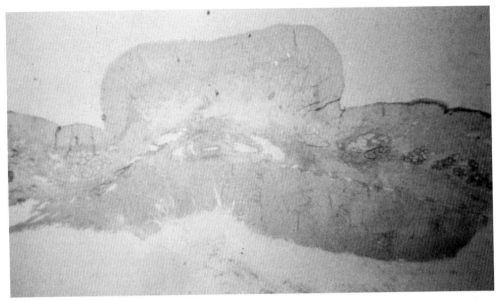

FIG. 3. Ligated canine varix at 24 hours (H & E stain, ×2). The raised necrotic area is the site of ligation. Note the presence of vascular channels and the inflammatory response in the submucosa. (From ref. 29, with permission.)

following treatment (13). Such ulcers appear associated with little risk of stricture formation.

Goff et al. (14) studied the effects of endoscopic ligation on esophageal motility and function by performing esophageal manometric examinations on patients who had undergone endoscopic ligation, on patients who had been treated with sclerotherapy, and on untreated controls who had esophageal varices. Patients treated with sclerotherapy had a greater incidence of stricture formation and less ability to relax the lower esophageal

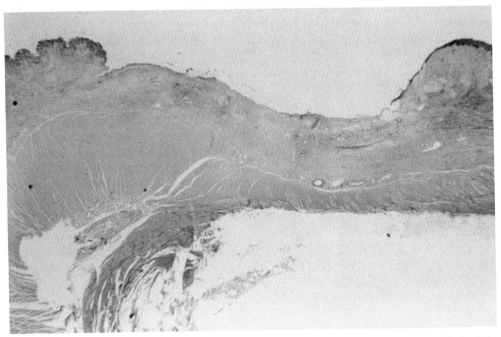

FIG. 4. Microscopic appearance of a ligated canine varix at 7 days (H & E stain, ×2). An intense inflammatory reaction is present in the submucosa and early reepithelialization is seen at the periphery of the ulcer. The muscularis propria is undisturbed. (From ref. 29, with permission.)

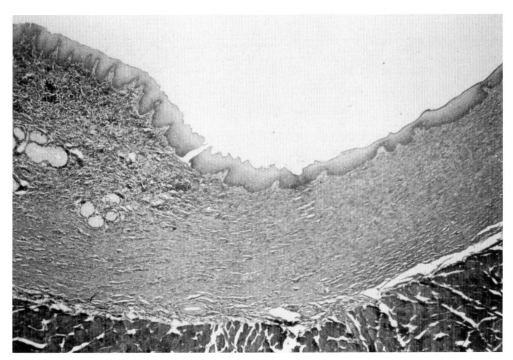

FIG. 5. Microscopic appearance of an endoscopically ligated varix at 52 days (×2). The treated site is reepithelialized and dense scar tissue has replaced the entire submucosa, obliterating both vascular channels and normal submucosal structures. The underling muscular wall is intact. (From ref. 29, with permission.)

sphincter; however, there were no persistent long-term differences between the three groups.

TECHNIQUE AND CLINICAL RESULTS OF ELASTIC BAND LIGATION

Technique

Patients with active upper gastrointestinal bleeding are stabilized and prepared as for routine emergent diagnostic endoscopic examination. Most receive intravenous sedation (usually meperidine and midazolam) and topical pharyngeal anesthesia. Complete survey examination of the esophagus, stomach, and duodenum is done. If varices are to be treated, an endoscopic overtube is inserted after completion of the survey examination. Overtube insertion is accomplished by using either the endoscope or an appropriately sized esophageal dilator as an obturator (15,16). The endoscope and attached ligating device is then inserted via the overtube.

The sequence of ligation treatment is predicated on the presence or absence of active bleeding. If a discrete site of active bleeding is identified, it should be ligated directly or, alternatively, ligation should be done immediately caudad and cephalad to the bleeding site

(Fig. 6). If active bleeding is present and no discrete bleeding site can be identified treatment is carried out as in the nonbleeding patient. Treatment begins with ligation of the largest most distal varix, usually at or just caudad to the gastroesophageal junction. Subsequent ligations are done at the same level or more cephalad until all variceal channels in the distal 5 to 7 cm of the esophagus are ligated at least once. Patients with bleeding from gastric fundal varices are probably best treated with a combination of ligation and sclerotherapy administered at the same sitting.

Combination treatment is performed by injection of sclerosant immediately following elastic band ligation of varices (17) (Fig. 7). Ligation of individual esophageal varices is first done near the gastroesophageal junction. Each variceal channel is ligated once. Intravariceal sclerotherapy is then done using 1 ml of sclerosant per varix at sites from 1 to 3 cm cephalad to the site of ligation. Combination treatment of gastric varices is done by first ligating the fundic varices, a task that usually requires the use of a retroflexed position (Fig. 8). After ligation has been done, from 1 to 5 ml of sclerosant is injected into the varix on the nonluminal side of the elastic band.

Following endoscopic ligation, patients are not given specific dietary restrictions. Those treated for bleeding gastric fundal varices are placed on the best available acid suppressing regimen to minimize the risk of auto-

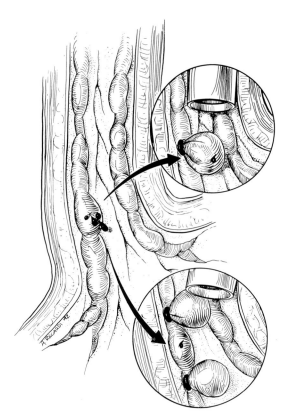

FIG. 6. Endoscopic ligation for active bleeding. If a discrete site of bleeding is identified the endoscopist may ligate the bleeding site directly *(top inset)* or ligate the varix both above and below the rent in the varix *(bottom inset).* If the site of bleeding in the distal esophagus cannot be discretely identified, all visible variceal tissue in the distal esophagus is ligated as in the elective setting. (From ref. 28, with permission.)

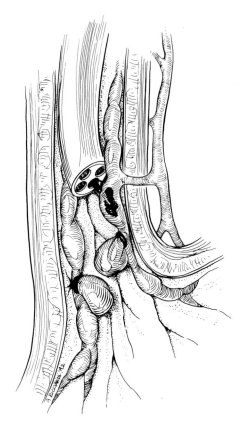

FIG. 7. Combined endoscopic ligation and low-volume sclerotherapy. After ligation of varices at the gastro-esophageal junction, 1 ml of sclerosant is injected into each varix at a distance of 1 to 2 cm cephalad to the ligation site. (From ref. 28, with permission.)

digestion of the ligated tissue with subsequent early slough and bleeding. Repeat ligation treatments aimed at eradication of varices are done at 7- to 14-day intervals until varices channels in the distal esophagus (or gastric fundus) are obliterated. Elective repeat treatments are done on an outpatient basis.

Results

Actively Bleeding Varices

One controlled trial of sclerotherapy versus endoscopic ligation and two uncontrolled studies suggest that elastic band ligation is effective treatment for actively bleeding varices. Our group treated 23 actively bleeding patients and achieved 72-hour control of hemorrhage in 96% (18). Rebleeding within 30 days occurred in 18% and overall survival was 61% at 9 months with all deaths occurring in Child class B and C patients.

Saeed et al. (19) treated ten actively bleeding patients

who had failed endoscopic sclerotherapy (mean 4.5 prior sclerotherapy sessions) and achieved early control in 90%. Rebleeding occurred in six patients by 90 days follow-up and was controlled again by ligation in five of the six. Survival was 67% at follow-up ranging to 22 months with all deaths occurring in Child class B and C patients.

A multicenter controlled trial treated 13 actively bleeding patients with sclerotherapy and 14 with elastic band ligation (20). Definitive control of active bleeding was 77% and 86%, respectively. These and the data above suggest elastic band ligation is equal to sclerotherapy for control of active bleeding.

Prevention of Recurrent Variceal Bleeding

Elastic band ligation was used to treat 146 consecutive cirrhotic patients with bleeding esophageal varices (21). Retreatment was done at 7- to 14-day intervals until distal esophageal varices were eradicated. A total of 114 patients survived initial hospitalization; 65 (57%) had 72 episodes of recurrent bleeding. Overall survival was 73%. Eighty percent of the patients who remained

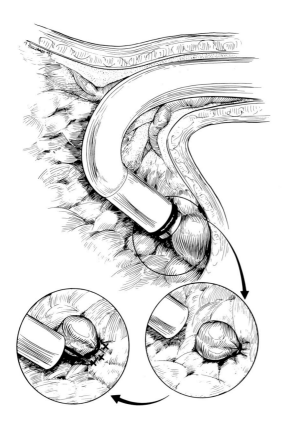

FIG. 8. Endoscopic elastic band ligation of gastric fundal varices. Treatment is done in a retroflexed position with initial ligation of all visible varices *(right inset).* After removing the ligating device from the endoscope, sclerosant is injected into the varix *(left inset).* Injections into the varix are done on the serosal side of the elastic band and sclerosant volume is limited to 5 ml per varix.

Four controlled trials comparing sclerotherapy with elastic band ligation are concluded or ongoing (5,12,20,22,23). Data from these trials are summarized in Table 1. Results to date support elastic band ligation as equal or superior to sclerotherapy in all outcome variables. Moreover, the new treatment appears to be associated with significantly fewer nonbleeding complications. The greater incidence of pulmonary complications in sclerotherapy treated patients in the multi-center study suggests a beneficial effect of ligation over sclerotherapy in this regard (20). Alternatively, fewer pulmonary complications in ligation patients may have resulted from prevention of tracheal aspiration by use of the endoscopic overtube, which in this trial was employed only in the group treated with ligation. The incidence of pulmonary complications (pneumonias) at interim analysis is similar in both the ligation and sclerotherapy arms of the Los Angeles study in which both cohorts were treated using an overtube, thus suggesting use of the overtube may prevent some pulmonary problems (22).

A trend toward fewer episodes of recurrent bleeding in patients treated with ligation has been observed in all of the controlled trial to date. This finding, along with fewer deaths from infection-related complications, contributed to improved survival in ligation treated patients in the multicenter trial. The lower incidence of recurrent bleeding in ligation treated patients may result from greater efficiency of ligation at eradication of varices. Fewer numbers of treatments (one to two fewer per patient) were required to eradicate varices in three of the four trials. This advantage of elastic band ligation may provide both outcome and economic advantages over sclerotherapy.

Combined Elastic Band Ligation and Sclerotherapy

Forty-six patients were enrolled in a pilot study of combination endoscopic ligation and low-volume sclerotherapy administered synchronously (17). Eradica-

in the study more than 30 days had varices eradicated from the distal esophagus with a mean of 5.5 treatment sessions. During the course of this study, there were four nonbleeding complications that required treatment: two esophageal strictures (single bougienage each), one meat impaction, and one patient with dysphagia that lasted for 36 hours.

TABLE 1. *Results from four prospective randomized trials comparing endoscopic ligation with endoscopic sclerotherapy*

Study	Patients	Therapy	Number rebled	Mean number Rx to eradicate[a]	% Survival	% Complications[b]
Multicenter (20)	65	ES	48%	5	55%*	22%*
	64	EVL	36%	4	72%*	2%*
El-Newihi et al. (22)	19	ES	37%	6*	95%	68%*
	20	EVL	25%	4*	95%	25%*
Westaby (24)	40	ES	53%	5*	NA	NA
	48	EVL	32%	3*	NA	NA
Young et al. (12)	13	ES	NA	6*	92%	15%
	10	EVL	NA	4*	90%	0

ES, endoscopic sclerotherapy; EVL, endoscopic variceal ligation.
[a] Mean number of treatments needed to eradicate esophageal varices.
[b] Nonbleeding complications requiring active treatment.
* $p < .05$.

tion of esophageal varices was accomplished with a mean of approximately two treatment sessions. Ulcerations at the site of ligation and sclerosant injection were seen in most patients within the first few days of treatment but resulted in few adverse effects. The overall rebleeding rate with mean follow-up of 8 months was 30%, with only one death resulting from hemorrhage. Serious complications associated with combination ligation sclerotherapy in this trial included one proximal esophageal perforation and two cases of spontaneous bacterial peritonitis.

Data from a French prospective randomized trial that compared endoscopic ligation with combined ligation and sclerotherapy confirmed findings in the above study and found eradication of varices could be accomplished with a mean of 1.2 combined ligation and sclerotherapy treatments in contrast to a mean of 4.4 treatments to eradicate using sclerotherapy alone (24). Hashizume et al. (25) described the use of endoscopic ligation as initial treatment followed by subsequent sclerotherapy. The design of this trial underscores an observation made by many who have used endoscopic ligation: smaller varices are harder to ligate than larger ones. Patients treated with this metachronous combination therapy were selected randomly and prospectively compared with a group treated by sclerotherapy alone. Most patients had not bled from varices and were treated to prevent a first bleed. The initial ligation treatment was followed at weekly intervals by sclerotherapy to obliterate residual varices. Patients treated with this regimen required less sclerosant to eradicate varices and had fewer complications such as renal and pulmonary insufficiency, fever, pain, and pleural effusion than those treated with sclerotherapy alone. It stands to reason that use of less sclerosant should result in fewer sclerosant-related complications and this group has taken advantage of thrombosis and venous stasis induced by elastic band ligation to enhance the effects and minimize complications of subsequent sclerotherapy. More efficient eradication of varices may be possible with combined ligation and sclerotherapy. Determination of the optimal combination of these methods and the best time sequencing (synchronous vs. metachronous treatment) is needed.

A small number of patients with bleeding gastric fundal varices have been treated with elastic band ligation and with combination ligation sclerotherapy (*unpublished data*). Initial attempts to treat gastric varices with ligation alone resulted in early rebleeding as the devitalized ligated tissue was rapidly autodigested in spite of optimal acid suppression. In subsequent cases, the use of sclerotherapy immediately following ligation (as described above) resulted in several gratifying responses with complete elimination of fundal varices. The small number of patients treated precludes drawing firm conclusions. I believe that some patients with

bleeding fundal varices can be controlled and successfully treated using endoscopic methods. On the other hand, when recurrent hemorrhage from fundal varices does occur, it is often torrential. Combined elastic band ligation and sclerotherapy is probably best used as an interim measure to halt acute bleeding while semi-elective preparations are made for more definitive control by either surgical or radiological shunt insertion.

Complications Associated with Elastic Band Ligation

Complications of elastic band ligation can be classified in two categories: those resulting from elastic band ligation and its subsequent tissue effects, and those from use of the overtube. Three published case reports describe mechanical complications caused by introduction of the overtube. These mishaps consisted of partial or complete esophageal perforations or trauma causing bleeding. Berkelhammer et al. (15) and Goldschmiedt et al. (16) concluded that overtube trauma was usually caused by "pinching" of the esophageal wall in the gap between the overtube and the endoscope when the latter was used as an obturator to facilitate introduction. The optimal solution to this problem is use of an esophageal dilator that completely fills the lumen of the overtube as the obturator to facilitate introduction into the esophagus.

Complications directly related to endoscopic ligation, in contrast to those from the overtube, are less common. Saltzman and Arora (26) report transient obstruction of the esophagus by boluses of ligated tissue. We observed one such case and concluded that a combination of the tissue boluses and distal esophageal spasm were to blame. The distal esophagus in our patient was tightly closed and an endoscope could not pass, but symptoms of dysphagia resolved without treatment. Transient distal esophageal spasm at the site of either ligation or sclerosant injection is not uncommon and may contribute to hemostasis in patients treated for active bleeding.

Johnson et al. (27) report bleeding from a ligation-induced esophageal ulcer. There is no question a finite risk of bleeding from such ulcers exists, but what is the magnitude of the risk? The controlled clinical trials comparing ligation with sclerotherapy have shown a trend toward a lower incidence of recurrent hemorrhage (from all causes) for patients treated with ligation. (12,20,22,23) The observed incidence of hemorrhage from treatment-induced ulcers in the multicenter trial was 6% and 8% for sclerotherapy- and ligation-treated patients, respectively—a similar risk of iatrogenic bleeding for each (20).

SUMMARY

Endoscopic elastic band ligation for bleeding esophageal varices is a new form of endoscopic treatment based on principles developed for elastic band ligation of internal hemorrhoids. Experimental studies have shown ligation results in replacement of submucosal structures, including varices, with scar tissue resulting in eradication of varices. Clinical studies have shown ligation results in consistent shallow ulceration at each treatment site. Such ulcers appear to have no greater propensity to bleed than ulcers induced by sclerotherapy and cause few esophageal strictures and no measurable effects on esophageal motility and function. Elastic band ligation appears equal in efficacy to sclerotherapy for control of active bleeding from esophageal varices. Ligation appears equal or superior to sclerotherapy for long-term prevention of recurrent variceal bleeding in all outcome variables and results in significantly fewer treatment-related complications. The combination of elastic band ligation with sclerotherapy, either synchronously or with metachronous application of the latter, may produce results superior to those obtainable with either treatment used alone.

REFERENCES

1. Blaisdell PC. Office ligation of internal hemorrhoids. *Am J Surg* 1958;96:401–404.
2. Barron J. Office ligation of internal hemorrhoids. *Am J Surg* 1963;105:563–567.
3. Greca F, Hares MM, Nevah E, et al. A randomized trial to compare rubber band ligation with phenol injection for treatment of hemorrhoids. *Br J Surg* 1981;68:250–252.
4. Russell TR, Donohue JH. Hemorrhoidal banding: a warning. *Dis Colon Rectum* 1985;28:291–293.
5. Gartell PC, Sheridan RJ, McGinn FP. Out-patient treatment of haemorrhoids: a randomized clinical trial to compare rubber band ligation with phenol injection. *Br J Surg* 1985;72:478–479.
6. Sim AJ, Murie JA, MacKenzie I. Three year follow up study on the treatment of first and second degree hemorrhoids by sclerosant injection or band ligation. *Surg Gynecol Obstet* 1983;157:534–536.
7. Stiegmann GV, Cambre T, Sun J. A new endoscopic elastic band ligating device. *Gastrointest Endosc* 1986;32:230–233.
8. Stiegmann GV, Sun JH, Hammond WS. Results of experimental endoscopic esophageal varix ligation. *Am Surg* 1988;54:105–108.
9. Egan J, Jensen DM, Hirabayashi K, et al. Randomized controlled study of endoscopic rubber band ligation and high volume sclerotherapy for actively bleeding gastric varices in dogs. *Gastrointest Endosc* 1991;37:239(abst).
10. Jensen DM, Weisz N, Hirabayashi K, et al. Randomized controlled study of rubber band ligation and sclerotherapy for active esophageal varix bleeding in dogs. *Gastroenterology* 1991;100:A92.
11. Jutabha R, Jensen D, Egan J, et al. Randomized prospective study of cyanoacrylate, sclerotherapy, or rubber band ligation for endoscopic hemostasis of bleeding canine gastric varices. *Gastrointest Endosc* 1992;38:235(abst).
12. Young M, Sanowski R, Rasche R. Comparison and characterization of ulcerations induced by endoscopic ligation of esophageal varices versus endoscopic sclerotherapy. *Gastrointest Endosc* 1993;in press.
13. Stiegmann GV, Goff JS, Sun JH, et al. Technique and clinical results of endoscopic variceal ligation (EVL). *Surg Endosc* 1989;3:73–78.
14. Goff JS, Reveille RM, Stiegmann GV. Endoscopic sclerotherapy versus endoscopic variceal ligation: esophageal symptoms, complications, and motility. *Am J Gastroenterol* 1988;83:1240–1244.
15. Berkelhammer C, Madhav G, Lyon S, et al. "Pinch" injury during overtube placement in upper endoscopy. *Gastrointest Endosc* 1993;in press.
16. Goldschmiedt M, Haber G, Kandel G, et al. A safety maneuver for placing overtubes during endoscopic variceal ligation. *Gastrointest Endosc* 1992;38:399–400.
17. Reveille RM, Goff JS, Stiegmann GV, et al. Combination endoscopic variceal ligation (EVL) and low volume sclerotherapy (ES) for bleeding esophageal varices: a faster route to variceal eradication? *Gastrointest Endosc* 1991;37:243(abst).
18. Stiegmann GV, Goff JS, Sun JH, et al. Endoscopic elastic band ligation for active variceal hemorrhage. *Am Surg* 1989;55:124–128.
19. Saeed Z, Michaletz P, Winchester C, et al. Endoscopic variceal ligation in patients who have failed sclerotherapy. *Gastrointest Endosc* 1990;36:572–574.
20. Stiegmann G, Goff J, Michaletz-Onody P, et al. Endoscopic sclerotherapy as compared with endoscopic ligation for bleeding esophageal varices. *N Engl J Med* 1992;326:1527–1532.
21. Goff JS. Endoscopic variceal ligation. *Can J Gastroenterol* 1990;4:639–642.
22. El-Newihi H, Migikovsky B, Laine L. A prospective randomized comparison of sclerotherapy and ligation for the treatment of bleeding esophageal varices. *Gastroenterology* 1991;100:A59(abst).
23. Westaby D. Prevention of recurrent variceal bleeding: endoscopic techniques. *Gastroenterol Endosc Clin North Am* 1992;2:121–136.
24. Koutsomanis D. Endoscopic variceal ligation combined with low volume sclerotherapy: a controlled study. *Gastroenterology* 1992;(102):A835(abst).
25. Hashizume M, Ohta M, Ueno K, et al. Endoscopic ligation of esophageal varices significantly reduces adverse effects of injection sclerotherapy. *Gastrointest Endosc* 1993;39:in press.
26. Saltzman J, Arora S. Complications of esophageal variceal band ligation. *Gastrointest Endosc* 1993;39:in press.
27. Johnson P, Campbell D, Antonson C, et al. Complications associated with endoscopic ligation of esophageal varices. *Gastrointest Endosc* 1993;in press.
28. Stiegmann GV. Endoscopic management of esophageal varices. In: Cameron JL ed. *Advances in surgery.* Chicago: Mosby Year Book, 1993;in press.
29. Stiegmann GV, Sun JH, Hammond W. Results of experimental endoscopic varix ligation. *Am Surg* 1988;54:113–118.

Advanced Therapeutic Endoscopy, 2nd Ed.,
edited by J. S. Barkin and C. A. O'Phelan.
Raven Press, Ltd., New York © 1994.

CHAPTER 11

Endoscopic Injection Sclerotherapy for Bleeding Esophageal and Gastric Varices

Rome Jutabha and Dennis M. Jensen

Various medical and surgical modalities are available for the treatment of bleeding and nonbleeding esophagogastric varices. These treatments include pharmacologic agents [vasopressin or vasopressin plus nitroglycerin (1), somatostatin (2,3), beta-blockers (4)], mechanical tamponade [Sengstaken-Blakemore or Linton tubes (5–7)], surgery [portosystemic shunting (8), devascularization and nondecompressive shunting (9), and liver transplantation (10–12)], angiography [transjugular intrahepatic portosystemic shunting (13)] and therapeutic endoscopy [rubber band ligation (14,15), injection sclerotherapy (16,17)] interventions. These different methods were originally developed and studied for control of esophageal variceal bleeding and more recently have been applied to gastric varices.

Endoscopic injection sclerotherapy was first introduced in 1939 by Crafoord and Frenckner (18) using a rigid esophagoscope, but did not gain widespread popularity until the advent of the flexible endoscope. Worldwide, endoscopic sclerotherapy is the most common primary therapy of bleeding esophageal varices during emergency or elective endoscopy. Therefore, this chapter focuses on the role of endoscopic injection sclerotherapy for the acute treatment of actively bleeding and nonbleeding esophagogastric varices as well as for obliteration of varices in long-term follow-up. The differences between esophageal and gastric varices will be reviewed in terms of their different prevalence, anatomic and histologic location, etiology, and natural history. Varices can occur in any segment of the gastroin-

testinal tract including the duodenum, jejunum, ileum, colon, and rectum (19–26). Ectopic varices are uncommon and account for less than 5% of all variceal bleeding and will not be discussed.

The following aspects of endoscopic injection sclerotherapy for esophagogastric varices will be reviewed: (a) advantages and drawbacks, (b) objectives of treatment, (c) efficacy of treatment, (d) injection technique and sclerosant regimen, and (e) side effects and complications. Data from the Center for Ulcer Research and Education (CURE) Hemostasis Research Group randomized trials of endoscopic injection sclerotherapy versus rubber band ligation (RBL) of esophagogastric varices will be summarized. Current CURE endoscopic injection techniques and sclerosant regimen will also be presented.

ESOPHAGEAL AND GASTRIC VARICES

Prevalence

Esophageal varices are more common than gastric varices. Gastric varices are usually associated with esophageal varices, but can occur as an isolated finding (27). The incidence of gastric varices in portal hypertensive patients with esophageal varices has been reported to be as low as 2% to as high as 100% (28). This wide variability is probably due to differences in patient populations and diagnostic criteria between series (29). In a study of 230 patients with esophageal and/or gastric varices using portal vein catheterization, gastric varices were present in 57% of patients (30). In a series of 568 patients with portal hypertension, 114 (20%) patients had primary (present on initial exam) gastric varices (28). Secondary gastric varices devel-

R. Jutabha and D. M. Jensen: Department of Medicine, Division of Gastroenterology, University of California, Los Angeles Center for the Health Sciences, Center for Ulcer Research and Education (CURE); and the West Lost Angeles Veterans Administration Medical Center, Los Angeles, California 90024-1684.

oped in 33 (6%) patients following sclerotherapy of esophageal varices.

Gastric varices account for 20% to 30% of esophagogastric variceal bleeding. In a series of 151 patients admitted with bleeding esophagogastric varices, 108 patients (72%) had bleeding esophageal varices and 33 patients (22%) had bleeding gastric varices documented by endoscopy (5). Gastric varices are five times more prevalent in bleeders than in nonbleeders, indicative of more advanced portal hypertension in gastric varices patients (28). Moreover, mortality related to bleeding gastric varices is disproportionately high. Therefore, although gastric varices are less common than esophageal varices, they are responsible for a significant proportion of variceal bleeding and mortality.

Anatomic and Histologic Location

Esophageal varices can be present throughout the entire length of esophagus, but are usually located in the distal 5 cm of esophagus. In elegant studies of the lower esophageal and upper gastric venous vasculature, Vianna et al. (31) utilized radiographic, morphometric, and corrosion cast techniques to delineate the histologic and functional anatomy of blood flow in the gastroesophageal region. The venous channels within this region of the esophagus are divided into two zones, the palisade and perforating zones. The palisade zone starts at the gastroesophageal junction (GEJ) and extends 2 to 3 cm up the esophagus. Blood flow in this zone is bidirectional, down into the gastric zone (portal system) and up into the perforating zone. The perforating zone extends 3 to 5 cm above the GEJ. Bleeding from esophageal varices most often occurs within this region. Therefore, treatments for active bleeding as well as elective esophageal variceal obliteration are targeted in this area. Esophageal varices in this area are located superficially in the lamina propria of the esophageal mucosa. Thus, deep injections are rarely required for adequate variceal sclerosis. In fact, deep injections are associated with higher complication rates and therefore should be avoided.

In contrast, gastric varices may involve any part of the stomach including the fundus, cardia, corpus, and antrum. Gastric varices occurring just below the GEJ are termed *junctional varices* (32). Massive gastric variceal bleeding can result in pooling of blood or clots, which will obscure large portions of the stomach. In addition, gastric varices often mimic normal rugal folds of the stomach. These factors can make localization of the bleeding gastric varix quite difficult. Gastric varices can sometimes be distinguished from rugal folds by air insufflation, which flattens rugal folds but not gastric varices. Endoscopic ultrasound more reliably establishes this diagnosis (33,34).

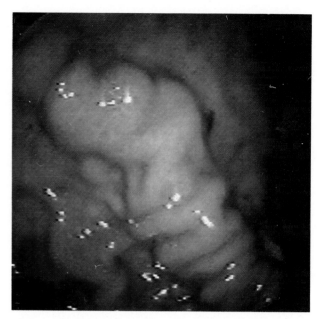

FIG. 1. Endoscopic appearance of fundal gastric varices with an adherent clot seen on turnaround.

Gastric varices are situated more deeply in the submucosa than esophageal varices. Gastric varices tend to be larger than esophageal varices and can become nodular or polypoid in appearance (Figs. 1 and 2). Therefore, deeper injections with larger amounts of sclerosants are often required for gastric varices to achieve adequate tamponade and variceal sclerosis as compared to esophageal varices. Also, gastric varices may widely branch and involve large areas of the stom-

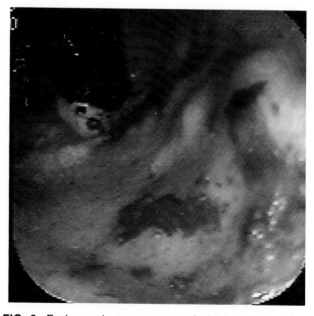

FIG. 2. Endoscopic appearance of giant gastric varices in the body of the stomach just above the angularis.

ach. Gastric varices are usually located in the gastric cardia or fundus (28,32), although in one series utilizing splenoportography, gastric varices were found more commonly along the lesser curvature of the stomach (35).

Etiology

Both esophageal and gastric varices develop as a consequence of portal hypertension. The causes of portal hypertension are multifactorial and can result from prehepatic, hepatic, and posthepatic pathology. The pathogenesis and natural history of portal hypertension and subsequent development of esophageal varices have been extensively studied and will not be discussed in this chapter (36,37).

In contrast, the pathogenesis of gastric varices is not well elucidated. Gastric varices can occur with esophageal varices in the setting of systemic portal hypertension, termed *primary varices*. Secondary gastric varices can subsequently develop following endoscopic injection sclerotherapy and obliteration of esophageal varices (28). Isolated gastric varices can develop as a result of segmental portal hypertension (in the absence of cirrhosis) due to splenic vein thrombosis related to pancreatic carcinoma or pancreatitis (38,39). Gastric varices are more common in segmental portal hypertension due to extrahepatic portal vein obstruction than in portal hypertension due to cirrhosis (28). This has been attributed to more direct transmission of portal hypertension to the short gastric and posterior gastric veins (28). For isolated gastric varices secondary to nonmetastatic disease causing splenic vein thrombosis, splenectomy cures segmental portal hypertension and is therefore the procedure of choice.

Natural History of Gastric Varices

Gastric varices develop as a result of advanced cirrhosis at a later stage of systemic portal hypertension than esophageal varices. Two large series of patients have reported the natural history of esophagogastric varices. Korula et al. (32) reported a series of 170 patients undergoing endoscopic sclerotherapy of gastroesophageal varices. Gastric varices were noted in 26 (15.3%) patients. Two distinct types of gastric varices were classified based on their differing anatomic location and responsiveness to sclerotherapy: (a) junctional varices were defined as varices near the gastroesophageal junction, no more than 2 cm below the squamocolumnar junction and diaphragmatic hiatus; and (b) fundal varices were defined as varices confined to the fundus with channels extending distal to the GEJ. Junctional and fundal gastric varices were found in 11.2% and 4.1% of patients, respectively. In compar-

ison to patients with esophageal varices, patients with fundal varices had a higher risk of rebleeding and of developing sclerotherapy-induced complications, and had decreased survival. Patients with junctional varices followed a similar course to patients with esophageal varices in terms of responsiveness to sclerotherapy and cumulative survival (32).

These results were supported by the most recent and largest endoscopic series of gastric varices to date of 568 patients with portal hypertension (28). Sarin et al. (28) prospectively followed and treated esophagogastric varices with endoscopic injection sclerotherapy. They classified gastric varices into four different types based on their anatomic location: gastroesophageal varices types 1 and 2, and isolated gastric varices types 1 and 2. Gastroesophageal varices are gastric varices found in association with esophageal varices, whereas isolated gastric varices are gastric varices occurring in the absence of esophageal varices (Fig. 3). Primary gastric varices that presented on initial endoscopy were also distinguished and compared to secondary varices that developed after sclerotherapy of esophageal varices.

Gastroesophageal varices extend from the esophagus to 2 to 5 cm below the GEJ along the lesser curvature. Gastroesophageal varices type 2 are more extensive than type 1 and extend beyond the GEJ into the fundus of the stomach. Gastroesophageal varices type

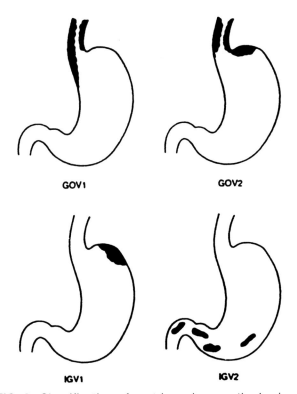

FIG. 3. Classification of gastric varices on the basis of location and relationship with esophageal varices. (Reprinted with permission, from ref. 28.)

1 are analogous to junctional varices in Korula et al.'s (32) classification. Isolated gastric varices type 1 are located in the fundus of the stomach and do not involve the cardia. Korula et al. termed these fundal varices. Isolated gastric varices type 2 or ectopic gastric varices can involve any other part of the stomach such as the body, antrum, or pylorus. Each type is said to have different natural histories and different responses to endoscopic sclerotherapy with combined paravariceal and intravariceal injections of absolute alcohol.

Gastroesophageal varices type 1 are the most common type, accounting for 75% of all primary gastric varices. They have a relatively benign course and require injection treatment only if they bleed or persist after 6 months following esophageal variceal bleeding. Gastroesophageal varices type 2 are more likely to bleed than gastroesophageal varices type 1 (55% versus 12%) and carry a slightly higher mortality. Sclerotherapy was effective for controlling active bleeding (70%) and for gastric variceal obliteration (54%). Isolated gastric varices type 1 are the rarest type of gastric varices occurring in only 1.6% of patients but they carry the highest risk of bleeding (73–78%). Because of this high risk of bleeding, Sarin et al. (28) recommended surgical therapy for this particular type of gastric varices. Isolated gastric varices type 1 occurred only as primary gastric varices. In contrast, isolated gastric varices type 2 or ectopic gastric varices are more often secondary (5%) than primary (0.5%), developing as a late consequence 1½ years after esophageal variceal obliteration. Bleeding from isolated gastric varices type 2 is said to be rare.

Gastric varices have a lower bleeding risk factor than esophageal varices (2.0 ± 0.5 versus 4.3 ± 0.4) (28). However, once bleeding occurs, gastric varices bleed more profusely, and require a greater number of transfusions than esophageal varices (4.8 versus 2.9 units). Furthermore, gastric variceal bleeding is more difficult to diagnose and control endoscopically. There is a higher mortality rate associated with gastric variceal bleeding than with esophageal variceal bleeding. The severity of liver dysfunction is the major determinant of survival in patients with either gastric and/or esophageal varices due to cirrhosis.

ENDOSCOPIC INJECTION SCLEROTHERAPY

Advantages and Drawbacks

Advantages of Endoscopic Injection Sclerotherapy

Over the past 15 to 20 years, numerous studies have confirmed the efficacy and safety of endoscopic injection sclerotherapy for acute hemostasis of bleeding esophageal varices as well as for decreasing the rate

TABLE 1. Efficacy of endoscopic injection sclerotherapy

Setting	Treatment goal	Degree of efficacy	
		Esophageal varices	Gastric varices
Prophylactic	Prevent first bleed	−	?
Emergency	Arrest active bleeding	+ + +	+ +
Elective	Prevent recurrent bleeding	+ +	+

−, not effective; +, slightly effective; + +, moderately effective; + + +, very effective; ?, efficacy unknown.

of rebleeding. Endoscopic injection sclerotherapy can achieve definitive hemostasis unlike pharmacologic and mechanical modalities, which are effective only in the short term (5,6,40). Surgical and radiologic treatments are highly dependent on the skill and experience of the surgeon or radiologist, and are usually performed only at large medical institutions. Portosystemic shunting is associated with a higher rate of encephalopathy. Moreover, these procedures are very costly in comparison to endoscopic injection sclerotherapy (41). Emergency sclerotherapy has been shown to save significantly more lives than medical therapy (42).

Endoscopic injection sclerotherapy has advantages of established efficacy and safety, low cost, ease of learning the technique, ease and rapidity of use, wide availability, and can be performed in the outpatient setting for elective (obliteration) treatment (Table 1). Additionally, sclerotherapy can also be combined with other medical or surgical therapies in selected patients. Some of the best results for survival in any randomized trial were in the Emory study when surgery was used as a backup or salvage for patients who failed sclerotherapy (43).

Drawbacks of Endoscopic Injection Sclerotherapy

The advantages of endoscopic injection sclerotherapy over other modalities for treatment of esophagogastric varices far outweigh the disadvantages. The few drawbacks of endoscopic injection sclerotherapy relate to potential complications of treatment. These complications include local effects (ulceration, bleeding, stricture, perforation) as well as systemic effects (bacteremia, sepsis, pleural effusion). These will be discussed in more detail later. For emergency sclerotherapy (to control active variceal bleeding) or elective sclerotherapy (to prevent rebleeding), the benefits of sclerotherapy far outweigh the risks if performed by a skilled endoscopist. However, patients treated with prophylactic sclerotherapy had poorer outcomes than the medically treated patients because of significant complications due to injection therapy (44,45).

Two randomized trials comparing rubber band ligation to sclerotherapy for esophageal varices concluded that variceal ligation was superior to sclerotherapy. The total number of endoscopies until variceal obliteration, the number of pulmonary complications, and the stricture rate were higher for the sclerotherapy group (14,15). However, most of these differences in results for sclerotherapy versus banding may be explained by differences in endoscopic techniques. These different factors include (a) the use of an overtube for variceal ligation that decreases the risk of pulmonary aspiration, as demonstrated in the Laine compared to the Stiegmann trials; (b) the very high incidence of esophageal stricture formation (almost 35%) in the Laine sclerotherapy series, which is much higher than other studies such as ours where the rate is less than 10%; (c) sclerotherapy sessions were not performed when postinjection ulcers were present in the Laine series; and (d) the injections of sclerosant were limited by volume (Stiegmann series) or other factors such as ulcers (Laine series) so that varix obliteration was slower. These nontherapeutic endoscopies were counted as part of the total number of endoscopies required for variceal obliteration.

In our experience, differences in outcomes between banding and sclerotherapy can be eliminated or significantly reduced by standardizing the techniques. Endotracheal intubation for airway protection in selected patients (with altered mental status, ongoing hematemesis, or respiratory compromise) will decrease the risk

of aspiration pneumonia. The number of endoscopies for varix obliteration is also reduced if sclerotherapy is continued with each endoscopy, unless confluent ulcers are present. The complication rate for postsclerotherapy strictures is less than 10% using our sclerosant treatment guidelines and schedule as outlined in Table 2. Furthermore, there is approximately a 20% advantage in efficacy of emergency sclerotherapy versus banding for hemostasis of severe acute bleeding from esophageal or gastric varices (46,47). Nevertheless, variceal ligation is a promising technique that is gaining widespread popularity, especially for elective cases.

Goals of Therapy

Prior to and during endoscopic treatment of esophagogastric varices, the patient must be resuscitated and stabilized. The objectives of endoscopic treatment for esophagogastric varices are (a) control of acute bleeding, (b) minimization of therapy-induced complications, and (c) prevention of further rebleeding episodes.

Patient Resuscitation and Stabilization

The importance of adequate resuscitation prior to diagnostic and therapeutic endoscopy cannot be overemphasized (48). Adequate intravascular volume replacement with IV fluids and blood products are vital to minimizing endoscopy-related mortality. The major-

TABLE 2. CURE endoscopic injection sclerotherapy technique for bleeding esophageal and gastric varices

	Esophageal varices	Gastric varices
Needle size (gauge)	25	25
Needle length (mm)	4–5	6–7
Sclerosant		
Agent	TES	TEE
Amount/injection (cc)	2	2–4
Maximum volume (cc)	<50[a]	<30[b]
Injection site		
Initial Rx	Bleeding focus	Bleeding focus
Concomitant Rx	Each EV at GEJ then 2.5 and 5.0 cm above GEJ	Two adjacent GV
Follow-up Rx	Residual EV in the distal 5 cm	Residual GV at previous Rx site
Adjuvant therapy (mg)	Ranitidine 150 b.i.d.	Omeprazole 20 q.d.–b.i.d.
Treatment interval (until obliteration)	1 week after initial Rx, then once every 2–3 weeks	1 week after initial Rx, then once every 2–3 weeks

[a] Maximum volume for esophageal refers to volume to inject all distal esophageal varices at GEJ and 2½ cm, and 5 cm above the GEJ during first sclerotherapy session.
[b] Maximum volume for gastric variceal sclerotherapy refers to the total volume to control the active bleeding of one gastric varix and to also inject the two adjacent gastric varices.
CURE, Center for Ulcer Research and Education; UCLA School of Medicine and the Wadsworth VA Medical Center; TES, equal volume mixture of 3% sodium tetradecyl sulfate, 98% ethanol, 0.9 normal saline; TEE, mixture of 5 cc of 3% sodium tetradecyl sulfate, 5 cc of 98% ethanol, ½ cc of 1:1,000 epinephrine; GEJ, gastroesophageal junction; EV, esophageal varices; GV, gastric varices.

ity of patients with bleeding esophagogastric varices have some degree of coagulopathy (prolonged prothrombin and partial thromboplastin times) related to decompensated liver disease as well as low platelet count secondary to hypersplenism. Thus, attempts should be made to correct or improve the underlying coagulopathy with fresh frozen plasma and the thrombocytopenia with platelet transfusions. Bleeding may diminish or stop completely following these measures. However, in many cases these steps may result in minimal improvement in these bleeding parameters because of primary fibrinolysis, low-grade disseminated intravascular coagulation, and hypersplenism.

Elective endotracheal or nasotracheal intubation with or without mechanical ventilation is recommended prior to emergency endoscopy for patients with massive bleeding, ongoing hematemesis, severe agitation, altered mental status, or impaired respiratory status. This will facilitate both the diagnostic and therapeutic endoscopies. Additionally, intubation protects the airway and minimizes the risk of aspiration pneumonia, which causes significant morbidity and mortality (15). The endotracheal or nasotracheal tube can be removed after the patient awakes from the premedication. In patients with hepatic encephalopathy, the use of long-acting benzodiazepines for sedation should be avoided due to the risk of exacerbating an already deteriorating mental status.

Other temporizing measures that may slow or stop variceal bleeding include balloon tamponade (5–7), somatostatin or octreotide (2,3), and intravenous vasopressin plus nitroglycerin (1). These therapies should be considered adjunctive and should not be instituted prior to endoscopic confirmation of variceal bleeding.

Control of Acute Bleeding

The primary goal of endoscopy is to first identify a definitive source for the bleeding episode. Because the most common cause of upper gastrointestinal (UGI) bleeding in patients with esophageal varices is nonvariceal in origin, other sources of UGI bleeding must be excluded prior to injection sclerotherapy (49,50). In our experience, ulcers, Mallory Weiss tears, and UGI angiomata are common nonvariceal sources of severe UGI hemorrhage in the cirrhotic patient with documented varices. Variceal bleeding stops spontaneously in greater than 50% of patients. But in those patients who continue to bleed, mortality is very high, approaching 70% to 80% in some series.

For patients with actively bleeding esophageal or gastric varices, we first control the active bleeding with intravariceal injections using a combination of agents. TES (tetradecyl sulfate, ethanol, and saline in equal volumes) is used for esophageal varices and TEE (te-

TABLE 3. *Injection solutions for esophagogastric varices*

Commonly used agents	Infrequently used agents
Sodium tetradecyl sulfate*	Cyanoacrylate
Ethanol*	Epinephrine*
Sodium morrhuate	Sodium linoleate
Polidocanol	Phenol-almond oil
Ethanolamine oleate	Thrombin
Dextrose	Liquid paraffin
Saline (for dilution)*	Fibrin-glue
	Sylnasol
	Diazepam
	Cefazolin
	Sodium ricindleate
	Quinine

* Plus various combinations of the above agents at different concentrations.

tradecyl sulfate, ethanol, and epinephrine) is used for gastric varices. In patients with esophageal variceal bleeding, we then inject all esophageal varices in the distal esophagus. For gastric variceal bleeding, we first control the active bleeding and then inject two adjacent nonbleeding gastric varices (46,47). The use of combination sclerosing agents is based on animal studies showing an increased hemostasis effect and fewer complications using a mixture of agents with different mechanisms of action than a very potent sclerosant as a single agent (51,52).

Potential mechanisms of acute hemostasis for various sclerosing agents include mechanical tamponade effect, esophageal and vascular smooth muscle spasm, and venous thrombosis (52) (Tables 3 and 4). Venous sclerosis results in eventual variceal obliteration. Cyanoacrylate is a unique hydrophilic tissue adhesive that spontaneously polymerizes immediately upon contact with water. Therefore, a lipid-based contrast agent, Lipiodol, is used to suspend and chase the cyanoacrylate to minimize polymerization within the injection syringe and catheter. A single intravariceal injection of cyanoacrylate can achieve immediate variceal hemostasis by mechanical plugging of the bleeding site with tissue adhesive (53). Specific injection techniques and sclerosants will be reviewed in detail later in this chapter.

Minimization of Therapy-Induced Complications

One must weigh the risks and benefits of different injection techniques and sclerosants in terms of their efficacy in achieving hemostasis and their associated complications. Ideally, an injection technique using an optimal sclerosant will yield high rates of definitive hemostasis and have few systemic side effects and local complications. The relationship between efficacy in achieving hemostasis and associated complications ap-

TABLE 4. *Proposed mechanism of sclerotherapy agents for gastric and esophageal varix hemostasis (52)*

Mechanism	Description	Agent
Tamponade: volume effect	Dependent upon varix size and volume injected	All solutions
Tamponade: gluing or polymerization	Plugs varix lumen and puncture sites	Cyanoacrylate
Vasoconstriction	Dependent upon deep location of gastric varices	Epinephrine and polidocanol
Primary venous thrombosis	Local activation of venous clotting	All agents except saline
Venous sclerosis	Dependent upon endothelial sclerosis and chemical inflammation	All agents except saline and epinephrine

pears inversely related for both injection technique and sclerosant. For example, combination sclerotherapy (intravariceal plus paravariceal injections) using high volumes of a potent sclerosant is effective for controlling acute bleeding. However, this method has high complication rates including ulceration and stricture formation (54).

The risk of secondary ulceration and rebleeding following endoscopic injection sclerotherapy of gastric varices was initially reported to be much higher than for esophageal varices (55). An exception to this may be intravariceal injection of cyanoacrylate glue (53,56,57). Cyanoacrylate has been used successfully in Europe and Canada for treating active gastric variceal bleeding as well for variceal obliteration. Unfortunately, it is not available for clinical use in the United States. In our experience, injection of nonbleeding gastric varices with sclerosant agents other than cyanoacrylate usually causes bleeding. Therefore, treatment of gastric varices without active bleeding or adherent clots should be avoided, in our opinion, unless the endoscopist is working in a country where cyanoacrylate is available.

Prevention of Rebleeding

Finally, the last goal of injection sclerotherapy of varices is to prevent rebleeding. Without further treatment to obliterate the varices, there is a 60% to 70% risk of rebleeding from persistent esophageal varices. This risk appears greatest following initial sclerotherapy and prior to variceal eradication. In other words, once a patient has experienced an initial variceal bleed, he or she continues to be at high risk for rebleeding; the risk for acute recurrent bleeding is highest within the first 24 to 72 hours of the initial bleed and decreases with time (58,59).

Different endoscopic and nonendoscopic criteria have been applied to assess the risk of rebleeding from esophageal varices such as red wale marking, cherry red spot, hematocystic spot, and diffuse redness [Japanese Research Society for Portal Hypertension (60)], and hepatic wedge pressure and portal pressure, respectively. Regardless of these signs or pressures,

once esophageal varices have been established as the bleeding site for severe UGI hemorrhage, endoscopic injection sclerotherapy is indicated for treatment of bleeding as well as nonbleeding esophageal varices to achieve acute hemostasis and to obliterate remaining varices in the distal esophagus.

The long-term risk of rebleeding remains high until esophageal varices are obliterated. Each recurrent episode of bleeding has significant mortality, especially in patients with severe liver disease, because these patients either have complications or further hepatic decompensation. The risk of rebleeding can be substantially reduced by follow-up endoscopic sclerotherapy sessions to obliterate residual varices (61). Unfortunately, prolonged survival has not been consistently demonstrated by sclerotherapy and variceal obliteration (62). Propranolol therapy for patients undergoing elective sclerotherapy can further decrease the risk of rebleeding and may increase survival (63).

Efficacy of Endoscopic Injection Sclerotherapy for Esophageal and Gastric Varices: Summary

Endoscopic injection sclerotherapy of esophagogastric varices can be performed in three different clinical situations based on the goal of treatment and the temporal relationship of the treatment to the acute bleeding episode (50) (see Table 1). We will summarize some of the recent literature on sclerotherapy for esophagogastric varices and then present our endoscopic sclerotherapy injection techniques.

Prophylactic sclerotherapy is undertaken prior to any bleeding episodes to prevent initial variceal bleeding. *Emergency* sclerotherapy is performed during the acute bleeding episode to arrest active variceal hemorrhage. Following acute hemostasis, *elective* or *serial* sclerotherapy is performed at 1 to 3 weekly intervals to obliterate remaining varices to prevent recurrent bleeding.

Prophylactic Sclerotherapy

Numerous randomized trials of prophylactic sclerotherapy versus medical therapy (no medications or beta-blockers) of esophageal varices have been reported in the literature and have been compiled in a recent metaanalysis (64). The results vary from negative to positive and are due to several differences between trials. These differences include (a) variable quality of the trials, (b) variable incidence of bleeding in the medical groups, (c) patient populations with different causes and degree of portal hypertension, and (d) diverse complication rates associated with sclerotherapy. The favorable results of prophylactic endoscopic injection sclerotherapy seen in early, poor quality trials were due to high bleeding rates among controls.

These results have not been duplicated in more recent, well-designed studies. A recent large Veterans Administration cooperative study compared prophylactic endoscopic injection sclerotherapy to control (sham sclerotherapy) in patients with alcoholic cirrhosis and esophageal varices (45). There were increased complication and mortality rates in the sclerotherapy group, yet no reduction in the rates of first esophageal variceal bleeding (45). Therefore, we do not recommend prophylactic endoscopic injection sclerotherapy of esophageal varices outside of a randomized controlled trial. If patients at higher risk for *de novo* variceal bleeding could be identified with endoscopic or other predictive factors for variceal bleeding, prophylactic endoscopic injection sclerotherapy may be beneficial for this select subgroup of patients. Further studies are warranted of these patients.

There are no data for prophylactic endoscopic injection sclerotherapy of gastric varices. However, due to high complication rates of secondary ulceration and rebleeding following endoscopic injection sclerotherapy of gastric varices with all agents besides cyanoacrylate, routine sclerotherapy of gastric varices is unlikely to be beneficial in primary prevention of bleeding (55). An exception to this rule may be seen with cyanoacrylate. It has been used successfully in Europe to obliterate gastric varices (53,56). This agent does not produce large treatment-induced ulcers as seen with sclerotherapy. However, delayed ulceration may be seen as late as 4 to 5 weeks following intravariceal injection resulting from extrusion of the cyanoacrylate cast (65). No randomized studies of prophylactic sclerotherapy versus other treatments for gastric varices have been reported.

hemostasis, decreased transfusion requirement, and decreased rebleeding rate (66–70). However, emergency sclerotherapy without follow-up serial sclerotherapy sessions does not improve acute mortality and may actually increase morbidity due to sclerotherapy-induced complications (68–70).

Endoscopic sclerotherapy has also been shown to be equal or superior to other nonendoscopic modalities for controlling active variceal bleeding. These treatments include intravenous vasopressin with or without nitroglycerin, somatostatin, beta-blockers, balloon tamponade (66), portosystemic shunting (43), devascularization and nondecompressive shunting (9), and esophageal transection (41,69). Emergency endoscopic injection sclerotherapy is the treatment of first choice for the acute hemostasis of actively bleeding esophageal varices in most hospitals in the world. As an alternative, endoscopic variceal band ligation appears to be a promising technique for both acute variceal hemostasis as well as obliteration (14,15). This technique is covered in detail in the chapter "Elastic Band Ligation" by Van Steigmann.

Initial reports of injection sclerotherapy for bleeding gastric varices were disappointing due to high rebleeding rates from treatment-induced ulcers (55). These bleeding episodes were associated with high mortality. Although all patients received histamine-2 receptor antagonists as prophylaxis for secondary bleeding ulcers, their poor outcomes were probably reflective of advanced liver disease and poor healing capacity. With the advent of more potent antisecretory agents (such as omeprazole), postsclerotherapy ulceration and rebleeding appears to be less problematic after either sclerotherapy or banding of gastric varices in our experience (46). Intravariceal cyanoacrylate injections are effective for acute hemostasis as well as for variceal obliteration. Because of its propensity to spontaneously polymerize, a great deal of experience and caution are needed in using this agent to avoid inadvertent damage to equipment and personnel.

We have recently reported a randomized series of patients treated with sclerotherapy versus rubber band ligation for active gastric variceal bleeding (46). Both methods could be used for acute hemostasis, but the failure rate of rubber band ligation for control of severe, active gastric variceal bleeding is about 20% in in our experience (46,47).

Emergency Sclerotherapy

The objective of emergency sclerotherapy is to stop active variceal bleeding. Numerous randomized trials comparing sclerotherapy to medical therapy for active esophageal variceal hemorrhage have demonstrated clear benefits of sclerotherapy in terms of definitive

Elective Sclerotherapy

The objective of elective or serial sclerotherapy is to obliterate residual varices and thereby prevent recurrent variceal bleeding. The risk of rebleeding from esophageal varices varies from 50% to 80% within 6 to 12 months of the initial bleed if no intervention is undertaken (70–72). In comparison to conventional medical therapy, sclerotherapy of esophageal varices can decrease the number of rebleeding episodes and can improve short-term survival related to bleeding (70–72). Two recent metaanalyses comparing shunt surgery, beta-blockers, or sclerotherapy to no preventive treatment demonstrated decreased variceal bleeding and mortality only in the sclerotherapy group (42,73).

Soehendra et al. (53) and Ramond et al. (56) reported successful obliteration of gastric varices using *n*-butyl cyanoacrylate. Sarin et al. (28) have reported successful obliteration of gastric varices by endoscopic injection sclerotherapy using absolute alcohol in patients with both primary and secondary gastric varices. Gastric varices frequently disappeared following endoscopic injection sclerotherapy and obliteration of esophageal varices in gastroesophageal varices type 1 (59%) and gastroesophageal type 2 (17%). In patients with diffuse gastric varices, they were less successful in controlling active bleeding and in obliterating varices.

Endoscopic Injection Sclerotherapy Technique

In this section the endoscopic injection techniques of the CURE Hemostasis Research Group are presented for esophageal and gastric varices (see Table 2). Also, some specific aspects of sclerotherapy are reviewed including endoscopes, sclerotherapy needle, sclerosants, injection location, treatment end point, treatment interval, adjunctive therapy, and treatment failure.

Our endoscopic hemostasis technique for esophageal variceal bleeding is to perform intravariceal injections using the free hand method using TES solution as a sclerosant. This sclerosant is a combination of equal volumes of tetradecyl sulfate (3%), ethanol (98%), and 0.9 normal saline solution so that the final concentrations are 1% tetradecyl, 33% ethanol, and 0.3 normal saline. The choice for this combination of agents is based upon results from laboratory studies of bleeding esophagogastric varices in a canine model (51). This solution had good hemostasis rates (75%) and low complication rates (less than 10% ulceration rate) following a single 2-cc injection. These results have been borne out in clinical studies of esophageal varices where the efficacy for control of acute bleeding is 100% and the stricture rate is only 7% with emergency sclerotherapy. In our recent CURE experiment, a mean of three sessions of sclerotherapy are required to obliterate esophageal varices.

The endoscopic treatment of bleeding gastric varices can prove to be more challenging to perform than esophageal varices because of several factors. Gastric variceal bleeding is usually more massive than esopha-geal variceal bleeding. In addition, it is often impossible to adequately lavage the stomach free of blood clots, which obscure large portions of the upper stomach where gastric varices tend to occur. Diagnosis and treatment of bleeding fundic varices must be performed in the retroflexed position and this can be very difficult with a stiff therapeutic endoscope in an actively bleeding patient.

Our current CURE endoscopic injection sclerotherapy protocol for gastric variceal bleeding include (a) combined sclerosing agents with different mechanisms of action, (b) epinephrine solution to minimize back bleeding from injection sites and to facilitate hemostasis, and (c) aggressive acid suppression with high-dose omeprazole to accelerate ulcer healing (52). Our sclerosing agent for gastric varix hemostasis is TEE (a mixture of 5 cc of 3.0% tetradecyl sulfate, 5 cc of 98% ethanol, and 0.5 cc of 1:1,000 epinephrine solution). The final concentration is 1.5% tetradecyl, 49% ethanol, and 1:20,000 epinephrine. High-volume sclerotherapy is used to treat actively bleeding gastric varices or those with an adherent clot during a severe UGI hemorrhage. The total volume of TEE needed for control of the actively bleeding gastric varices has been less than 20 cc, although multiple injections are often required. Since this agent has been used for gastric varix hemostasis, both active gastric varix bleeding and secondary bleeding induced by the injection needle puncture have been controlled in all patients with sclerotherapy (46). After hemostasis of the actively bleeding gastric varix, we inject two adjacent nonbleeding gastric varices to attempt obliteration and decrease the risk of rebleeding. Following gastric varix sclerotherapy, omeprazole 20 mg b.i.d. is given orally. Since this agent has been available, severe bleeding from sclerotherapy-induced gastric ulcers has been infrequently noted as a complication. This medication is continued until the three gastric varices are obliterated. In CURE studies, we are able to obliterate bleeding gastric varices in a mean of three to four sclerotherapy sessions.

Endoscope

A two-channel therapeutic endoscope is recommended for treatment of bleeding esophagogastric varices during an emergency (Fig. 4). This facilitates simultaneous suctioning of the bleeding area (which is critical for adequate diagnostic visualization prior to treatment) and endoscopic treatment. Once an injection sclerotherapy needle has been placed in one of the suction channels, the other channel remains patent for continued suctioning and irrigation. Irrigation is through a third small channel via syringe. Suction channels on two different sides of the endoscope also facilitate treatment of varices of different sides of the

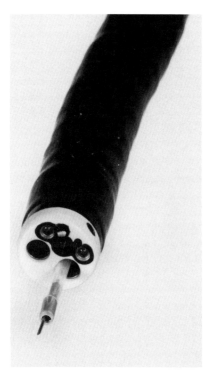

FIG. 4. Large double channel (with two 3.8-mm channels) therapeutic endoscope with a sclerotherapy needle.

esophageal or gastric lumen. A sclerotherapy catheter can be placed down either suction channel to reach the varix. We prefer video therapeutic endoscopes. Drawbacks of therapeutic endoscopes compared to smaller diameter single channel endoscopes are (a) therapeutic endoscopes are less well tolerated by patients and require more premedication, thus they are usually reserved for emergency endoscopic injection sclerotherapy for active bleeding; (b) they are less flexible and more difficult to retroflex, thus visualization of the gastroesophageal junction, cardia, and fundus may be limited; and (c) treatment of esophagogastric varices may be difficult in these areas.

Sclerotherapy Needle

For endoscopic injection sclerotherapy of esophageal varices a 4- to 5-mm retractable needle is preferred. Catheters are disposable and inexpensive. Longer needles have been associated with higher rates of bacteremia and should be avoided for treatment of esophageal varices. Gastric varices are more deeply situated in the submucosa compared to esophageal varices and require a longer needle (6–7 mm) for intravariceal injection.

Sclerosant

Numerous agents have been applied for injection sclerotherapy (see Table 3). An even larger number of

laboratory studies and clinical trials have been performed to assess the relative acute and long-term efficacy and safety of different agents. Sarin and Kumar (54) have reviewed various aspects of sclerosing agents for variceal sclerotherapy.

It is difficult to determine the optimal sclerosing agent from these experimental results because of many variables such as heterogeneous patient populations, multiple combinations of agents, different dilutions and concentrations, varying amounts of agents injected, and differing locations of injections. In general, most clinical studies have compared only two different agents (74). For these reasons, previous studies are unable to answer the question of which agent is the ideal sclerosant. The choice of sclerosing agents is usually based on individual preference and institutional availability. Relative cost is also an important factor in selecting an agent.

We have studied the relative efficacy and safety of different agents for esophageal and gastric variceal hemostasis and obliteration in a canine model of portal hypertension (52,75–78). Various agents have different proposed mechanisms of action as shown in Table 4. We prefer to use agents that have more than one mechanism of action. In blinded studies, these are more effective and safer than single agents for hemostasis of esophageal or gastric varices (52,78).

Most of the commonly used sclerosants, such as tetradecyl sulfate and ethanol, result in vascular endothelial damage, thrombus formation, and eventual variceal obliteration (79). Epinephrine has been demonstrated to be very effective for acute gastric variceal hemostasis but ineffective for gastric variceal obliteration (52). The combination of epinephrine with a potent sclerosing agent would presumably result in a very effective agent for both acute gastric variceal hemostasis and variceal obliteration. Based on these laboratory study results, we currently use a combination of agents with different mechanisms of action for variceal injection. We are performing additional blinded randomized, controlled studies of different combinations of agents in our canine model of portal hypertension. In clinical trials, we are currently using TES and TEE for esophageal and gastric varices, respectively.

Injection Location

Placement of injections for actively bleeding esophagogastric varices is dependent on convention. In the United States, therapeutic endoscopists prefer intravariceal injections. In Europe, paravariceal injections or combination (intravariceal plus paravariceal) injections are often preferred. This distinction may not be as important as previously thought because up to 25%

to 35% of intended intravariceal injections actually result in paravariceal injection (80). Each technique has been shown to be effective for acute hemostasis as well as for variceal obliteration.

In the case of active bleeding from either esophageal or gastric varices, we perform initial injections distal, proximal and adjacent to the bleeding site. Once active bleeding has been controlled, all other nonbleeding distal esophageal varices are injected starting at the GEJ, then 2.5 and 5.0 cm above the GEJ. For gastric varices, we inject the two adjacent nonbleeding varices with two to three distal and proximal injections.

Treatment End Point

There are few data regarding initial treatment end point. With active variceal bleeding, the primary goal of therapy is to achieve acute hemostasis without inducing treatment complications. Overly aggressive injection sclerotherapy can be as hazardous as persistent variceal bleeding. Excessive amounts of sclerosant or number of injections generally will not increase the hemostasis rate but can exacerbate bleeding and increase the complication rate. With our sclerosing agents, successful intravariceal injections will cause blanching of the varix. In our treatment scheme, injections should be discontinued once active bleeding has ceased and distal or adjacent varices have been injected without exceeding a total of 50 to 60 cc of TES for esophageal varices or 25 to 30 cc of TEE for gastric varices (see Table 2). If bleeding persists despite maximal injection therapy, rubber band ligation or other nonendoscopic methods should be considered (see Treatment Failure, below).

During elective follow-up endoscopy for sclerotherapy, it is often difficult to determine whether a varix is completely obliterated. Various techniques have been used to assess varix patency. Intravariceal injections that cause bleeding indicate varix patency. Difficulty injecting a varix or raising a bleb indicates thrombosis. Endoscopic ultrasound with Doppler studies will help distinguish patent versus occluded varices. In most cases, successful sclerotherapy will flatten varices, stigmata such as veins-on-veins will disappear, and the varix will lose its bluish color. After esophageal variceal obliteration, we perform surveillance endoscopy and injection of new esophageal varices every 1 to 2 years.

Treatment Interval

Treatment intervals have ranged from 4 to 5 days to every 3 weeks. The advantage of early follow-up and retreatment is early eradication of varices, thereby shortening the high-risk period for rebleeding (81,82).

The disadvantage is increased complications associated with more frequent treatment such as unhealed ulcerations or strictures postsclerotherapy. Endoscopy at 3-week intervals usually allows time for these ulcers to completely heal. However, this treatment schedule requires more time to completely eradicate varices, thus increasing the chances of rebleeding between treatments before variceal obliteration. Our injection schedule is to perform the first two sessions within 1 week of each other. Subsequent sessions can then be scheduled at 2- to 3-week intervals until all esophageal varices in the distal esophagus are obliterated or the three gastric varices are flat. We do not withhold sclerotherapy injections when posttreatment ulcers are present. Rather we inject varices adjacent to the ulcers. Distal esophageal strictures are not a contraindication for endoscopic injection sclerotherapy and are usually dilated prior to sclerotherapy. Esophageal varices distal and proximal to the stricture are then injected.

Adjunctive Therapy

Esophageal and gastric ulcers occur very frequently following endoscopic injection sclerotherapy. These ulcers are usually uncomplicated and heal spontaneously within 1 to 3 weeks. However, they can be large and deep and cause secondary bleeding, stricture formation, or perforation. Factors implicated in these complications are (a) treatment timing and indication (emergency hemostasis has higher complication rates than elective sclerotherapy), (b) technique related factors (too deep injection, too frequent sessions, or paravariceal approach), (c) sclerosants (excessive amount, strength, or concentration of sclerosant), and (d) host factors (poor nutritional and metabolic status, gastric acidity, decompensated liver disease).

Gastric acidity has been implicated in increased tissue damage as well as delayed healing following endoscopic injection sclerotherapy, especially in the stomach. Different antisecretory therapies and topical agents have been evaluated to minimize acid-induced tissue injury and to accelerate healing of secondary ulcers following endoscopic injection sclerotherapy of esophagogastric varices. These antisecretory agents include H2-receptor antagonists such as cimetidine (Tagamet), ranitidine (Zantac), and omeprazole (Prilosec) (65,83). Sucralfate (Carafate) was reported to decrease the size of esophageal ulcers following endoscopic injection sclerotherapy of esophageal varices, but it did not accelerate the overall healing rate as compared to placebo (84). After emergency sclerotherapy of patients with bleeding esophageal or gastric varices, we empirically treat them with continuous IV infusion

H2-blockers and then omeprazole 20 mg po b.i.d. as soon as they are taking fluids.

Treatment Failure

As previously discussed, prophylactic sclerotherapy of previously nonbleeding esophagogastric varices may increase the overall morbidity and mortality due to treatment-induced complications relative to the risks of the first variceal bleeding episode. Therefore, prophylactic sclerotherapy of esophagogastric varices is not indicated outside of a study protocol.

For the infrequent situation of continued or increased bleeding from esophagogastric varices after endoscopic injection sclerotherapy by a skilled endoscopist, additional endoscopic or nonendoscopic interventions are needed to slow down or stop ongoing bleeding. We have used combination therapy (such as rubber band ligation and additional sclerotherapy) to achieve hemostasis of bleeding esophageal or gastric varices, which initially failed sclerotherapy alone. Also, several nonendoscopic treatments might be considered. First, balloon tamponade and/or intravenous infusion of vasopressin (with or without nitroglycerin), or intravenous somatostatin can be applied as a temporizing measure. Repeat endoscopy and injection sclerotherapy can then be performed within 24 hours. Second, surgical intervention such as a decompressive shunt operation or devascularization procedure may be feasible in some patients. However, these operations have high morbidity and mortality when performed in the emergent setting, especially in patients with severe liver disease. The third and most commonly used procedure is radiologic shunting via a transjugular intrahepatic portosystemic shunt (TIPS) procedure. TIPS can be performed to control active esophagogastric variceal bleeding and prevent early rebleeding up to about 6 months (13,85).

The TIPS procedure was initially applied as a temporizing measure prior to liver transplantation for controlling variceal bleeding that had failed sclerotherapy. The indications are currently being widely expanded. However, high cost, the need for a highly skilled radiologist, and frequent stent occlusion and rebleeding within 6 months limit its widespread use and role as definite long-term treatment of bleeding esophageal or gastric varices. Moreover, there are no randomized controlled trials comparing TIPS to endoscopic hemostasis or other well-established treatments for controlling active variceal bleeding. Endoscopic injection sclerotherapy remains the initial treatment of choice for control of active variceal hemorrhage in most hospitals.

Repeat serial sclerotherapy is very effective for obliterating esophageal varices. Patients with persistent esophageal varices in the distal 5 cm of the esophagus usually fail obliteration therapy because of poor compliance and failure to return for repeat sclerotherapy sessions, in our experience. Other factors contributing to poor results include suboptimal injection technique (such as inadequate amounts of sclerosant or failure to inject all distal varices), continued alcohol intake in patients with alcoholic cirrhosis, and end stage or severely decompensated liver disease of various etiologies. When patient reliability and compliance are in question, TIPS or surgical shunting may be the best alternative for decreasing the risk of recurrent variceal bleeding. Liver transplantation is the only definitive treatment that can improve survival in severely decompensated liver disease.

Side Effects and Complications

Complications of endoscopic injection sclerotherapy can be categorized as either local or systemic (Table 5). Fever, retrosternal discomfort, and transient dysphagia are the most common acute complaints following endoscopic injection sclerotherapy. These are due to the local inflammatory response and usually resolve spontaneously within 24 to 48 hours (86–88). In rare

TABLE 5. Complications of endoscopic injection sclerotherapy

Local esophageal complications
  Ulceration
  Perforation
  Stricture
  Intramural hematomas
  Motility disturbance
Systemic complications
  Pulmonary
    Infiltrate
    Effusion
    Adult respiratory distress syndrome
  Cardiac
    Bradyarrhythmia
    Transient coronary spasm
    Pericarditis
    Pleural effusion
  Central nervous system
    Spinal cord infarction
  Vascular
    Digital ischemia and gangrene
    Portal vein thrombosis
    Mesenteric vein thrombosis
  Infectious
    Bacteremia
    Septicemia
    Peritonitis
    Abscesses (brain, perinephric, esophageal)
  Blood coagulation disorders
    Disseminated intravascular coagulation
    Prolongation of prothrombin time and partial thromboplastin time
    Decrease fibrinogen

instances, this local inflammation may become more generalized and progress to mediastinitis, pericarditis, and cardiac tamponade (89).

Esophageal eschars and ulcers usually develop within 1 week after sclerotherapy, being noted in up to 80% to 90% of patients within 48 hours of injection. Many therapeutic endoscopists consider these postsclerotherapy eschars or ulcers to be an anticipated effect of adequate sclerosis, and not a complication (50). The risk factors associated with esophageal ulcers are highly concentrated sclerosants (such as absolute alcohol), large volumes of sclerosants, deep injections, serial injections in close proximity along the same varix, and frequent sclerotherapy sessions before complete healing of previous ulcers. Esophageal strictures develop much more frequently following injection sclerotherapy than after rubber band ligation (14).

Esophageal perforation represents one of the most serious and life-threatening complication of sclerotherapy. Perforation is reported in 1% to 4% of patients usually within 2 to 14 days after injection. Risks factors associated with perforation include Child's class C patients, deep injections, and large volumes of potent sclerosants. In a metaanalysis of seven randomized trials evaluating the effect of serial endoscopic variceal sclerotherapy on long-term survival, complications of esophageal stricture, esophageal perforation, bleeding due to ulceration and pneumonia were 11.8%, 4.3%, 12.7%, and 6.8%, respectively (62).

In a recent multicenter study of 1,192 patients treated with endoscopic variceal sclerotherapy, one or more clinically relevant complications were evaluated. These were defined as confluent esophageal ulcer (8.6% incidence), esophageal wall necrosis (0.2%), submucosal hematoma (0.3%), bleeding esophageal ulcer (6%), bleeding from injection site (3%), esophageal stenosis (7%), and death (0.9%), and these occurred in 222 patients for an overall complication rate of 18.6% (90). The severity of liver disease was directly related to the incidence of complications. Emergency sclerotherapy had the highest complication rate compared to elective or prophylactic treatments. A rare autopsy case of spinal cord paralysis has been reported following esophageal sclerotherapy (91).

SUMMARY AND CONCLUSIONS

At this time, prophylactic sclerotherapy cannot be recommended for treatment of previously nonbleeding esophageal varices because potential benefits are offset by posttreatment complications. Until better prognostic measures are developed to select out high-risk patients who are most likely to bleed and thus most likely to benefit from therapy, prophylactic sclerotherapy should not be performed outside of a study protocol.

Prophylactic treatment of gastric varices has not been studied in randomized controlled trials. We suggest that future trials should compare prophylactic injection sclerotherapy to minimally invasive methods with low morbidity, such as no treatment (control) or treatment with beta-blockers. These safety issues must be answered prior to embarking on studies to compare two invasive and potentially deleterious modalities for prophylactic therapy of gastric varices.

Emergency endoscopic injection sclerotherapy is a well-established treatment for acute esophageal variceal hemostasis. Injection sclerotherapy is highly effective and is very safe when performed by a skilled therapeutic endoscopist. It should be considered the gold standard for comparing and assessing new treatment modalities for controlling active esophageal variceal bleeding. Likewise, serial injection sclerotherapy is both safe and effective for esophageal variceal obliteration to prevent rebleeding. Rubber band ligation is a promising technique for esophageal variceal hemostasis and obliteration, especially for elective cases. Emergency treatment of severe, active variceal hemorrhage with current single shot banding devices will result in a failure rate of approximately 20% for banding. This compares to less than a 5% failure rate with sclerotherapy for active variceal bleeders in our experience.

Several series of injection therapy using absolute alcohol and cyanoacrylate have demonstrated both safety and efficacy for acute hemostasis and obliteration of bleeding gastric varices. Treatment-induced complications such as rebleeding from postinjection ulcers may be reduced with aggressive antisecretory therapy such as high-dose omeprazole. Further studies of combined injection agents with different mechanisms of action are warranted. Combination endoscopic treatments such as injection sclerotherapy in the acute setting (for acute hemostasis) followed by rubber band ligation in the elective setting (for variceal obliteration) should also be considered.

It is important to remember that all current treatment modalities for patients with esophagogastric varices secondary to end stage liver disease, with the exception of orthotopic liver transplantation, do not alter the natural history of the underlying liver disease. Ultimately, long-term survival is dependent upon the extent and degree of hepatic decompensation.

ACKNOWLEDGMENTS

The CURE results and studies included were funded in part by NIH grants NIDDK R01-33273 (Dr. Jensen), NIDDK 41301 (CURE CORE Grant), a VA Merit Review Research Grant (Dr. Jensen), and an American Society of Gastrointestinal Endoscopy Career Development Award (Dr. Jutabha).

REFERENCES

1. Grace ND. In: McDermont WY, Bothe A, eds. *Surgery of the liver*. Boston: Blackwell, 1988;303–314.
2. Jenkins SA. *Drug* 1992;44(suppl 2):36–55,70–72.
3. Kravetz D, Bosch J, Teres J, et al. *Hepatology* 1984;4:442–446.
4. Conn HO, Grace ND, Bosch J, et al. *Hepatology* 1991;13:902–912.
5. Panes J, Teres J, Bosch J, Rodes J. *Dig Dis Sci* 1988;33:454–459.
6. Minocha A, Richards RJ. *J Clin Gastroenterol* 1992;14:36–38.
7. Correia PJ, Alves MM, Alexandrio P, et al. *Hepatology* 1984;4:885–888.
8. Rypins EB, Sarfeh IJ. *Surg Clin North Am* 1990;70:395–405.
9. Inokuchi K and Cooperative Study Group of Portal Hypertension of Japan. *Hepatology* 1990;12:1–6.
10. Henderson JM. *Gastroenterol Clin North Am* 1992;21:197–213.
11. Reyes J, Iwatsuki S. *Adv Surg* 1992;25:189–208.
12. Iwatsuki S, Starzl TE, Todo S, et al. *Surgery* 1988;104:697–705.
13. Richter GM, Noeldge G, Roessle M, et al. *Radiology* 1990;174:1027–1030.
14. Laine L, El-Newihi HM, Migikovsky B, Sloane R, Garcia F. *Ann Intern Med* 1993;119:1–7.
15. Stiegmann GV, Goff JS, Michaletz-Onody PA, et al. *N Engl J Med* 1992;326:1527–1532.
16. Stray N, Jacobsen C, Rosselow A. *Acta Med Scand* 1982;211:125–129.
17. Pacquet K, Oberhammer E. *Endoscopy* 1978;10:7–12.
18. Crafoord C, Frenckner P. *Acta Otolaryngol (Stockh)* 1939;27:422.
19. Barbish AW, Ehrinpreis MN. *Am J Gastroenterol* 1993;88:90–92.
20. Kunisaki T, Someya N, Shimokawa Y, et al. *Endoscopy* 1973;5:101–104.
21. Richter RM, Pochaczevsky R. *Arch Surg* 1967;95:269–273.
22. Shearburn WE, Cooper DR. *Arch Surg* 1966;93:425–427.
23. Foutch PG, Sivak MV. *Am J Gastroenterol* 1984;79:756–760.
24. Izsak EM, Finlay JM. *Am J Gastroenterol* 1980;73:131–136.
25. Hosking SW, Johnson AF, Smart HL, Triger DR. *Lancet* 1989;1:349–352.
26. Chawla Y, Dilawari JB. *Gut* 1991;32:309–311.
27. Sarin SK, Sachdev G, Nanda R, Misra SP, Broor SL. *Br J Surg* 1988;75:747–750.
28. Sarin SK, Lahoti D, Saxena SP, Murthy NS, Makwana UK. *Hepatology* 1992;16:1343–1349.
29. Sarin SK, Kumar A. *Am J Gastroenterol* 1989;84:1244–1249.
30. Wantanabe K, Kimura K, Matsutani S, Ohto M, Okuda K. *Gastroenterology* 1988;95:434–440.
31. Vianna A, Hayes PC, Moscoso G, et al. *Gastroenterology* 1987;93:876–879.
32. Korula J, Chin K, Ko Y, Yamada S. *Dig Dis Sci* 1991;36:303–309.
33. Bedford RA, Catalano MF, Carey WD, et al. *Gastrointest Endosc* 1993;39:#2230.
34. Bresnahan J, Vanagunas A, Srivastava A, Nemeck A. *Gastrointest Endosc* 1993;39:#2231.
35. Mathur SK, Dalvi AN, Someshwar V, Supe AN, Ramakantan R. *Br J Surg* 1990;77:432–435.
36. Vargo JJ, Sivak MV. In: Sugawa C, Schuman BM, Lucas CE, eds. *Gastrointestinal bleeding*. New York: Igaku-Shoin, 1992;449–477.
37. Bosch J, Pizcueta P, Feu F, Fernandez M, Garcia-Pagan JC. *Gastroenterol Clin North Am* 1992;21:1–14.
38. Mullan FJ, McKelvey STD. *Postgrad Med J* 1990;66:401–403.
39. Madsen MS, Petersen TH, Sommer H. *Ann Surg* 1986;204:72–77.
40. Burroughs AK. *J Hepatol* 1991;13:1–4.
41. Triger DR, Johnson AG, Brazier JE, et al. *Gut* 1992;33:1553–1558.
42. Pacquet KJ, Feussner H. *Hepatology* 1985;5:580–583.
43. Henderson JM, Kutner MH, Millikan WJ, et al. *Ann Intern Med* 1990;11:262–269.
44. Gregory P, Hartigan P, Amodeo D, et al. *Gastroenterology* 1987;92:A1414.
45. The Veterans Affairs Cooperative Variceal Sclerotherapy Group. *N Engl J Med* 1991;324:1779–1784.
46. Jensen D, Kovacs T, Randall G, et al. *Am J Gastroenterol* 1993;88:1510.
47. Jensen D, Kovacs TOG, Randall G, et al. *Gastrointest Endosc* 1993;39:279(abst).
48. Freeman ML. *Gastrointest Endosc Clin North Am* 1991;1:209–239.
49. Westaby D, Hayes PC, Gimson AES, et al. *Hepatology* 1989;9:274.
50. Matloff DS. *Gastroenterol Clin North Am* 1992;21:103–117.
51. Jensen DM, Machicado GA, Silpa ML. *Endoscopy* 1986;18(suppl 2):18–22.
52. Jutabha R, Jensen DM, See J, Hirabayashi K, Machicado G. *Gastrointest Endosc* 1993;39:280.
53. Soehendra N, Nam V Ch, Grimm H, Kempeneers I. *Endoscopy* 1986;18:25–26.
54. Sarin SK, Kumar A. *Am J Gastroenterol* 1990;85:641–649.
55. Trudeau W, Prindiville T. *Gastrointest Endosc* 1986;32:264–268.
56. Ramond MJ, Valla D, Mosnier JF, Degott C, Bernuau J, Rueff B, Benhamou JP. *Hepatology* 1989;10:488–493.
57. Loperfido S. *Endoscopy* 1987;19:87.
58. Burroughs AK, Mezzanotte G, Philips A, et al. *Hepatology* 1989;9:801.
59. Smith JL, Graham DY. *Gastroenterology* 1982;82:968.
60. Beppu K, Inokuchi K, Koyanagi N, et al. *Gastrointest Endosc* 1981;27:213–218.
61. Sarles HE, Sanowski RA, Talbert G. *Am J Gastroenterol* 1985;80:595–599.
62. Infante-Rivard C, Esnaola S, Villeneuve J-P. *Gastroenterology* 1989;96:1087.
63. Vinel J, Lamouliatte H, Cales P, et al. *Gastroenterology* 1992;102:1760–1763.
64. Pagliaro L, Amico GD, Sorensen TIA, et al. *Ann Intern Med* 1992;117:59–70.
65. Jensen DM, Jutabha R, Egan J, Hirabayashi K, Machicado GA. *Gastroenterology* 1992;102:A90.
66. Barsoom MS, Bolous FL, El-Rooby AA, et al. *Br J Surg* 1982;69:76–78.
67. Yassin YM, Sherif SM. *Br J Surg* 1983;70:20–22.
68. Larson A, Cohen H, Zweiban B, et al. *JAMA* 1986;255:447–500.
69. Burroughs AK, Hamilton G, Phillips A, et al. *N Engl J Med* 1989;321:857–862.
70. Copenhagen Esophageal Varices Sclerotherapy Project. *N Engl J Med* 1984;311:1594.
71. Soderlund C, Ihre T. *Acta Chir Scand* 1985;151:449.
72. Westaby D, Williams R. *Scand J Gastroenterol* 1984;suppl 102:71.
73. Pagliaro L, Burroughs AK, Sorensen TIA, et al. *Gastroenterol Int* 1989;2:71.
74. Kitano S, Iso Y, Yamaga H, Hashizume M, Higashi H, Sugimachi K. *Br J Surg* 1988;75:751–753.
75. Jensen DM, Machicado GA, Tapia JI, Kauffman G, Franco P, Beilin D. *Gastroenterology* 1983;84:573–579.
76. Jutabha R, Jensen DM, Egan J, Hirabayashi K, Machicado GA. *Gastrointest Endosc* 1992;38:235.
77. Jensen DM, Silpa ML, Tapia JI, Beilin DB, Machicado GA. *Gastroenterology* 1983;84:1455–1461.
78. Jutabha R, Jensen DM, See J, Machicado G, Hirabayashi K. *Gastroenterology* 1993;104:A113.
79. Suzuki N, Nakao A, Nonami T, Takagi H. *Gastroenterol Jpn* 1992;27:309–316.
80. Rose JDR, Crane MD, Smith PM. *Gut* 1983;24:946–949.
81. Sarin SK, Sachdev G, Nanda R, et al. *Gut* 1986;27:210.
82. Westaby D, Melia W, MacDougall B, et al. *Gut* 1984;25:129.
83. Egan J, Jensen DM, Hirabayashi K, Machicado GA. *Gastroenterology* 1991;100:A58.
84. Paquet KJ, Koussouris P, Keinath R, Rambach W, Kalk JF. *Am J Med* 1991;91(suppl 2A):147S–150S.
85. LaBerge JM, Ring EJ, Gordon RL, et al. *Radiology* 1993;187:413–420.
86. Heaton ND, Howard ER. *Gut* 1993;34:7–10.
87. Reilly JJ, Schade RR, Van Theil DS. *Am J Surg* 1989;147:85–88.
88. Stringer MD, Howard ER, Mowat AP. *J Pediatric Surg* 1989;24:438–442.
89. Tahibian N, Schwartz JT, Smith JL, Graham DY. *Surgery* 1987;102:546–547.
90. Zambelli A, Arcidiacono PG, Arcidiacono R, et al., and New Italian Endoscopic Club. *Gastroenterology* 1993;104:1023.
91. Seidman E, Weber AM, Morin CL, et al. *Hepatology* 1984;4:950–954.

Advanced Therapeutic Endoscopy, 2nd Ed.,
edited by J. S. Barkin and C. A. O'Phelan.
Raven Press, Ltd., New York © 1994.

CHAPTER 12

Techniques and Results for Control of Gastrointestinal Bleeding: Injection Therapy

John G. Lee and Joseph W. Leung

The 1989 National Institutes of Health (NIH) consensus conference on therapeutic endoscopy and bleeding ulcers recommended endoscopic hemostatic therapy in patients at high risk for rebleeding and death, i.e., those with large blood loss, active bleeding, or endoscopic stigmata of recent hemorrhage. Multipolar electrocoagulation (MPEC) commercially available as BICAP probe and heat probe were deemed most promising techniques for endoscopic hemostatic therapy. While injection therapy seemed to be effective for hemostasis, there were insufficient data to make any formal recommendations. Since then injection treatment for bleeding ulcers has become increasingly popular due to its simplicity, low cost, portability, and excellent hemostasis achieved. Thus far, a number of randomized clinical trials have unequivocally demonstrated the safety and efficacy of injection therapy for peptic ulcer bleeding.

MECHANISM OF INJECTION TREATMENT

Epinephrine and absolute alcohol are most frequently used for injection therapy in the United States. Other agents including 1% polidocanol, ethanolamine, and sodium tetradecyl sulfate have different properties but similar hemostatic potential.

Chung et al. (1) used laser Doppler flowmetry and reflectance spectrophotometry to study the effect of epinephrine injection in the rat stomach (1). A submucosal injection of 1:10,000 dilution epinephrine decreased the local gastric blood flow for the duration of the 2 hours measured. Also, the autoregulatory escape

from vasoconstriction that was evident on topical application was not observed with submucosal injection. The hemostatic effect of epinephrine is also enhanced by the promotion of platelet aggregation. Lastly, the large volumes injected contribute toward local tamponade of the bleeding vessel. Up to 10 ml of epinephrine can be injected safely with few systemic complications other than transient tachycardia because most of it is metabolized by the liver in a first-pass effect. In some cases 20 ml of epinephrine has been injected without complications.

Absolute alcohol obliterates the vessel by rapid dehydration and tissue fixation. One percent polidocanol induces bowel wall spasm and acute edema with subsequent inflammation and sclerosis (2). Tissue damage ranging from ulceration to perforation is directly related to the volume of sclerosant injected. Thus, we suggest limiting absolute alcohol injections to a total volume of 1 to 2 ml and polidocanol to 10 ml to avoid perforation.

According to Randall et al. (2), absolute ethanol, TEC (mixture of 1% tetradecyl sulfate, 32% ethanol, and 0.3 normal saline), and polidocanol, but not epinephrine, induced hemostasis of dog serosal arteries. Whittle et al. (3) compared normal saline (NS), hypertonic saline (HS), 1:10,000 epinephrine in NS and HS, 1:20:000 in HS and thrombin cocktail (mixture of thrombin, cephapirin, and 1% tetradecyl) as hemostatic agents in dog serosal vessels. Normal saline caused significant reduction in blood flow but no hemostasis, thus supporting local tamponade as a factor in reducing blood loss. Epinephrine solutions induced reductions of from 30% to 75% in blood flow, but the hemostatic rates were similar among the three solutions tested. Rutgeerts et al. (4) found contact thermocoagulation to be superior to injection treatment for

J. G. Lee and J. W. Leung: Division of Gastroenterology, Duke University Medical Center, Durham, North Carolina 27710.

the control of experimentally created bleeding ulcers in dog stomachs. However, in the clinical setting injection treatment is as efficacious as contact thermocoagulation. This disparity between *in vitro* and *in vivo* data is due perhaps to a lack of fibrosis at the base of an acute experimental ulcer or possible intrinsic differences between the canine and human gastric mucosa. Thus, extrapolation of animal experimental data to the clinical setting could be misleading.

TECHNIQUE OF INJECTION TREATMENT

Injection therapy is performed with a disposable 25- or 23-gauge sclerotherapy needle that protrudes 5 mm beyond the plastic sheath. In chronic ulcers, a more rigid metal sheath sclerotherapy needle may aid in penetrating the fibrotic ulcer base. Face shield and a stopcock-equipped syringe should always be used to prevent possible splash injuries.

A forceful irrigation is sometimes required to clean the ulcer for optimal visualization. Contact thermocoagulation devices have a built-in washing apparatus; for injection therapy, a modified Water Pik fitted with a stopcock and a plastic catheter can be inserted through the biopsy channel to provide a continuous jet of water at 500 ml/min (5). Alternatively, manual irrigation can be delivered through a double-lumen catheter (Hemoject Injection Catheter; Microvasive, Watertown, MA) (6). We believe that the modified Water Pik system is preferable because it delivers a greater continuous flow and can be operated using a foot switch. Both devices can be used with any endoscopes having a biopsy channel size >2.8 mm. Finally, videoendoscopy facilitates the coordination between the endoscopist and the assistant during therapeutic procedures.

We inject around 10 ml of 1:10,000 dilution epinephrine in 0.5- to 1-ml aliquots into and around the bleeding vessel. If heavy bleeding impedes proper visualization, initial injections in the vicinity of the vessel often slow the bleeding enough to allow its identification. For ulcers with active oozing underneath an adherent blood clot, we inject into and around the clot at the base of the ulcer without removing the clot. We do not routinely inject nonbleeding vessels and blood clots. It is important to control the depth of injection especially in the duodenum to avoid perforation and the possibility of peritoneal injection.

Mucosal edema, blanching, and cessation of bleeding signifies a successful injection. Recurrent bleeding can be safely controlled with a repeated epinephrine injection. However, injection of sclerosants should be limited to one session. If this fails to control the bleeding the patients should be taken to surgery.

RESULTS

The end points of clinical studies assessing endoscopic hemostatic therapy are mortality, rebleeding, emergency surgery, transfusion requirement, and hospital stay (Table 1). Numerous controlled randomized studies have established the benefits of injection therapy with regard to all end points except mortality. However, the inability of hemostatic therapy to influence mortality rate may be due to a type II error. For example, 418 to 4,190 patients (for 10–100% patient eligibility) per group would be needed to demonstrate a reduction in mortality from 10% to 5% using a 1-tailed t-test with an α of 0.05 and a β of 0.8 (7). Such a study would be difficult if not impossible to perform. To date, the best evidence for reduction in mortality after endoscopic injection therapy in nonvariceal upper gastrointestinal bleeding is offered by a recent metaanalysis (8).

CHOICE OF AGENTS: SINGLE AGENT OR COMBINATION?

We inject epinephrine alone for bleeding ulcers (Fig. 1). Others have used epinephrine followed by injection of a sclerosant, contact thermocoagulation, or laser. However, the superiority of combination therapy has not been confirmed by randomized controlled trials. On the contrary, it appears that epinephrine alone is as efficacious as combination therapy for bleeding ulcers.

Chung and colleagues (9) compared injection of 1:10,000 dilution epinephrine (0.5- to 1-ml increments to a maximum of 20 ml) to epinephrine plus absolute alcohol (0.5–1 ml into the vessel) in 72 patients with active ulcer bleeding. Hemostasis was achieved in 95% and 91% of these patients with no differences in transfusion requirement, hospital stay, and emergency surgery. Other studies comparing epinephrine to epinephrine plus 3% sodium tetradecyl sulfate or polidocanol in bleeding vessels did not demonstrate any advantages to combination therapy (10,11). Likewise, the addition of neodymium:yttrium-aluminum garnet (Nd:YAG) laser treatment did not seem to enhance the efficacy of epinephrine injection (11,12). No randomized trials have addressed whether epinephrine injection followed by thermocoagulation yields superior results.

Therefore, in cases of active peptic ulcer bleeding, existing evidence supports the use of epinephrine alone as the initial hemostatic treatment. Theoretically, epinephrine injection alone may be less effective in nonbleeding ulcers since it does not have intrinsic thrombogenic properties. Thus, it seems advisable to follow epinephrine injection with a sclerosant or thermocoagulation to obliterate the nonbleeding vessel.

TABLE 1. *Results of endoscopic injection therapy versus thermocoagulation*

Author	Year	#	Trial design	Treatment methods	Initial hemostasis	Rebleed	Emergency surgery	Death
Chung et al.	1991	68	PR	EPI	65 (96%)	11 (17%)	14 (20%)	3
		64		HP	53 (83%)	6 (11%)	14 (22%)	6
Laine	1990	29	PR	ETOH	14/14 (100%)	3 (10%)	(7%)	3
		31		MPEC	10/12 (83%)	2 (6%)	(6%)	3
Waring et al.	1991	31	PR	ETOH	30 (97%)	7 (23%)	2 (7%)	7
		29		MPEC	27 (93%)	7 (25%)	6 (22%)	14
Lin et al.	1990	46	PR	ETOH	31 (68%)	2 (7%)	2 (4%)	0
		45		HP	44 (98%)	8 (18%)	3 (7%)	2
Choudari et al.	1992	60	PR	EPI + Ethanolamine	58 (97%)	8 (13%)	7 (12%)	2
		60		HP	57 (95%)	9 (15%)	7 (12%)	3

EPI, epinephrine; ETOH, alcohol; HP, heater probe; MPEC, multipolar electrocoagulation; NR, not reported; PR, prospective randomized.

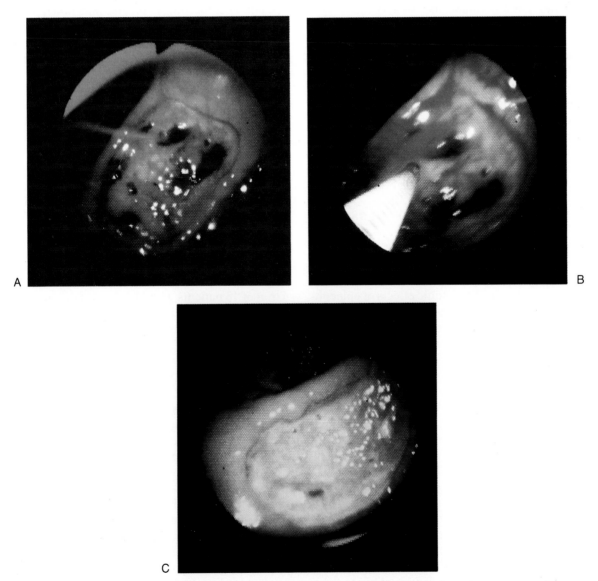

FIG. 1. A: Ulcer with a bleeding artery is identified. **B:** The bleeding has slowed to an ooze after the initial injection of 1:10,000 dilution epinephrine. Further injections to a total dose of 10 ml achieves immediate hemostasis. **C:** Repeat endoscopy in 24 hours reveals a healing ulcer. The *black spot* identifies the "visible vessel."

INJECTION TREATMENT VERSUS CONTROLS

Rebleeding rate (reduced from 43% to 5%), transfusion requirement, and hospital stay but not mortality were significantly improved with injection of epinephrine and 1% polidocanol in 113 patients with active ulcer bleeding and nonbleeding visible vessels (13). On the other hand, Pascu and coworkers (14) observed a reduction in mortality with absolute alcohol injection treatment. Unfortunately, this reduction in mortality seemed to be due to an increased mortality from emergency surgery in the control group. Balanzo et al. (15) found a significant reduction in rebleeding rate (44% to 19%) and transfusion requirements from 2.86 units to 1.63 units. The rate of emergency surgery did not differ because three patients with rebleeding underwent injection therapy rather than surgery.

Chung et al. (16) used a different approach in a randomized trial of epinephrine injection versus conservative management in patients with active ulcer bleeding. Because of difficulty in defining rebleeding, all patients with recurrent hematemesis, shock, and melena after endoscopic treatment, or transfusion requirement greater than 8 units after endoscopy underwent surgery. While the mortality was unchanged, there were significant decreases in emergency surgery (41% to 15%), transfusion requirement, and hospital stay.

RANDOMIZED STUDIES: INJECTION VERSUS THERMOCOAGULATION

Only a few published randomized trials have compared injection therapy to noncontact thermocoagulation. In these studies the hemostatic effects of epinephrine were similar to that of epinephrine plus Nd:YAG laser and microwave thermocoagulation (11,17). On the other hand, a large number of randomized trials have been performed comparing MPEC and heat probe against injection therapy.

Laine (18) compared MPEC with absolute alcohol injection in patients with active bleeding and nonbleeding visible vessels. The treatment induced bleeding in 35% of patients from each group, but this was controlled with continued treatment in all patients. Overall, the two methods were equally effective. There was one perforation in the MPEC group. Similar results were obtained by Waring et al. (19) in a study comparing MPEC treatment to absolute alcohol injection.

Another study compared alcohol injection and heat probe therapy to conservative treatment in 137 patients, 26% to 33% of whom had arterial bleeding (20). If the alcohol injection (0.3- to 0.5-ml aliquots for a total volume of 1–2 ml) did not stop the bleeding in 5 minutes, the heat probe set at 15 to 30 J was applied until cessation of bleeding. Both heat probe and alcohol injection treatments decreased the hospital stay, emergency surgery, and mortality (not significant), but heat probe treatment produced superior hemostasis. However, the design of the trial may have been biased against the results of alcohol injection.

Chung et al. (21) randomized 132 patients with arterial bleeding to receive either epinephrine injection or heat probe treatment. Contrary to the above results, the initial hemostasis proved to be superior with injection treatment (96% versus 83%). There were no differences in hospital stay, emergency surgery, or transfusion requirement. Two patients in the heat probe group perforated after repeat therapy. These authors also concluded that injection treatment is technically easier to perform.

Choudari et al. (22) randomized 120 patients with major ulcer bleeding to receive injection treatment with epinephrine plus ethanolamine or heat probe. The rates of hemostasis, hospital mortality, transfusion requirement, and hospital stay were similar between the two groups.

INJECTION TREATMENT FOR NONPEPTIC ULCER NONVARICEAL BLEEDING

Dieulafoy's disease, Mallory-Weiss tear, and bleeding neoplasm have all been successfully treated using injection therapy. While there are no randomized controlled trials in these areas, the cumulative clinical experience by different groups present convincing arguments for injection therapy. Epinephrine injection (mean volume of 2.5 ml) followed by contact thermocoagulation achieved 95% hemostasis in a prospective trial of 18 patients with Dieulafoy's disease (23). Absolute alcohol, hypertonic glucose solution, and polidocanol also appear to be effective in Dieulafoy's disease (24,25).

Injection therapy has also been advocated for bleeding from Mallory-Weiss tears. Patients with stigmata of recent bleeding and those with portal hypertension seem particularly suitable for injection therapy (26,27). Gastrointestinal bleeding from mucosal tumors may respond favorably to injection therapy (28). Finally, injection therapy appears to be an effective means of controlling postpolypectomy and sphincterotomy bleeding (29,30).

We recommend epinephrine injection (0.5–1.0 ml per injection to a maximum of 10 ml) plus contact thermocoagulation for Dieulafoy's disease. Most cases of Mallory-Weiss tears should not be treated. Exceptions include active bleeding, patients at high risk for recurrent bleeding (on anticoagulation, persistent nausea and vomiting, portal hypertension), and the elderly. The agent of choice is epinephrine injected in 0.5- to 1-ml increments for a maximum dose of 5 to 10 ml.

Bleeding from neoplasms can be similarly treated using the same doses as for peptic ulcers. Since these lesions often have a necrotic base, contact thermocoagulation or sclerotherapy should be avoided to decrease the risk of perforation. Postpolypectomy bleeding should be treated using the same doses of epinephrine as for peptic ulcers. For postsphincterotomy bleeding, it seems prudent to limit the total dose of epinephrine to 5 ml in order to avoid papillary edema or infiltration into the pancreas. Special care should also be taken to avoid injections and thermocoagulation near the pancreatic orifice to minimize the risk of pancreatitis.

REPEAT THERAPY

Although randomized controlled trials have not addressed whether repeat hemostatic therapy improves outcome, some investigators have routinely performed repeat endoscopy and therapy. Favorable results in these studies have been attributed in part to the repeat therapy, but since other studies have shown similar results without repeat intervention, this alone does not explain the excellent hemostasis achieved with injection therapy.

COMPLICATIONS

Complications from injection therapy are rare with only a few cases of perforation reported in the literature (29,31,32). An interim analysis of their results by Chung et al. (*personal communication*) suggest that ulcers heal more slowly after injection therapy with sclerosant or absolute alcohol injection.

CONCLUSION

Available information from randomized controlled studies indicate that injection therapy is superior to conservative management and equal to MPEC or heat probe for the treatment of bleeding ulcers. Injection therapy entails less rebleeding, shorter hospital stay, less need for emergency surgery, and lower hospital costs, but mortality is unchanged. We recommend injection treatment as the initial hemostatic therapy because it is cheap, effective, and easy to perform. An injection of 10 to 20 ml of 1:10,000 dilution epinephrine into and around the bleeding vessel is highly effective. In cases of nonbleeding vessels, we recommend epi-

nephrine injection followed by a sclerosant or thermocoagulation to obliterate the vessel. Repeat endoscopic hemostatic therapy can be performed safely and effectively with epinephrine and may contribute to improved outcome.

REFERENCES

1. Chung SCS, Leung JWC, Leung FW. *Dig Dis Sci* 1990;35(8):1008–1011.
2. Randall GM, Jensen DM, Hirabayashi K, Machicado GA. *Gastroenterology* 1989;96:1274–1281.
3. Whittle TJ, Sugawa C, Lucas CE, et al. *Gastrointest Endosc* 1991;37:305–309.
4. Rutgeerts P, Geboes K, Vantrappen G. *Gastroenterology* 1989;97:610–621.
5. Chung SCS, Leung JWC. *Endoscopy* 1987;19:47.
6. Laine L. *Gastrointest Endosc* 1992;38(5):594–596.
7. Benjamin SB. *Gastrointest Endosc* 1990;36(5):S56–S61.
8. Cook DJ, Guyatt GH, Salena BJ, Laine LA. *Gastroenterology* 1992;102:139–148.
9. Chung SCS, Leung JWC, Leong HT, Lo KK, Griffin SM, Li AKC. *Gastrointest Endosc* 1990;36:194.
10. Chung SCS, Leung HT, Chan ACW, Yung MY Leung JWC, Li AKC. *Gastrointest Endosc* 1992;38:231.
11. Rutgeerts P, Vantrappen G, Broeckaert L. Coremans G, Janssens J, Hiele M. *Lancet* 1989;1:1164–1166.
12. Loizou LA, Bown SG. *Gut* 1991;32:1100–1103.
13. Panes J, Viver J, Forne M, Garcia-Olivares E, Marco C, Garau J. *Lancet* 1987;2:1292–1294.
14. Pascu O, Draghici A, Acalovchi I. *Endoscopy* 1989;21:53–55.
15. Balanzo J, Sainz S, Such J, et al. *Endoscopy* 1988;20: 289–291.
16. Chung SCS, Leung JWC, Steele RJC, Crofts TJ, Li AKC. *Br Med J* 1988;296:1631–1633.
17. Panes J, Viver J, Forne M. *Gastrointest Endosc* 1991;37:611–616.
18. Laine L. *Gastroenterology* 1990;99:1303–1306.
19. Waring JP, Sanowski RA, Sawyer RL, Woods CA, Foutch PG. *Gastrointest Endosc* 1991;37(3):295–298.
20. Lin HJ, Lee FY, Kang WM, Tsai YT, Lee SD, Lee CH. *Gut* 1990;31:753–757.
21. Chung SCS, Leung JWC, Sung JY, Lo KK, Li AKC. *Gastroenterology* 1991;100:33–37.
22. Choudari CP, Rajgopal C, Palmer KR. *Gut* 1992;33:1159–1161.
23. Stark ME, Gostout CJ, Balm RK. *Gastrointest Endosc* 1992;38: 545–550.
24. Lin HJ, Lee FY, Tsai YT, Lee SH, Lee CH, Kang WM. *J Clin Gastroenterology* 1989;11:507–510.
25. Pointner R, Schwab G, Konigsrainer A, Dietze O. *Gastroenterology* 1988;94:563–566.
26. Kovacs TOG, Jensen DM. In: Jensen DM, ed. *Gastrointest Endosc Clin North Am*. Philadelphia: WB Saunders, 1991;1: 387–400.
27. Di Felice G. *Surg Endosc* 1991;5:24–27.
28. Randall CM, Jensen DM. In: Jensen DM, ed. *Gastrointest Endosc Clin North Am*. Philadelphia: WB Saunders, 1991;1: 401–427.
29. Asaki S, Nishimura T, Satoh A, Goto Y. *Tohoku J Exp Med* 1983;140:339–352.
30. Sherman S, Hawes RH, Nisi R, Lehman GA. *Gastrointest Endosc* 1992;38:123–126.
31. Chester JF, Hurley PR. *Endoscopy* 1990;22:287–288.
32. Dell 'Abate P, Spaggiari L, Carboynani P, Soliani P, Karake I, Foggi E. *Endoscopy* 1991;23:352–353.

Advanced Therapeutic Endoscopy, 2nd Ed.,
edited by J. S. Barkin and C. A. O'Phelan.
Raven Press, Ltd., New York © 1994.

CHAPTER 13

Techniques and Results for Control of Gastrointestinal Bleeding: Bipolar/Multipolar Electrocoagulation and Heater Probe

Loren Laine

A variety of endoscopic modalities for the treatment of gastrointestinal bleeding are available. The thermal methods of endoscopic hemostasis can be divided into contact methods (monopolar electrocoagulation, bipolar/multipolar electrocoagulation, and heater probe) and noncontact methods [yttrium-aluminum garnet (YAG) and argon laser]. The National Institutes of Health (NIH) Consensus Conference on therapeutic endoscopy and bleeding ulcers concluded that the two "most promising techniques" of endoscopic hemostasis, based on clinical efficacy and safety, were bipolar/multipolar electrocoagulation and heater probe (1). This chapter provides a summary of the experimental background, equipment, technique, clinical trials, and complications of bipolar/multipolar electrocoagulation and the heater probe.

EXPERIMENTAL BACKGROUND

Bipolar electrocoagulation works by completion of an electrical circuit between two electrodes on the tip of a probe, as contrasted with monopolar electrocoagulation in which the circuit is completed between an electrode on the probe tip and a patient (ground) electrode. The maximum temperature achieved with bipolar electrocoagulation is 100°C. As the temperature rises toward 100°C, tissue water evaporates. Once the tissue is dry, the electrical flow is dramatically reduced because of high tissue resistance (2). Unlike the monopolar generator, the bipolar generator output is too low

L. Laine: Division of Gastrointestinal and Liver Diseases, Department of Medicine, University of Southern California School of Medicine, Los Angeles, California 90033.

to drive electrons across the region of desiccated tissue, effectively shutting off the bipolar probe at 100°C and preventing severe tissue injury.

While bipolar electrocoagulation generates electrical energy that is converted to thermal energy in the tissue, the heater probe uses the direct generation of thermal energy for hemostasis. The maximum temperature achieved by the heater probe is 250°C, although Jensen reports that the temperature at the probe-tissue interface does not exceed 100°C (3).

Bipolar electrocoagulation and the heater probe are effective in coagulating virtually 100% of arteries up to 2 mm in diameter in a canine model (4). This size is important because Swain et al. (5) have shown that arteries in gastric ulcers with visible vessels that rebleed average 0.7 mm with a range of 0.1 to 1.8 mm. The ability to compress a bleeding vessel with the bipolar or heater probe before heat delivery (coaptive coagulation) appears to be the reason for superior hemostatic efficacy—especially in arteries larger than 0.5 mm in diameter (2). Mean hemostatic bond strengths as high as 1,200 to 1,500 mm Hg have been reported with bipolar/multipolar electrocoagulation and the heater probe (6,7).

EQUIPMENT

Bipolar/Multipolar Electrocoagulation

In the past the BICAP was the sole form of bipolar/multipolar electrocoagulation commercially available and the published clinical trials of bipolar/multipolar electrocoagulation have employed the BICAP. Newer forms of bipolar probes have recently been introduced.

The BICAP probe is a multipolar probe: it has three pairs of electrodes on its side and tip. Electrocoagulation can be performed (the electrical circuit will be completed) as long as any pair of electrodes is in contact with the tissue. This allows for tangential application of the BICAP probe. The newer bipolar probes (e.g., Gold Probe, BiCOAG Probe) have the bipolar electrodes in a parallel spiral pattern along the length of the active portion of the probe. This also allows for tangential application.

A comparison of the BICAP and Gold probes in an experimental setting (8) revealed that the only significant difference between the two was that the Gold probe was stiffer. Since force of application is a factor in determining depth of coagulation (see below), the greater stiffness of the Gold probe may allow better coagulation, especially when the tip of the endoscope cannot be placed near the bleeding lesion (i.e., when a greater length of the probe must be extended outside of the endoscope) or when the probe is applied tangentially. However, the BICAP probes have recently been stiffened and allow a force of application similar to that of the Gold probes.

The bipolar generators require the operator to determine the watt setting to be used (1 to 10 = 5 to 50 W) and the time of electrocoagulation [1- or 2-second pulses or continuous (electrical energy generated as long as the operator depresses the foot pedal)].

Heater Probe

The heater probe has a silicone chip in the tip that generates heat for delivery to the adjacent tissue. Unlike the bipolar generators, which require the operator to determine the watts and seconds to be delivered, the heater probe is a computer-controlled unit that delivers a predetermined amount of energy from 5 to 30 joules (joules are watt-seconds). A 30-joule pulse will take approximately 5 to 8 seconds to be delivered (3).

Bipolar probes provide irrigation via a central channel while heater probes have water jets spaced around the side of the probe tip. Thus, irrigation can be delivered while the probe is applied to the bleeding tissue when using the heater probe but not the bipolar probe.

TECHNIQUE

Bipolar/Multipolar Electrocoagulation

Important variables in the use of bipolar electrocoagulation include (a) appositional pressure applied to the bleeding lesion, (b) watt setting (1 to 10 or 5 to 50 W on the BICAP generator), (c) duration of electrocoagulation, and (d) size of the probe (2.3 vs. 3.2 mm). Several investigators have evaluated the effect of these parameters in bipolar/multipolar electrocoagulation.

Johnston et al. (2) found that ten or less 2-second pulses at 25 W (equivalent to a setting of 5 on the 50-W BICAP generator) successfully coagulated all canine mesenteric arteries 0.25 to 1.5 mm in diameter as long as sufficient force was used to occlude the exposed arteries; if lighter application was used, treatment was not successful. Swain et al. (9) found that a strong force of application produced a greater surface area of coagulation than a weak force.

Jensen et al. (10), assessing BICAP watt settings of 1 to 9 in a beef liver model, reported that a midrange setting of 5 produced the greatest depth of coagulation; in a follow-up abstract (11), these authors indicated that the greatest coagulation depths for both BICAP and Gold probes occurred at watt settings of 3 and 5. In both reports, "firm tamponade" was used, but this parameter was not evaluated or quantified further.

Harrison and Morris (6) reported that a 20-second pulse duration with the BICAP produced a significantly greater hemostatic bond strength than a 2-second treatment, but they used 500 g in applying the probe tip—markedly higher than is achieved in clinical practice. Morris et al. (12) also have reported that the large (3.2 mm) BICAP probe is more effective in coagulating canine arterial hemorrhage than is the small (2.3 mm) probe. This difference was seen primarily in the larger arteries, 1.5 mm or more in diameter.

Laine (8) recently evaluated the parameters of application force, watt setting, and treatment duration together in an encapsulated beef liver model in an attempt to determine which combination of parameters is most effective. The first question to address is how much force can be applied with the bipolar probe placed through the biopsy channel of the endoscope. The maximal appositional force is just over 100 g (8,13), and this number decreases significantly as the tip of the endoscope is moved further from the bleeding lesion or the probe is applied tangentially. The maximal force of application for the bipolar probe is achieved when the tip of the endoscope is en face and as close as possible to the bleeding lesion.

Increasing the force of application (from 0 to 50 to 100 g) significantly increased the depth of coagulation, and an increasing duration of coagulation (up to 10 or 14 seconds) was also associated with a greater depth of coagulation (8). Interestingly, lower watt settings of 3 (15 W) produced the greatest depths of coagulation—when combined with forceful application (100 g) and prolonged coagulation (14 seconds or seven consecutive 2-second pulses). Presumably, higher watt settings approach 100°C more quickly than low settings, leading to more rapid tissue desiccation and an earlier shutdown of thermal energy production.

In summary, the optimal technique for bipolar electrocoagulation should include (a) use of the large 3.2-mm probe, (b) positioning of the tip of the endoscope en face as close as possible to the bleeding lesion, (c) lower watt settings of 3 to 5 (15 to 25 W), and (d) prolonged periods of coagulation. Multiple 2-second pulses given in rapid succession appear to be as effective as a single long pulse of identical duration (8).

Heater Probe

Johnston et al. (2) reported that the heater probe successfully coagulated all canine mesenteric arteries ≤1.5 mm in size with <10 pulses at 30 joules if the vessel was completely occluded with the probe; coagulation of the artery was unsuccessful if only light touch with the probes was used. In contrast, Swain et al. (9) reported that the heater probe delivered the same amount of thermal energy and produced similar areas of coagulative necrosis in experimental canine gastric ulcers at low and high application forces and at different angles (0°, 45°, and 90°). Johnston et al. (7) reported mean hemostatic bond strengths in canine mesenteric arteries of 1,336 mm Hg for 120 joules of heater probe and 1,459 mm Hg with 240 joules. Similarly, Jensen et al. (10) reported that increasing the time of heater probe coagulation with 30 joule pulses from 14 to 28 to 42 seconds increased the depth of coagulation in an experimental beef liver model (2.1 to 3.7 to 4.6 mm) with an accompanying increase in sticking noted.

At present, the recommendations for use of the heater probe by Jensen (3) are firm tamponade of a bleeding ulcer with four 30-joule pulses given per tamponade station before repositioning the probe. Jensen suggests two to three 20-joule pulses per tamponade station with a moderate force of application for bleeding Mallory-Weiss tears and only one to two 10-joule pulses with gentle pressure for angiomas.

CLINICAL TRIALS

Evaluation of clinical trials of endoscopic hemostasis requires assessment of the clinical and endoscopic criteria used by the investigators as well as the hemostatic technique employed. Clinical characteristics such as hemodynamic instability, bright red blood per os and per rectum, and significant transfusion requirements all indicate a large, acute bleeding episode and are associated with an increased morbidity and mortality. Although increasing age and the presence of concurrent illness are not clearly predictive of further bleeding, they are associated with an increased mortality (1).

The appearance of an ulcer crater at endoscopy provides perhaps the best prognostic information available. Patients with active bleeding or a nonbleeding visible vessel have the worst prognosis: in our experience at the University of Southern California, (USC), emergency surgery is required in almost two-thirds of patients with actively bleeding ulcers and one-third of those with ulcers containing nonbleeding visible vessels (14–16). On the other hand, patients with a clean-based ulcer almost never rebleed or require emergency surgery and those with stigmata of recent hemorrhage such as flat pigmented spots or adherent clots also have a relatively low rate of rebleeding and emergency surgery (16).

Clinical trials of endoscopic hemostasis should include patients with clinical and endoscopic findings indicating a significant risk of persistent or recurrent bleeding. These patients are the ones most likely to benefit from intervention. Low-risk patients should not be included because hemostatic therapy is unlikely to improve outcome in a group that rarely rebleeds or requires intervention. Significant differences therefore will be unlikely in trials that include a number of low-risk patients. The NIH Consensus Conference Panel also agreed that endoscopic therapy should be used only in patients at high risk for persistent or recurrent bleeding and death—those with clinical evidence of a large initial blood loss and with endoscopic evidence of active bleeding or a nonbleeding visible vessel (pigmented protuberance) in an ulcer crater (1).

Bipolar/Multipolar Electrocoagulation

Two prospective, controlled trials from USC have shown multipolar electrocoagulation (BICAP) to be effective (14,17). Only patients with major upper gastrointestinal tract hemorrhage were eligible (bloody nasogastric aspirate, melena, or hematochezia; unstable vital signs, transfusion requirements of ≥2 units of blood in 12 hours, or a drop in hematocrit of at least 6% in 12 hours). The first study examined patients with active bleeding at endoscopy (defined as persistent bleeding for at least 5 minutes of observation) (14). Forty-four patients were included, and the results are shown in Table 1. The second study included 75 pa-

TABLE 1. *Multipolar electrocoagulation for active upper gastrointestinal hemorrhage (14)*

	Sham therapy (N = 23)	Electrocoagulation (N = 21)
Blood transfusions (units)	5.4 ± 0.9*	2.4 ± 0.9
Emergency surgery	57%*	14%
Hospital days	7.2 ± 1.1*	4.4 ± 0.8
Hospital charges ($)	7550 ± 1480*	3420 ± 750
Mortality	13%	0

* $p < .05$ for sham therapy vs. multipolar electrocoagulation.

TABLE 2. *Multipolar electrocoagulation for ulcers with nonbleeding visible vessels (17)*

	Sham therapy (N = 37)	Electro-coagulation (N = 38)
Rebleeding	41%*	18%
Blood transfusions (units)	3.0 ± 0.6	1.6 ± 0.3
Emergency surgery	30%*	8%
Hospital days	6.2 ± 0.7*	4.3 ± 0.4
Hospital charges ($)	5730 ± 650*	3790 ± 410
Mortality	0	3%

* $p < .05$ for sham therapy vs. multipolar electrocoagulation.

tients with ulcers containing nonbleeding visible vessels (Table 2) (17). Overall, these two studies show a significant benefit for multipolar electrocoagulation in all parameters except mortality.

Four controlled trials of multipolar electrocoagulation from the United Kingdom have not been as positive (4,18–20). The largest of the four trials did show a decrease in further bleeding and a trend toward lower transfusion requirements in the patients treated with multipolar electrocoagulation (20), but the other three trials showed no benefit for multipolar electrocoagulation treatment.

Analysis of the clinical and endoscopic entry criteria for these trials and the hemostatic technique may provide an explanation for the differences in results between the USC and the British studies. Stringent clinical criteria were not used in the British studies; rather, any patient with upper gastrointestinal hemorrhage or symptoms suggestive of upper gastrointestinal hemorrhage was eligible. In addition, three of the four studies included many patients with minor stigmata of recent hemorrhage (18–20), while in the fourth trial, ~90% of the patients had nonbleeding visible vessels and the remainder had lesser stigmata (4). Thus, these studies were not limited to patients with a high risk of further bleeding.

Disparate techniques also may help explain at least some of the variability between the USC and British studies. Laine (14,17), using a "scorched earth" technique, applied the large (3.2 mm) BICAP probe with the maximal force possible to the vessel and the immediately surrounding area and treated for prolonged periods (mean >40 seconds). In contrast, the investigators with less successful results applied coagulation for mean durations of less than 20 seconds (4,6,18) and did not report how forcefully they applied the probes to the bleeding sites. In addition, three of the four British studies used the small (2.3 mm) probes.

Preliminary results from a United States trial (21) that included only patients with active bleeding and nonbleeding visible vessels showed significantly better hemostasis with multipolar electrocoagulation than

with no endoscopic treatment, but no significant improvement in other parameters (including further bleeding). However, after altering their technique (from 1- to 2-second pulses at a setting of 8- to 10- to 14-second pulses at a setting of 5) (10) and then employing a stiffer probe (22) these investigators have noted extremely good results with bipolar electrocoagulation.

Heater Probe

Jensen et al. (21) have presented data in abstract form showing excellent results for heater probe in a prospective, controlled trial of patients with ulcers and active bleeding or nonbleeding visible vessels (Table 3). Patients had significant benefits in terms of further bleeding, transfusion, and need for surgery as compared to a control group receiving no endoscopic therapy. A recent unblinded controlled study of patients with active bleeding or nonbleeding visible vessels from Taiwan also reported significant benefit of heater probe in hemostasis, emergency surgery, hospital stay, and, importantly, mortality (23).

Two controlled trials from Europe have reported no significant benefit with heater probe (24,25), while a third reported borderline significance ($p = .05$) for rebleeding but no improvement in any other parameter (26). Two of these last three studies included only patients with high-risk stigmata (24,26) and 80% of patients in the third study also had active bleeding or a nonbleeding visible vessel (25). It is possible that small sizes may have diminished the chance to show small significant differences; for example, the largest of the three studies (a total of 99 patients in control and heater probe groups) had a 95% confidence interval for the difference in rebleeding of −34% to 4% in favor of heater probe (25).

TABLE 3. *Comparison of multipolar electrocoagulation, heater probe, and no endoscopic treatment for ulcers with active bleeding or nonbleeding visible vessels (21)*

	Control (N = 32)	Electro-coagulation (N = 30)	Heater probe (N = 32)
Hemostasis (active)	20%	90%*	93%*
Further bleeding	72%	44%	22%*
Surgery for bleeding	41%	33%	3%*
Blood transfusions (units)	3.5	3.7	1.3
Mortality	9%	3%	3%

* $p < .05$ vs. control.

COMPARISON OF BIPOLAR/MULTIPOLAR ELECTROCOAGULATION AND HEATER PROBE IN THE EXPERIMENTAL SETTING

Bipolar/multipolar electrocoagulation and the heater probe are reported to be equally safe and effective in coagulating canine mesenteric arteries (2) and canine gastric ulcers (27). In addition, Johnston et al. (2) found that bipolar electrocoagulation and the heater probe were significantly more effective than the YAG laser in coagulation of canine arteries 0.5 mm in diameter or greater.

Swain et al. (9) compared four thermal probes (dry and liquid monopolar, multipolar, and heater probe) in experimental canine gastric ulcers and found that the multipolar and heater probes were safest based on the incidence of full-thickness damage. The multipolar and heater probes were comparable in all categories except that multipolar electrocoagulation required 10.3 ± 7.6 pulses to achieve hemostasis versus 5.3 ± 2.3 pulses needed for the heater probe ($p < .02$). The authors therefore concluded that the heater probe was more effective than bipolar/multipolar electrocoagulation.

Although a number of differences exist between bipolar/multipolar electrocoagulation and the heater probe, the possibility of a difference in the hemostatic bond strength generated by the two methods may be the most important to consider. An abstract from 1985 (7) states that the heater probe produces bond strengths significantly greater than those produced by multipolar electrocoagulation in 1-mm canine mesenteric arteries (~1400 versus ~800 mm Hg). In contrast, Michaletz and Judge (13) reported mean coaptive bond strengths of 1,154 mm Hg for multipolar electrocoagulation and 863 mm Hg for the heater probe (difference not statistically significant). Harrison and Morris (6) have recently shown that multipolar electrocoagulation produces a median bond strength of 1,160 mm Hg (range 500 to 2,000 mm Hg) with a single prolonged application of 20 seconds. No studies have evaluated the maximal force of application that can be applied with the heater probe, but differences in the appositional force could explain variable results with these devices. Even if differences in hemostatic bond strength do exist between bipolar/multipolar electrocoagulation and the heater probe, it seems doubtful that they are of clinical significance since all the values reported are well above arterial pressure.

PROSPECTIVE, RANDOMIZED CLINICAL COMPARISONS OF BIPOLAR/MULTIPOLAR ELECTROCOAGULATION, HEATER PROBE, AND OTHER HEMOSTATIC MODALITIES

Three prospective trials provide a comparison of bipolar/multipolar electrocoagulation and the heater

TABLE 4. *Comparison of multipolar electrocoagulation, YAG laser, and heater probe for actively bleeding ulcers (28)*

	Electro-coagulation (N = 30)	YAG laser (N = 30)	Heater probe (N = 31)
Primary hemostasis	93%	93%	94%
Rebleeding	10%	10%	19%
Blood transfusions (units)	2.0	1.0	2.0
Emergency surgery	7%	7%	13%
Hospital days	5	4	4
Hospital charge ($)	70	200	50
Mortality	7%	0	0

probe. Hui et al. (28), studying only patients with actively bleeding ulcers, reported rebleeding in <10% of patients treated with multipolar electrocoagulation and 19% of those treated with the heater probe; surgery was required for 7% of the electrocoagulation group and 15% of the heater probe group (differences not statistically significant) (Table 4). In contrast, a preliminary report from Jensen et al. (21) comparing multipolar electrocoagulation, the heater probe, and no endoscopic treatment showed the heater probe to be significantly better than no treatment in terms of hemostasis, further bleeding, and rate of surgery, while electrocoagulation was significantly better than no endoscopic treatment only in hemostasis (Table 3). As mentioned earlier, since changing their technique, these investigators have had much improved results with multipolar electrocoagulation. A recent abstract reported better results with bipolar electrocoagulation (Gold probe) than the heater probe, but since patients in the heater probe group were sicker at entry, the authors concluded that the two devices were comparable (22).

Two studies comparing multipolar electrocoagulation and injection therapy with absolute ethanol are available. In the first study (29), all patients had clinical evidence of major upper gastrointestinal hemorrhage and endoscopic findings of an ulcer with active bleeding or a nonbleeding visible vessel. Results with both forms of treatment were excellent and no significant differences were seen (Table 5). Fewer than 10% of patients in each group required urgent surgery for bleeding. Waring et al. (30) also found no significant differences between multipolar electrocoagulation and injection therapy: 20% of injected patients and 25% of patients given electrocoagulation rebled; surgery was performed in 6% of patients treated with injection versus 20% of those treated with multipolar electrocoagulation.

Multipolar electrocoagulation has been compared to

TABLE 5. *Comparison of multipolar electrocoagulation and injection of absolute ethanol for ulcers with active bleeding or nonbleeding visible vessels (29)*

	Electro-coagulation (N = 31)	Injection (N = 29)
Further bleeding	6%	10%
Blood transfusions (units)	1.8 ± 0.6	1.3 ± 0.4
Surgery for bleeding	6%*	7%
Hospital days	5.8 ± 0.9	7.2 ± 2.5
Hospital charges ($)	7160 ± 1630	8520 ± 2960
Deaths	3%	3%

* One additional patient had emergency surgery for a perforated duodenal ulcer 9 days after treatment.

the YAG laser in three trials (28,31,32), although all patients received injection therapy with epinephrine before thermal treatment in one of the trials (32). No significant differences were seen in any parameter between the groups treated with multipolar electrocoagulation and YAG laser in any of the three studies (Table 4). Heater probe and YAG laser have been compared in two studies (25,28), and neither study showed significant differences between the modalities.

Several studies have compared heater probe with injection therapy. Lin et al., in two trials, reported that heater probe provides better initial hemostasis than alcohol injection. Their first trial (33) allows no further comparisons to be drawn because of study design. Their second trial (23) does report better "ultimate hemostasis" with heater probe but no significant differences in the important parameters of transfusions, emergency surgery, hospital stay, and mortality. Chung et al. (34) compared epinephrine injection with the heater probe and Choudari et al. (35) compared epinephrine/polidocanol injection therapy with heater probe. Both studies reported comparable results for the two treatments. Finally, preliminary results from two small studies also showed no significant differences between heater probe and injection therapy (24,36).

COMPLICATIONS

Although the relatively limited tissue injury caused by bipolar/multipolar electrocoagulation and the heater probe makes these devices among the safest hemostatic methods available, full-thickness injury can occur in the canine model (13), and ulcers develop within 2 days after application to normal gastric mucosa in man (15). Thus, ulcers may be increased in size with endoscopic hemostatic treatment. Surprisingly, however, Chung et al. (34) reported that ulcers healed at a normal rate despite heater probe therapy: 88%

healed at 4 weeks compared to 92% healed after epinephrine injection therapy.

Induction of bleeding and perforation are the two major complications to evaluate in endoscopic hemostatic therapy. Bleeding may be induced by multipolar electrocoagulation in up to 35% of patients with nonbleeding visible vessels (17,29), but it almost always can be controlled at the same endoscopy with continued electrocoagulation treatment (17,29).

Perforation has been reported immediately after multipolar electrocoagulation for upper gastrointestinal hemorrhage in only one patient (this 81-year-old woman was treated conservatively without surgery and had an uncomplicated recovery) (4). Two cases of delayed perforation [4 days (32) and 9 days (29) after multipolar electrocoagulation for bleeding ulcers] also have been reported. Perforation may be slightly more common with heater probe (25,26,34), albeit still very rare. Chung et al. (34) reported perforation in 2 of 64 patients treated with heater probe. Both of these patients developed their perforation after receiving retreatment with the heater probe at 24 hours (only 4 of the 64 patients received a second treatment). Thus, endoscopists should be wary when considering retreatment of bleeding ulcers with the heater probe.

SUMMARY

Experimental data show that bipolar/multipolar electrocoagulation and the heater probe are effective in achieving hemostasis in vessels of the size encountered in bleeding peptic ulcers in man. Data from clinical trials indicate that bipolar/multipolar electrocoagulation and the heater probe are effective in improving outcome in patients at high risk for persistent or recurrent bleeding—those with clinical evidence of major hemorrhage and endoscopic evidence of active bleeding or a nonbleeding visible vessel in an ulcer. Bipolar/multipolar electrocoagulation, the heater probe, and injection therapy should be considered roughly comparable in safety and efficacy for the treatment of nonvariceal upper gastrointestinal bleeding.

REFERENCES

1. NIH Consensus Development Conference. Therapeutic endoscopy and bleeding ulcers. *JAMA* 1989;262:1369–1372.
2. Johnston JH, Jensen DM, Auth D. Experimental comparison of endoscopic yttrium-aluminum-garnet laser, electrosurgery, and heater probe for canine gut arterial coagulation: importance of compression and avoidance of erosion. *Gastroenterology* 1987; 92:1101–1108.
3. Jensen DM. Endoscopic coagulation therapy. Part A: Heater probe. In: Sugawa C, Schuman BM, Lucas CE, eds. *Gastrointestinal bleeding.* New York: Igaku-Shoin, 1992;298–313.
4. Brearley S, Hawker PC, Dykes PW, Keighley MRB. Per-endoscopic bipolar diathermy coagulation of visible vessels using a

3.2 mm probe—a randomized clinical trial. *Endoscopy* 1987;19: 160–163.

5. Swain CP, Storey DW, Bown SG, et al. Nature of the bleeding vessel in recurrently bleeding gastric ulcers. *Gastroenterology* 1986;90:595–608.

6. Harrison JD, Morris DL. Does bipolar electrocoagulation time affect vessel weld strength? *Gut* 1991;32:188–190.

7. Johnston J, Rawson S, Namihira Y. Experimental comparison of heater probe and BICAP for endoscopic treatment of gastrointestinal bleeding. *Gastrointest Endosc* 1985;31:155–156(abst).

8. Laine L. Determination of the optimal technique for bipolar electrocoagulation treatment: an experimental evaluation of the BICAP and Gold probes. *Gastroenterology* 1991;100:107–112.

9. Swain CP, Mills TN, Shemesh E, et al. Which electrode? A comparison of four endoscopic methods of electrocoagulation in experimental bleeding ulcers. *Gut* 1984;25:1424–1431.

10. Jensen D, Kirabayashi K, CURE Hemostasis Research Group. A study of coagulation depths with BICAP and heater probe to improve endoscopic hemostasis of bleeding peptic ulcers. *Gastrointest Endosc* 1989;35:181(abst).

11. Jensen DM, Kirabayashi K. A comparative study of coagulation depths and efficacy of arterial coagulation for Gold probe. *Am J Gastroenterol* 1989;84:1161(abst).

12. Morris DL, Brearley S, Thompson H, Keighley MRB. A comparison of the efficacy and depth of gastric wall injury with 3.2- and 2.3-mm bipolar probes in canine arterial hemorrhage. *Gastrointest Endosc* 1985;31:361–363.

13. Michaletz PA, Judge D. Microwave energy compared with heater probe and BICAP in canine models of peptic ulcer hemorrhage. *Gastroenterology* 1989;97:676–684.

14. Laine L. Multipolar electrocoagulation in the treatment of active upper gastrointestinal hemorrhage: a prospective controlled trial. *N Engl J Med* 1987;316:1613–1617.

15. Laine L, Weinstein WM. Multipolar electrocoagulation (MPEC)-induced gastric injury in man: a prospective study. *Gastrointest Endosc* 1988;34:178–179.

16. Laine L, Cohen H, Brodhead J, Cantor D, Garcia F, Mosquera M. Prospective evaluation of immediate versus delayed refeeding and prognostic value of endoscopy in patients with upper gastrointestinal hemorrhage. *Gastroenterology* 1992;102: 314–316.

17. Laine L. Multipolar electrocoagulation in the treatment of peptic ulcers with nonbleeding visible vessels: a prospective, controlled trial. *Ann Intern Med* 1989;110:510–514.

18. Goudie BM, Mitchell KG, Birnie GG, Mackay C. Controlled trial of endoscopic bipolar electrocoagulation in the treatment of bleeding peptic ulcers. *Gut* 1984;25:A1185(abst).

19. Kernohan RM, Anderson JR, McKelvey ST, Kennedy TL. A controlled trial of bipolar electrocoagulation in patients with upper gastrointestinal bleeding. *Br J Surg* 1984;71:889–891.

20. O'Brien JD, Day SJ, Burnham WR. Controlled trial of small bipolar probe in bleeding peptic ulcers. *Lancet* 1986;1:464–467.

21. Jensen DM, Machicado GA, Kovacs TOG, et al. Controlled randomized study of heater probe and BICAP for hemostasis of severe ulcer bleeding. *Gastroenterology* 1988;94:A208(abst).

22. Jensen DM, Kovacs TOG, Freeman M, et al. A multicenter randomized prospective study of gold probe versus heater probe for hemostasis of very severe ulcer or Mallory-Weiss bleeding. *Gastroenterology* 1991;100:A92(abst).

23. Lin HJ, Lee FY, Kang WM, Tsai YT, Lee SD, Lee CH. Heat probe thermocoagulation and pure alcohol injection in massive peptic ulcer haemorrhage: a prospective, randomised controlled trial. *Gut* 1990;31:753–757.

24. Avgerinos A, Rekoumis G, Argirakis G, Gouma P, Papadimitriou N, Karamanolis D. Randomized comparison of endoscopic heater probe electrocoagulation, injection of adrenalin and no endoscopic therapy for bleeding peptic ulcers. *Gastroenterology* 1989;96:A18(abst).

25. Matthewson K, Swain CP, Bland M, Kirkham JS, Bown SG, Northfield TC. Randomized comparison of Nd YAG laser, heater probe, and no endoscopic therapy for bleeding peptic ulcer. *Gastroenterology* 1990;98:1239–1244.

26. Fullarton GM, Birnie GG, Macdonald A, Murray WR. Controlled trial of heater probe treatment in bleeding peptic ulcers. *Br J Surg* 1989;76:541–544.

27. Jensen DM, Tapia JI, Machicado GA, et al. Endoscopic heater and multipolar probes for treatment of bleeding canine gastric ulcers. *Gastrointest Endosc* 1982;28:151(abst).

28. Hui WM, Ng MMT, Lok ASF, Lai CL, Lau YN, Lam SK. A randomized comparative study of laser photocoagulation, heater probe, and bipolar electrocoagulation in the treatment of actively bleeding ulcers. *Gastrointest Endosc* 1991;37:289–304.

29. Laine L. Multipolar electrocoagulation versus injection therapy in the treatment of bleeding peptic ulcers: a prospective, randomized trial. *Gastroenterology* 1990;99:1303–1306.

30. Waring JP, Sanowski RA, Woods CA, et al. Bicap versus injection sclerotherapy for bleeding ulcers: a randomized, controlled study. *Am J Gastroenterol* 1989;84:1172(abst).

31. Goff JS. Bipolar electrocoagulation versus Nd-YAG laser photocoagulation for upper gastrointestinal bleeding lesions. *Dig Dis Sci* 1986;31:906–910.

32. Rutgeerts P, Vantrappen G, Van Hootegem P, et al. Neodymium-YAG laser photocoagulation versus multipolar electrocoagulation for the treatment of severely bleeding ulcers: a randomized comparison. *Gastrointest Endosc* 1987;33:199–202.

33. Lin HJ, Tsai YT, Lee SD, et al. A prospectively randomized trial of heat probe thermocoagulation versus pure alcohol injection in nonvariceal peptic ulcer hemorrhage. *Am J Gastroenterol* 1988; 83:283–286.

34. Chung SCS, Leung JWC, Sung JY, Lo KK, Li AKC. Injection or heat probe for bleeding ulcer. *Gastroenterology* 1991;100: 33–37.

35. Choudari CP, Rajgopal C, Palmer KR. Comparison of endoscopic injection therapy versus the heater probe in major peptic ulcer haemorrhage. *Gut* 1992;33:1159–1161.

36. Rutgeerts P, Gevers AM, Hiele M, Broeckaert L, Kums R, Vantrappen G. Randomized trial comparing injection of ethanol, injection of epinephrine and heater probe for control of active bleeding from peptic ulcers. *Gastrointest Endosc* 1992;38: 241(abst).

Advanced Therapeutic Endoscopy, 2nd Ed.,
edited by J. S. Barkin and C. A. O'Phelan.
Raven Press, Ltd., New York © 1994.

CHAPTER 14

Endosonographic Evaluation of Submucosal Lesions of the Gastrointestinal Tract

Michael L. Kochman and Robert H. Hawes

Until recently, endoscopists have been confined to direct visual inspection and biopsy forceps "palpation" in the evaluation of submucosal lesions. The development of endoscopic ultrasound (EUS) now enables the endoscopist to examine these lesions more thoroughly. The ultrasound evaluation of submucosal lesions involves the assessment of its internal echoarchitecture and careful tracing of the echo layers of the gut wall to determine which layer gives rise to the lesion.

Submucosal tumors (SMTs) are often incidental findings found during the performance of endoscopic or barium examinations. The incidence has been estimated to be about 0.36% (1). Occasionally, large submucosal lesions may cause symptoms that lead to their discovery. Benign and malignant neoplasms of the gastrointestinal tract wall, extraluminal neoplasms, large extrinsic vessels, intramural vessels, and luminal indentation caused by adjacent organs including the liver and spleen can all be causes of SMTs (Table 1). The endoscopic appearance rarely yields an exact diagnosis, and standard biopsy techniques are usually insufficient to obtain histologic material for diagnosis. Each of these lesions has characteristic endosonographic findings that help determine its origin and in many instances lead to the exact diagnosis. This chapter reviews the endosonographic principles associated with imaging SMTs, the typical endosonographic patterns associated with the most common lesions, and suggests which tissue sampling techniques may be useful to confirm the diagnosis and to aid in the clinical management of these lesions.

M. L. Kochman: Department of Medicine, Division of Gastroenterology, University of Pennsylvania, Philadelphia, Pennsylvania 19104.

R. H. Hawes: Department of Medicine, Division of Gastroenterology/Hepatology, Indiana University School of Medicine, Indiana University Hospital and Outpatient Center, Indianapolis, Indiana 46202-5000.

ENDOSCOPIC AND RADIOLOGIC APPEARANCE OF SUBMUCOSAL LESIONS

Endoscopic recognition of submucosal lesions is relatively simple, while endoscopic determination of their etiology can be quite difficult. The topography may vary but, by definition, all are covered by mucosa. In some instances, the overlying mucosa may be eroded or ulcerated. Mucosal irregularity may be the result of mechanical trauma or of the primary process itself. It is important to recognize that routine biopsy seldom yields a diagnosis and that no endoscopic appearance is pathognomonic for a particular tumor. A "pillow" sign may be present, which could be suggestive of a lipoma or a cyst. Some SMTs deform or disappear with air insufflation, such as lymphatic cysts, varices, and

TABLE 1. *Extrinsic and intrinsic submucosal lesions of the gastrointestinal tract*

Extrinsic	Intrinsic
Spleen	Leiomyoma
Liver	Leiomyoblastoma
Splenic remnant	Leiomyosarcoma
Lymphadenopathy	Lipomas
Abscesses	Liposarcoma
Endometriosis	Varices
Pancreas	Ménétrier's disease
Cysts	Pancreatic rest
Pancreatic pseudocysts	Cysts
Vascular—aortic arch,	Carcinoid
splenic artery	Schwannoma
	Neurogenic tumors
	Lymphangioma/
	lymphatic cysts
	Granular cell tumors
	Neuroendocrine tumors
	Lymphoma

thickened folds. In some cases, such as varices, mucosal biopsy attempts may be hazardous. Because most routine biopsies are nondiagnostic, special techniques can be employed such as multiple biopsies from the same spot ("tunneling"), which may yield diagnostic tissue.

With barium contrast studies, submucosal lesions typically appear as an area of indentation into the lumen of the gastrointestinal tract, with smooth overlying mucosa. Little specific information concerning the etiology of the tumor can be obtained from these studies. Other radiologic exams can provide useful information. Computed tomography (CT) scans, for instance, may aid in the differentiation of the extrinsic press versus intrinsic submucosal lesions. Rosch et al. (2) examined the ability of three imaging modalities to assess 34 endoscopically identified submucosal lesions. EUS imaged all 34, while 11 out of 13 were found by barium studies and only 16 of 24 were imaged by CT.

EUS EVALUATION OF SUBMUCOSAL LESIONS

Imaging Principles

Endosonography typically portrays the gastrointestinal wall as consisting of five echo layers (3): the first (hyperechoic) layer corresponds to the balloon-mucosal interface, the second (hypoechoic) corresponds to the deep mucosa, the third (hyperechoic) corresponds to the submucosa, the fourth (hypoechoic) corresponds to the muscularis propria, and the fifth (hy-

perechoic) corresponds to the serosa or adventitial interface (Fig. 1). The high resolution of endosonography allows for the differentiation of submucosal lesions that are intrinsic to the gut wall from adjacent structures that cause an extraluminal press. This distinction is an important one, for it will aid in limiting the differential diagnosis of the lesion and will direct the next steps in the evaluation process.

The imaging of SMTs can be difficult but is usually rewarding. Small lesions may be difficult to find, especially in a large cavity like the stomach. It can be frustrating and time-consuming to search for a small submucosal lesion with the echoendoscope. The usual practice is to perform a standard forward viewing endoscopy prior to EUS, to localize the lesion of interest and carefully note its anatomic position and its distance from the incisors. In some instances, a mark in the mucosa with a small biopsy bite or saline injection adjacent to the SMT may aid in subsequent localization with the echoendoscope. The ultrasound endoscope is then introduced and the tip positioned adjacent to the lesion of interest. It is important not to compress the lesion as this will cause difficulties with wall layer determination. One must be cognizant that the focal point of the Olympus 7.5 MHz transducer is approximately 3 cm, while the 12 MHz transducer has a focal length of 2.5 cm (Olympus Corp., Lake Success, NY). In contrast, the Pentax/Hitachi system, which scans at 5 and 7.5 MHz has a variable focal length (Pentax, Orangeburg, NY; Hitachi, Conshohocken, PA). This means that the best imaging resolution of a lesion will occur when the distance between the transducer and the le-

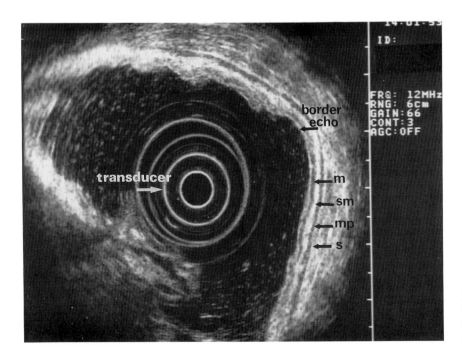

FIG. 1. Normal five-layer pattern of the GI tract wall demonstrated in the stomach. SM, submucosa; MP, muscularis propria; S, serosa.

sion matches the focal length. When trying to examine submucosal lesions in the stomach, it is helpful to instill 300 to 600 cc of water to allow coupling of the ultrasound waves between the transducer and stomach wall. This permits imaging of the lesion without having to excessively inflate the balloon, which can distort the anatomy and adversely affect interpretation of the images. Despite concerns about the installation of this volume of water during endosonography, aspiration has not been reported with this technique. Proper examination of the lesion involves evaluation of size and internal echo characteristics including density and homogeneity.

The hallmark of an intramural submucosal tumor is the disruption or expansion of one of the echo layers with preservation of the other layers. The key to imaging with EUS is to position the lesion at the focal distance from the transducer and then, using various transducer positions, trace the wall layers up to and around the tumor. One must determine from which layer the mass arises because this is one of the keys in determining its origin.

Intrinsic Versus Extrinsic Lesions

When a "bulge" is encountered in the gastrointestinal (GI) tract during endoscopy, it is not always apparent whether the mass originates from the gut wall or represents a press from an adjacent structure. A typical example is a patient referred for a "submucosal" mass in the fundus of the stomach and on endosonographic examination it turns out to be an external press from the spleen. This differentiation is easily made with endoscopic ultrasound. If the lesion arises from outside the wall of the GI tract, one can normally discern an intact five-layer wall structure between the gut lumen and the mass. This differentiation may become more difficult if the extrinsic mass is malignant and is actually invading the gut wall from the outside. In these cases, the epicenter of the mass is usually well outside the gut wall and this manifests a different pattern than seen if the tumor arises from within the gut wall.

Vessels

Varices are the most frequently encountered vessels that may simulate the appearance of a submucosal tumor. Varices course through the third hyperechoic layer (submucosa) and are seen as round or linear, homogeneously anechoic structures (Fig. 2). Usually, as a transducer is moved back and forth across vessels, they are noted to elongate and become serpiginous. If a varix contains organized clot, there may be some diffuse echoes within it. Occasionally aberrant or aneurysmal arteries or veins may be found in uncommon locations. These will tend to be more linear than varices and can usually be traced to a larger vessel. Rösch et al. (4) reported on the findings in 15 patients with submucosal lesions that were subsequently demonstrated by endosonography to be splenic vessels. They found that only 2 of 15 patients had evidence of portal hypertension. They additionally studied 10 patients with portal hypertension and were unable to demonstrate any gastric compression by the endoscopic or

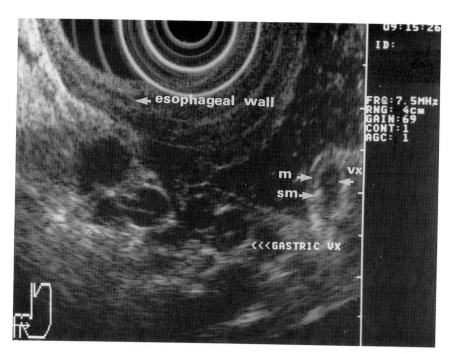

FIG. 2. Endoscopic ultrasound view of gastric varices. Note their location in the submucosa (SM). The transducer in this view is in the distal esophagus and the image is looking through the esophageal wall into the fundus. M, mucosa; VX, varix.

endosonographic examinations. They concluded that the normal vascular structures, in addition to varices, may cause gastric submucosal lesions.

ENDOSCOPIC ULTRASOUND FINDINGS IN SPECIFIC SUBMUCOSAL LESIONS

Smooth Muscle Tumors

Smooth muscle tumors are the most commonly encountered of the submucosal tumors. They account for approximately 1% of all gastrointestinal tumors (5). They may come to medical attention as incidental findings due to nonsteroidal anti-inflammatory drug (NSAID)-induced bleeding or present with abdominal pain or symptoms of obstruction (6). They are the most commonly encountered benign tumor of the esophagus and small bowel and account for nearly 50% of benign gastric tumors (7–9). Less than 3% of all leiomyomas are in the colon (10). Endoscopically they typically have a smooth surface, although larger smooth muscle tumors may have an overlying ulcerated area. This may be due to mechanical forces and local trauma. Esophageal leiomyomas rarely bleed, in contrast to gastric or duodenal leiomyomas. These lesions are usually firm when "palpated" with biopsy forceps.

Leiomyomas most often arise from the muscularis propria, although they may rarely arise from the muscularis mucosa (Fig. 3). Histologically they are smooth muscle tumors. They are typically well contained within a defined area, though they lack a capsule. Their echo texture is usually homogeneous but they may occasionally be inhomogeneous if large (11,12). They are typically hypoechoic but may appear anechoic, partic-

ularly if the gain on the ultrasound console is turned down (Fig. 4). They may contain areas of hyperechoic reflectors that appear to correspond with hyaline degeneration. The hypoechoic cystic appearance that may be seen in some larger leiomyomas or leiomyosarcomas represents liquefaction necrosis (11). As the size of a leiomyoma increases the likelihood of malignancy increases.

It is not possible to differentiate a leiomyoma from its malignant counterpart by endoscopic examination. Tissue may be obtained to confirm the diagnosis; techniques for obtaining this are discussed later in this chapter. Various techniques have been used to endoscopically remove leiomyomas including endoscopic enucleation or snare polypectomy, which allows for pathologic examination of the entire tumor (13,14).

In contrast to leiomyomas, leiomyosarcomas are extremely uncommon and account for less than 0.25% of gastric tumors and a similarly low proportion of tumors of the small bowel (10). They typically are found in patients who are older than 50 (15). At the time of presentation approximately 30% of leiomyosarcomas may be shown to have metastases (5). Multiple leiomyomas should increase the suspicion of a leiomyosarcoma. On histologic examination spindle cells with mitoses and abnormal nuclei may be seen, though at times the only clue, prior to resection, of the malignant nature of the tumor is its behavior. It tends to be larger than a leiomyoma and is usually inhomogeneous and may contain irregular hypoechoic areas. It has been suggested that all smooth muscle tumors with irregular hypoechoic areas be considered leiomyosarcomas until proven otherwise (10). They may have irregular margins and extend through the outermost echo layer or demon-

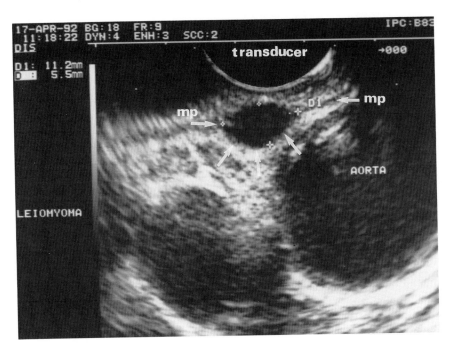

FIG. 3. Endoscopic ultrasound view of leiomyoma. Note that it is contiguous with the muscularis propria (MP). This image was obtained with the Pentax FG-32UA, linear array echoendoscope.

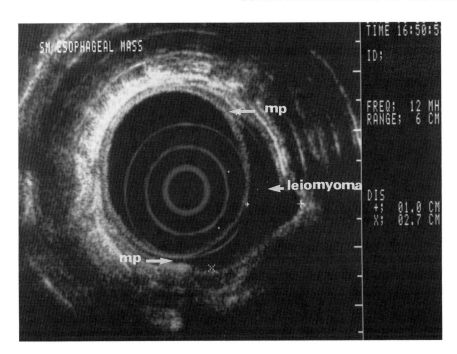

FIG. 4. Endoscopic ultrasound demonstrating an esophageal leiomyoma. This smooth muscle tumor is anechoic but its origin from the muscularis propria (MP) is evident.

strate frank invasion of adjacent organs. When malignancy is proven or suspected surgical removal is recommended.

Lipomas

Lipomas are common gastrointestinal tumors and may account for up to 6% of all GI tumors (16). Most are found in the colon, although 20% may be found in the small intestine and less than 5% in the stomach. Lipomas are the second most common benign tumor in the colon with an incidence of approximately 0.25%. They are usually solitary and are rarely found in the esophagus. Less than 3% of benign gastric tumors are lipomas (17). Gastric lipomas present with bleeding in greater than 50% of cases and less frequently with abdominal pain (18). In the small intestine, lipomas may account for up to 20% of the benign tumors and they rarely (<6%) are a source of bleeding (19). The bleeding is thought to be secondary to necrosis of the overlying mucosa. When acutely bleeding, if viewed endoscopically, they may be confused with smooth muscle tumors or carcinomas.

The diagnosis of lipomas is usually relatively uncomplicated. Endoscopically they are usually smooth, well-defined, submucosal masses with normal overlying mucosa that may have a yellowish tint. They may occasionally be pedunculated or contain a central ulceration. When lipomas are grasped with biopsy forceps they "tent," and when closed biopsy forceps are pushed into them they indent or "cushion" (20). These signs are a reflection of the soft semiliquid fat contained within the lesion. By EUS examination, lipomas

are located in the third layer (submucosa) and characteristically have a homogeneous, hyperechoic echo pattern with smooth outer margins (Fig. 5) (21). Rarely they may be located in subserosa. The endosonographic appearance is often sufficient for the diagnosis because most other SMTs that are located in the submucosa are typically hypoechoic. Histologically they are encapsulated and are well differentiated. Typically they are asymptomatic and do not require excision, although if they present with gastrointestinal bleeding, removal is advocated (16).

Liposarcomas are extremely rare tumors. Very few reports exist in the literature and it appears that they are not a practical consideration when evaluating a lipoma (22). Computed tomography may be of value to help evaluate suspicious lesions for evidence of malignancy (23).

Pancreatic Rest

Pancreatic rests are usually found in the duodenum or stomach. Their location is variable in that 75% are submucosal and roughly 25% are found in the muscularis propria (22). Thus, by EUS examination they may be seen to arise in the second, third, or fourth wall layer. They are echo variable, although they are usually relatively hypoechoic (Fig. 6) and may contain tubular anechoic structures (ducts) (24). They occasionally may be noted to have a central hypoechoic area.

Metastatic Disease

It is important to recognize that malignancies may present as a submucosal tumor. This may be as a result

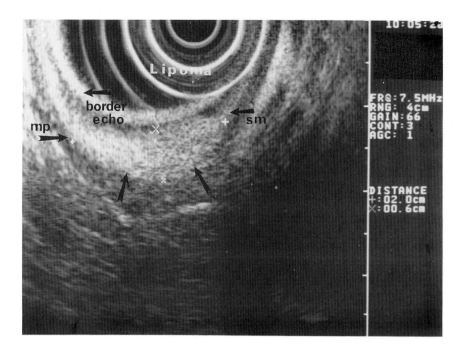

FIG. 5. Endoscopic ultrasound demonstrating a gastric lipoma. Note that it is hyperechoic and located in the submucosa (SM). MP, muscularis propria.

of predominant submucosal spread of a gastrointestinal carcinoma or may be due to metastatic disease. Tumors most likely to metastasize in this manner are melanoma, breast carcinoma, esophageal carcinoma, and colon carcinoma. Metastatic carcinomas typically disrupt the muscularis propria and invade the submucosa and are detected as a hypoechoic mass by EUS. Endoscopically, they appear as a raised area with or without central ulceration. In the majority of cases the primary is known beforehand. Most submucosal metastatic tumors are seen in the stomach, occurring in up to 2%

of patients with known malignancies. Rarely, the spindle cell variant of lung cancer may be difficult to discern from leiomyomas.

Cysts

Submucosal gastrointestinal cysts are rare. Duplication cysts are extremely rare and they may account for less than 2% of all esophageal tumors but 10% of all duplication cysts are esophageal (22,25). They may be

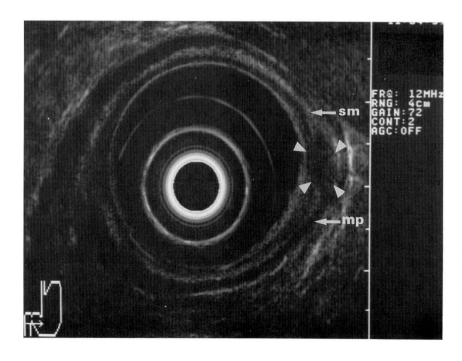

FIG. 6. Endoscopic ultrasound from the antrum showing a slightly hypoechoic mass in the submucosa (SM). The tumor was visualized with a standard endoscope and visually guided FNA was performed revealing cells consistent with a pancreatic rest. MP, muscularis propria.

found anywhere along the gastrointestinal tract. The majority of cysts found in the stomach are congenital benign cysts or duplication cysts. Cysts are usually anechoic well-demarcated structures located in the third layer (submucosa) of the wall (26). Occasionally the cysts may be demonstrated to contain septa, seen most often in the colon. Cysts are usually circular or oval, but almost invariably have smooth borders.

Neuroendocrine Tumors

The majority of these tumors, other than the carcinoid variety, are generally found in the duodenal wall in the submucosal layer. In Zollinger-Ellison syndrome, approximately 15% of the tumors are extrapancreatic. Insulinomas are almost exclusively located in the pancreas (99%) but somatostatinomas and glucagonomas can be found in the duodenum (22).

Carcinoids are relatively rare, accounting for 1.5% of all gastrointestinal tumors, and may be found anywhere along the GI tract. They account for 20% of small bowel malignancies. Over 60% are seen in the ileum and appendix, up to 25% in the hindgut including the rectum, and less than 4% are found in the stomach or duodenum (22). Gastric carcinoids make up about 3% of all gastric tumors and total 3% of all carcinoids (27). The vast majority of these are out of the reach of the currently available echoendoscopes, although up to 9% may be found in the duodenum (28). They may range in size from 4 mm nodules to 2 cm submucosal masses. They occasionally ulcerate and may present with gastrointestinal bleeding. Less than 40% of the time standard endoscopic biopsies yield the diagnosis due to their submucosal nature.

Carcinoids are of intermediate echo density and are located in the submucosa, although they may rarely erode through the overlying mucosa. The prognosis appears to be related to the size and location of the carcinoid. Carcinoids less than 1 cm in size rarely metastasize (<5%) and may be treated with careful local snare resection. If the carcinoid is larger than 2 cm a surgical resection may be needed, as over 60% may be shown to be metastatic. If shown not to be metastatic at the time of diagnosis, appendiceal and rectal carcinoids rarely metastasize, and may be treated with local resection.

Rare Submucosal Tumors

The following tumors are extremely rare gastrointestinal tumors for which little endosonographic data are available.

Neurogenic tumors are extremely rare lesions that in total make up about 3% of small bowel tumors. The vast majority of these tumors are benign and they ap-

pear to come to medical attention due to gastrointestinal bleeding, although obstructive symptoms may occur. The most common neurogenic tumor is the neurofibroma. They are most common in the jejunum and are reported to undergo malignant change in 10% to 15% of cases. Schwannomas are the second most common neurogenic small bowel tumors. Most symptoms are nonspecific, although the most common complaint is gastrointestinal bleeding (29). These lesions are commonly seen in the muscularis propria. Neurilemomas, which are composed of benign Schwann cells, are encapsulated. They are reported to have a mixed echo pattern and may be located in the submucosa or muscularis propria.

Granular cell tumors, also referred to as granular cell myoblastomas, are uncommonly found in the gastrointestinal tract. Controversy exists surrounding their origin, although recent data indicate that they are of neural origin and not derived from smooth muscle (30). About 33% of the tumors may be found in the esophagus and they account for about 1% of benign esophageal tumors (31). They may exhibit malignant behavior with lymph node metastases, although they are less aggressive than leiomyosarcomas and have characteristic histologic findings that differentiate them (32). It has been reported that granular cell tumors larger than 4 cm or that demonstrate growth should be considered potentially malignant. They are found in the submucosal layer and appear hypoechoic with a smooth border. Generally, they have the same echo pattern as the leiomyoma. They tend to be larger and may have central necrosis or calcification. There are no reliable endosonographic criteria to differentiate them from leiomyomas or leiomyosarcomas.

The rarest neurogenic tumor appears to be the paraganglioma. They commonly present with bleeding and may have ulcerated overlying mucosa and are almost exclusively found in the duodenum (>85%) (33). They may range in size from 1 to 4 cm. On EUS examination they are solid and inhomogeneous and appear to arise from the submucosa (34). They are not accompanied by adenopathy, although some feel that they are neoplastic lesions. Typically they are slightly less echogenic than surrounding fat.

Eosinophilic granulomas and fibrovascular polyps are typically submucosal and may have a mixed echo pattern. They are inflammatory lesions and are not associated with eosinophilic gastritis or systemic eosinophilia.

Gastric vascular hamartomas are another extremely rare SMT and account for only 0.01% of all gastric tumors (35). They usually present with bleeding and may be associated with leiomyomas. They are usually found in the stomach and are contained within the submucosa.

ENDOSCOPIC ULTRASOUND RESULTS IN THE EVALUATION OF SUBMUCOSAL TUMORS

The largest reported experience with submucosal lesions is that of Yasuda et al. (36). They evaluated upper gastrointestinal lesions in 308 patients. They determined that of 210 lesions that met the criteria as submucosal tumors, 89 were varices and 9 lesions ultimately were shown to be lymphoma. Their experience revealed leiomyomas to be the most prevalent of the submucosal tumors, accounting for 60 patients. Twenty-eight patients had cysts and 24 cases of aberrant pancreas were found. The authors felt that endosonography was a useful imaging technique that had the ability to provide unique information concerning submucosal lesions. Additionally, they felt that endosonography was sufficient by itself for the diagnosis of lipomas and cysts.

Caletti et al. (37) reported their prospective experience in the evaluation of 25 submucosal gastric tumors and found that endosonography was useful in making the diagnosis in 24 cases. In the majority of cases, they utilized surgical correlation and standard radiologic imaging techniques to confirm their endosonographic impressions. Caletti et al. were able to image 24 of the lesions with the only failure being a small antral lesion. They found 11 patients to have extrinsic compression; 6 were due to normal anatomic variants, while in 5 it was due to a pathologic extraluminal process. One patient was found to have a malignant-appearing, inhomogeneous submucosal mass and loss of layer integrity. This was subsequently demonstrated to be a submucosal cancer that was not suspected by prior evaluation. Ten patients were found to have homogeneous, hypoechoic lesions arising from the fourth layer that were diagnosed as leiomyomas by their endosonographic pattern. Seven were subsequently confirmed to be leiomyomas by surgery. One patient had a hyperechoic lesion arising from the submucosal layer that was diagnosed as a lipoma and confirmed by surgery. One patient with cirrhosis had a fundal polypoid mass and endosonography revealed the mass to be echo free with septa of the appearance of gastric varices. Caletti et al. concluded that endosonography allows for the correct discrimination between extrinsic and intrinsic lesions and allows for initial evaluation of size, location, and probable origin of SMTs.

A multicenter experience with submucosal tumors was tabulated and reported by Boyce et al. (38). Ninety-one patients were included in this study. Twenty-eight of the patients had esophageal lesions, 15 (54%) of which were leiomyomas. They were reported to be typically smooth, nearly round hypoechoic lesions that arose from the muscularis propria. Gastric lesions were seen in 55 patients. Twenty (36%) leiomyomas were found and this included two leiomyosarcomas. Eight

duodenal lesions were evaluated, which included two lipomas. In the 50 patients in whom pathologic or angiographic follow-up was available, endosonography established the correct diagnosis in 48.

Tio et al. (12) reviewed their results of EUS examinations compared with surgical pathology in patients with either suspected esophageal leiomyomas or leiomyosarcomas. They found that benign smooth muscle tumors are typically hypoechoic with sharply demarcated borders and arise from the fourth layer of the wall. These were not associated with penetration into surrounding organs and were not accompanied by lymphadenopathy. In contrast they found that the malignant smooth muscle tumors, either leiomyosarcoma or leiomyoblastoma, tended to have poorly defined margins accompanied by lymphadenopathy or extension into adjacent organs. Inhomogeneity in echo pattern or fistula formation may be associated with malignant smooth muscle tumors but these signs of malignancy are not reliable. In their series, tumors larger than 4 cm were likely to exhibit changes suggestive of malignancy. It should be noted, however, that with smooth muscle tumors greater than 4 to 5 cm in size, the pattern of the back wall of the tumor may be difficult to assess due to poor penetration of the echoes. The authors suggested that tumors less than 4 cm in size, without endosonographic evidence for malignancy, may be followed at 3-month intervals, although there are no data concerning outcome or the cost-effectiveness of this approach.

Yasuda et al. (39) reported that of the 50 SMTs they studied, 34 were leiomyomas and 3 were leiomyosarcomas. Importantly, none of the 10 smooth muscle tumors found in the esophagus or the single duodenal tumor were malignant. Of the 26 smooth muscle tumors found in the stomach, 3 were suspected to be malignant and were shown to be leiomyosarcomas at surgery. Thirty of the smooth muscle tumors arose from the muscularis propria, while 4 appeared to arise from the muscularis mucosae. All of the leiomyosarcomas arose from the muscularis propria in this series.

HISTOLOGICAL DIAGNOSIS IN SUBMUCOSAL TUMORS

The echoarchitecture and layer of origin can often allow for an educated guess as to the histology of a submucosal tumor. It must be remembered, however, that EUS is not equivalent to histology and in certain cases it may be important to confirm an EUS impression with actual tissue sampling. There are a number of techniques that can be utilized to obtain tissue (Table 2).

One of the primary advantages of EUS is its ability to differentiate a solid submucosal tumor from a blood

TABLE 2. *Biopsy techniques*

Jumbo biopsy
    Standard technique
    Tunnel technique
Fine needle aspiration (FNA)
    Endoscopic directed
    Real-time ultrasound directed
Snare polypectomy
    Standard technique
    "Strip" biopsy technique

vessel (particularly a varix) or extraluminal compression. The techniques described should not be applied to varices or aberrant vessels, and when using these biopsy techniques the endoscopist should be certain that he/she is not sampling a vascular structure.

Jumbo forceps can obtain larger tissue samples than conventional forceps but are usually ineffective in providing adequate sampling of submucosal tumors. In a recent study of tissue sampling techniques in neuroendocrine tumors (located in submucosa), jumbo biopsy forceps alone identified only 1 of 11 neuroendocrine tumors (40). Jumbo forceps in conjunction with the "tunneling" technique may allow adequate sampling in some SMTs, particularly lipomas. However, there is some concern about bleeding when this type of "excavation" is undertaken.

Polypectomy snares have been successfully utilized to obtain deep biopsies, particularly in cases of enlarged gastric folds. It is known from experience with removing gastric polyps with snare and cautery, that large ulcers are created that have potential for significant bleeding. The perceived risk of this type of biopsy has limited its utilization. In a recent study of snare biopsy in submucosal neuroendocrine tumors, four of six tumors were identified with snare polypectomy. However, of the 12 cases where this technique was employed, one nodule was excessively damaged by cautery and the histopathology was uninterpretable, one sample was dropped in the small bowel lumen and could not be retrieved, and one snare removal resulted in a duodenal perforation (40). Another group has also recently reported a duodenal perforation after snare biopsy of a neuroendocrine tumor (41).

Recently, the Japanese have begun reporting on a "strip" biopsy technique that they have utilized for removal of early gastric cancer (42). This technique involves injection of saline in the submucosa under the early gastric cancer and then utilization of a polypectomy snare to remove the raised lesion. The Japanese have reported excellent success with this technique without significant complications. This technique may hold promise in small submucosal lesions, particularly in the stomach. Lightdale (*personal communication*) at Memorial Sloan-Kettering has reported on one case

of successful removal of a duodenal gastrinoma with this technique.

Caletti et al. (43) have recently reported on the results of their guillotine-type needle for sampling submucosal tumors. This needle is a catheter-based system that can be passed down the biopsy channel of a standard therapeutic upper endoscope and obtains a core of tissue. Caletti et al. report a 90% success rate in 21 patients without any significant complications. This needle is not commercially available in the United States. Despite Caletti et al.'s positive initial experience there are some reservations about the safety of this method if it were more widely utilized. Its greatest role is likely to be with leiomyomas. If applied to esophageal leiomyomas it may cause problems for the surgeon if the patient comes to surgical resection. When removing esophageal leiomyomas, the surgeon attempts to enucleate the tumor using an extraesophageal approach without disrupting the mucosa. Sometimes, aggressive biopsy attempts cause inflammation and subsequent fibrosis that "tacks" the tumor to the mucosa and may expose the patient to the risk of tearing the mucosa during the enucleation process. Because of this potential hazard, aggressive "tunneling" techniques and possibly the Caletti needle should be avoided in esophageal leiomyomas.

With the exception of the Caletti needle, the techniques for tissue sampling mentioned above are primarily intended for lesions in the submucosa. Leiomyomas, which arise from the muscularis propria, and extrinsic lesions are not amenable to these techniques. Many feel that fine needle aspiration (FNA) offers the safest and most successful method of tissue sampling (40,44). FNA can be performed under endoscopic guidance for lesions arising from the gut wall. We have utilized the Saccamano needle (Microvasive, Watertown, MA), which is 200 cm long and has a 13 mm long, 23-gauge needle. Under endoscopic guidance, the needle is thrust into the lesion and then is moved back and forth within the lesion as the assistant aspirates with a 10-cc syringe. In our experience, this technique was successful in obtaining diagnostic tissue in five of seven (71%) cases of intramural lesions, nine of nine (100%) cases of tumors arising from outside the gut wall, and three of four (75%) cases of gastric ulcer. Leiomyomas are the most difficult lesion to successfully obtain tissue from and in our series we were successful in two of four (50%) cases. With leiomyomas, the cells are more adherent and thus more difficult to dislodge and aspirate. Additionally, interpretation is considerably more difficult and an expert cytopathologist is required. In our series, patients underwent EUS prior to FNA. In the cases of the leiomyomas, the endoscopic ultrasound pattern was consistent with a smooth muscle tumor, but determining the precise histologic grade (leiomyoma, leiomyoblastoma, leiomyo-

TABLE 3. *Summary table of submucosal tumors*

Tumor	GI location and distribution	Internal echo characteristics	Layer	Unique features	Recommended tissue sampling technique	Management
Leiomyoma	Esophagus, stomach, duodenum—most common; colon/rectum—rare	Hypoechoic, sharply defined margins, may appear anechoic	4th, rarely 2nd	May have hyperechoic reflectors, >4 cm increased probability of malignancy	Needle cytology, guillotine biopsy—stomach	Benign, surgical or endoscopic removal if symptomatic
Leiomyosarcoma	Esophagus, stomach, duodenum colon/rectum—rare	Hypoechoic, may be inhomogeneous, may have poorly defined margins	4th	Hypoechoic cystic areas, irregular outer margins—suggestive of malignancy	Needle cytology, guillotine	Malignant, surgical removal
Lipoma	Esophagus—rare, stomach <5%, small intestine—20%, colon/rectum >60%	Hyperechoic, homogeneous, smooth margins	3rd	>50% gastric lipomas bleed, <5% may be demonstrated to be subserosal	Needle cytology to confirm diagnosis	Benign, endoscopic or surgical removal if symptomatic
Liposarcoma	See Lipoma	Hyperechoic, inhomogeneous, may be invasive	3rd	Tend to be larger than 4 cm	Needle cytology	Malignant, surgical removal
Pancreatic rest	Stomach, duodenum—most common; esophagus, colon/rectum—rare	Echo-variable, relatively hypoechoic, may contain tubular anechoic structures	3rd or 4th	Variable layer: 75%—submucosal, 25%—muscularis propria	Needle cytology	Benign
Eosinophilic granulomas, fibrovascular polyps	Esophagus, stomach, duodenum, colon, rectum	Mixed echo pattern, hypoechoic	3rd	Not associated with systemic eosinophilia, inflammatory lesions	Needle cytology	None unless symptomatic
Gastric vascular hamartomas	Esophagus, stomach, duodenum, colon, rectum	Not reported	3rd	Usually found because of bleeding, may be associated with leiomyoma	Needle cytology	Benign, endoscopic or surgical removal if symptomatic

Lesion	Location	EUS appearance	Layer	Comments	Diagnosis	Treatment
Fibromas	Esophagus, stomach, duodenum, colon, rectum	Hypoechoic	2nd, 3rd		Needle cytology	Benign, endoscopic or surgical removal if symptomatic
Cysts	Esophagus, stomach, duodenum, colon, rectum	Anechoic, smooth borders, may have septa	3rd	EUS appearance diagnostic, may contain septa, most benign	Needle cytology if clinically warranted	Endoscopic treatment or surgical removal if symptomatic
Granular cell tumor (myoblastoma)	Esophagus—33%, stomach, duodenum, colon, rectum	Hypoechoic, smooth border, may have lymph node metastasis	4th	May have the same EUS appearance as a leiomyoma or leiomyosarcoma	Needle cytology	Malignant—surgical removal
Miscellaneous neurogenic tumors (schwannoma, neurofibroma, neurilemoma, ganglioneuroma, maparaganglioma	Esophagus, stomach, duodenum >85%, colon, rectum	Mixed echo pattern, inhomogeneous	3rd or 4th	Bleeding most common symptom, most are considered benign	Needle cytology	Endoscopic or surgical removal if symptomatic or malignant
Carcinoid	Esophagus, stomach/duodenum <10% ileum/appendix—60%, colon/rectum—25%	Intermediate echo density, well demarcated	3rd	Rectal rarely metastatic, <5% of carcinoids smaller than 10 mm are metastatic	Needle cytology	Surgical removal, endoscopic removal if in rectum
Other endocrine tumors	Duodenum—majority	Homogeneous, intermediate echo density, well demarcated	3rd		Needle cytology	Surgical or endoscopic removal, would avoid snare technique
Duplication cysts	Esophagus—10%, stomach, duodenum, colon, rectum	Homogeneous, anechoic, well demarcated	3rd	EUS appearance diagnostic, usually incidental findings in adults	Benign	Endoscopic treatment if symptomatic, surgical if recurrent

sarcoma) is potentially problematic. We concluded from our study that the combination of EUS and endoscopically directed FNA provided a very high diagnostic yield in patients with submucosal lesions.

The Olympus endoscopic ultrasound system is capable of obtaining excellent images of submucosal or extrinsic lesions and, in the former cases, can usually localize the layer of origin. Due to the type of radial sector scan that is obtained with this system, real-time ultrasound-directed biopsy is not possible. Thus, if FNA is to be performed, one must use a standard therapeutic forward viewing endoscope and rely on visible landmarks to direct the needle catheter. Additionally, if the lesion is deep (in the muscularis propria or outside the GI tract wall), the needles available can be too short to allow sufficient penetration and cytologic specimens are inadequate.

Recently, the Pentax and Hitachi corporations have teamed to introduce an endoscopic ultrasound system with a design that is fundamentally different than the Olympus system. The Pentax/Hitachi system utilizes a series of piezoelectric elements mounted in a rectangular configuration on a curved surface. Rows of elements are electronically activated in a sequence and provide a sector scan along the axis of the endoscope.

A biopsy channel is incorporated into the instrument that will accommodate a specially designed aspiration needle (Wilson-Cook, Winston-Salem, NC). The needle exits the distal tip of the ultrasound endoscope at an angle along the long axis of the scope. Thus, the needle can be traced in real time as it is advanced out of the scope and into the tissue. This system shows great promise for ultrasound-directed FNA. With this system, one can confirm in real time that the aspiration needle is within the target tissue, and thus reliable lesion sampling is possible. This technique is not required in small, submucosal lesions, which can be adequately sampled using the technique described earlier. However, this technique is particularly useful with deep lesions in the muscularis propria and with lesions outside the GI tract wall (45). In these cases, the ability to confirm that the needle is in the target lesion and readjust under "direct vision" is a major advantage. Additionally, deeper lesions require a longer needle, which may be more dangerous. Directing them with real-time ultrasound imaging may allow for greater safety. This ultrasound technology is quite new and difficult to learn and therefore there is not a great deal of experience with this technique. However, preliminary experience looks very promising and it likely will find increased utilization in the future.

CONTROVERSIES CONCERNING MANAGEMENT OF SUBMUCOSAL LESIONS

Many submucosal tumors are incidental findings and once they have been determined to be benign may be left alone (Table 3). If symptoms occur, if the lesion is malignant, or if it is capable of malignant degeneration, surgical removal is usually indicated. Many lesions requiring excision will need a laparotomy but the development of innovative minimally invasive endoscopic procedures may obviate traditional surgery. Snare polypectomy and cyst drainage have been used to treat submucosal lesions (14,21,46). Major complications, including perforation and severe hemorrhage, may occur with these procedures. To decrease the likelihood of hemorrhage during the resection of a polypoid SMT, it may be prudent to undertake an EUS examination to ensure that a large vessel is not present (47). Endosonographers must be prudent and have sufficient experience to be able to diagnose vascular lesions and to differentiate submucosal from extraluminal lesions before embarking on these potentially dangerous techniques.

As a general rule most lesions less than 3 cm with smooth margins will likely be benign. Larger lesions, especially those containing inhomogeneous areas or irregular borders should raise the suspicion for malignancy. The presence of perilesional lymph nodes is highly suggestive of malignancy. In these cases, surgical removal is recommended.

PATHOLOGICAL DIAGNOSIS

The characterization of a SMT is best made by a combination of endosonography and, if indicated, fine needle aspiration cytology. The need for histology in leiomyomas in stressed because as Caletti et al. (43) reported in their series, of 18 leiomyomas diagnosed by endosonography, 2 were determined to be leiomyosarcomas when biopsied. Interpretation of FNA samples, especially in leiomyomas, requires an expert cytopathologist. If one is not available, referral to a specialized center can be recommended. We feel that efforts should be made in most nonvascular submucosal tumors to obtain tissue confirmation.

FOLLOW-UP

The follow-up for an extrinsic submucosal lesion is clearly dependent upon the etiology of the mass effect. Historically, benign defined causes of SMTs do not require follow-up if they are not symptomatic, malignant, or capable of degenerating into malignancies.

Pancreatic rests and leiomyomas are two lesions that are commonly encountered and engender concern because of the possibility of being malignant or of malignant degeneration (24,48). We recommend that if these lesions are diagnostic possibilities, tissue be obtained to establish a diagnosis. Leiomyomas less than 3 cm in diameter can probably be followed unless causing symptoms. The interval for reexamination and cost-effectiveness of this approach have not been established.

In summary, endoscopic ultrasound has provided a useful adjunct to endoscopy in the evaluation of submucosal lesions. Methods are available to obtain histologic confirmation when indicated.

REFERENCES

1. Hedenbro JL, Ekelund M, Wetterberg P. Endoscopic diagnosis of submucosal gastric lesions. *Surg Endosc* 1991;5:20–23.
2. Rosch T, Lorenz R, Dancygier H, et al. Endosonographic diagnosis of submucosal upper gastrointestinal tract tumors. *Scand J Gastroenterol* 1992;27(1):1–8.
3. Kimmey MB, Martin RW, Haggitt RC, et al. Histologic correlates of gastrointestinal ultrasound images. *Gastroenterology* 1989;96:433–441.
4. Rosch T, Lorenz R, Wichert A, et al. Gastric fundus impression caused by splenic vessels: detection by endoscopic ultrasound. *Endoscopy* 1991;23:85–87.
5. Senewiratne S, Strong R, Reasbeck PG. Smooth muscle tumors of the upper gastrointestinal tract. *Aust N Z J Surg* 1987;82(5):419–420.
6. Stalikowicz R, Eliakim R, Ligumsky M, et al. Drug induced bleeding of gastric leiomyoma. *Am J Gastroenterol* 197;82(5):419–420.
7. Morrissey K, Cho ES, Gray GF, et al. Muscular tumors of the stomach. *Ann Surg* 1973;178(2):148–155.
8. Reid BJ. Benign nonepithelial tumors. In: Yamada T, ed. *Textbook of gastroenterology*. Philadelphia: JB Lippincott, 1991.
9. Serraf A, Klein E, Schneebaum S, et al. Leiomyomas of the duodenum. *J Surg Oncol* 1988;39:183–186.
10. Lee FI. Gastric leiomyomas and leiomyosarcoma. *Postgrad Med J* 1979;55:575–578.
11. Nakzawa S, Yoshino J, Nakamura T, et al. Endoscopic ultrasonography of gastric myogenic tumor. *J Ultrasound Med* 1989;8:353–359.
12. Tio TL, Tytgat GNJ, den Hartog Jager FCA. Endoscopic ultrasonography for the evaluation of smooth muscle tumors in the upper gastrointestinal tract: an experience with 42 cases. *Gastrointest Endosc* 1990;36:342–350.
13. Fujisaki J, Mine T, Akimoto K, Yoshida S, Hasegawa Y, et al. Enucleation of a gastric leiomyoma by a combined laser and snare electrocutting technique. *Gastrointest Endosc* 1988;34(2):128–130.
14. Kadakia SC, Kadakia AS, Seargent K. Endoscopic removal of colonic leiomyoma. *J Clin Gastroenterol* 1992;15(1):59–62.
15. Lindsay PC, Ordonez N, Raaf JH. Gastric leiomyosarcoma. *J Surg Oncol* 1981;18:399–421.
16. Agha FP, Dent TL, Fiddian-Green RG, et al. Bleeding lipomas of the upper gastrointestinal tract. *Am Surg* 1985;51:279–285.
17. Johnson DCI, DeGennaro VA, Pizzi WF et al. Gastric lipomas. *Am J Gastroenterol* 1981;75:299–301.
18. Chu AG, Clifton JA. Gastric lipoma presenting as peptic ulcer. *Am J Gastroenterol* 1983;78(10):615–618.
19. Michel LA, Ballet T, Collard JM, et al. Severe bleeding from submucosal lipoma of the duodenum. *J Clin Gastroenterol* 1988;10(5):541–545.
20. DeBeer RA, Shinya H. Colonic lipomas. *Gastrointest Endosc* 1975;22(2):90–91.
21. Nakamura S, Lida M, Suekane H, et al. Endoscopic removal of gastric lipoma: diagnostic value of endoscopic ultrasonography. *Am J Gastroenterol* 1991;86(5):619–623.
22. Fenoglio-Preiser CM, Lantz PE, Listrom MB, Davis M, Rilke FO, eds. *Gastrointestinal pathology: an atlas and text*. New York: Raven Press, 1989;36.
23. Heiken JP, Forde KA, Gold RP. Computed tomography as a definitive method for diagnosing gastrointestinal tract lipomas. *Radiology* 1982;142:409–414.
24. Minamoto T, Ueda H, Ooi A, et al. A limitation of endoscopic ultrasound: an unusual case of early gastric cancer overlying a pancreatic rest. *Am J Gastroenterol* 1991;86(5):622–626.
25. VanDam J, Rice TW, Sivak MV. Endoscopic ultrasonography and endoscopically guided needle aspiration for the diagnosis of upper gastrointestinal tract foregut cysts. *Am J Gastroenterol* 1992;87(6):762–765.
26. VanDam J, Zuccaro G, Sivak MV. Endosonographic diagnosis of a submucosal gastric cyst. *J Ultrasound Med* 1992;11:61–63.
27. Purcell R, Singh I, Lewis E, Muzac A. Gastric carcinoid presenting with massive upper gastrointestinal bleeding. *NY State J Med* 1988;2:80–81.
28. Gencsi E, Lux E, Kaduk B, et al. Upper gastrointestinal bleeding as an unusual presentation of duodenal carcinoid. *Endoscopy* 1986;18:105–107.
29. Hesselfeldt-Nielsen J, Geerdsen JP, Pedersen VN. Bleeding schwannoma of the small intestine. *Acta Chir Scand* 1987;153:623–625.
30. Seo IS, Azzarelli B, Warner TF, et al. Multiple visceral and cutaneous granular cell tumors. Ultrastructural and immunocytochemical evidence of Schwann cell origin. *Cancer* 1984;53(10):2104–2110.
31. Orlowska J, Pachlewski J, Gugulski A, et al. A conservative approach to granular cell tumors of the esophagus. *Am J Gastroenterol* 1993;88(2):311–315.
32. Plantinga ER, Mravunac M, Joosten HJ. Gastric leiomyoblastoma. *Acta Chir Scand* 1979;145(8):571–574.
33. Cohen T, Zweig SJ, Tallis A, et al. Paraganglioneuroma of the duodenum. *Am J Gastroenterol* 1981;75:197–203.
34. Smithline AE, Hawes RH, Kopecky KK, et al. Gangliocytic paraganglioma, a rare cause of upper gastrointestinal bleeding. *Dig Dis Sci* 1993;38(1):173–177.
35. Taylor TV, Torrance HB. Haemangiomas of the gastrointestinal tract. *Br J Surg* 1974;61(3):236–238.
36. Yasuda K, Cho E, Nakajima M, et al. Diagnosis of submucosal lesions of the upper gastrointestinal tract by endoscopic ultrasonography. *Gastrointest Endosc* 1990;36(2):S17–S20.
37. Caletti G, Zani L, Bolondl L, Brocchi E, et al. Endoscopic ultrasonography in the diagnosis of gastric submucosal tumor. *Gastrointest Endosc* 1989;35:413–418.
38. Boyce GA, Sivak MV, Rosch T, Classen M, et al. Evaluation of submucosal upper gastrointestinal tract lesions by endoscopic ultrasound. *Gastrointest Endosc* 1991;37:449–454.
39. Yasuda K, Nakajima M, Kawai K. Endoscopic ultrasonography in the diagnosis of submucosal tumor of the upper digestive tract. *Scand J Gastroenterol* 1986;21(S123):59–67.
40. Benya RV, Metz DC, Hijazi UM, et al. Fine needle aspiration cytology of submucosal nodules in patients with Zollinger-Ellison syndrome. *Am J Gastroenterol* 1993;88(2):258–265.
41. Straus E, Raufman JP, Samuel S, et al. Endoscopic cure of the Zollinger-Ellison syndrome: removal of duodenal gastrinoma from the proximal limb of a gastrojejunostomy. *Gastrointest Endosc* 1992;38(6):709–711.
42. Fujimori T, Nakamura T, Hirayama D, et al. Endoscopic mucosectomy for early gastric cancer using modified strip biopsy. *Endoscopy* 1992;24:187–189.
43. Caletti GC, Brocchi E, Ferrari A, et al. Guillotine needle biopsy as a supplement to endosonography in the diagnosis of gastric submucosal tumors. *Endoscopy* 1991;23:251–254.
44. Wiersema MJ, Hawes RH, Tao LC. Endoscopic ultrasonograpy as an adjunct to fine needle aspiration cytology of the upper and lower gastrointestinal tract. *Gastrointest Endosc* 1992;38(1):35–39.
45. Wiersema MJ, Kochman ML, Chak A, et al. Real-time endoscopic ultrasound guided FNA of a mediastinal lymph node. *Gastrointest Endosc* 1993;39(3):429–431.
46. Yu JP, Luo HS, Wang XZ. Endoscopic treatment of submucosal lesions of the gastrointestinal tract. *Endoscopy* 1992;24:190–193.
47. Tio TL, Tytgat GN. Endoscopic ultrasonography of an arteriovenous malformation in a gastric polyp. *Endoscopy* 1986;18(4):156–158.
48. Jeng KS, Yang KC, Kuo SHF. Malignant degeneration of heterotopic pancreas. *Gastrointest Endosc* 1991;37(2):196–198.

Advanced Therapeutic Endoscopy, 2nd Ed.,
edited by J. S. Barkin and C. A. O'Phelan.
Raven Press, Ltd., New York © 1994.

CHAPTER 15

Significance of Endosonography in Diagnosing and Staging Colorectal Lesions

Thian Lok Tio

The history of ultrasound (US) in medicine started immediately after World War II with Dussik's work in Austria on the evaluation of the human brain, which he called "the way to hyperphonography of the brain" (1). In 1950 an American physician J. J. Wild introduced US for the measurement of tissue changes and in 1952 he reported the first use of transrectal US (2,3). It took, however, almost two decades for further clinical application to be employed in Europe and Japan (4,5). Urologists established transrectal and transurethral US for the evaluation of prostate gland diseases. In 1972 a Dutch physicist reported the use of miniature echoprobe for intracardiac scanning, followed in 1976 by a German gastroenterologist using a miniature catheter echoprobe through the biopsy channel of a gastroscope with A-mode imaging technology (6,7). At the end of 1970s, Hisanaga, a Japanese cardiologist, Di Magno, an American gastroenterologist, and Strohm, a German gastroenterologist, reported independently the use of a flexible echoendoscope for transesophageal and transgastric imaging in the field of cardiology and gastroenterology (8–10).

During the next decade many reports were published concerning the clinical use of so-called endosonography (ESG), which includes the use of an echoendoscope and a flexible non-optic and miniature catheter echoprobe. In 1986 Tytgat and I (11) published the first atlas of transintestinal endosonography during the World Congress of Gastroenterology in Sao Paolo, Brazil. Recently, for teaching purposes I have published a video laser disk entitled "Atlas of Endosonography" (12).

This chapter describes the value of ESG in the diagnosis and staging of colorectal lesions.

INSTRUMENTS

The widely used standard instrument is a rigid non-optic echoprobe with a small echoprobe attached at the tip of the rigid shaft. The scanning device of the echoprobe can be sectorial, radial, or linear-array. In the case of a tight stenosis, there is a sector scanning vaginal probe, in which a sector echoprobe is attached longitudinally to the shaft. In the case of rectal stenosis a flexible small caliber echoprobe can be used, which is usually used for transesophageal US. A laparoscopic flexible echoprobe is also suitable for transrectal US. Recently, an echocolonoscope has become available, in which an echoprobe is attached to the tip of a forward-viewing colonoscope (Fig. 1). The diameter of the echoprobe and endoscope is 15 mm and the length of the instrument is 130 cm. Currently, a miniature catheter echoprobe has also become available, which can be inserted through the biopsy channel of an endoscope for endoscopic-guided ESG (Fig. 2).

INVESTIGATION TECHNIQUE

Non-Optic Transrectal ESG

The technique of investigation is similar to that of rectoscopy. Phosphate enema or another cleaning procedure is necessary to eliminate feces from the rectum to prevent artifacts on ESG images. The patient can be positioned in the left-lateral decubital or supine position. Rectal digital examination is recommended to dilate the sphincter and to examine the rectum. Then the

T. L. Tio: Division of Gastroenterology, Department of Medicine, Georgetown University Medical Center, Washington, DC 20007.

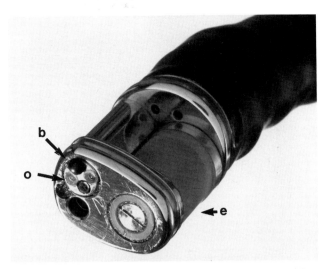

FIG. 1. An Olympus echocolonoscope (CF-UM3) with a small echoprobe *(e)* attached beyond forward-viewing optics *(o)* and parallel to the biopsy channel *(b)*.

rigid or flexible instrument is inserted into the rectum as deeply as possible. In the case of resistance due to a stenosis, further insertion into the proximal part should be avoided because of the risk of perforation. Then the instrument is slowly withdrawn under continuous ESG images until the target lesion is visualized. Careful assessment of the lesion is necessary to obtain the maximal extent of the target lesion. For topographic anatomical orientation the prostate gland or uterus or urine bladder and the coccygeal bone can be used as landmarks. The latter should be placed at 6 o'clock and automatically the prostate gland or uterus and the urine bladder will be found at the contralateral part between 10 and 2 o'clock. At the level of distal rectum the pelvic floor muscles can be seen as hypoechoic muscle bundles adjacent to the rectal lumen. The levator ani muscles are seen adjacent to the rectal wall and form as symmetrical arch muscles between the coccyx and the prostate gland or the uterus. At the sphincter level the internal sphincter muscle is seen as local thickening of the muscularis propria. The external sphincter is seen immediately adjacent to the internal sphincter.

Endoscopic ESG

The technique of investigation for endoscopic ESG is comparable with standard colonoscopy. For rectal lesions an echogastroscope, echoduodenoscope, or echocolonoscope can be used. For proximal suprarectal lesions, however, only an echocolonoscope should be used because of its forward-viewing optics; an echogastroscope or echoduodenoscope is not suitable because of the lateral-viewing optics. The target lesion should be found endoscopically and the echoprobe should be placed accordingly. By using an echocolonoscope the echoprobe should be advanced approximately 1 cm beyond the target because the transducer is located 1 cm distally to the optics. However, this is not necessary when using an upper echoendoscope, because the position of the transducer can be controlled endoscopically. In the case of an extramural lesion, the tip of the instrument should be inserted proximally to the lesion using the information gathered by standard colonoscopy or x-ray examination. An echocolonoscope has a sector image of approximately 330° because of the biopsy channel, which hinders a full-size image of 360°. In contrast, an upper echoendoscope has a 360° radial image because the biopsy channel is placed beyond the transducer. The ESG orientation is similar to that obtained with a non-optic echoprobe.

Endoscopic-Guided ESG

The technique of investigation is comparable with colonoscopy. The lesion must be found endoscopically. Then the miniature probe is inserted through the biopsy channel to the target under endoscopic control. For clear ultrasonic imaging the space between the transducer and the lesion should be filled with water to achieve an acoustic window. This can be accomplished by removing the miniature probe from the biopsy channel, subsequently filling the colorectal lumen with water. Recently, a miniature echoprobe covered with a balloon has become available, which allows clear imaging by filling the balloon with water. The penetration of the transducer varies from 1 to 3 cm

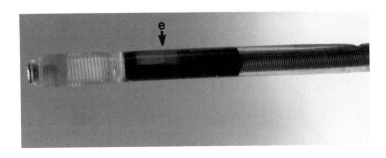

FIG. 2. An Olympus miniature catheter-like echoprobe *(e)*, which can be inserted through a biopsy channel of large caliber endoscope.

depending on the frequency employed. Therefore, a miniature echoprobe is only suitable for the assessment of limited mural abnormality or a small lesion directly adjacent to the colorectal wall.

INDICATIONS

During the last decade indications for the use of ESG, which include rectal and perirectal diseases not accurately diagnosed by endoscopy, computed tomography (CT), and transabdominal US, have been generally accepted by many investigators, particularly in Europe. The most important indications of ESG are listed as follows:

1. Cancer staging and follow-up
2. Staging and follow-up of colorectal non-Hodgkin's lymphoma (NHL)
3. Differential diagnosis of villous adenoma versus advanced cancers
4. Diagnosing and staging of submucosal abnormalities
5. Diagnosing of perirectal fistulas and abscesses.

RESULTS

Staging and Follow-Up of Colorectal Cancers

The interpretation of colorectal wall structures is comparable to those of gastrointestinal wall (11,12). In essence, the colorectal wall is imaged as five distinct individual layers: the mucosa, submucosa, muscularis propria, and the perirectal fat tissue (Fig. 3). The mus-

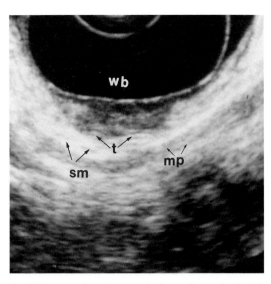

FIG. 4. ESG reveals a hypoechoic pattern limited in the first and second layer (mucosa) without pentration into the third layer (submucosa) compatible with a T1-mucosal carcinoma.

cularis propria of the rectal wall may appear as a thick muscle bundle, which sometimes can be seen as two separate layers—the internal circular layer and the outer longitudinal layer surrounded by a hyperechoic fat tissue without a serosal overlying layer. In the colon, however, there is an overlying serosal layer that is difficult or even impossible to distinguish from the perirectal fat tissue. Carcinoma is visualized as a hypoechoic pattern destructing partially or totally the normal wall architecture, depending on the depth of tumor infiltration. Regional lymph nodes are seen as a hyperechoic or hypoechoic pattern, which can readily be distinguished from the more hyperechoic fat tissue (13,14).

According to the definition published in our initial results, a metastatic lymph node is imaged as a hypoechoic pattern with distinct boundaries. Occasionally, direct penetration of tumor into adjacent lymph nodes can be seen, which is strongly suggestive of malignancy. A benign lymph node can be seen as a hyperechoic pattern with no clearly defined borders, and may be difficult to differentiate from the surrounding fat tissue (15).

Recently, the depth of tumor infiltration has been used as the main criterion for the staging of colorectal cancer, replacing the longitudinal length of the tumor. The definition of regional lymph nodes has been revised. In our series involving 91 cases with colorectal cancer, the accuracy of ESG in staging rectal and colonic cancers was 81% and 93%, respectively (16). ESG was accurate in staging almost all categories except for T2 cancers (Figs. 4–8), due to the presence of peritumoral inflammation after irradiation or an associated peritumoral abscesses (16). Overstaging and understaging occurred in 13% and 2%, respectively. For

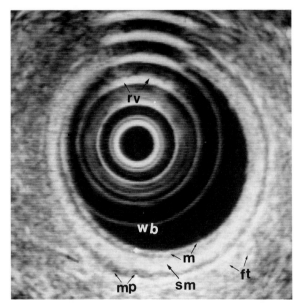

FIG. 3. ESG image reveals five distinct layers architecture of normal rectal wall. m, mucosa; sm, submucosa; mp, muscularis propria; pf, perirectal fat; wb, water-filled balloon; rv, reverberation phenomena due to the biopsy channel.

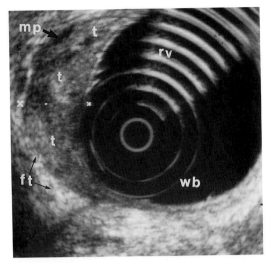

FIG. 5. ESG obtained with an echocolonoscope reveals a semicircumferential hypoechoic transmural pattern *(t)* penetrating the muscularis propria *(mp)* into the perirectal fat tissue *(ft)*. Note the tumor thickness of 2 cm without penetration into the prostate gland. The finding is consistent with a T3 rectal carcinoma.

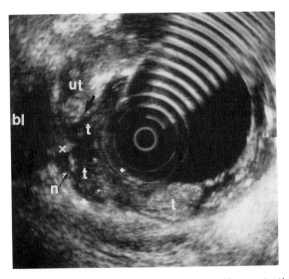

FIG. 6. ESG reveals an exophytic tumor *(t)* penetrating *(arrows)* through the perirectal fat tissue *(ft)* into the adjacent uterus *(ut)*. Note a small hypoechoic lymph node with clearly defined borders *(n)* suspicious of malignancy. The urine bladder *(bl)* is seen as an anechoic cavity adjacent to the uterus.

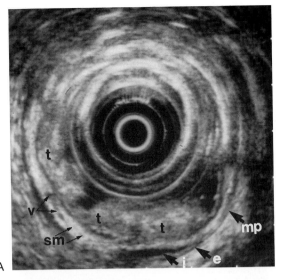

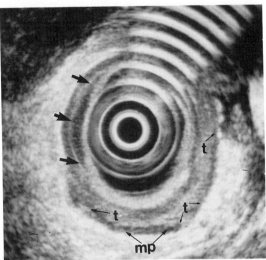

FIG. 7. A: ESG obtained with an echocolonoscope reveals a hypoechoic exophytic tumor located in the mucosa without penetration into the submucosa *(sm)*. Note a small dilated vein in the submucosa. The muscularis propria *(mp)* is seen as an internal *(i)* and external *(e)* layer. The finding is consistent with a villous adenoma. **B:** ESG obtained with an echocolonoscope reveals a semicircular hypoechoic tumor *(t)* with penetration *(thin arrows)* into the muscularis propria *(mp)*, strongly suspicious for malignancy. Note there is an area *(thick arrows)* showing that the tumor is limited to the submucosa *(sm)*. The latter may be consistent with villous adenoma without malignant degeneration.

the staging of regional lymph node metastasis the accuracy of ESG was 70%, the sensitivity 94%, and the specificity 55%. Correlation between ESG and histology using the Duke classification was less accurate: for rectal cancers the accuracy for Duke classes A, B, and C were 48%, 50%, and 96%, respectively; for colonic cancers, 67%, 46%, and 91%, respectively. The overall accuracy was only 67%. Staging of distant metastasis was excluded because liver metastases and

peritoneal dissemination could not be employed due to the limited penetration depth of US. Therefore, abdominal US or CT is necessary for complete staging.

In a Japanese series, ESG has been proven to be accurate in staging colorectal cancers. The accuracy for tumor staging was 84.9% (17). T2 carcinomas were correctly diagnosed in all 13 cases. The discrepancy between the Japanese series and our results was attributed to the absence of peritumoral inflammation or ab-

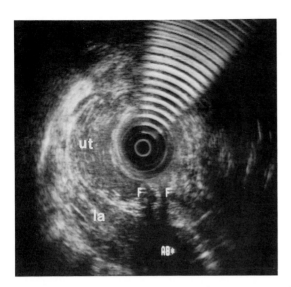

FIG. 8. ESG obtained with an echocolonoscope at the level of rectum reveals two fistulous tracts *(F)* communicating with an anechoic abscess cavity *(ab)*. Note the fistulas and abscess are located at the level of pelvic floor muscle. The lesions are partially destructing the unilateral levator ani musculature *(la)*. Reverberation *(rv)* phenomena occupy approximately 30° of the 360° image due to the biopsy channel. ut, uterus.

scesses. The accuracy in diagnosing regional lymph nodes in their series was only 38%. In another Japanese series involving 164 cases—preoperative staging compared to the histology of resection specimen—the accuracy for the tumor staging was 83% (18). The sensitivity and specificity in the diagnosis of regional lymph node metastasis were only 68% and 70%, respectively. The overall accuracy for the Duke staging was 62%, which is similar to that of our results. In an American series involving 45 cases, the accuracy of ESG in staging tumor categories and regional lymph node metastasis was 89% and 79%, respectively (19). In two German series involving 209 patients the authors reported an accuracy of tumor staging of 90% (20,21).

Staging of Rectal NHL

Primary gastrointestinal NHL is rare. The stomach is the predilection site. ESG has been reported to be the most accurate diagnostic imaging technique for the staging of gastric NHL (22). Recently, mucosa-associated lymphoid tissue lymphoma (MALTOMA) has been increasingly used as the predicting factor for the prognosis (23,24). On ESG rectal NHL is seen as a hypoechoic intramural or transmural infiltration similar to that of gastric NHL. There are only a few cases reported, indicating its rarity (11). Some authors believe that ESG facilitates the differentiation of gastric NHL from gastric cancers (25). This, however, is speculative because such differentiation cannot be made

based solely on the echo pattern. The histology remains the gold standard for the diagnosis.

Differential Diagnosis Between Villous Adenomas and Advanced Cancers

The differential diagnosis between villous adenomas and advanced cancers can be very difficult by endoscopy because the biopsy specimen may be taken at an inappropriate site, one that may not represent the malignant degenerated area. On ESG the diagnosis of villous adenoma is made based on the echo pattern located only on the mucosa level if the biopsy specimen does not represent a carcinoma. Intraepithelial or intramucosal carcinoma, however, cannot be distinguished from a villous adenoma with ESG because both have an abnormality localized in the mucosa. Evidence of lymph nodes suspicious for metastasis found by ESG can be taken into consideration for malignancy. Advanced cancers, however, can be distinguished from villous adenomas using the depth of tumor infiltration as the criterion. The minimum criterion for malignancy should be penetration into the muscularis propria, which represents a T2 carcinoma. Transmural infiltration is almost always suspicious for malignancy except if peritumoral infiltration or abscesses are present, which cannot be ruled out based on ESG findings.

Recently, transrectal ESG has been reported to be helpful in defining the malignant degeneration of villous adenoma (26). In the near future ESG-guided aspiration cytology should be employed routinely to reduce the risk of a false-positive or false-negative diagnosis. In our previous series of endoscopically diagnosed villous adenoma involving 81 cases who underwent transrectal ESG for cancer screening (26), the final diagnosis was made based on the histology of surgical resection specimen, or 5 months' follow-up after laser ablation in 39 cases. ESG made a correct diagnosis of carcinomatous degeneration in 9 of 12 patients (sensitivity 75%). A false-negative diagnosis occurred in the remaining 3 patients. In 46 of 54 cases—all treated with laser therapy—ESG diagnosed correctly a villous adenoma (specificity 85%). In the remaining 8 cases ESG misinterpreted malignancy due to the disrupted muscularis propria. Seven of these patients had previous surgery or laser therapy, which led to the disruption of the underlying structure beyond the lesion. Because of the high predictive value for a negative diagnosis (villous adenoma, 94%), transcolorectal ESG should be recommended for the evaluation of villous adenomas to detect malignancy, especially if nonsurgical treatment such as endoscopic polypectomy or laser ablation is considered.

Diagnosing and Staging of Submucosal Abnormalities

ESG has considerable clinical importance for the diagnosis of submucosal lesions because endoscopy can visualize only mucosal abnormalities, whereas ESG can see through the mucosa to identify the cause of abnormalities. Clinically, the most common submucosal tumors in the gastrointestinal tract are leiomyomas, leiomyoblastomas or leiomyosarcomas, carcinoids, endometriosis, and recurrent cancers after resection (27,28). The diagnosis of recurrent rectal cancer with ESG has been reported by many surgeons who used transrectal ESG in follow-up of patients after resection surgery. A recurrent carcinoma can be seen as a local thickening of the muscularis propria or a limited intrasubmucosal tumor, which may lead to the diagnosis of leiomyoma if a preoperative ESG is not performed and a comparison between a preoperative and postoperative ESG cannot be done. In such cases, ESG-guided aspiration cytology is essential to diagnose the malignant nature of the disease because endoscopy and biopsy may be negative. A differential diagnosis between an extramural mass and a submucosal tumor can be made by ESG based on the location of abnormalities. In one special case of ovarian cancer involving the perisigmoidal colon found by ESG the final histology of the resection specimen revealed an additional primary sigmoid cancer—multisynchronous cancers.

Recently, a case report of localized colitis cystica profunda in the rectum has been published (29). The lesion was described as a hypoechoic cystic lesion located in the submucosa, whereas the muscularis propria was intact. The diagnosis of malignancy was therefore unlikely. The histology of endoscopic resected specimen confirmed the diagnosis of colitis cystica profunda. ESG has also been reported to be useful in staging gastrointestinal carcinoids (5 gastric, 7 duodenal, and 17 rectal) by determining the depth of involvement and the presence of lymph node metastases (30). Carcinoid was described as an oval or round hypoechoic tumor with smooth margins located in the submucosa. The overall accuracy for the assessment of tumor's depth and lymph node metastases was 75%. In the near future ESG-guided aspiration cytology should become a routine procedure to obtain a tissue diagnosis (31,32).

Diagnosis and Staging of Perirectal Fistulas and Abscesses

The diagnosis of perianal or perirectal fistulas or abscesses can be made by visual inspection if a skin lesion is present. This, however, may represent only the tip of the iceberg because the primary lesion may be deeply buried in the perirectal space. Incidentally, the radiologist can diagnose a fistula during barium enema study by the presence of a communication between the fistula and the colorectum. Fistulography has been used for the assessment of fistulas. This, however, is often painful and may be associated with the risk of infection due to the dissemination of infected content. Transrectal ESG has been reported to be accurate in the assessment of fistulas and abscesses because of the clear imaging of the abnormality and its adjacent structures. A fistula is visualized as a hypoechoic or anechoic duct-like structure adjacent to the lumen or within the perirectal floor. An abscess is seen as a hypoechoic or anechoic cavity located in the perirectal space, which is often associated with a fistula. The involvement of pelvic floor musculature (33,34), the sphincter muscles, the urine bladder, the vagina, or the scrotum may be found, in the case of rectovaginal fistula, which may lead to dyspareunia. In some cases transvaginal ESG has been reported to be more accurate than the transrectal approach. Transrectal ESG has also been reported to be valuable in the evaluation of patients with Crohn's disease. The most powerful capability of ESG is to image the sphincter muscles—the internal sphincter and the external sphincter of the anus—and the pelvic floor musculature, which are essential in understanding the normal and pathological anatomy (33,34).

CONCLUSIONS

Transcolorectal ESG has been rapidly developed due to the advanced technology of US, particularly since the development of the rigid echoprobe and the echoendoscope. Cancer staging has become the most important indication for daily clinical work. Distinction between a villous adenoma and an advanced cancer is clinically important because of the different strategy of treatment. A villous adenoma can be treated with local resection—endoscopically or surgically. An advanced cancer, however, should be resected surgically if possible. In nonresectable cases, down-staging can be designed using radiotherapy. This, however, requires accurate monitoring with ESG.

Recently, surgeons have been advocating endoscopic colectomy, which requires adequate patient selection by ESG. In diagnosing perirectal fistulas and abscesses, a rigid transrectal instrument is more suitable than an echoendoscope due to the easy handling of the instrument and the cost-benefit ratio. In the case of suprarectal lesion, however, an echocolonoscope is the choice of instrument due to its capability of identifying mural and extramural lesions and of performing a therapeutic approach if necessary. In the case of limited mural abnormality the use of miniature probe during regular colonoscopy will become the trend in the future because it is easy to handle and it is not a time-consuming procedure.

REFERENCES

1. Dussik KT, Dussik F, Wyt L. Auf dem Weg zur Hyperphonographie des Gehirnes. *Wien Med Wochenschr* 1947;97:425–429.
2. Wild JJ. The use of ultrasonic pulses for the measurement of biological tissue changes. *Surgery* 1950;27:183–187.
3. Wild JJ, Reid JM. Echographic tissue diagnosis. Proceedings of the 4th annual conference on ultrasonic therapy, Detroit, August 1955.
4. Watanabe H, Kato H, Tanaka M, Terasawa Y. Diagnostic application of ultrasonotomography for the prostate. *Jpn J Urol* 1968;59:273–277.
5. Holm HH, Northeveld AA. Transurethral ultrasonic scanner. *J Urol* 1974;111:238–248.
6. Bom N, Lancee CT, van Egmond FC. An ultrasonic intracardiac scanner. *Ultrasonics* 1972;10:72–76.
7. Lutz H, Rosch W. Transgastroscopic ultrasonography. *Endoscopy* 1976;8:203–205.
8. Hisanaga K, Hisanaga A. A new real-time sector scanning system of ultra-wide angle and real-time recording to entire cardiac images: transesophagus and transchest methods. *Ultrasound Med* 1978;4:391–401.
9. Strohm WED, Philip F, Hagenmuller F, Classen M. Ultrasonic tomography by means of ultrasonic fiberendoscope. *Endoscopy* 1980;12:241–244.
10. Di Magno EP, Buxton JL, Regan PT. The ultrasonic endoscope. *Lancet* 1980;1:629–631.
11. Tio TL, Tytgat GNJ. *Atlas of transintestinal ultrasonography*. Aalsmeer, The Netherlands: Mur-Kostverloren, 1986.
12. Tio TL. *Atlas of endosonography: interactive videodisc program*. New York: Olympus, 1992.
13. Tio TL, Tytgat GNJ. Endoscopic ultrasonography in the assessment of intra- and transmural infiltration of tumors in the esophagus, stomach and papilla of Vater and in the detection of extraesophageal lesions. *Endoscopy* 1984;16:203–210.
14. Kimmey MB, Martin RW, Haggitt RC, Wang KY, Franklin DW, Silverstein WF. Histologic correlates of gastrointestinal ultrasound images. *Gastroenterology* 1989;96:433–441.
15. Tio TL, Tytgat GNJ. Endoscopic ultrasonography in analyzing peri-intestinal lymph node abnormality. *Scand J Gastroenterol* 1986;21(suppl 123):158–163.
16. Tio TL, Coene PP, van Delden OM, Tytgat GNJ. Colorectal carcinoma: preoperative TNM classification with endosonography. *Radiology* 1991;179:165–170.
17. Shimizu S, Tada M, Kawai K. Use of endoscopic ultrasonography for the diagnosis of colorectal tumors. *Endoscopy* 1990;22:31–34.
18. Cho E, Nakajima M, Yasuda K, Ashihara T, Kawai K. Endoscopic ultrasonography in the diagnosis of colorectal invasion. *Gastrointest Endosc* 1993;39:521–527.
19. Boyce G, Sivak MV, Lavery IC, Facio VW, Church JM, Milson J, Petras R. Endoscopic ultrasonography in the preoperative staging of rectal carcinoma. *Gastrointest Endosc* 1992;38:468–471.
20. Feifel G, Hildebrandt U, Dhom G. Assessment of depth of invasion in rectal cancer by endosonography. *Endoscopy* 1987;19(2):64–67.
21. Heintz A, Buess G, Junginger T. Endorectal Sonographie zur Beurteilung der Infiltrationstiefe von Rektumtumoren. *Dtsch Med Wochenschr* 1990;115:1083–1087.
22. Tio TL, den Hartog Jager FCA, Tytgat GJN. Endoscopic ultrasonography of non-Hodgkin lymphoma of the stomach. *Gastroenterology* 1986;91:401–408.
23. Cogliatti SB, Schmid U, Schumacher URS, Eckerd F, Hansmann ML, Heddrich J, Takahashi H, Lennert K. Primary B-cell gastric lymphoma: a clinicopathological study of 145 patients. *Gastroenterology* 1991;101:1159–1170.
24. Radaszkiewicz T, Dragosics B, Bauer P. Gastrointestinal malignant lymphoma of the mucosa-associated lymphoid tissue: factors relevant to prognosis. *Gastroenterology* 1992;102:1628–1638.
25. Bolondi L, Casanova P, Caletti EC, Grigioni W, Zani L, Barbara L. Primary gastric lymphoma versus gastric carcinoma: endoscopic US evaluation. *Radiology* 1987;65:821–826.
26. Hulsman FC, Tio TL, Mathus-Vliegen E. Colorectal villous adenoma: transrectal US in screening for invasive malignancy. *Radiology* 1992;185:193–196.
27. Tio TL, Tytgat GNJ, den Hartog Jager FCA. Endoscopic ultrasonography for the evaluation of smooth muscle tumors in the upper gastrointestinal tract: our experience with 42 cases. *Gastrointest Endosc* 1990;36:342–350.
28. Tio TL, Tytgat GNJ. Comparison of blind transrectal ultrasonography with endoscopic ultrasonography in assessing rectal and perirectal diseases. *Scand J Gastroenterol* 1986;21(suppl):104.
29. Hulsman FJH, Tio TL, Reeders JWA, Tytgat GNJ. Transectal US in the diagnosis of localized colitis cystica profunda. *Radiology* 1991;181:201–203.
30. Yoshikane H, Tsukamoto Y, Niwa Y, Goto H, Hase S, Mizutani K, Nakamura T. Carcinoid tumors of the gastrointestinal tract: evaluation with endoscopic ultrasonography. *Gastrointest Endosc* 1993;39:375–383.
31. Tio TL, Sie LH, Tytgat GNJ. Endosonography and cytology in diagnosis and staging pancreatic body and tail carcinoma. *Dig Dis Sci* 1993;1:59–64.
32. Vilmann P, Jacobsen GK, Henriksen FW, Hancke S. Endoscopic ultrasonography with guided fine needle aspiration biopsy in pancreatic disease. *Gastrointest Endosc* 1992;38(2):172–173.
33. Tio TL, Mulder CJJ, Weijers OB, Sars PRA, Tytgat GNJ. Endosonography of perianal and perirectal fistulas and/or abscesses in Crohn's disease. *Gastrointest Endosc* 1990;4:331–336.
34. Van Outryve MJ, Pelckmans PA, Michielsen PR, Van Maerice YM. Value of transrectal ultrasonography in Crohn's disease. *Gastroenterology* 1991;101:1171–1177.

Advanced Therapeutic Endoscopy, 2nd Ed.,
edited by J. S. Barkin and C. A. O'Phelan.
Raven Press, Ltd., New York © 1994.

CHAPTER 16

Role of Endoscopic Ultrasound in Benign and Malignant Colorectal Lesions

Ulrich Hildebrandt

The first flexible ultrasound instrument was completed in 1953 by John Wild, the pioneer of endosonography (1). Because of technical shortcomings it was never used clinically, but it inspired further effort to develop the technique. Twenty years later, Lutz introduced an A-mode ultrasonic probe that could be passed down the biopsy channel of an endoscope (2), and in 1980, Hisanaga and Hisanaga (3) performed echocardiography using an ultrasonic transducer attached to the tip of a flexible fiberoptic endoscope.

Di Magno et al. (4) and Strohm et al. (5) reported on the endoscopic ultrasonic tomography of the upper gastrointestinal tract and adjacent organs and a comprehensive overview of endosonography in gastroenterology has been published by Tio (6). In 1983 Alzin et al. (7), Dragsted and Gammelgaard (8), and Hildebrandt et al. (9) reported on the application of endorectal ultrasound in rectal cancer.

An ultrasound colonoscope became available in 1989. This chapter describes the equipment and the technique of colorectal sonography, and discusses benign and malignant findings and their impact on treatment decisions.

EQUIPMENT

Until 1989 exclusively rigid probes had been available for endosonography. They were either inserted blindly into the rectal lumen or through a rectoscope. Sector scanners are superior to linear scanners. The superiority of 360° sector scanners lies in the fact that the rectum and its surroundings can be scanned continuously by simply drawing back the endosonic probe.

U. Hildebrandt: Department of General Surgery, University of Saarland, Homburg Saar, Germany.

The usual frequency of the transducer head is 7.5 MHz. It represents a compromise between resolution and penetration depth. Rigid probes cannot usually be inserted deeper than 15 cm, but by passing it through a rectoscope the tip of the probe can be positioned at 20 cm (10). The examination is, however, likely to be more uncomfortable at this level. There are a number of rigid probes marketed for ultrasound examination of the rectum and we use the B. and K. Medical (Naerum, Denmark) instrument. Since 1990 we use the Olympus ultrasound colonoscope CF Type UM 3 to evaluate lesions that are situated farther than 15 cm from the anal verge. The endoscopic and ultrasonic features of the instrument are specified in Table 1.

METHOD OF EXAMINATION

Endorectal sonography is performed with the patient in the lithotomy position. Prior to examination, the pa-

TABLE 1. *Main specifications of the Olympus ultrasound colonoscope CF Type UM 3*

Endoscopic function	
Optical system	Angle of view: forward
Distal end	Outer diameter: 17.4 mm
Flexible portion	Outer diameter: 13.7 mm
Working length	1033.0 mm
Biopsy channel	Inner diameter: 2.8 mm
Ultrasonic function	
Display mode	B-mode
Scanning method	Mechanical radial scanning
Scanning direction	At right angle to direction of insertion
Scanning angle	300° sector
Frequency	7.5 MHz
	12.0 MHz
Focusing point	25.0 mm (12.0 MHz)
	30.0 mm (75 MHz)

tient's rectum is evacuated with an enema. The total length of the rigid probe with the transducer fitted on the end is 24 cm. The transducer rotates mechanically. The reflections of the transmitted ultrasonic waves are received at a 90° angle. Scanning radially to the longitudinal axis of the rectal probe, it provides a 360° display of the rectum and the surrounding tissues (11). The ultrasonic probe is inserted via the rectoscope, which is introduced into the rectum as far as possible. Following insertion of the probe, the rubber balloon that is attached over the transducer is filled with approximately 60 ml of degassed water. During simultaneous withdrawal of the probe and the rectoscope, the region of interest is scanned in a continuous fashion.

ENDOSONOGRAPHIC CHARACTERISTICS OF THE COLORECTAL WALL

Endosonographically the normal colorectal wall appears as two dark hypoechoic and three white hyperechoic lines when a 7.5- or 12.0-MHz transducer is used (Fig. 1). The inner white line represents the borderline of the reflected ultrasound beam. If a water-filled balloon is used for acoustic interfacing, the balloon is identical with the borderline reflection (12). The innermost hypoechoic black line represents the mucosa. The middle hyperechoic line is identical with the submucosa. The outer hypoechoic black line represents the muscularis propria. The outermost hyperechoic white line represents the serosa where the bowel is covered with it, or it represents the borderline to the mesorectal or mesocolic fat. The thickness of the sonographically appearing lines is nearly the same for all five layers in the intact colonic wall. The typical five-layer structure is characteristic throughout the

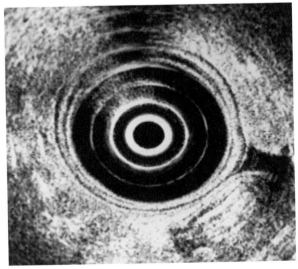

FIG. 1. Endosonogram of the normal colorectal wall (12.0 MHz).

gastrointestinal tract and the interpretation of the different layers is uniform (13,14).

ENDOSONOGRAPHIC ANATOMY OF THE PELVIC FLOOR

The pelvic diaphragm, which consists of the levator ani and coccygeus muscles, forms the pelvic floor. With the probe in the anal canal endosonography can demonstrate that the muscle sheet stretches between the pubis anteriorly and the coccyx posteriorly. The obturator internus muscle is seen as a hypoechoic band in front of the hyperechoic pubic ramus. The puborectalis muscle forms a sling at the junction of the rectum and the anal canal. The junctional area is endosonographically characterized by a thickening of the wall. The internal and external anal sphincters can be differentiated. The mucosa of the anal canal appears hyperechoic. The internal sphincter is hypoechoic. The next hyperechoic and relatively hypoechoic structures are the external sphincter together with the conjoined longitudinal muscle.

ENDOSONOGRAPHIC RELATIONS TO THE COLORECTUM

Anteriorly in the male the rectum is related to the base of the bladder, the seminal vesicles, and the prostate. The endosonographic appearance of the bladder depends on how full it is. The rectovesical septum, which is closely associated with the prostate, represents a potential cleavage plane between the rectum and the prostate. Another landmark is the seminal vesicles, which extend to both sides of the prostate. In the female the anterior relation of the rectum is the vagina. Tumors penetrating into the posterior wall of the vagina are clearly visualized endosonographically in varying shapes and sizes, depending on the age of the patient. Blood vessels are hypoechoic. Mostly vessels have a typical bright reflection of the echo. Veins can be differentiated from arteries by their sonographic appearance in different planes. The endosonographic continuity of hypoechoic vessels is the criterion used to differentiate them from hypoechoic lymph nodes.

ENSOSONOGRAPHY IN BENIGN COLORECTAL DISEASE

Anorectal Abscesses

For the five types of anorectal abscesses—perianal, ischiorectal, submucosal, intersphincteric, and supralevator—the treatment differs. Therefore, it is important to distinguish them. The perianal abscess, the most common of the five types, is situated superficially lateral to the anal verge. Clinically it presents as an area of erythema, induration, or fluctuance. Despite the absence of fluctuance or significant induration, endosonography may help to establish an abscess already present.

Ischiorectal abscess mostly presents as a large erythematous induration of the buttock. The evaluation of the extension of the abscess cavity by endosonography may affect the choice of incision.

The sonographic appearance of a submucosal abscess is characteristic.

Due to the inflammatory reaction the mucosa is thickened. The hypoechoic muscularis propria and the hypoechoic abscess form an integrated whole. Intraluminal drainage is the therapy of choice in masses with that specific endosonographic appearance.

An intersphincteric abscess occurs between the internal and external sphincter of the anus. Ultrasound examination demonstrates the intact mucosa and the abscess between the two sphincters.

Colorectal Adenomas

Adenomas by definition are benign. Due to their relationship with the subsequent development of cancer, their sonographic imaging is of some interest. They may be as small as 1 mm or larger than 7 cm, pedunculated or sessile. The aim of preoperative endosonography of adenomas is to evaluate whether carcinoma is visible on ultrasound. Generally, the larger the adenoma, the greater the likelihood of malignant change. Polypoid adenomas under 1 cm in diameter have been shown to have a 1% incidence of malignant change, while villous adenomas have a 10% risk of malignancy. Among adenomas larger than 2 cm, malignant change occurs in 35% of polypoid lesions and in 50% of villous adenomas. There are a number of technical problems in scanning adenomas. The water-filled balloon will squash and distort the anatomy of a polyp. On some occasions it is helpful to fill the rectum with water first and scan the adenoma with little water in the balloon. With endosonography adenomas have the following appearances:

1. Flat adenomas are sonographically characterized by a circumscribed thickening of the inner hypoechoic layer representing the mucosa.
2. Polypoid adenomas have a heterogeneous echo pattern: therefore, transformation into a malignant lesion cannot be assessed by endosonography. Carcinoma in situ and severe dysplasia will be impossible to detect (Fig. 2).
3. If there is a sizable T1 carcinoma arising within adenoma, it may be visible by a large hypoechoic area in a relatively hyperechoic adenoma.

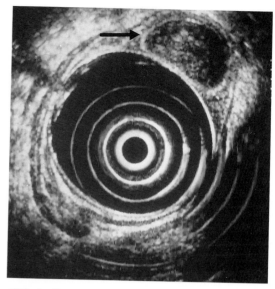

FIG. 2. Endosonogram of a polypoid adenoma.

4. Both an adenoma and a T1 carcinoma have the sonographic criterion that the outer hypoechoic layer representing the muscularis propria is intact. Hence, a tumor with an intact muscle layer can be assessed for malignancy only by histological examination.

These criteria are the same for examination with the rigid or with the flexible instrument.

The endosonographic definition of a sessile adenoma of the colorectum that cannot be removed endoscopically has the following implications for treatment:

1. Adenomas of the rectum are excised in full thickness by the transanal endoscopic microsurgical (TEM) technique.
2. Adenomas of the colon are resected by the minimally invasive technique of laparoscopic surgery (Figs. 3 and 4).

Since we are at the beginning of the new surgical era, that of endoscopic minimally invasive surgery, diagnostic endosonography will be invaluable for the differentiation of colorectal adenomas.

ENDOSONOGRAPHIC DIFFERENTIATION OF MUCOSAL AND TRANSMURAL NONSPECIFIC INFLAMMATORY BOWEL DISEASE

Inflammation of the gut can be classified as that of known cause, which is mostly infective, and that of unknown cause, or nonspecific inflammatory bowel disease. The two types of nonspecific inflammation, ulcerative colitis and Crohn's disease, have points of similarity and difference, and can be distinguished from one another on anatomical grounds. The term *in-*

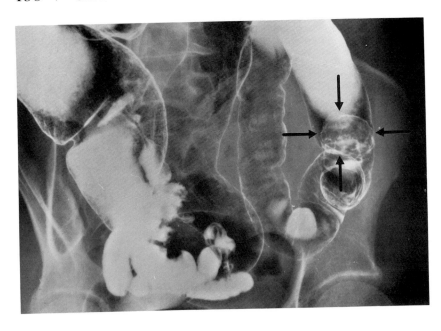

FIG. 3. Roentgenographic findings of a polypoid adenoma in the sigmoid colon (arrows).

determinate colitis describes the situation in which the two disorders may overlap in their macroscopic features.

The indication for surgical treatment of inflammatory bowel disease is essentially failure of medical treatment. If a colectomy is indicated it is necessary to know, from a surgical point of view, whether it is an ulcerative colitis or a Crohn's colitis. In those patients in whom the disease affects only the mucosa of the colon, as it is in ulcerative colitis, restorative proctocolectomy with an ileal reservoir is the surgical procedure of choice. An accurate differential diagnosis of ulcerative colitis and Crohn's disease can readily be made by endoscopy in about 80% to 90% of cases. In a prospective study of 357 patients, the endoscopic signs were accurate in 89% of the patients with a 4% error rate and 7% of patients with an indeterminate diagnosis (15). The significance of biopsy was evaluated prospectively in 146 patients in whom the diagnosis of Crohn's disease of the colon was established by clinical, laboratory, endoscopic, and radiologic criteria. Histologic findings were diagnostic of Crohn's disease in 24.7%, consistent with Crohn's disease in 54.8%, and nondiagnostic of Crohn's disease in 20.5% (16). Despite the complementary findings of endoscopy and biopsy, about 10% of cases do not have the standard macroscopic and microscopic features of ulcerative colitis or Crohn's colitis. In a prospective study we determined the value of ultrasonic colonoscopy in the differentiation of mucosal and transmural inflammation in patients with nonspecific inflammatory bowel disease.

ENDOSONOGRAPHIC TECHNIQUE

Fifty-seven patients with nonspecific inflammatory bowel disease were investigated. In addition to the standard diagnostic investigations, including endoscopy, biopsy, and radiology, the patients were examined with the ultrasound colonoscope (Fig. 5) and the disease was classified with respect to mural or transmural inflammation. The endoscopic appearance was recorded on videotape at insertion, and the ultrasonic appearance of the colonic wall was recorded during withdrawal of the instrument (17).

When the mucosa showed signs of inflammation but ultrasonography revealed the five-layer structure of the colonic wall, this was classified as mucosal inflammation. Inflammatory signs in combination with loss

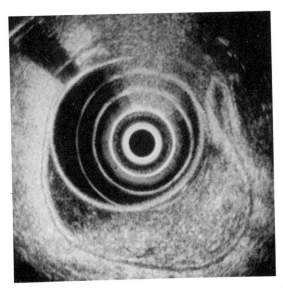

FIG. 4. Endosonogram of the adenoma demonstrating the intact muscle layer. The tumor was removed by laparoscopic colon resection.

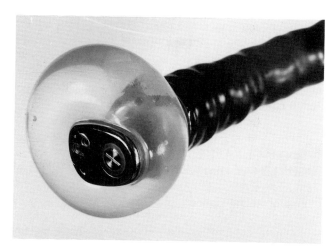

FIG. 5. Tip of the Olympus ultrasound colonoscope CF type UM 3. The transducer is surrounded by a water-filled balloon for acoustic interfacing.

of the ultrasonic five-layer structure was classified as transmural inflammation. In 30 of the 57 patients the colon was resected for various reasons, such as failure of medical treatment and stenosis. In these 30 patients preoperative endoscopic and ultrasonic findings were compared with the findings on examination of cross sections of the excised specimen.

ENDOSONOGRAPHIC CHARACTERISTICS

Ulcerative Colitis

Endosonographically the five-layer structure is uninterrupted throughout the length of the colon (Fig. 6).

In comparison to the normal colon wall the submucosa appears thicker. This phenomenon can be explained physically. Epithelial destruction of the mucosa permits the transmission of more sound energy, which is reflected at the submucosa. The higher amount of reflected sound energy at the level of the submucosa results in thickening of this layer on the ultrasound image. The same happens with edema of the mucosa. The edematous mucosa transmits more sound energy, which is reflected at the submucosal level. Thus, the thickening of the submucosa seen on ultrasonography is a typical sign of mucosal inflammation.

Crohn's Colitis

Discontinuous interruptions or loss of the five-layer structure corresponding to the anatomical variations of transmural inflammation were found (Figs. 7 and 8). Segments of normal five-layered bowel were interspersed with abnormal areas. Thickening of the colonic wall and merging of the mucosa with the submucosa into one layer is one of the various ultrasonic appearances. In other cases the whole colon wall appears as one layer with a thin hyperechoic margin. A typical sign of transmural inflammation is deep longitudinal ulcers with loss of the mucosa and submucosa. On ultrasonography the bare muscle layer was seen as one hypoechoic layer with a hyperechoic margin. The endosonographic criteria for mucosal and transmural inflammation are summarized in Table 2.

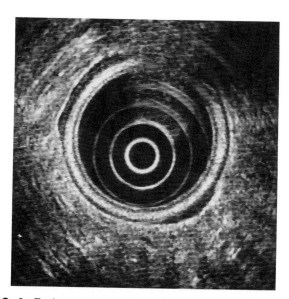

FIG. 6. Endosonogram of ulcerative colitis demonstrating the five-layer structure with thickening of the middle hyperechoic layer corresponding to the submucosa.

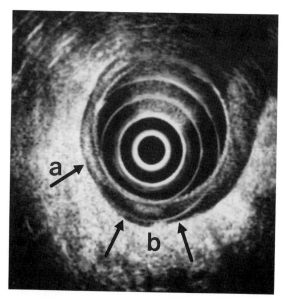

FIG. 7. Endosonogram of Crohn's colitis. The *arrows* indicate a circumscribed section with five layers **(a)** and a section where the colonic wall appears as one layer due to transmural inflammation **(b)**.

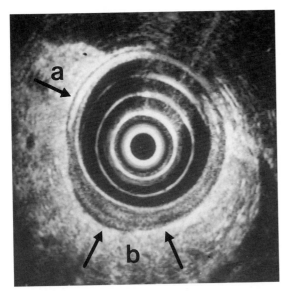

FIG. 8. Endosonogram of Crohn's colitis. Intact five-layer structure **(a)** and transmural inflammation with merging of the individual layers **(b)**.

TABLE 2. *Endosonographic definition of ulcerative and Crohn's colitis*

Mucosal inflammation (ulcerative colitis)	Transmural inflammation (Crohns colitis)
Five-layer structure of the colonic wall Thickening of the submucosa	Sectional interruption of the five-layer structure Less than five layers depending on the degree of transmural inflammation

FINDINGS ON SURGERY AND COMPARISON WITH CLINICAL RESULTS

Endosonography alone attributed the 30 cases either to mucosal or transmural inflammation. This was consistent with the histopathological result in 12 cases of mucosal inflammation. In one case the pathologist found features of both ulcerative and Crohn's colitis. By endoscopy three cases were estimated as ulcerative and two as indeterminate colitis. Histologically four of

TABLE 3. *Comparison of endoscopy, endosonography, and pathology in 30 patients with nonspecific inflammatory bowel disease*

	Ulcerative colitis	Crohn's colitis	Pathologic features of both	Indeterminate colitis
Endoscopy	15	13	–	2
Endosonography	12	18	–	–
Pathology	12	17	1	–

the five undiagnosed cases were revealed to be Crohn's colitis and the fifth had features of both. The resuts are compared in Table 3.

In conclusion, patients suspected of having transmural nonspecific inflammation of the colon can be excluded from ileoanal pouch reconstruction.

ENDOSONOGRAPHY IN MALIGNANT COLORECTAL DISEASE

Staging of Rectal Cancer

Just as surgical principles for the resection of breast and anal cancers have been recently challenged and effectively revised, the treatment of rectal cancer is currently undergoing scrutiny and change. By aggressive anterior approaches that resect adequate proximal and lateral mesorectum the surgeon is capable of obtaining oncologic results equivalent to abdominoperineal resection. Functional results using a wide variety of restorative procedures with anastomoses as low as the dentate line are generally quite acceptable. The philosophy of rectal cancer surgery has been expressed by Mason (18): "No two patients with rectal cancer are ever exactly alike. It must follow, therefore, that no single orthodox standard operation can be the best treatment for every patient with carcinoma of the rectum."

With the advent of rectal endosonography it has been possible to stage the cancer prior to therapy decisions. Parallel to the new staging modality more sophisticated sphincter-sparing operative techniques have been developed. By endosonography the levator ani muscles as well as the external and internal anal sphincter can be exactly exhibited. Hence it is possible to define how close the tumor extends to these structures.

Assessment of Tumor Penetration Depth

The endosonographic assessment of penetration depth within and through the rectal wall follows the TNM staging system. A tumor that is confined to the submucosa is classified as stage ES T1 (Fig. 9). ES T2 means confinement to the muscle layer (Fig. 10), and ES T3 means penetration through the wall (Fig. 11). The accuracy of the endosonographic prediction of tumor penetration depth ranges from 87% to 95% (Table 4). Most of the misinterpretations of sonographic tumor staging are due to an accompanying peritumorous inflammation causing overstaging. Our own results are based on 204 patients with primary rectal cancer. The tumor penetration depth T was predicted with a sensitivity of 96% and specificity of 89%.

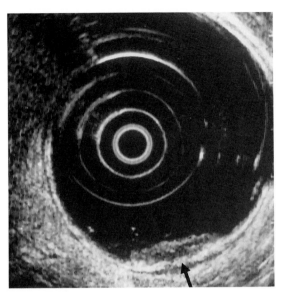

FIG. 9. Endosonogram of rectal cancer stage ES T1. The submucosa *(arrow)* is not infiltrated.

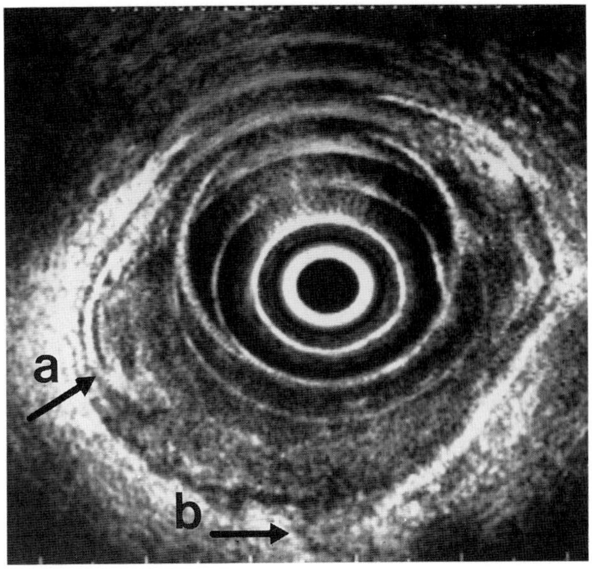

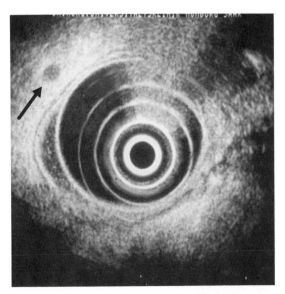

FIG. 11. Endosonogram of rectal cancer stage ES T3. The tumor penetrates through the submucosa **(A)** and through the muscle layer **(B).**

Evaluation of Lymph Nodes

Endosonographically lymph nodes appear with different echo patterns. Based on sonographic characteristics two main groups can be differentiated: hypoechoic and hyperechoic lymph nodes. On the basis of the different echo patterns a prospective study was established to evaluate the endosonographic prediction of a tumor stage ES N1. Lymph nodes were defined as follows: hyperechoic lymph nodes (Fig. 12) represent nonspecific inflammatory changes, and hypoechoic lymph nodes (Fig. 13) represent lymph node metasta-

TABLE 4. *Accuracy of endosonographic assessment of tumor penetration depth ES T in rectal cancer*

ES T	Accuracy (%)
Accarpio et al. (21)	94
Beynon et al. (22)	90
Boscaini and Montori (13)	91
Glaser et al. (23)	88
Hildebrandt and Feifel (12)	88
Orrom et al. (24)	95
Romano et al. (25)	87

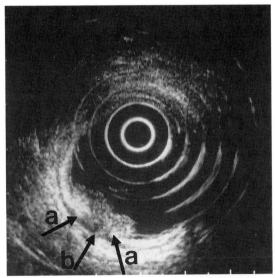

FIG. 10. Endosonogram of rectal cancer stage ES T2. The penetration through the submucosa is indicated by *arrows* **(A).** The tumor penetrates the muscle layer **(B).**

FIG. 12. Endosonogram of a hyperechoic lymph node *(arrow)* representing nonspecific inflammation.

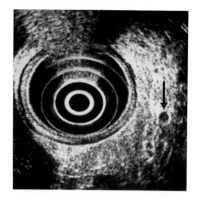

FIG. 13. Endosonogram of a hypoechoic lymph node *(arrow)* representing a lymph node metastasis.

ses. A total of 113 patients with rectal cancer were scanned with 7.5 MHz and entered the study (14). Following operation the histopathological findings were compared with the preoperative assessment of ES NO or ES N1. Nonspecific inflammatory lymph nodes were predicted with a specificity of 83%. Lymph node metastases were predicted with a sensitivity of 72%.

Our current policy in staging lymph nodes is the following: If lymph nodes are not visible by ultrasound, the probability of lymph node metastases will be very low. Hyperechoic lymph nodes visualized by ultrasound are due to nonspecific inflammatory changes. Hypoechoic lymph nodes are highly suggestive of lymph node metastases. Besides the exclusively hypoechoic or hyperechoic lymph nodes, which can be identified as such by endosonography, there are others that represent no characteristic echo patterns and create difficulties for differentiation. This fact and the occurrence of micrometastasized lymph nodes that are not detectable by ultrasound explain in part the specificity of 83% and the relatively low sensitivity of 72%. If the results obtained with endosonography are measured with conventional imaging modalities such as CT, the accuracy rate is significantly higher (19) (Table 5). Accurate preoperative staging is a clue to the correct therapeutic strategy.

TABLE 5. *Specificity and sensitivity of CT and ES in the evaluation of lymph nodes*

	Specificity (%)	Sensitivity (%)
CT		
Dixon et al. (26)	96	39
Grabbe et al. (27)	91	34
Rifkin and Wechsler (28)	91	67
ES		
Beynon et al. (29)	77	68
Hildebrandt (20)	83	72
Saitoh et al. (30)	82	73

If an experienced rectal endosonographer has carried out the examination and the assessment is correct for depth of invasion and lymph node involvement, how does endosonography influence management?

Management by Endosonographic Tumor Stage

Stage ES T1 NO

These tumors are confined to the submucosa, where lymph node involvement has been excluded by endosonography. If situated in the lower rectum and if abdominoperineal excision would be the alternative, these patients can be treated by local excision (20).

Stage ES T2 NO

Here the tumor has extended into the muscularis propria. The risk of lymph node involvement is 10% to 20%. Some of these involved nodes will be detected by endosonography. In older patients without nodal involvement a local excision could be employed if abdominoperineal excision is the alternative. In younger patients sphincter-saving procedures such as low anterior resection and intersphincteric excision with or without colonic reservoir is the appropriate therapy.

Stages ES T2 N1 and ES T3 NO

ES T2 N1 tumors are treated by a sphincter-saving procedure such as low anterior resection or intersphincteric excision with colonic reservoir. ES T3 NO tumors are managed depending on the depth of tumor growth. Deep invasion within the lower third of the rectum implicating insufficient lateral excision of the tumor and mesorectum indicates abdominoperinal excision. Slight invasion instead with the expectation of lateral clearance indicates one of the sphincter-saving procedures.

Stages ES T3 N1 and ES T4

In this group, which has the worst prognosis, survival rates have not improved in the last 30 years. While surgery remains the definitive treatment, there must be further assessment of the role of adjuvant therapy in the hope of improving survival rates. By identifying involved nodes, selection for radiotherapy could be more accurate and its effect in this particular group assessed. Infiltration into adjacent organs staged as ES T4 will clearly identify patients suitable for preoperative radiotherapy or those who are candidates for en bloc resection of invaded structures.

REFERENCES

1. Wild JJ, Reid JM. Diagnostic use of ultrasound. *Br J Phys Med* 1956;11:248–264.
2. Lutz H, Rösch W. Transgastroscopic ultrasonography. *Endoscopy* 1976;8:203–205.
3. Hisanaga K, Hisanaga A. High speed rotating scanner for trans-oesophageal cross-sectional echocardiography. *Am J Cardiol* 1980;46:837.
4. Di Magno EP, Buxton JL, Regan PT. The ultrasonic endoscope. *Lancet* 1980;1:629–631.
5. Strohm WD, Philipp I, Hagenmüller F, Classen M. Ultrasonic tomography by means of an ultrasonic fiberendoscope. *Endoscopy* 1980;12:241–244.
6. Tio TL. *Endosonography in gastroenterology.* Berlin: Springer-Verlag, 1988.
7. Alzin H, Kohlberger E, Schwaiger R, Alloussi S. Valeur d'écho-graphie endorectale dans la chirurgie du rectum. *Ann Radiol* 1983;26:334–336.
8. Dragsted J, Gammelgaard J. Endoluminal ultrasonic scanning in the evaluation of rectal cancer: a preliminary report of 13 cases. *Gastrointest Radiol* 1983;8:367–369.
9. Hildebrandt U, Feifel G, Zimmermann FA, Goebbels R. Significant improvement in clinical staging of rectal carcinoma with a new intrarectal ultrasound scanner. *J Exp Clin Cancer Res* 1983;2(suppl):53.
10. Hildebrandt U, Feifel G, Schwarz HP, Scherr O. Endorectal ultrasound: instrumentation and clinical aspects. *Int J Colorect Dis* 1986;1:203–207.
11. Feifel G, Hildebrandt U, Dhom G. Assessment of depth of invasion in rectal cancer by endosonography. *Endoscopy* 1987;19:64–67.
12. Hildebrandt U, Feifel G. Endorectal sonography. *Surg Annu* 1990;22:169–183.
13. Boscaini M, Montori A. Transrectal ultrasonography: interpretation of normal intestinal wall structure for the preoperative staging of rectal cancer. *Scand J Gastroenterol* 1986;21(suppl 123):82–98.
14. Hildebrandt U, Klein T, Feifel G, Schwarz HP, Schmitt RM. Endosonography of pararectal lymph nodes: in vitro and in vivo evaluation. *Dis Colon Rectum* 1990;33:863–868.
15. Pera A, Bellando P, Caldera D. Colonoscopy in inflammatory bowel disease. *Gastroenterology* 1987;92:181–185.
16. Pötzi R, Walgram M, Lochs H. Diagnostic significance of endo-scopic biopsy in Crohn's disease. *Endoscopy* 1989;21:60–62.
17. Hildebrandt U, Kraus J, Ecker K, Schmid T, Schüder G, Feifel G. Endosonographic differentiation of mucosal and transmural nonspecific inflammatory bowel disease. *Endoscopy* 1992;24:(suppl):297–390.
18. Mason AJ. The spectrum of selective surgery. *Proc R Soc Med* 1976;69:237–244.
19. Kramann B, Hildebrandt U. Computed tomography versus en-dosonography in the staging of rectal carcinoma: a comparative study. *Int J Colorect Dis* 1986;1:216–218.
20. Hildebrandt U. Local curative treatment of rectal cancer. *Int J Colorect Dis* 1991;6:74–76.
21. Accarpio G, Scopinaro G, Clandiani F, Davini D, Mallarini G, Saita S. Experience with local rectal cancer excision in light of two recent preoperative diagnostic methods. *Dis Colon Rectum* 1987;30:296–298.
22. Beynon J, Roe AM, Foy DM. Preoperative staging of local inva-sion in rectal cancer using endoluminal ultrasound. *J R Soc Med* 1987;80:23–24.
23. Glaser F, Schlag P, Herfarth C. Endorectal ultrasonography for the assessment of invasion of rectal tumours and lymph node involvement. *Br J Surg* 1990;77:883–887.
24. Orrom WJ, Wong WD, Rothenberger DA, Jensen LL, Goldberg SM. Endorectal ultrasound in the preoperative staging of rectal tumors. *Dis Colon Rectum* 1990;33:654–659.
25. Romano G, De Rosa P, Vallone G, Rotaondo A, Grassi R, Santi-angelo ML. Intrarectal ultrasound and computed tomography in the pre- and postoperative assessment of patients with rectal carcinoma. *Br J Surg* 1985;72(suppl):117–119.
26. Dixon AK, Kelsey FI, Morson BC, Nicholls RJ, Mason AY. Preoperative computed tomography of carcinoma of the rectum. *Br J Radiol* 1981;54:655–659.
27. Grabbe E, Lierse W, Winkler R. The perirectal fascia: morphol-ogy and use in staging of rectal carcinoma. *Radiology* 1983;143:241–246.
28. Rifkin MD, Wechsler RI. A comparison of computed tomogra-phy and endorectal ultrasound in staging rectal cancer. *Int J Colorect Dis* 1986;1:219–223.
29. Beynon J, Mortensen NJ, Foy DM, Channer JL, Rigby HS, Virgee J. Preoperative assessment of mesorectal lymph node involvement in rectal cancer. *Br J Surg* 1989;6:276–279.
30. Saitoh N, Okui K, Sarashina H, Suzuki M, Arai T, Nunomura M. Evaluation of echographic diagnosis of rectal cancer using intrarectal ultrasonic examination. *Dis Colon Rectum* 1986;29:234–242.

Advanced Therapeutic Endoscopy, 2nd Ed.,
edited by J. S. Barkin and C. A. O'Phelan.
Raven Press, Ltd., New York © 1994.

CHAPTER 17

New Techniques for the Endoscopic Removal of Foreign Bodies

Marios Pouagare and *Patrick G. Brady

Foreign bodies of the upper or lower gastrointestinal tract are common problems that may result in significant morbidity and mortality. Rigid endoscopy and surgery were the procedures of choice for removal of gastrointestinal foreign bodies up until the early 1970s. Like many other aspects of gastroenterological practice, flexible fiberoptic endoscopy has revolutionized the management of gastrointestinal foreign bodies. The first reports (1,2) of removal of foreign bodies with flexible fiberoptic endoscopes appeared in 1972. Since then, improvements in flexible fiberoptic endoscopes and videoendoscopes, and the development of various accessories, such as foreign body forceps, snares, overtubes, and cylindrical tip attachments, have made endoscopic removal the procedure of choice for dealing with gastrointestinal foreign bodies (3–6). In this chapter we discuss the endoscopic removal of foreign bodies from both the upper and lower gastrointestinal tracts.

ANATOMIC CONSIDERATIONS

Foreign bodies tend to become impacted at areas of physiologic or pathologic narrowing. Before entering the esophagus, the foreign object must pass through the hypopharynx. Pointed objects may become impacted at this level, usually in the valleculae or the piriform sinuses. Below the hypopharynx, areas of narrowing are found in the esophagus, at the pylorus, the ileocecal valve, and the anus.

The esophagus has four areas of physiologic narrow-

ing. The most proximal is the upper esophageal sphincter located approximately 15 cm from the incisor teeth in adults. Two areas of physiologic narrowing occur in the mid-esophagus related to compression by the aortic arch at 23 cm and the left main stem branches at 27 cm. The most distal point of narrowing occurs at the diaphragmatic hiatus at 40 cm. An enlarged left atrium can result in compression of the distal third of the esophagus creating another area of narrowing.

Once a foreign body traverses the esophagus, it usually passes through the remainder of the gastrointestinal tract without difficulty. The pylorus, the ligament of Treitz, the ileocecal valve, and the anus are potential areas of impaction. Anomalies such as a Meckel's diverticulum, annular pancreas, or duodenal diaphragm can become sites of impaction. Pathologic processes such as benign or malignant stricture and diverticula can also become sites of impaction.

FOREIGN BODIES OF THE UPPER GI TRACT

Types of Foreign Bodies

Foreign bodies can be classified as true foreign bodies that are naturally foreign to the gastrointestinal tract, and food-related foreign bodies. True foreign bodies should be characterized as sharp or dull, pointed or blunt, and toxic or nontoxic. Their length and width should be measured. These features, along with the location of the true foreign body, determine whether endoscopic removal is indicated. Coins, toys, nails, and safety pins are the most frequently seen foreign bodies in children. Iatrogenic foreign bodies include dental instruments, nebulizer parts, suction and endotracheal tubes, and biopsy instruments. Button

M. Pouagare and P. G. Brady: Department of Medicine, James A. Haley Veterans Administration Hospital, Tampa, Florida 33612; and *University of South Florida College of Medicine, Tampa, Florida 33612.

batteries are the most commonly encountered toxic foreign body.

The most common type of food-related foreign body is the impacted meat bolus. The majority of patients presenting with a meat bolus impaction have an underlying esophageal stenosis (5,7). Endoscopic evaluation of the esophagus is thus mandatory in these patients even if the bolus passes spontaneously. Denture wearers are at particular risk for ingestion of fish and chicken bones due to their impaired oral sensation.

Clinical Presentation

Patients who have swallowed a foreign body may present with a wide range of signs and symptoms. Many patients give a clear history of the ingestion episode. However, some patients are unaware of the ingestion episode or are unwilling or unable to provide the information to the physician. A careful history and a high index of suspicion, especially for the groups of patients listed in Table 1, is needed in arriving at a correct diagnosis.

Esophageal foreign bodies may cause odynophagia, dysphagia, or complete esophageal obstruction with regurgitation and sialorrhea. Infants and younger children may present only with refusal to take feedings or with chronic pulmonary aspiration. Impaction of a meat bolus at or immediately below the upper esophageal sphincter compresses the adjacent trachea, resulting in respiratory obstruction. This is commonly called "café coronary" or "steakhouse syndrome." Respiratory symptoms including stridor, coughing, and choking are common presenting complaints in children because their soft tracheal rings are easily compressed by the esophageal foreign body.

Objects that lodge at the level of the aortic arch can perforate the esophagus, resulting in an aortoesophageal fistula. This rare complication may initially present with a self-limited herald bleed, only to be followed later by massive, exsanguinating hemorrhage. Recently, a case of an esophageal-carotid artery fistula due to a penetrating fish bone has been reported (8). This patient died due to massive bleeding.

TABLE 1. *People most prone to present with a foreign body in the upper gastrointestinal tract*

Children
Persons with esophageal disease
Denture wearers
Mentally retarded
Persons with psychiatric disease
Alcoholics
Prisoners
Drug smugglers and/or abusers

Retained gastric foreign bodies may be asymptomatic or they may present with dyspepsia, early satiety, obstruction, perforation, or hemorrhage. Delays of weeks, or rarely years, may occur before a patient presents with symptoms relating to foreign body ingestion. A long-standing foreign body may result in free perforation, abscess formation, or injury to adjacent solid organs or vascular structures due to migration of the object. Toxic foreign bodies can cause acute or chronic toxic reactions. Copper, lead, and nickel poisoning has been reported after retention of metallic foreign bodies.

Physical examination is important in detecting early complications. Subcutaneous emphysema indicates perforation of the hypopharynx or esophagus. Peritoneal signs indicate perforation of the stomach or intestine.

Radiographic Evaluation

The first diagnostic study that should be obtained is a plain radiograph. Plain films of the neck, chest, and abdomen should be taken in the posteroanterior and lateral projections. A flat object, such as a coin, is usually oriented in the frontal plane when it is in the esophagus, and in the sagittal plane when it is in the trachea. Subcutaneous air, pneumomediastinum, pneumothorax, or plural effusion suggest esophageal perforation. Free air under the diaphragm or in the retroperitoneum suggest gastric or intestinal perforation.

Many foreign bodies are radiopaque and can be easily seen on plain radiographs. However, many others are not radiopaque, such as objects made out of glass, wood, or plastic. Even thin metallic objects such as aluminum can tops are not radiopaque. Careful examination of soft-tissue films may be helpful. Xeroradiography is an excellent technique for visualizing the soft tissues of the neck and may show foreign bodies not evident on plain films. Contrast studies may be required for detecting radiolucent foreign bodies or for determining perforation.

When looking for a radiolucent foreign body, a small amount of thin barium should be used to minimize the risk of aspiration. When looking for perforation, a small amount of Gastrografin or other water-soluble agents should be used because they are readily reabsorbed from the mediastinum, pleural space, or peritoneum. Contrast studies, however, are unnecessary and undesirable in patients with food bolus impaction. The presence of barium in the esophagus complicates removal of the food bolus because it obscures endoscopic visualization. The use of Gastrografin is contraindicated in food bolus impactions because it is extremely hypertonic and causes a severe chemical pneumonitis if aspirated into the lung. Use of barium-impregnated cotton balls is never indicated because it only adds one more foreign body to be removed.

Therapy

Indications for Removal

All foreign bodies impacted in the esophagus should be removed. The impaction of a meat bolus at or just below the cricopharyngeus with tracheal compression and resultant respiratory obstruction, the so-called café coronary, is a true emergency. Esophageal obstruction at lower levels requires prompt but not emergency treatment. The majority of rounded objects initially found in the lower third of the esophagus pass spontaneously (9). Thus, a 12-hour period of observation is permissible in this situation. Blunt objects impacted higher in the esophagus must be removed earlier due to sialorrhea and potential for pulmonary aspiration. Early removal of meat bolus impaction is recommended, even when the bolus is located in the distal third of the esophagus, because delay allows softening, which makes extraction difficult.

Not all foreign bodies in the stomach need to be removed (Table 2). Blunt foreign bodies that can pass through the pylorus and negotiate the fixed duodenal angles need not be removed. Murat and colleagues (10) recommended removal of foreign bodies that are more than 6 cm in length in children and more than 13 cm in length in adults. Plastic bag clips, although not sharp or pointed, need to be removed because they can attach to the mucosa with potential severe complications (11,12). Toxic foreign bodies should also be removed.

Blunt gastric foreign bodies can be managed conservatively initially. The recommended period of observation varies widely in the literature from 2 days to indefinitely (13). We recommend removal if a blunt foreign body has not traversed the pylorus in 2 weeks (6). Usually gastric foreign bodies greater than 2 cm in diameter cannot traverse the pylorus and one may elect to re-move these earlier. However, coins as large as quarters and even a Susan B. Anthony dollar (diameter of 2.5 cm) have been observed to pass spontaneously (6). Blunt foreign bodies in the duodenum should be removed if they have not progressed in 1 week (10,14).

Management

Over the past two decades, flexible endoscopy has become the preferred method of removal of foreign bodies. Successful removal depends on proper preparation and proper selection of instruments. A variety of foreign body removal accessories are available for use with flexible endoscopes such as rubber-clad forceps, alligator forceps, rat-toothed forceps, three-pronged forceps, snares, and baskets (Fig. 1). Hennig and Seuberth (15) reported the design of a special snare for the extraction of foreign bodies. Their snare has two distinguishing features: (a) a special handle that allows rotation of the snare through 360° so that the foreign body can be grasped from any angle, and (b) the inside surface of the snare is covered by tiny studs that allows better grasping of the foreign body.

Duplication of the foreign body and simulation of removal are highly recommended. It is important to test the available grasping instruments on a duplicate of the foreign body to determine which instrument is best suited to grasping and manipulating it. A Kelly clamp and a laryngoscope should always be available when removing a foreign body so that any object inadvertently dropped in the hypopharynx can promptly be retrieved.

When extracting esophageal foreign bodies, the endoscope must be inserted under direct visualization to avoid inadvertently striking the foreign object and further impacting it or causing it to penetrate the esophageal wall. In the following subsections we describe the flexible endoscopic techniques for removing various foreign objects from the upper gastrointestinal tract.

Meat Bolus Impaction

A meat bolus should be extracted within several hours of impaction, before it softens. If it is extracted early enough, even a large bolus can often be extracted in one piece. Once the bolus has softened, multiple passages of the endoscope are usually necessary to extract it in small pieces with repeated insertions and withdrawals of the endoscope through an overtube that is left in place. A recently described technique by Saeed and colleagues (16) may considerably simplify the removal of a meat bolus impaction in the esophagus. The technique is based on modifying the endoscope into a direct-vision suction device. This is accomplished by attaching to the tip of the endoscope

TABLE 2. Indications for removal of foreign bodies from the upper gastrointestinal tract

Esophageal foreign bodies
  All foreign bodies
Gastric and duodenal foreign bodies
  Sharp or pointed objects
  Toxic foreign bodies
  Plastic bag clips
  Long objects:
    6 cm in children
    13 cm in adults
  Blunt objects after:
    2 weeks observation in the stomach
    1 week observation in the duodenum

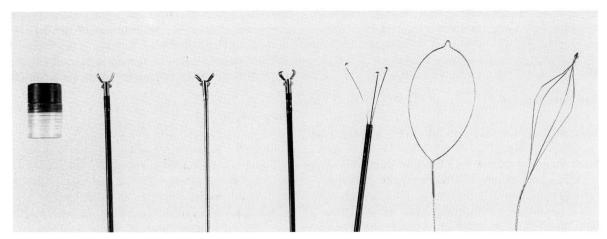

FIG. 1. Foreign body removal accessories for use with flexible endoscopes. From left to right are pictured a drum tip, an alligator forceps, a rubber-clad forceps, a rat-toothed forceps, a three-pronged forceps, a polypectomy snare, and a basket.

the drum tip, or end-hood, for variceal rubber band ligation (Fig. 2). The modified endoscope is passed through the overtube and under direct vision the impacted bolus is suctioned into the drum. It is removed by withdrawing the endoscope through the overtube. Saeed and colleagues reported the successful use of this method in seven patients. The authors had the opportunity to use this method in six cases of meat bolus impaction. In five out of the six cases the new method significantly reduced the time spent in removing the meat bolus. In one case, the suction technique had to be aborted and the removal completed with a polypectomy snare. Overall, we feel that the suction technique is an important addition to our armamentarium in the endoscopic removal of meat bolus impactions.

Another novel technique for treating meat bolus impactions is the use of laser. Klein (17) reported one case during which neodymium:yttrium-aluminum garnet (Nd:YAG) laser was used to burn the center of an impacted meat bolus causing it to fall into the stomach. Since this technique carries with it the added expense and the potential complications of laser therapy, it is not recommended.

Coins

Coins cannot be removed with the standard endoscopic biopsy forceps because the small jaws of this instrument easily slip off the metallic surface. However, coins can be easily removed when necessary by use of an alligator forceps or snare. Once firmly grasped, the coin and endoscope are removed simultaneously under direct vision guidance. In the esophagus, the coin should be rotated so that it lies in the coronal plane, which is the widest plane of the cervical esophagus and the hypopharynx.

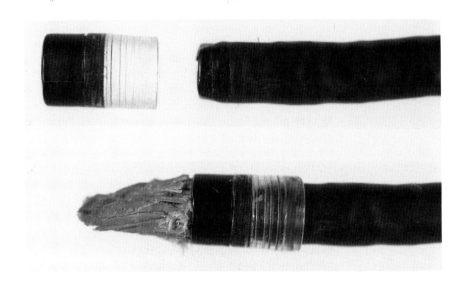

FIG. 2. Top: Endoscope and drum tip before attachment. **Bottom:** Piece of meat suctioned into the drum tip.

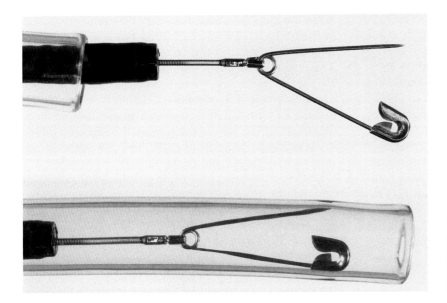

FIG. 3. Top: An opened safety pin grasped with a foreign body forceps before withdrawal through an overtube. **Bottom:** The safety pin totally withdrawn into the overtube to avoid exposing mucosal surfaces to its sharp point.

Coins located in the esophagus should be removed promptly. However, once they pass into the stomach emergency extraction is not necessary. We generally allow 2 weeks for the coin to pass through the pylorus before endoscopically removing it from the stomach. Once past the pylorus, coins usually traverse the small intestine and colon without difficulty.

Sharp and Pointed Foreign Bodies

These objects should be removed with the sharp point trailing to avoid mucosal laceration or perforation. If the object is pointed at both ends (e.g., a toothpick), the proximal sharp end must be completely covered by the grasping forceps. If the object has a single pointed end and is directed cephalad, it can be carried into the stomach and turned so that the pointed end trails before it is removed.

The use of a protective plastic overtube should be considered when sharp or pointed foreign bodies are being removed (18). For use in the stomach, an overtube should be at least 60 cm long, whereas shorter overtubes suffice for esophageal use. The overtube is first loaded over the endoscope up to the control handle, the endoscope is then inserted in the usual manner, and the overtube is advanced over it as needed. When the foreign body is being withdrawn, the overtube remains in place, thus protecting the mucosal surface (Fig. 3).

An alternative to the use of an overtube for removal of sharp gastric foreign bodies is the use of a protective hood (Fig. 4). The hood can be made out of the condom part of an external urinary catheter and attached with silk suture to the tip of the endoscope (19). When not in use, the hood is folded backward. A parachute suture is affixed to the leading edge of the hood and grasped by biopsy forceps passed through the biopsy channel. This prevents the hood from totally everting onto the endoscope during insertion. The hood is unfolded over the tip by pulling the endoscope through the esophagogastric junction after releasing the parachute suture. The hood can be unfolded before or after the foreign object is grasped.

Tuen and coworkers (20) reported using an end-hood attached to the tip of the endoscope in the removal of

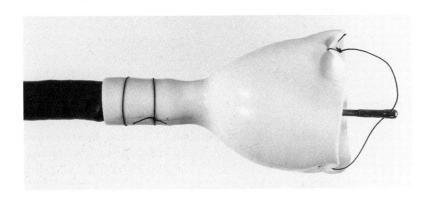

FIG. 4. Protective hood attached to the endoscope and the parachute suture grasped by the biopsy forceps.

ingested parts of a broken glass thermometer. The end-hood was made by cutting the tip of a 32F Argyle chest drainage catheter and attaching it to the distal end of the endoscope. The broken pieces of the glass thermometer were maneuvered into the end-hood and kept there by applying suction. This technique is similar to the technique described by Saeed and colleagues (16) for the removal of meat bolus impaction.

If a pointed object, such as a toothpick or bone, is wedged across the lumen and gentle manipulation fails to disimpact it, then an attempt should be made to transect the object before removal. Farr and Pratt (21) reported the use of suture removal scissors (Olympus FS-1K) through the endoscope to transect a chicken bone wedged across the lumen of the esophagus.

Elongated Foreign Bodies

Long objects are associated with a high incidence of perforation because they are unable to negotiate the fixed curves of the duodenum. Objects longer than 6 cm in children and 13 cm in adults need to be removed from the stomach and duodenum (Table 2). The snare is the grasping instrument of choice. The snare should be placed close to the cephalad end of the object so that during withdrawal the long axis of the object may align itself with the long axis of the esophagus. If the object is elongated and stiff, it may be difficult to withdraw through the hypopharynx. In these cases, we suggest tilting the patient's head backward and moving the neck forward, to create a straight passage from the cervical portion of the esophagus to the mouth, and extracting the object with the aid of a Kelly clamp.

Toothbrushes are special elongated foreign objects since they never pass spontaneously and always need to be removed (22,23). When the bristle end is in the fundus, the toothbrush is first moved into the antrum and then the bristles closest to the tip are grasped with forceps and pulled through the gastroesophageal junction. If the toothbrush is lying with its handle end in the fundus, a closed biopsy forceps can then be passed through the hole at the end of the handle, opened, and then pulled through the gastroesophageal junction. If there is no hole at the end, the end of the handle needs to be grasped with a snare and pulled through the gastroesophageal junction.

Button Batteries

Batteries can cause injury by direct corrosive action, low voltage burn, pressure necrosis, and release of toxic substances. The National Button Battery Ingestion Hotline and Registry was established in 1982 to collect data and provide emergency consultation service (202-625-3333). A total of 2,382 cases of battery ingestion were reported between 1983 and 1990 (24), the majority (2,320) being button batteries. The vast majority of patients had a relatively benign course. There were no deaths, and only two patients required long-term treatment, both involving injury to the esophagus requiring repeated dilations. A significant decline in both surgical and endoscopic intervention occurred during the 7-year period. Endoscopic intervention has declined from 13.1% to 2.1% and surgical intervention from 2.0% to 0.4%.

Batteries lodged in the esophagus should be removed emergently. Removal should be done endoscopically under direct visualization. Foley catheters or magnet catheters are not recommended. These two techniques increase the risk of dropping the battery in the hypopharynx and the patient aspirating it.

Batteries that have passed beyond the esophagus need not be retrieved unless the patient develops signs or symptoms of gastrointestinal injury or the battery fails to go through the pylorus within 48 hours. Ipecac is contraindicated because it is rarely successful and because it may result in movement of the battery from the stomach to the esophagus, necessitating emergent retrieval.

Patients that have ingested mercuric oxide cells should be followed more closely due to the greater likelihood that these cells will split in the gastrointestinal tract. If the cell is observed to split, blood and urine mercury levels should be checked and chelation therapy initiated if levels are in the toxic range.

Cocaine

Packages of cocaine are intentionally ingested to prevent detection by customs agents or police. These packages can cause obstruction or acute cocaine poisoning if they break. McCarron and Wood (25) have described three types of cocaine packages: Type 1 includes condoms, finger cots, and balloons. These packages are highly susceptible to breakage. Type 2 consists of five to seven layers of tubular latex and are less susceptible to breakage. Type 1 and 2 packages are seen as round densities on x-ray, sometimes surrounded by a gas halo. Type 3 consists of cocaine paste in aluminum foil covered with three to five layers of tubular latex. They are more resistant to breakage. Type 3 packages are smaller and usually not seen on x-ray. Type 1 packages should be removed surgically. Type 2 and 3 may be treated medically if (a) no broken containers have been passed or demonstrated on x-ray, (b) the patient is asymptomatic, (c) there is no gastrointestinal obstruction, (d) time lapsed since ingestion is less than 24 to 48 hours. Endoscopic removal should not be attempted since rupture of the package during removal can and has occurred (26).

Gastric Bezoars

There are two main types of gastric bezoars, phytobezoars, and trichobezoars. Phytobezoars are usually found in patients with delayed gastric emptying. Surgical vagotomy (27) and diabetic gastroparesis are the most common causes. Ingestion of vegetable matter, such as citrus fruit, fruit skins, vegetables, and seeds by patients with delayed gastric emptying may result in the formation of gastric phytobezoars. A special type of phytobezoars is the persimmon bezoar or diospyrobezoar that result from the ingestion of unripened persimmons. These berries contain a juice that has large amounts of pectin and gum. These components form a coagulum in the acid environment of the stomach. Unripe persimmons are one of the few materials that can form a bezoar in a normal stomach after a single ingestion.

Trichobezoars, or hair balls, form in the stomach of habitual hair swallowers, usually young women with otherwise normal stomachs.

The type of therapy employed for gastric bezoars depends on the type of bezoar. Phytobezoars can be treated in various ways: (a) mechanical fragmentation with biopsy forceps or snare (28,29), or with water jet generated by a water pick adapted to the biopsy channel (30), (b) endoscopic injection of cellulase (31), or acetylcysteine into the bezoar, (c) cellulase (32) or papain (33) given orally. Papain should be reserved for persimmon bezoars that are resistant to mechanical disruption because papain is a proteolytic enzyme that has an ulcerogenic potential.

Trichobezoars are more difficult than phytobezoars to treat. Small trichobezoars may be removed endoscopically with a foreign body forceps or snare. Larger trichobezoars are more difficult to manage endoscopically and many times require surgery. Soehendra (34) reported the successful endoscopic treatment of a large trichobezoar measuring 15 cm × 7 cm using a combination of Nd:YAG laser and Dormia basket. Extracorporeal shock wave lithotripsy (ESWL) has been recently used to treat a gastric bezoar (35) after failed endoscopic removal.

Miscellaneous Foreign Bodies

A technique has been described for the removal of large objects with a hole that cannot be grasped with a foreign body forceps or snare (36). This technique entails grasping a silk thread with a biopsy forceps that has been passed through the biopsy channel of an endoscope. The forceps is then retracted into the end of the biopsy channel and the thread is brought along the outside of the endoscope. The entire apparatus is passed into the stomach, and the forceps is inserted through the hole in the foreign body. The forceps is then opened, and the thread is regrasped and retracted into the biopsy channel to form a closed loop that holds the foreign body (Fig. 5). Then the entire assembly is withdrawn together.

FOREIGN BODIES OF THE LOWER GI TRACT

Types of Foreign Bodies

Lower GI tract foreign bodies can be divided into two major groups: those that have been ingested and those that have been inserted through the anal canal. The majority of ingested foreign bodies will pass

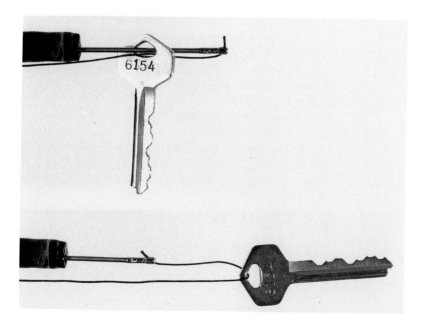

FIG. 5. Top: Removal of a foreign body with a large hole. The silk thread grasped with a biopsy forceps is passed through the hole. **Bottom:** After opening the forceps the silk thread is regrasped to form a complete loop. The endoscope and the foreign body can now be withdrawn simultaneously.

through the gastrointestinal tract spontaneously, but occasionally, even though the foreign body managed to traverse the esophagus, pylorus, and duodenum, it may impact at the ileocecal valve, appendix, anus, or sites of pathologic narrowing. Foreign bodies are inserted into the rectum for a number of reasons: (a) for diagnostic and therapeutic purposes such as rectal thermometers and enema tube sheaths that have not been removed prior to administration of the enema; (b) sexual pleasure such as rubber phalluses, vibrators, and bottles; and (c) by accident.

Clinical Presentation

The clinical presentation of patients that have ingested a foreign body has been discussed earlier. The clinical presentation of patients that have inserted a foreign body through the anal canal varies considerably. The patient may be completely asymptomatic or may present with abdominal pain, rectal pain, rectal bleeding, or urinary tract symptoms. Physical examination may be unrevealing or the patient may have peritoneal signs if intraperitoneal perforation has occurred. Low-lying foreign objects can be palpated on digital rectal examination. Foreign bodies that have migrated proximally can sometimes be palpated on abdominal examination.

Radiographic Evaluation

Plain x-rays of the abdomen, including upright and lateral views, should be obtained in all patients to confirm the location of the foreign body and to help exclude intra- and retroperitoneal perforation. If perforation is suspected but not confirmed by plain radiographs, a Gastrografin enema should be performed.

Therapy

Ingested Foreign Bodies

The majority of ingested foreign bodies that reach the colon will pass spontaneously. Thus a period of observation is warranted in the asymptomatic patient with a colonic foreign body that is not sharp or pointed. If the patient develops symptoms (37) or if there is failure of spontaneous elimination within 7 days, then the foreign body should be removed (38). Pointed or sharp foreign objects should be removed without delay because of an increased risk of perforation (39,40).

The instrument of choice for the removal of ingested colorectal foreign bodies is the colonoscope or flexible sigmoidoscope, depending on the exact location of the foreign body. Good visibility is essential and thus the patient's colon should be prepared appropriately. For rectal or sigmoid foreign bodies, two Fleet enemas can be used. More proximal foreign bodies require a more thorough colon preparation. If there are no signs or symptoms of obstruction, an oral electrolyte lavage preparation should be used. If partial colonic obstruction is suspected, then tap water enemas can be used to prepare the colon. Strong peristaltic stimulants should be avoided in all cases. As with the removal of foreign bodies of the upper GI tract, a variety of foreign body forceps and snares are available for use with the colonoscope.

Inserted Foreign Bodies

For the management of inserted foreign bodies, it is helpful to classify them as low lying (distal to the rectosigmoid junction) and high lying (at or proximal to the rectosigmoid junction). They can be further subdivided into sharp objects, large rounded objects, and glass bottles. The broken rectal thermometer is an example of a sharp inserted foreign body. If perforation is not present, proctosigmoidoscopy with removal of any glass fragments under direct visual control is recommended. Perforation requires prompt surgical repair, since delay can be associated with mortality rates as high as 70% (41).

Large rounded foreign bodies include vibrators, plastic phalluses, fruits, vegetables, balls, broomsticks, and rubber hoses (4,42). If the distal end of the object is rounded and can be grasped with a snare or foreign body forceps, extraction with a flexible sigmoidoscope is possible (43). When this is not possible, anesthesia to relax the anal sphincter and extraction with an operative proctoscope and specially designed grasping forceps is required (44). Local anesthesia is sufficient to achieve complete relaxation of the anal sphincter. Lidocaine 0.5% or bupivacaine 0.5% can be injected through a 25- or 27-gauge needle into the subdermal and submucosal tissue of the perianal area and anal canal to achieve anesthesia. If the anus cannot be adequately dilated to remove the foreign body, a lateral internal sphincterotomy will relieve the stenosis (45). Following removal of the foreign body, complete proctosigmoidoscopy should be performed to exclude mucosal lacerations, perforation, or a missed second foreign body.

Glass bottles require special care during removal to avoid fracture. If the open end of a wide-mouthed glass bottle is directed cephalad, it will create a suction effect, drawing mucosa into the mouth of the bottle. Care must be taken to overcome this suction effect before the bottle can be extracted (4). There are various methods of accomplishing this. Two or more Foley cathe-

RECTAL OR COLONIC FOREIGN BODY

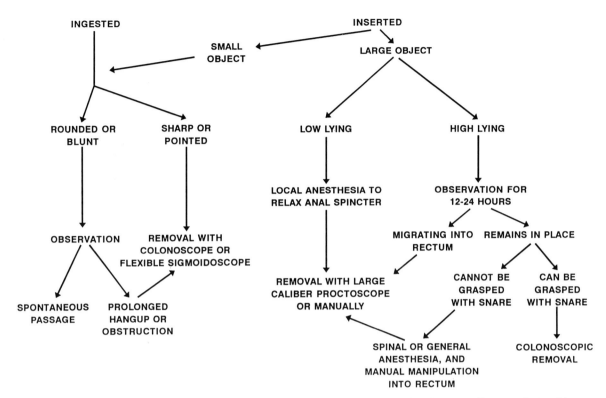

FIG. 6. Algorithm for the management of rectal and colonic foreign bodies. (From ref. 4, with permission.)

ters can be introduced around the object, and after inflation of the balloons air can be injected proximal to the opening of the bottle. Another method to overcome the suction effect is to insert a flexible sigmoidoscope past the bottle and insufflate air.

Patients with large high-lying foreign bodies can be observed for 12 to 24 hours during which time the foreign body usually descends into the rectum. If the foreign body fails to migrate during this period of observation, colonoscopy should be performed if the object has a surface that can be grasped. If not, then the patient can be placed in the lithotomy position under general or spinal anesthesia, and the object can be manipulated into the rectal ampulla by abdominal palpation. If this fails, laparotomy will be necessary.

The management of colorectal foreign bodies is summarized in Fig. 6.

REFERENCES

1. Maimon HN, Milligan FD. Removal of a foreign body from the stomach. *Gastrointest Endosc* 1972;18:163–164.
2. Gelzayed EA, Jetly K. Fiberendoscopy: removal of a retained sewing needle from the stomach. *Gastrointest Endosc* 1972;18:161–162.
3. Webb WA. Foreign bodies of the upper gastrointestinal tract. In: Taylor MB, ed. *Gastrointestinal emergencies*. Baltimore: Williams & Wilkins, 1992.
4. Brady PG. Foreign bodies of the lower GI tract. In: Taylor MB, ed. *Gastrointestinal emergencies*. Baltimore: Williams & Wilkins, 1992.
5. Brady PG. Esophageal foreign bodies. *Gastroenterol Clin North Am* 1991;20(4):691–701.
6. Brady PG. Endoscopic removal of foreign bodies. In: Silvis SE, ed. *Therapeutic gastrointestinal endoscopy*. New York: Igaku-Shoin, 1990.
7. Vizcarrondo FJ, Brady PG, Nord HJ. Foreign bodies in the upper gastrointestinal tract. *Gastrointest Endosc* 1983;29:208.
8. Yang CY. The management of ingested foreign bodies in the upper digestive tract: a retrospective study of 49 cases. *Singapore Med J* 1991;32:312–315.
9. Spitz L. Management of ingested foreign bodies in childhood. *Br Med J* 1971;4:469–472.
10. Murat J, Vuillard P, Petua J, et al. A propos de 108 observations de corps étrangers deglutis du tube digestif a l'exclusion de l'oesphage. *Lyon Chir* 1969;65:379–388.
11. Guindi MM, Troster MM, Walley VM. Three cases of an unusual foreign body in small bowel. *Gastrointest Radiol* 1987;12:240–242.
12. D'Auria DA, Naidorf T, Hashmi MA, Levine SM. Endoscopic excision of a foreign body in the pyloric channel. *Gastrointest Endosc* 1990;36(4):406–408.
13. Bendig DW, Mackie GG. Management of smooth-blunt gastric foreign bodies in asymptomatic patients. *Clin Pediatr* 1990;29(11):642–645.
14. Pellerin D, Fortier-Beaulieu M, Guegnen J. The fate of swallowed foreign bodies: experience of 1250 instances of sub-dia-

phragmatic bodies in children. *Prog Pediatr Radiol* 1969;2: 286–302.

15. Hennig AE, Seuberth K. Endoscopic removal of foreign bodies using a newly developed extractor. *Endoscopy* 1988;20:70–72.

16. Saeed ZA, Michaletz PA, Feiner SD, et al. A new endoscopic method for managing food impaction in the esophagus. *Endoscopy* 1990;22:226–228.

17. Klein I. Resourceful management of esophageal food impaction. *Gastrointest Endosc* 1990;36:80.

18. Werth RW, Edwards C, Jennings WC. A safe and quick method for endoscopic retrieval of multiple gastric foreign bodies using a protective sheath. *Surg Gynecol Obstet* 1990;171:419–420.

19. Garrido J, Barkin JS. Endoscopic modification for safe foreign body removal. *Am J Gastroenterol* 1985;80:957–958.

20. Tuen HH, Lai ECS, Fan ST. Endoscopic retrieval of ingested broken glass in the esophagus and stomach by end-hood and suction technique. *Gastrointest Endosc* 1989;35:357–358.

21. Farr CM, Pratt W. The scissors approach to a chicken bone lodged in the esophagus. *Gastrointest Endosc* 1989;35:357.

22. Chinitz MA, Bertrand G. Endoscopic removal of toothbrushes. *Gastrointest Endosc* 1990;36:527–530.

23. Kirk AD, Bowers BA, Moylan JA, Meyers WC. Toothbrush swallowing. *Arch Surg* 1988;123:382–384.

24. Litovitz T, Schmitz BF. Ingestion of cylindrical and button batteries: an analysis of 2,382 cases. *Pediatrics* 1992;89(4):747–757.

25. McCarron MM, Wood JD. The cocaine ''body packer'' syndrome. Diagnosis and treatment. *JAMA* 1983;250:1417–1420.

26. Suarez CA, et al. Cocaine-condom ingestion. Surgical treatment. *JAMA* 1977;238:1391–1392.

27. Tebar JC, Campos RR, Paricio PP, et al. Gastric surgery and bezoars. *Dig Dis Sci* 1992;37:1694–1696.

28. McKechnie JC. Gastroscopic removal of a phytobezoar. *Gastroenterology* 1972;62:1047–1051.

29. Brady PG. Gastric phytobezoars consequent to delayed gastric emptying. *Gastrointest Endosc* 1978;24:159–161.

30. Madsen R, Skibba RM, Galvan A, et al. Gastric bezoars. A technique of endoscopic removal. *Dig Dis Sci* 1978;23:717–719.

31. Gold MH, Patterson TE III, Green GI. Cellulase bezoar injection: a new endoscopic technique. *Gastrointest Endosc* 1976;22: 200–202.

32. Pollard HB, Block GE. Rapid dissolution of phytobezoar by cellulase enzyme. *Am J Surg* 1968;116:933–936.

33. Dann D, Rubin S, Passman H, et al. The successful medical management of a phytobezoar. *Arch Intern Med* 1959;103: 598–601.

34. Soehendra N. Endoscopic removal of a trichobezoar. *Endoscopy* 1989;21:201.

35. Benes J, Chmel J, Jodl J, et al. Treatment of a gastric bezoar by extracorporeal shock wave lithotripsy. *Endoscopy* 1991;23: 346–348.

36. Dunkerly RC, et al. Fiberendoscopic removal of large foreign bodies from the stomach. *Gastrointest Endosc* 1974;21:170–171.

37. Bermam JH, Radhakrishnan J, Kraut JR. Button gastrostomy obstructing the ileocecal valve removed by colonoscopic retrieval. *J Pediatr Gastroenterol Nutr* 1991;13:426–428.

38. Viceconte G, Viceconte GW, Bigholo G, et al. Endoscopic removal of foreign bodies in the large bowel. *Endoscopy* 1982;14: 176–177.

39. Alberti-Flor JJ, Hernandez ME, Ferrer JP, et al. Endoscopic removal of an impacted colonic foreign body (fish bone) complicated by a pelvic abscess. *Gastrointest Endosc* 1992;38:100–102.

40. Callon RA, Brady PG. Toothpick perforation of the sigmoid colon: an unusual case associated with *Erysipelothrix rhusiopathiae* septicemia. *Gastrointest Endosc* 1990;36:141–143.

41. Lau JTK, Ong GB. Broken and retained rectal thermometers in infants and young children. *Aust Paediatr J* 1981;17:93–94.

42. Obrador A, Gaya J, Pueyo J, Dolz C. Colonoscopic removal of a long piece of lawn hose. *Gastrointest Endosc* 1988;34:286–287.

43. Kantorian JC, Riether RD, Sheets JA, et al. Endoscopic retrieval of foreign bodies from the rectum. *Dis Colon Rectum* 1987;30:902–904.

44. Berci G, Morgenstern L. An operative proctoscope for foreign-body extraction. *Dis Colon Rectum* 1983;26:193–194.

45. Kingsley AN, Abcarian H. Colorectal foreign bodies. Management update. *Dis Colon Rectum* 1985;28:941–944.

Advanced Therapeutic Endoscopy, 2nd Ed.,
edited by J. S. Barkin and C. A. O'Phelan.
Raven Press, Ltd., New York © 1994.

CHAPTER 18

Percutaneous Endoscopic Gastrostomy: Advances in Technique, Prevention, and Management of Complications

P. Gregory Foutch

In 1980 Gauderer et al (1) reported their initial experience with percutaneous endoscopic gastrostomy (PEG), and this important innovation has significantly altered our approach to sick patients in need of long-term enteral alimentation. Experience with PEG over the past decade has enhanced our understanding of the potential risks and complications associated with the procedure. This chapter focuses on advances in methods of PEG placement as well as on prevention, recognition, and management of important complications.

CANDIDATES FOR PEG

In general, PEG is well suited for patients with a functional gastrointestinal tract who have a potential for extended survival ($\geq$4 weeks) and who are unable or unwilling to consume sufficient protein and calories to meet metabolic demands (2). Usual candidates include individuals with impaired deglutition because of a neurological disease (i.e., stroke, anoxic encephalopathy, dementia, brain tumor) or head and neck cancer (3–5). However, PEG may be important in the nutritional management of patients with facial trauma, severe cardiac or respiratory failure, or other catabolic conditions. Stellato and Gauderer (6) showed that PEG could be effective for long-term gastric decompression in selected individuals with various complex intraabdominal processes. PEG has also been evaluated for use and shown to be effective in certain high-risk pa-

tients including those with cancer, those with a tracheostomy, and sick patients managed in an intensive care setting (7–9). A few investigators have put the PEG to creative use. A nasobiliary drainage catheter was rerouted out through a PEG in a patient with cholangiocarcinoma to serve as convenient access to the bile duct for intraluminal radiation therapy (10). PEG has been used to manage a difficult patient with gastric volvulus and assist in the placement of esophageal stents (11,12). Some investigators have connected an external biliary drain to a PEG to internalize bile flow through the stomach or duodenum (13–15). The principles of PEG were successfully applied to a dilated colon in two individuals who had percutaneous endoscopic cecostomy for decompression (16).

CONTRAINDICATIONS TO PEG

To optimize the uncomplicated success of the procedure it is important that certain safety precautions be taken before placement of the PEG (Table 1). Maximum intragastric air insufflation must be achieved for required apposition of the stomach to the abdominal wall (it should be possible to push on the abdomen with a finger and clearly indent the stomach as viewed

P. G. Foutch: Department of Medicine, Division of Gastroenterology, University of Arizona College of Medicine, Tucson, Arizona 85724; and Division of Gastroenterology, Desert Samaritan Hospital, Mesa, Arizona 85202.

TABLE 1. *Mandatory safety precautions taken before placement of the PEG*

Maximum intragastric air insufflation of the stomach
Transillumination of the abdominal wall with the endoscopic light
Indirect finger compression on the gastric wall
Selection of a safe gastrocutaneous fistulous tract

through the endoscope). Endoscopic transillumination of the abdominal wall must be demonstrated to guide precise placement of the percutaneous catheter (2). Selection of a "safe" gastrocutaneous fistulous tract using a fluid-filled syringe and 22-gauge needle enhances the safety and technical success of the procedure (17) (see "Gastrocolocutaneous Fistulae," below). Failure to successfully complete any of these safety maneuvers can result in complications. Therefore, PEG is contraindicated in any patient in whom one or more of these maneuvers fail.

Transillumination of the abdominal wall with the endoscopic light or indirect finger compression on the stomach may not be possible in obese patients or those with massive hepatomegaly. The procedure is inadvisable for patients with sepsis, large ascites, or diffuse inflammatory, infectious, or neoplastic disease involving the walls of the abdomen or anterior stomach. Gastrointestinal obstruction or proximal small bowel fistulae contraindicate all forms of enteral feeding. The invasive nature of the technique requires correction of any significant coagulation defect beforehand. Nutritionally depleted patients with conditions that prohibit gastric endoscopic intubation, including obstructing esophageal lesions refractory to dilation, must be managed by other means.

When PEG tubes are placed adhesions form between the stomach and abdomen to support the gastrocutaneous fistula. The union of these structures prevents leakage of gastric contents into the peritoneal cavity. Patients likely to pull out the catheter prematurely before adhesions form are at high risk for gastric leakage and peritonitis and are probably better served by a surgical gastrostomy (18). In this circumstance the sutured attachment between the abdominal wall and stomach is secure and probably safer for these individuals. PEG is not contraindicated in patients who have had prior abdominal surgery, although the technical success rate may be lower in those who have had a partial gastric resection (17,19). A PEG can be placed in individuals with a ventriculoperitoneal shunt as long as the exact location of the shunt is known and it is clear that the device will not be damaged by the procedure (4).

METHODS OF PEG PLACEMENT

Three methods of PEG placement have been described. The original technique reported by Gauderer et al. (1) requires percutaneous puncture of the stomach with a cannula, which serves as a conduit for passage of a suture. The suture is endoscopically snared, brought out the patient's mouth, and tied to the feeding tube. Hand traction is applied to the abdominal end of the suture, which pulls the catheter down the esophagus into the stomach and out through the abdomen (pull-string method). The endoscope is reinserted to inspect placement of the device to insure that excessive traction on the internal bolster of the catheter against the gastric mucosa has been avoided. Over the years minor modifications in technique and tube design and construction have occurred but the basic approach has remained unchanged and is popular among clinicians. Experience with this method is extensive (5,20–29). Cumulative results (Table 2) show that the procedure can be performed successfully in almost all cases and the associated rates for procedure-related mortality (0.5%) and major (2.8%) and minor (8.7%) complications are low.

A second method for PEG placement involves pushing a feeding catheter into position over a guidewire (push-wire method) (3). The wire is inserted into the stomach through a transabdominal Seldinger cannula and endoscopically snared and brought out through the

TABLE 2. *Cumulative success, morbidity, and mortality rates for PEG placement performed by the pull-string method*

Investigator, date of report (ref.)	Patients N	Success %	Morbidity Minor %	Morbidity Major %	Mortality %
Gottfried and Plumser, 1984 (20)	24	100	0	0	0
Strodel et al., 1983 (21)	45	96	9	7	0
Plumeri et al., 1983 (22)	46	100	7	0	0
Griffin et al., 1984 (23)	16	100	44	0	0
Thatcher et al., 1984 (24)	16	81	19	0	0
Ponsky et al., 1985 (25)	306	100	4	2	0
Kirby et al., 1986 (26)	55	93	24	9	0
Stern, 1986 (27)	100	100	4	1	1
Larson et al., 1987 (5)	314	95	13	3	1
Sangster et al., 1988 (28)	155	100	8	3	1.3
Grant, 1988 (29)	125	98	5	4	0
Total	1,202	98	8.7	2.8	0.5

TABLE 3. *Cumulative success, morbidity, and mortality rates for PEG placement performed by the push-wire and introducer methods*

Investigator, date of report (ref.)	Patients N	Success %	Morbidity		Mortality %
			Minor %	Major %	
Push-wire method					
Kozarek et al., 1986 (30)	15	100	7	7	0
Hogan et al., 1986 (31)	20	100	5	15	5
Stiegmann et al., 1988 (32)	23	100	4	17	0
Foutch et al., 1988 (3)	118	96	12	4	0.8
Total	176	97	10	7	1
Introducer method					
Russell et al., 1984 (33)	28	100	11	0	0
Kozarek et al., 1986 (30)	15	87	13	0	0
Deitel et al., 1988 (34)	28	100	4	0	0
Miller et al., 1989 (35)	316	96	4	2	0.6
Total	387	96	8	0.5	0.2

patient's mouth. The PEG catheter is pushed over the oral end of the wire until it emerges through the abdominal wall. An assistant grasps the emerging catheter tip and pulls it out through the body wall until the internal bolster of the catheter is brought down into the stomach. The endoscope is then reinserted to precisely seat the device. Although this method of PEG placement has broad appeal, published experience is limited (Table 3) (3,30–32).

Both the pull-string and push-wire methods involve two passes of the gastroscope to safely complete the procedure as well as per os insertion of the feeding catheter. Contamination of the gastrostomy tube with oropharyngeal bacteria contributes to the risk of peristomal infection. The introducer technique was developed to avoid these disadvantages (33). A dilator with a peel-away sheath is percutaneously inserted into the stomach over a guidewire with endoscopic observation. The wire and dilator are removed and a balloon-tip catheter that serves as the gastrostomy tube is inserted through the sheath, which is peeled away and removed. The inflated balloon anchors the catheter in place and tension on the tube brings the stomach into apposition with the body wall. Results to date show a high technical success rate for this method, with an acceptable rate of complications (Table 3) (30,33–35). Premature rupture of the balloon with leakage of gastric contents and peritonitis has been a problem in some series (35).

It is unknown if one method is superior to another. Only a limited number of comparative studies have been performed and individual patient treatment groups have been small. Kozarek et al. (30) compared the push-wire and introducer methods in 30 patients. Complication rates between the two groups were simi-

lar but the push-wire method was easier to complete. Deitel et al. (34) compared the pull-string and introducer methods in 56 subjects. Technical success rates were 100% for each group but the latter method was faster (16 minutes versus 27 minutes, $p < .001$) and associated with fewer wound infections (0% versus 21%). Hogan et al. (31) prospectively evaluated PEG placement by the pull-string and push-wire methods in 40 patients. Procedure times, estimates of ease of insertion of the gastrostomy tube, and morbidity and mortality rates for the two methods were similar. These data do not permit firm conclusions regarding the preeminence of a particular technique. All the methods appear to be safe when performed by experienced operators and technical success rates are high (Tables 2 and 3).

COMPLICATIONS OF PEG

Cumulative results from large series show that PEG can be performed safely in the vast majority of patients (Tables 2 and 3). Minor complications are reported in 8.0% to 10% (mean, ~8.0%) of subjects. More significant problems occur in 1.0% to 7.0% (mean, ~3.0%) of individuals and the procedure-related mortality rate is less than 1.0% (mean, ~0.5%). Aspiration, peritonitis, hemorrhage, peristomal wound infections, and gastrocolic fistulae account for the majority of major complications (Table 4). Slow migration of the device out of the stomach has been observed in a few instances (36–38). Although placement of a PEG is safe and serious adverse events are uncommon, occurrence of a significant complication results in death in nearly 25% of cases (Table 4). This observation reflects the generalized debilitated condition of sick patients requiring

TABLE 4. *Types of major complications associated with PEG and subsequent outcome reported from seven large series evaluating 1433 patients[a]*

Type of complication	Patients, N	Mortality per complication
Aspiration	7	4/7 (57%)
Peritonitis	13	4/13 (31%)
Gastric perforation (no peritonitis)	3	0
Hemorrhage	6	0
Peristomal infections	4	0
Gastrocolic fistula	3	0
Other		
Laryngospasm during the procedure	1	1/1 (100%)
Unnecessary laparotomy	3	0
Total	40/1,433 (2.8%)	9/40 (23%)

[a] Data derived from series reported in the last 7 years evaluating 100 patients or more (3,5,25,27–29,35).

PEG and their intolerance to serious adverse events. Since aspiration and peritonitis account for approximately 90% of procedure-related deaths (Table 4), it is likely that the incidence of PEG-related mortality could be reduced further by placing emphasis on prevention and early recognition of these two potentially devastating complications.

Bronchopulmonary Aspiration

Bronchopulmonary aspiration of gastric contents can occur during the PEG procedure or at any point afterward as a consequence of tube feeding (3,5,28,29,35). Larson et al. (5) observed episodes of fatal aspiration occurring within 24 hours of the procedure in 2 of 299 patients (0.7%) (5). Grant (29) reported aspiration in 2 of 125 (1.6%) subjects and attributed both events directly to the PEG procedure (29). These individuals were successfully treated with intravenous antibiotics. Several factors account for the relatively high incidence of procedure-related aspiration in patients undergoing PEG. The majority of treated patients are elderly and have CNS disease or other conditions that impair reflexes that protect the airway. Also, the PEG is placed with the patient in the supine position with the head of the bed elevated, and the stomach is intentionally overinflated—factors that collectively augment the incidence of this complication.

Effective prevention of bronchopulmonary aspiration requires knowledge of factors that increase the risk. Consequently, the procedure should be completed in a timely fashion and oversedation should be avoided. The gastrointestinal assistant should maintain a clear airway for the patient at all times. We put the PEG to gravity drainage for 12 to 24 hours after placement to decompress the stomach (3) because a transient postprocedure ileus may adversely affect a small percentage of individuals (3,5). It is important to document the presence of bowel sounds before initiating feeding. Despite implementation of these preventative measures, aspiration will still occur in a small proportion of patients. Fever, leukocytosis, respiratory symptoms, and an infiltrate on chest radiography are suggestive. When diagnosed, broad-spectrum antibiotics should be prescribed immediately. Prompt recognition and appropriate treatment is effective for the majority of patients (3,29,35).

Nearly all data on risk for bronchopulmonary aspiration associated with gastrostomy tube feeding have been obtained in the acute care setting. Relatively little information exists regarding aspiration after discharge of tube-fed patients to extended care facilities. Cogen and Weinryb (39) detected probable or possible cases of aspiration pneumonia in 23% of 107 patients fed through a gastrostomy tube in a skilled nursing facility, and 85% of these individuals had PEGs in place. No association could be made between aspiration and age or mental status of the patient or method of feeding (intermittent or continuous). A history of pneumonia (presumably due to aspiration) antedating placement of the gastrostomy tube did identify individuals at increased risk. Approximately 6% of patients ultimately died as a consequence of this complication.

Taylor et al. (40) performed a population-based cohort study on 97 patients having PEG placed between 1982 and 1988. Follow-up continued for 2 years or until death of the patient. Fifty-four patients (56%) had 179 episodes of pneumonia after placement of the feeding tube. Pneumonia was the most common cause of death in this series of patients. These data suggest that aspiration among patients managed with a PEG is a common event.

Chronic care of tube-fed patients should include measures to prevent aspiration. Patients should be fed with the head of the bed elevated at least 30°, with the position maintained for a minimum of 1 hour after the feeding has stopped. Regular assessment of gastric residual volumes and aggressive medical treatment of gastroesophageal reflux should be considered routine aspects of long-term care.

It has been suggested that placement of a percutaneous endoscopic jejunostomy (PEJ) catheter may prevent aspiration in patients initially managed with a PEG (41), but the weight of evidence does not support this claim (42,43). The incidence of aspiration in PEJ patients is 17% to 60% (42–44), and this is a disturbing observation since aspiration is the major indication for this method of feeding. However, available studies were not designed to distinguish between aspiration of oropharyngeal secretions and feeding solutions. Huxley et al. (45) showed that 70% of patients with depressed consciousness aspirate their oropharyngeal secretions. Placement of a PEJ in such patients could not be expected to favorably affect the natural history of this problem. Also, the position of the PEJ catheter when aspiration occurs is seldom known. Consequently, the incidence of bronchopulmonary aspiration of feeding solution for patients with PEJ catheters maintained correctly within the jejunum has not been precisely defined. It is possible that failure to prevent aspiration may be due to the inability to maintain the catheter in proper position or the presence of unabated oropharyngeal aspiration—the clinical course of which is unaffected by the feeding tube.

Peritonitis

Peritonitis occurs in 0% to 1.2% of PEG patients and is one of the potentially fatal complications of the procedure (3,5,27–29,35). This serious side effect can occur by one of several mechanisms.

Premature removal of the catheter is the most common cause of peritonitis (3,28,35). Tube dislodgment in general occurs in 0.8% to 3.4% of PEG patients (3,5,28,29), although these figures usually apply to the acute care setting only. The incidence of catheter displacement may be highest for individuals having PEGs inserted by the introducer method, which uses a balloon-tipped catheter for the gastrostomy tube (35). Deflation or rupture of the balloon allows the stomach to move away from the abdominal wall, leaving the catheter tip in the peritoneal cavity. Solid-tipped catheters may erode through the gastric wall if tension applied to the external portion of the device is excessive. In any case, removal of a PEG before firm adhesions form between stomach and abdominal wall results in gastric perforation with the potential for peritonitis and death, especially if diagnosis is delayed.

Other mechanisms accounting for peritonitis are less common but all depend on leak of gastric contents into the abdominal cavity. Larson et al. (5) stripped off the internal crossbar of a de Pezzer catheter on four separate occasions when the device was pulled through an esophageal stricture. In two of these cases the catheter was unknowingly pulled through the stomach and left in the peritoneal cavity. Sangster et al. (28) inadvertently pulled one limb of an internal crossbar on a de Pezzer catheter through the stomach during the initial placement of the PEG and an intraabdominal leak occurred. If the stomach is not brought into apposition with the parietal surface of the abdominal wall when the PEG is inserted it is possible for gastric contents to leak out around the catheter and soil the peritoneal cavity. Miller et al. (35) observed this complication in

1 of 330 PEGs (0.3%). Perforation of a gastric ulcer unrelated to the PEG was a cause of peritonitis in one patient (28).

Because peritonitis results in a fatal outcome in approximately one-third of PEG patients (Table 4) it is important that great care be taken to avoid this complication. Early tube displacement appears to be the most troublesome problem. For this reason excessive tension on the catheter should be avoided that otherwise may lead to tissue necrosis and extrusion of the tube (3). Also, there is concern regarding use of balloon-tipped catheters for the initial gastrostomy tube (46). These devices are prone to deflate or rupture in the acidic environment of the stomach (47). In one series, balloon failure occurred in 11 of 330 cases (3.3%) (35). The product manufacturer subsequently replaced latex with Silastic balloons in an effort to reduce the risk of complications but it is unknown if this modification is efficacious. No matter which device is employed (balloon- or solid-tipped catheters) it is important to endoscopically confirm correct placement of the catheter at the conclusion of the procedure.

Consequences of displaced tubes and subsequent management depend on timing of the event in relation to initial placement of the PEG. Catheter dislodgment is usually a minor problem if the gastrocutaneous fistulous tract is mature. In this case gastric contents will leak out on the skin surface. We frequently use a gastrostomy button as a replacement device in this instance and have reported success with this approach (48). When catheter displacement occurs prior to maturation of the gastrocutaneous fistulous tract and the event is promptly recognized, it is usually sufficient to insert a nasogastric tube for suction and administer broad-spectrum antibiotics and observe the patient over several days (49). The PEG procedure can usually be repeated at a later date if the patient's clinical course is uneventful. However, presence of fever, leukocytosis, diminished bowel sounds, and abdominal pain and tenderness suggest peritonitis and warrant laparotomy.

Buried Bumper Syndrome

Excessive traction applied to the PEG over an extended period shortens the gastrocutaneous fistulous tract, causes ischemic necrosis of the gastric epithelium, and allows the internal bolster to slowly erode through the stomach wall (38). Over a period of weeks as the PEG gradually migrates anteriorly, it may come to lie partially or completely outside the stomach, embedded in the abdominal wall as the excavated gastric site heals and reepithelializes behind it. This complication has been termed the buried bumper syndrome and has occurred almost exclusively with the Sacks-Vine gastrostomy tube (36–38,50–52). The design (internal crossbar with blunt edges) and composition of these catheters may be important predisposing factors. The problem has been recognized within 5 days to 11 months after placement of the device but in most cases difficulties became apparent after 3 to 4 months of use (36–38,50–52).

Immobility of the gastrostomy tube, fixation to an area of induration on the abdominal wall, and resistance to flow through the PEG associated with leakage around the tube are diagnostic signs (51). Evaluation with a lateral abdominal x-ray will show the tube tip and internal bolster lying in the soft tissues between the gastric air bubble and skin surface (36). At endoscopy, the PEG may not be visible and there may be no trace of its exit from the stomach (36,52). In some instances, a small mucosal dimple or ulceration may be the only sign marking the previous PEG site, or the end of the device but not the crossbar may still be present in the gastric lumen (37,38,51).

Treatment requires removal of the tube. In most instances, this is achieved by incising skin over the internal bolster and carefully dissecting it out. Purulent material may be expressed from the wound but it is safe to reuse the existing tract for placement of a second catheter using antibiotic prophylaxis. In an effort to prevent the buried bumper syndrome, we recommend that the internal bolster from the gastrostomy tube not be brought into direct contact with the gastric mucosa (3), but rather leave a space of 2 to 3 mm. Behrle et al. (50) observed the syndrome in 2 of 12 patients managed with a Sacks-Vine gastrojejunostomy tube. They postulated that the bowed jejunal tube in the stomach directed increased back pressure at a focal point beneath the internal bolster of the gastrostomy tube. This effect led to pressure necrosis and outward migration of the PEG. They recommend using gastrostomy rather than gastrojejunostomy tubes whenever possible.

Hemorrhage

Hemorrhage occurring as a complication of PEG is an uncommon event and among large series has been reported in 0% to 2.5% of cases (3,5,27–29). Gastric ulcers located beneath the internal bolster are the most common cause and probably result from either simple frictional abrasion of the mucosa caused by movement of the PEG or excessive traction on the device, pressure necrosis, and ischemia. Cappell (53) reported two cases of profuse bleeding from erosions in the distal esophagus. Bleeding occurred immediately after the procedure and was presumably due to traumatic placement of the PEG.

Presenting symptoms usually include nausea, vomiting, abdominal pain, hematemesis, or melena. Aspiration of gastric contents through the PEG will show

blood. Endoscopy is mandatory for precise diagnosis. Ulcerations beneath the internal bolster can be missed, so it is important to push the PEG inward during the endoscopic examination to lift it off the mucosa in an effort to expose the lesion. The device should be secured in this position if an ulcer is present and H2-blocker therapy prescribed. This treatment approach has been successful in all reported cases (3,54).

Gastric ulcers and associated bleeding can probably be prevented by avoiding direct contact between the internal bolster and gastric mucosa when the PEG is initially placed. Measures employed to prevent the buried bumper syndrome are probably effective in preventing bleeding ulcers as well.

Sick patients managed with a PEG have a high incidence of concomitant acid peptic disease at the time when the device is placed. Scott et al. (55) and Wolfsen et al. (56) endoscopically diagnosed gastric or duodenal ulcers in 16% and 14% of PEG patients, respectively. Scott et al. observed that bleeding following placement of the feeding catheter was more likely due to a preexisting peptic ulcer rather than a complication from the PEG. These data support the importance of thorough diagnostic upper endoscopy prior to placement of a PEG to detect unsuspected ulcers that could bleed at a later date.

Peristomal Wound Infections

Peristomal wound infection occurs in 5% to 30% of PEG patients and is the most common procedure-related side effect (2,57). The majority of infections are minor and easily treated with antibiotics alone or in combination with incision and drainage of the wound. More serious infections are uncommon yet can be difficult to manage.

Necrotizing fascitis is a rapidly progressive infectious process characterized by primary involvement of fascia and subcutaneous tissue, extensive undermining of skin, sparing of muscle, and severe systemic toxic manifestations (58). At least seven cases involving the abdominal wall have been reported following placement of a PEG and three of these individuals (43%) have died (18,59–64). The pathogenesis for infection in this particular setting has not been clearly defined. However, since the mouth and pharynx are colonized with bacteria and the feeding tube is pulled through the oropharynx and out the abdominal wall, it is likely that minor infections as well as those resulting in necrotizing fascitis are due to contamination of the catheter with oropharyngeal bacteria and local spread of these organisms into the surrounding soft tissues. No cases of fascitis have been reported among patients having PEGs placed by the introducer method—a technique where the catheter is directly inserted through the abdominal wall and not pulled through the pharynx. The majority of infections reported to date have been polymicrobial with gram-negative organisms and staphylococcal and streptococcal species isolated most often. All have occurred within 9 days after placement of the device.

Risk factors for necrotizing fasciitis in general include diabetes mellitus, atherosclerosis, alcoholism, malnutrition, immunosuppression, and age over 50 years (58,65,66). Fever and leukocytosis are common presenting features and occur within days after placement of the PEG. Edema, erythema, ecchymosis, induration, crepitance, and bullae may appear at or in a location on the abdominal wall or flank remote from the gastrostomy site. Pus can sometimes be expressed from the gastrocutaneous fistulous tract (60). Plain abdominal radiographs will show fluid and gas in the subcutaneous tissues of the abdominal wall and computed tomography (CT) can confirm this observation (59–61). Sepsis with rapid deterioration in the clinical status of the patient usually follows the onset of initial signs and symptoms. Necrotizing fasciitis is fatal unless recognized early. Treatment includes broad-spectrum antibiotics, aggressive surgical debridement of all devitalized tissue, closure of the gastrostomy, and nutritional support provided by either an enteral (jejunostomy) or parenteral route. This management approach has been successful in the majority of instances.

Peristomal wound infections are preventable if certain precautions are taken. It is appropriate to shave the patient's abdomen and disinfect the skin with a povidone-iodine solution prior to placement of the catheter. Some investigators attempt to reduce oropharyngeal bacterial contamination by having patients gargle with an antibiotic solution (41,60), but this preventative measure may be unnecessary. Our own incidence of peristomal wound infection was 0% among 118 patients and we administer a single dose of a cephalosporin before the procedure without an antibiotic gargle (3). In a randomized controlled trial, Jain et al. (67) showed that 1 g of cefazolin administered 30 minutes prior to the procedure reduced the incidence of peristomal wound infections from 28.6% to 7.4% (67). Importantly, no patient in the treated group developed a wound abscess that required surgical drainage, whereas three of eight individuals who did not receive antibiotic prophylaxis and developed a purulent discharge required incision and drainage. At least four individuals with necrotizing fasciitis following PEG placement did not receive antibiotic prophylaxis and three of these individuals died (59,60,62–64).

There should be an adequate exit site for the gastrostomy tube from the skin. Bacteria and gastric secretions can become trapped in the soft tissues if the skin incision is small and totally occupied by the catheter. We make a skin incision that is several millimeters

larger than the diameter of the gastrostomy tube. Direct contact between the internal bolster and gastric epithelium should be avoided when the device is placed and the external retention disk should be loosely applied to the skin to avoid ischemic necrosis not only of the stomach wall but the soft tissues of the abdominal wall as well. Breakdown of these tissues may augment the risk for infection (59,63). The stoma should be left open to air and cleansed daily with hydrogen peroxide. We usually apply a povidone-iodine ointment to the stoma for the first 7 days after the procedure. Finally, a PEG should not be placed in patients with concurrent infection. Forty-three percent of individuals with necrotizing fasciitis had a coexistent infection when the PEG was placed (64). In such instances, persistent elevation in temperature may be erroneously attributed to an extraneous infection and not recognized as an early sign of an abdominal wall abscess or necrotizing fasciitis. Also, Korula and Rice (62) suggest that bacteremia from other sites of infection may contribute to development of necrotizing fasciitis, especially in association with ischemic necrosis of the soft tissues of the abdominal wall and impaired host defense mechanisms.

Gastrocolocutaneous Fistulae

On occasion, the colon can be interposed between the abdominal wall and stomach when the PEG is placed. If this relationship is not recognized, then it is possible to insert the device through the bowel and stomach causing a gastrocolocutaneous fistula. At least ten cases have been reported in the literature, all occurring within 14 days to 1 year after insertion of the PEG (25,35,68–72). The fistula frequently becomes manifest when the original catheter is replaced with a new device. In this instance, the replacement tube is reinserted through the colocutaneous tract into the colon but not the stomach. Tube feeding is then delivered directly into the large bowel causing diarrhea. In some cases, patients presented with fecal emesis with their original catheter in place (71). A definitive diagnosis can usually be made by injection of barium or Gastrografin through the PEG, which will show the catheter tip in the colon. The gastrocolic and colocutaneous fistula will usually close spontaneously within 7 to 10 days after the PEG is removed (25,70,72). If not, takedown of the fistula is indicated, which can be performed in conjunction with a surgical gastrostomy.

By taking certain precautions it is possible to avoid this complication. With the patient supine on the endoscopic table, elevating the head of the bed at least 30° above the horizontal will tend to displace the transverse colon in the caudad direction and away from the site chosen for PEG placement. Endoscopic transillumination of the abdominal wall and indirect finger compression on the stomach at the site are useful measures and when completed successfully suggest the absence of interposed structures between body wall and stomach. However, we showed that these safety maneuvers by themselves may not be 100% reliable in predicting a safe procedure, especially in patients with prior abdominal surgery (17).

One-third of patients with gastrocolocutaneous fistulae reported to date have had prior laparotomy, including partial gastrectomy in one case. Therefore, we advocate establishing a "safe" gastrocutaneous fistulous tract prior to placement of the PEG. This maneuver is performed by thrusting a 22-gauge, 1½-inch needle attached to a 20 cc saline loaded syringe through the preselected PEG site into the gastric lumen. The barrel on the syringe is retracted as the needle is slowly advanced through the abdominal wall. Safe tracts are determined by simultaneous air return in the aspirating syringe and endoscopic visualization of the intragastric needle. Failure to visualize the needle tip with the endoscope at the precise point when gas bubbles are aspirated back into the syringe suggests presence of a bowel loop located anterior to the stomach. Inability to aspirate gas and failure to see the needle indicate incomplete apposition of the stomach to the abdominal wall. We have seen this on one occasion in a patient with a Billroth II gastrectomy. In this case, absence of the pyloric sphincter allowed for uncontrolled air loss into the small bowel, preventing maximum air insufflation of the stomach, and dense adhesion probably prevented anterior migration of the gastric remnant. Failure to complete any of the usual safety maneuvers, including determination of a safe gastrocutaneous fistulous tract, is an absolute contraindication to placement of a PEG.

Pneumoperitoneum

Pneumoperitoneum has been observed following PEG in 36% to 38% of patients (73,74). In most cases, this finding is created by endoscopic intragastric air insufflation in association with the percutaneous puncture of the stomach, which allows leakage of gas. It is not known why free intraabdominal air accumulates in some individuals but not others. Multiple percutaneous needle punctures of the stomach, prolonged procedure time, excessive air insufflation, elevated intragastric pressure, and incomplete apposition of the stomach to the abdominal wall may be predisposing factors, but this is unproven.

Pneumoperitoneum is a common radiographic finding following PEG placement that follows a benign course in the vast majority of patients. Affected individuals fail to develop fever, leukocytosis, or pain. Di-

agnostic tests and therapeutic interventions are unnecessary. On occasion, pneumoperitoneum may occur in association with a serious intraabdominal complication. However, in these cases clinical signs (fever, leukocytosis, peritoneal signs) and symptoms (pain, abdominal distention) suggest a pathological condition, and measures to exclude a gastric perforation or leak and associated peritonitis are warranted.

Gastroesophageal Reflux

Data are conflicting regarding the influence of PEG on gastroesophageal reflux disease (GERD). There is obvious concern that intragastric delivery of feeding formula in recumbent patients may increase the risk of this adverse event. However, results from large series of PEG patients seldom include acid reflux as an important complication (3,5,25,35). Data are available that indicate individuals with preexisting GERD may continue to reflux when PEG feedings are initiated (75) and this problem may predispose patients to aspiration pneumonia (76).

Johnson et al. (77) prospectively evaluated seven patients undergoing PEG to determine the influence of the procedure on gastroesophageal reflux. Reflux episodes decreased in six of seven subjects, and lower esophageal sphincter pressure increased and reflux scores decreased after the procedure in all patients. Anterior apposition of the gastric wall attained during placement of the PEG may favorably alter the angle of His, have a gastropexy-like effect, and accordingly increase lower esophageal sphincter pressure and decrease reflux (77). However, these favorable effects may not be sustained, as one patient restudied within 2 days after PEG did not maintain the initial post-PEG improvement at 4 weeks. Grunow et al. (78) determined pH scores in ten children before and after PEG. None had abnormal pH scores before the procedure, but in six children scores became abnormal afterward and three (30%) developed symptoms. These data suggest that children not refluxing before PEG placement may have a propensity for the complication afterward. Specific mechanisms accounting for gastroesophageal reflux in these individuals were not determined and it was not possible to accurately predict which patients were at greatest risk.

Fundoplication has been standard therapy for children with severe gastroesophageal reflux, especially those with brain injury (79). Elevation of the head of the bed, slow continuous infusion of the feeding formula, and H2-blocker therapy may be effective in adults (75). There are no reports to date on omeprazole for reflux in this setting, but at least on theoretical grounds this medication might be useful for resistant cases.

REFERENCES

1. Gauderer MWL, Ponsky JL, Izant RJ Jr. Gastrostomy without laparotomy: a percutaneous endoscopic technique. *J Pediatr Surg* 1980;15:872–875.
2. Foutch PG, Haynes WC, Bellapravalu S, et al. Percutaneous endoscopic gastrostomy (PEG): a new procedure comes of age. *J Clin Gastroenterol* 1986;8:10–15.
3. Foutch PG, Woods CA, Talbert GA, et al. A critical analysis of the Sacks-Vine gastrostomy tube: a review of 120 consecutive procedures. *Am J Gastroenterol* 1988;83:812–815.
4. Ponsky JL, Gauderer MWL. Percutaneous endoscopic gastrostomy: indications, limitations, techniques and results. *World J Surg* 1989;13:165–170.
5. Larson DE, Burton DD, Schroeder KW, et al. Percutaneous endoscopic gastrostomy: indications, success, complications and mortality in 314 consecutive patients. *Gastroenterology* 1987;93:48–52.
6. Stellato TA, Gauderer MWL. Percutaneous endoscopic gastrostomy for gastrointestinal decompression. *Ann Surg* 1987; 205: 119–122.
7. Stellato TA, Gauderer MWL. Percutaneous endoscopic gastrostomy in the cancer patient. *Am Surg* 1988;54:419–422.
8. Slezak FA, Kofol WH. Combined tracheostomy and percutaneous endoscopic gastrostomy. *Am J Surg* 1987; 154:271–273.
9. Kelly KM, Lewis B, Gentili DR, et al. Use of percutaneous gastrostomy in the intensive care patient. *Crit Care Med* 1988; 16:62–63.
10. Foutch PG, Steinway D, List A, et al. Gastrostomy-biliary drainage in a patient with bile duct cancer: a basis for multimodality treatment. *Gastrointest Endosc* 1989; 35:341–343.
11. Eckhauser ML, Ferron JP. The use of dual percutaneous endoscopic gastrostomy (DPEG) in the management of chronic intermittent gastric volvulus. *Gastrointest Endosc* 1985;31:340–342.
12. Foutch PG, Talbert G, Sanowski RA. Nonoperative traction method for placement of esophageal stents: a new use for the percutaneous endoscopic gastrostomy. *Gastrointest Endosc* 1988; 34:259–262.
13. Ponsky JL, Aszodi A. External biliary-gastric fistula: a simple method for recycling bile. *Am J Gastroenterol* 1982; 77:939–940.
14. Foutch PG, Sawyer RL, Sanowski RA. The biliogastric shunt: a method for simultaneous internal diversion of bile and enteric feeding in patients with cancer. *Gastrointest Endosc* 1989;35:440–442.
15. Shike M, Gerdes H, Botet J, Coit D, Ciaburri D. External biliary duodenal drainage through a percutaneous endoscopic duodenostomy. *Gastrointest Endosc* 1989;35:104–105.
16. Ponsky JL, Aszodi A, Perse D. Percutaneous endoscopic cecostomy: a new approach to nonobstructive colonic dilation. *Gastrointest Endosc* 1986;32:108–111.
17. Foutch PG, Talbert GA, Waring JP, et al. Percutaneous endoscopic gastrostomy in patients with prior abdominal surgery: virtues of the safe tract. *Am J Gastroenterol* 1988; 83:147–150.
18. Ditesheim JA, Richards W, Sharp K. Fatal and disastrous complications following percutaneous endoscopic gastrostomy. *Am Surg* 1989;55:92–96.
19. Stellato TA, Gauderer MWL, Ponsky JL. Percutaneous endoscopic gastrostomy following previous abdominal surgery. *Ann Surg* 1984;200:46–50.
20. Gottfried EB, Plumser AB. Endoscopic gastrojejunostomy: a technique to establish small bowel feeding without laparotomy. *Gastrointest Endosc* 1984;30:355–357.
21. Strodel WE, Eckhauser FE, Lemmer JH, Knol JA, Dent TL. Endoscopic percutaneous gastrostomy. *Contemp Surg* 1983;23:17–23.
22. Plumeri PA, Wesner NN, Cohen NN. Percutaneous endoscopic gastrostomy. *Pa Med* 1983;86:57–58.
23. Griffin RA, Hung CT, Mitchell RD. Percutaneous endoscopic gastrostomy—its applicability to clinical practice. *Gastrointest Endosc* 1984;30:150(abst).
24. Thatcher BS, Ferguson DR, Paradis K. Percutaneous endoscopic gastrostomy: a preferred method of feeding tube gastrostomy. *Am J Gastroenterol* 1984;79:748–750.
25. Ponsky JL, Gauderer MWL, Stellato TA, et al. Percutaneous approaches to enteral alimentation. *Am J Surg* 1985; 149:102–105.
26. Kirby DF, Craig RM, Tsang TK, Plotnick BH. Percutaneous endoscopic gastrostomies: a prospective evaluation and review of the literature. *JPEN* 1986;10:155–159.
27. Stern JS. Comparison of percutaneous endoscopic gastrostomy with surgical gastrostomy at a community hospital. *Am J Gastroenterol* 1986;81:1171–1173.
28. Sangster W, Cuddington GD, Bachulis BL. Percutaneous endoscopic gastrostomy. *Am J Surg* 1988;155:677–679.
29. Grant JP. Comparison of percutaneous endoscopic gastrostomy with stamm gastrostomy. *Ann Surg* 1988;207:598–603.
30. Kozarek RA, Ball TJ, Ryan JA. When push comes to shove: a comparison between two methods of percutaneous endoscopic gastrostomy. *Am J Gastroenterol* 1986;81:642–646.
31. Hogan RB, DeMarco DC, Hamilton JK, Walker CO, Polter DE. Percutaneous endoscopic gastrostomy—to push or pull. *Gastrointest Endosc* 1986;32:253–258.
32. Stiegmann G, Goff J, VanWay C, et al. Operative versus endoscopic gastrostomy: preliminary results of a prospective randomized trial. *Am J Surg* 1988;155:88–92.
33. Russell TR, Brotman M, Norris F. Percutaneous gastrostomy: a new simplified and cost-effective technique. *Am J Surg* 1984; 148:132–137.
34. Deitel M, Bendago M, Spratt EH, Burul CJ, To TB. Percutaneous endoscopic gastrostomy by the pull and introducer methods. *CJ Surg* 1988;31:102–104.
35. Miller RE, Castlemain B, Lacqua FJ, et al. Percutaneous endoscopic gastrostomy: results in 316 patients and review of literature. *Surg Endosc* 1989;3:186–190.
36. Fay DE, Luther R, Gruber M. A single procedure endoscopic technique for replacing partially extruded percutaneous endoscopic gastrostomy tubes. *Gastrointest Endosc* 1990; 36:298–300.
37. Kaplan DS, Fried MW. Migration of PEG tubes. *Am J Gastroenterol* 1989;84:1590–1591.
38. Klein S, Heare BR, Soloway RD. The buried bumper syndrome: a complication of percutaneous endoscopic gastrostomy. *Am J Gastroenterol* 1990;85:448–451.
39. Cogan R, Weinryb J. Aspiration pneumonia in nursing home patients fed via gastrostomy tubes. *Am J Gastroenterol* 1989; 84:1509–1512.
40. Taylor CA, Larson DE, Ballard DJ, et al. Predictors of outcome after percutaneous endoscopic gastrostomy: a community-based study. *Mayo Clin Proc* 1992;67:1042–1049.
41. Strodel WE, Ponsky JL. Complications of percutaneous gastrostomy. In Ponsky JL, ed: *Techniques of percutaneous gastrostomy.* New York: Igaku-Shoin, 1988;63–78.
42. DiSario JA, Foutch PG, Sanowski RA. Poor results with percutaneous endoscopic jejunostomy. *Gastrointest Endosc* 1990;36:257–260.
43. Wolfsen HC, Kozarek RA, Ball TJ, et al. Tube dysfunction following percutaneous endoscopic gastrostomy and jejunostomy. *Gastrointest Endosc* 1990;36:261–263.
44. Kaplan DS, Murthy UK, Linscheer WG. Percutaneous endoscopic jejunostomy: long-term follow up of 23 patients. *Gastrointest Endosc* 1989;35:403–406.
45. Huxley EJ, Viroslav J, Gray WR, et al. Pharyngeal aspiration in normal adults and patients with depressed consciousness. *Am J Med* 1978;64:564–568.
46. Foutch PG. Nonsurgical gastrostomy: x-ray or endoscopy. *Am J Gastroenterol* 1990;85:1560–1562.
47. Banerjee B, Moore J. Complication of the Russell PEG method. *Gastrointest Endosc* 1989;35:132–133.
48. Foutch PG, Talbert GA, Gaines JA, et al. The gastrostomy button: a prospective assessment of safety, success and spectrum of use. *Gastrointest Endosc* 1989;35:41–44.
49. Ponsky JL. Percutaneous endoscopic stomas. *Surg Endosc* 1989;69:1227–1236.
50. Behrle KM, Dekovich AA, Ammon HV. Spontaneous tube extrusion following percutaneous endoscopic gastrostomy. *Gastrointest Endosc* 1989;35:56–68.
51. Schwartz HI, Goldberg RI, Barkin JS, et al. PEG feeding tube

migration impaction in the abdominal wall. *Gastrointest Endosc* 1989;35:134–135.

52. Shallman RW, Norfleet RG, Hardache JM. Percutaneous endoscopic gastrostomy feeding tube migration and impaction in the abdominal wall. *Gastrointest Endosc* 1988;34:367–368.

53. Cappell MS. Esophageal bleeding after percutaneous endoscopic gastrostomy. *J Clin Gastroenterol* 1988;10:383–385.

54. Patel PH, Hunter W, Willis M, et al. Upper gastrointestinal hemorrhage secondary to gastric ulcer complicating percutaneous endoscopic gastrostomy. *Gastrointest Endosc* 1988;34:288–289.

55. Scott JS, Edelman DS, Unger SW. Percutaneous endoscopic gastrostomy: a mandate for complete diagnostic upper endoscopy. *Am Surg* 1989;55:85–87.

56. Wolfsen HC, Kozarek RA, Ball TJ, et al. Value of diagnostic upper endoscopy preceding percutaneous gastrostomy. *Am J Gastroenterol* 1990;85:249–251. .

57. Jonas SK, Neimark S, Panwalker AP. Effect of antibiotic prophylaxis in percutaneous endoscopic gastrostomy. *Am J Gastroenterol* 1985;80:438–441.

58. Janevicius RV, Hann SE, Batt MD. Necrotizing fascitis. *Surg Gynecol Obstet* 1982;154:97–102.

59. Cave DR, Robinson WR, Brothschi EA. Necrotizing fascitis following percutaneous endoscopic gastrostomy. *Gastrointest Endosc* 1986;32:294–296.

60. Greif JM, Ragland JJ, Ochsner MG, et al. Fatal necrotizing fascitis complicating percutaneous endoscopic gastrostomy. *Gastrointest Endosc* 1986;32:292–294.

61. Haas DW, Sharmaraja P, Morrison JG, et al. Necrotizing fascitis following percutaneous endoscopic gastrostomy. *Gastrointest Endosc* 1988;34:487–488.

62. Korula J, Rice HE. Necrotizing fascitis and percutaneous endoscopic gastrostomy. *Gastrointest Endosc* 1987; 33:335–336.

63. Martindale R, Witte M, Hodges G, et al. Necrotizing fascitis as a complication of percutaneous endoscopic gastrostomy. *JPEN* 1987;11:583–585.

64. Foutch PG. Complications of percutaneous endoscopic gastrostomy and jejunostomy: recognition, prevention and treatment. *Gastrointest Endosc Clin North Am* 1992;2:231–248.

65. Fisher JR, Conway MJ, Takeshita RT, et al. Necrotizing fascitis: importance of roentgenographic studies for soft tissue gas. *JAMA* 1979;241:803–806.

66. Rouse TM, Malangoni MA, Schulte WJ. Necrotizing fasciitis: a preventable disaster. *Surgery* 1982;92:765–771.

67. Jain NK, Larson DE, Schroeder KW, et al. Antibiotic prophylaxis for percutaneous endoscopic gastrostomy: a prospective, randomized, double-blind clinical trial. *Ann Intern Med* 1987; 107:824–828.

68. Bui HD, Dang CV, Schlater T, et al. A new complication of percutaneous endoscopic gastrostomy. *Am J Gastroenterol* 1988;83:448–451.

69. Fernandes ET, Hollabaugh R, Hixon SD, et al. Late presentation of gastrocolic fistula after percutaneous gastrostomy. *Gastrointest Endosc* 1988;34:368–369.

70. Saltzberg DM, Anand K, Juvan P, et al. Colocutaneous fistula: an unusual complication of percutaneous endoscopic gastrostomy. *JPEN* 1987;11:86–87.

71. Stefan MM, Holcomb GW III, Ross AJ III. Cologastric fistula as a complication of percutaneous endoscopic gastrostomy. *JPEN* 1989;13:554–556.

72. van Gossum A, Desmarez B, Cremer M. A colo-cutaneous-gastric fistula: a silent and unusual complication of percutaneous endoscopic gastrostomy. *Endoscopy* 1988;20:161.

73. Plumser AB, Gottfried EB, Clair MR. Pneumoperitoneum after percutaneous endoscopic gastrostomy. *Am J Gastroenterol* 1984;79:440–441.

74. Strodel WE, Lemmer J, Eckhauser F, et al. Early experience with endoscopic percutaneous gastrostomy. *Arch Surg* 1983; 118:449–453.

75. Hollands MJ, Fletcher JP, Young J. Percutaneous feeding gastrostomy. *Med J Aust* 1989;151:328–331.

76. Patel PH, Thomas E. Risk factors for pneumonia after percutaneous endoscopic gastrostomy. *J Clin Gastroenterol* 1990;12: 389–392.

77. Johnson DA, Hacker JF III, Benjamin SB, et al. Percutaneous endoscopic gastrostomy effects on gastroesophageal reflux and the lower esophageal sphincter. *Am J Gastroenterol* 1987; 82: 622–624.

78. Grunow JE, Al-Hafidh AS, Tunell WP. Gastroesophageal reflux following percutaneous endoscopic gastrostomy in children. *J Pediatr Surg* 1989;24:42–45.

79. Gauderer MWL, Stellato TA. Gastrostomies: evolution, techniques, indications and complications. *Curr Probl Surg* 1986;23: 657–719.

Advanced Therapeutic Endoscopy, 2nd Ed.,
edited by J. S. Barkin and C. A. O'Phelan.
Raven Press, Ltd., New York © 1994.

CHAPTER 19

Percutaneous Endoscopic Jejunostomy: Indications, Techniques, and Evaluation

Gustavo A. Calleja and Jamie S. Barkin

Enteral feeding via percutaneous endoscopic gastrostomy (PEG) has substantial advantages over nasogastric tubes, which predispose the patient to sinusitis, require frequent replacement after inadvertent removal, and are uncomfortable and unattractive. However, aspiration pneumonia has been reported at rates ranging from 40% to 56% in patients who are fed via nasogastric tubes as well as PEGs (1,2). The mechanism of this aspiration is unclear. It may be (a) related to an abnormal swallowing mechanism, which leads to aspiration of oropharyngeal contents, or (b) secondary to gastroesophageal (GE) reflux, as patients with a prior history of either aspiration pneumonia or GE reflux are at greatest risk for aspiration pneumonia after PEG placement (2,3). Surgical jejunostomy has been shown to protect patients from aspiration; therefore, percutaneous endoscopic jejunostomy (PEJ) has been developed as an alternative to PEG in patients with a history of aspiration pneumonia or those with significant GE reflux (4,5). An additional advantage of PEJ placement is that some designs permit the combined functions of gastric drainage and jejunal feedings (6). Clinical settings in which this is likely to be useful include partial mechanical obstruction of the stomach or functional motility disorders, such as with diabetes mellitus and postoperative nonfunctioning gastrojejunostomy (7), which preclude gastric feeding but potentially allow for jejunal feeding, and patients with a tracheoesophageal fistula.

TECHNIQUE AND EQUIPMENT

Percutaneous endoscopic jejunostomy was initially described by Ponsky and Aszodi (5) in 1984 using a

modification of their previously described technique for PEG placement. Various jejunostomy kits are commercially available, eliminating the need for tube modification (Table 1).

There are many variations in the characteristics and features of these PEJ tubes. Their value is largely untested in controlled studies. Thus, a longer PEJ tube might seem a better choice to prevent reflux of feedings. However, this is untested, and a longer tube may be more likely to clog. A few generalizations are possible. A larger diameter jejunostomy tube is less prone to clogging. The gastric port included with many kits cannot be added to an existing jejunostomy tube that does not have one. This is a desirable feature, as it does not impede the function of the jejunal tube and may be needed at some point to aspirate gastric contents or to infuse medications directly into the stomach, which helps to prevent jejunostomy tube clogging. The selection of "push" or "pull" placement technique, that is, the selection of a tube placed over a guidewire or grasped at the tip, is dependent on the preference of the endoscopist.

All these PEJ tubes are made of polyurethane, are radiopaque, and many have weighted tips. They are intended for use with the respective manufacturer's PEG systems. The tips of jejunostomy tubes designed for placement by the "pull" technique have an attached silk suture (or other feature) that can be grasped to pull it beyond the pylorus.

The initial phase of PEJ insertion is placement of a PEG using the standard technique described elsewhere in this book. The "pull" placement method begins with passage of the jejunostomy tube through the gastrostomy tube into the stomach. The optimal length to which to cut the gastrostomy tube is undefined; however, a shorter PEG tube will lengthen the portion of the jejunostomy tube that passes into the stomach and

G. A. Calleja and J. S. Barkin: Division of Gastroenterology, Mount Sinai Medical Center, Miami Beach, Florida 33140.

TABLE 1. *PEJ kits by manufacturer*

Brand	Model	PEG size	PEJ length	PEJ size external/ internal	Features
Bard	000319	20 Fr	27 inch	9 Fr/6 Fr	A, T, S, W
	00732	20 Fr	35 inch	9 Fr/6 Fr	A, T, G, F
Biosearch	17-1009	16 or 20 Fr	35 inch	9 Fr/7 Fr	O, T, G, F
	17-1012	20 Fr	35 inch	12 Fr/10 Fr	O, T, G, F
	17-5009	20 Fr	35 inch	9 Fr/7 Fr	A, T, G, F
	14-7222	16 Fr	27 inch	8 Fr/6 Fr	O, T, S, W
	14-7226	12 Fr	27 inch	12 Fr/10 Fr	O, T, S, W
	17-3022	22 Fr-included	35 inch	9 Fr/7 Fr	A, T, G, F
	17-3024	24 Fr-indicated	35 inch	9 Fr/7 Fr	A, T, G, F
	17-2009	Replacement for 17-3022 and 3024	35 inch	9 Fr/7 Fr	A, T, G, F
Corpak	30-7368	20 Fr	36 inch	8 Fr/6 Fr	A, T, Gr, W, P
	30-7361	20 Fr	36 inch	10 Fr/8 Fr	A, T, Gr, W, P
	30-1438	20 Fr	43 inch	8 Fr/6 Fr	A, G, F, P
	30-1431	20 Fr	43 inch	10 Fr/8 Fr	A, G, F, P
	30-7366	16 Fr-pediatric	36 inch	6 Fr/4 Fr	A, T, Gr, W, P
Medical Innovations Corporation (MIC)	200-14	Replaces a PEG	20 inch	14 Fr/9 Fr	O, G, F
	200-16	Replaces a PEG	20 inch	16 Fr/11 Fr	O, G, F
	200-18	Replaces a PEG	20 inch	18 Fr/13 Fr	O, G, F
	200-20	Replaces a PEG	20 inch	20 Fr/15 Fr	O, G, F
	200-22	Replaces a PEG	20 inch	22 Fr/16 Fr	O, G, F
	200-24	Replaces a PEG	20 inch	24 Fr/18 Fr	O, G, F
	200-12LV	Replaces a PEG	20 inch[a]	12 Fr/7 Fr	O, G, F
	250-16	Replaces a PEG	20 inch	16 Fr/10 Fr	A, T, S, W
	250-18	Replaces a PEG	20 inch	18 Fr/12 Fr	A, T, S, W
	250-22	Replaces a PEG	20 inch	22 Fr/14 Fr	A, T, S, W
	210-16	Replaces a PEG	22 inch	6 Fr/3 Fr	A, T, G
	210-18	Replaces a PEG	22 inch	7 Fr/4 Fr	A, T, G
	210-20	Replaces a PEG	22 inch	8 Fr/5 Fr	A, T, G
	210-22	Replaces a PEG	22 inch	9 Fr/5 Fr	A, T, G
	210-24	Replaces a PEG	22 inch	9 Fr/5 Fr	A, T, G
	210-26	Replaces a PEG	22 inch	10 Fr/6 Fr	A, T, G
	210-28	Replaces a PEG	22 inch	12 Fr/8 Fr	A, T, G
	210-30	Replaces a PEG	22 inch	14 Fr/9 Fr	A, T, G
	210-16LV	Replaces a PEG	10 inch	6 Fr/3 Fr	A, T, G
	210-18LV	Replaces a PEG	10 inch	7 Fr/4 Fr	A, T, G
Ross	167	14–22 Fr	30 inch	9 Fr/6 Fr	O[b], T, W, S
	168	18, 22 Fr	30 inch	12 Fr/9 Fr	O[b], T, W, S
	169	18 Fr	30 inch	9 Fr/6 Fr	A, T, W, S
Sandoz	087001	22 Fr	26 inch	9 Fr/6 Fr	A, T, W, S
	087002	22 Fr	26 inch	12 Fr/9 Fr	O, T, W, S
	085001	28 Fr	26 inch	12 Fr/9 Fr	A, T, W, S
	085101	28 Fr	26 inch	12 Fr/9 Fr	A, G, F, P
	087101	22 Fr	26 inch	9 Fr/6 Fr	A, G, F, P
Wilson-Cook	PEGJ-12-24	24 Fr	25 inch	12 Fr/8 Fr	A, G, F, P

[a] Can be cut to desired length.
[b] Y connector to PEG is available to allow gastric aspiration.
O, Single lumen (no gastric aspiration); A, gastric aspirating port; T, weighted tip; S, suture string on tip; Gr, grip tip; G, guidewire placement; F, flow-through tip; W, wire stylet; P, plug keeps air in stomach during placment.

beyond. Once within the gastric lumen, the silk suture is grasped with a polypectomy snare or an "alligator" grasping forceps that has been passed through the endoscope. The aim of this approach is to guide the tube through the pylorus and into the small intestine.

Many different guiding techniques have been utilized, and they range from blindly pushing the grasping instrument with the attached tube through the pylorus into the duodenal bulb, to visually guided passage of the jejunal tube along with the endoscope through the pylorus and into the jejunum. We prefer the latter. Once the instrument is past the pylorus, Gottfried and Plumser (8) describe a technique of releasing the suture from the grasp of the alligator forceps, regrasping the jejunal tube at the level of the pylorus, and repetitively advancing the jejunal tube through the pylorus. Problems associated with this method include possible difficulty releasing the suture, which may be caught in the teeth of the forceps; difficulty regrasping the jejunal tube; the propensity for the jejunal tube to kink upon itself, remain in, and, on occasion, to knot in the duodenum; and tube displacement back into the stomach. In addition, when feedings are initiated in the duodenum, the pylorus does not prevent reflux back into the stomach, thus allowing GE reflux and aspiration. The techniques that have been developed to overcome this problem involve placement of the jejunal tube more distally. This is accomplished by passage of the tube and forceps along with the endoscope through the pylorus and into the distal duodenum. Once there, the grasping tool is advanced further into the duodenal lumen, and then the feeding tube is disengaged from the grasping device. Subsequently, the endoscope is removed, leaving the jejunal feeding tube in place. However, frequently there is "sticking" of the PEJ tube to the endoscope resulting from friction between the two, which results in the PEJ "following" the scope back into the stomach upon withdrawal of the endoscope. This problem can be minimized by using a wire stylet within the jejunal tube, thus theoretically keeping the jejunal tube more rigid and as straight as possible during withdrawal of the endoscope; doing so decreases the amount of contact between the two, which is what predisposes the tube to sticking.

Placement of the PEJ tube into the small intestine can also be accomplished by an over the wire "push" method, utilizing a modified Seldinger technique as first described by Lewis et al. (9). They passed a bronchoscope via the gastrostomy site, through the pylorus and into the duodenum. Then a 0.35-mm guidewire was passed through its biopsy channel and advanced into the small bowel past the ligament of Treitz under endoscopic and fluoroscopic guidance. The bronchoscope was withdrawn, and placement of the wire was confirmed radiologically. A jejunal feeding tube was then passed over the wire under fluoroscopic guidance. A pediatric gastroscope can be placed through a surgical gastrostomy; however, endoscopic gastrostomies needed to be dilated with Savary dilators to allow passage of the endoscope. The commercial evolution of this technique involves peroral passage of the endoscope, through which a forceps is passed to grasp a guidewire that is inserted through a PEG (10,11). Alternatively, the endoscopic forceps can be passed outward through the PEG to grasp the guidewire outside the body and then pull it back into the gastric lumen. In both techniques the wire is then guided into the small bowel, and the jejunal tube is passed over it after removal of the endoscope.

MacFadyen et al. (12) have recently described favorable results with a third technique. A biopsy forceps was introduced through a PEG, snared endoscopically and pulled out the patient's mouth. The endoscope was reinserted alongside the forceps and advanced into the fourth portion of the duodenum or jejunum. A 0.035-inch guidewire was then passed through the endoscope into the small bowel, and an 8-French nasobiliary tube (NBT) was passed over the wire. These were left in place and the endoscope withdrawn. The proximal end of the NBT was then grasped extraorally by the biopsy forceps. The biopsy forceps and NBT were pulled back into the stomach and out the PEG. The externalized NBT was then fastened to the PEG, leaving the distal portion in the small bowel.

A fourth technique described more recently utilized a hybrid of the second and third techniques (13). A steerable biliary glidewire, which had been introduced via a PEG, was grasped and guided into the duodenum. A 40-cm biliary catheter with a stiffening cannula was passed over the glidewire, which was then released. The catheter's rigidity permitted blind passage of the slippery, torqueable glidewire for an additional 10 to 15 cm. After removal of the biliary catheter, a 12-French J-tube was passed over the glidewire, into the jejunum.

Patients who have undergone partial or total gastrectomy can undergo PEJ placement directly into the efferent limb utilizing a variant of standard PEG technique (14). Initially, the efferent limb is identified endoscopically by the relative absence of bile. The endoscope is passed into this limb, and an area is located on the abdominal wall where the light is intensely and discretely visible, and where, as in PEG placement, there is excellent one-to-one correlation between fingertip pressure exerted on the abdominal wall and indentation observed intraluminally. The PEJ tube is then inserted in a manner similar to PEG placement (15). PEJ tube placement using this technique was successful in 9 of 11 of Shike et al.'s (16) patients (82%), with the two failures secondary to the inability to obtain good one-to-one visualization, indicating that no portion of the jejunum was sufficiently close to the abdominal wall. This technique has also been utilized for direct catheter placement into the jejunum in patients with intact stomachs (16). This technique requires peroral passage of an enteroscope distal to the ligament of Treitz, at which point a site with good transluminal light concentration is located on the abdominal wall, and a standard PEG technique is used. This procedure was successful in five of six patients, with the one failure again attributed to lack of one-to-one visualization. A swift stab is required to introduce the sheathed stylet into the bowel lumen. This quick action is to prevent movement and laceration of the targeted jejunum or of an adjacent loop, or insertion of the catheter into the abdominal cavity. The procedure is technically more difficult and further clinical experience is warranted before widespread use of the technique can be endorsed.

Once the site of a PEJ placed directly into the jejunum has matured, it may be converted into a skin-level jejunostomy or "button" (17). The technique involves endoscopic snaring and removal of the jejunal tube, leaving a jejunocutaneous fistula. The endoscope is then reintroduced to observe the skin-level button as it traverses into the jejunal lumen (18). The button, which is similar to those utilized as replacement devices in patients with PEGs, is especially cosmetically appealing for the ambulatory patient.

COMPLICATIONS

Most complications are not unique to PEJ placement and are related to placement of the PEG portion of this two-stage procedure. However, there appears to be a higher incidence of tube dysfunction with a PEJ than with a PEG (19). Complications that are associated with the PEG portion occur in up to 35% of patients (20), and are listed in Table 2.

Aspiration still remains a common and serious complication in patients with a PEJ (3,8,9,19–24). It occurs in 11% to 100% of PEJ patients and has a mortality rate ranging from 2.8% to 50% (20–22). While prevention of aspiration was the initial goal of PEJ, it seems that it has not been entirely achieved. However, its incidence may be overestimated because it is defined broadly as either a pre- or postmortem demonstration of feeding solution in the bronchial tree or the presence of an unexplained infiltrate on chest x-ray associated with leukocytosis and fever (20,21). This definition fails to discriminate between two etiologies of aspiration—one is aspiration of refluxed gastric secretions and feeding solution, which might be preventable, and the other is aspiration of oropharyngeal secretions (22), which is not prevented by the placement of a PEJ. In addition, PEJs tend to be placed in patients who are thought to be at greatest risk for aspiration (19,20), including debilitated patients with a depressed mental status (8) or those who have had a prior episode of aspiration prior to PEJ placement (20,21,25).

TABLE 2. *PEG complications*

Wound infection and cellulitis, early or late
Abdominal wall abscess
Intraperitoneal leakage of gastric contents/peritonitis
Erosion/migration of the internal crossbar through the gastric wall
Gastric ulceration beneath the internal crossbar, resulting in bleeding
Bleeding at the site of insertion
PEG occlusion, breakage, removal
Leakage around PEG site

Other factors that may predispose to aspiration include (a) underlying diseases such as diabetes mellitus with gastroparesis, which may have prompted the placement of the PEJ (19); (b) PEJ malpositioning or its migration into the stomach, which may occur in up to 50% of cases (21); and (c) placement of the PEJ in the duodenum (24). DiSario et al. (20) have reported a 60% rate of aspiration with duodenal placement, which fails to prevent aspiration because (a) the pylorus will not prevent backwash into the stomach of intraduodenal feedings; (b) the proximal feeding holes of a jejunostomy tube may lie within the stomach; and (c) tubes placed in the duodenum may not only fail to progress distally into the jejunum, but they may also regress or be displaced proximally into the stomach (9,24). Fortunately, if they do not regress into the stomach, they tend to migrate distally. Gottfried found that 81% of tubes placed only into the second portion of the duodenum migrated distal to the ligament of Treitz within 24 hours (8). It is noteworthy that the position of the PEJ was not ascertained after the occurrence of aspiration in any of these studies.

Initial testing of a method to secure the jejunal tube to the mucosa of the small bowel using an endoscopic clip fixing device (26) offers the potential to clarify this issue further. However, this method does not offer a permanent solution to the problem of migration of the PEJ, since mucosal clips are sloughed within a matter of weeks. Reflux and aspiration of gastric secretions, which range from 400 to 1660 ml per day, may occur despite PEJ placement, especially in patients with poor gastric emptying due either to mechanical obstruction or gastroparesis (6). Furthermore, this problem may be exacerbated by placement of a PEG, which has been shown to decrease gastric emptying (27).

Studies to specifically evaluate the effect of PEJ placement on gastroesophageal reflux will require esophageal pH monitoring before and after placement. Nonetheless, the data suggest that continuous suction applied to a gastric port may be especially beneficial in the patient with a PEJ who has poor gastric emptying. Routine use of this feature has the potential to reduce the risk of aspiration of feeding solutions, whether they enter the stomach indirectly by refluxing from the duodenum or directly by tube migration into the stomach. The latter would become evident by the large volume of feeding solution recovered via the port. The ability to suction gastric secretions through the gastric port of many commercially available PEJs is an advantage not shared by surgical feeding jejunostomies, which may also be complicated by aspiration (25).

Malposition of the jejunal tube can occur in 35% to 39% of patients either because its initial placement was not correct or because of later migration (20,21). PEJ malposition into the duodenum, stomach, and esophagus can be detected radiographically; however, this is not usually a routine procedure (20,21). Dislodgment of the PEJ from the PEG portion, sometimes with total extrusion of the PEJ, ranges from 8.3% to 59% of cases (8,20,21,23). Use of adhesive glue between the PEG and PEJ has been utilized without success (23). It is hoped this problem will be eliminated with future PEJ designs.

Tube clogging is the most common problem seen with feeding via PEJ as well as via PEG. It occurs in up to 45% of PEJs (8,9,19–21,23). This is more frequent than with PEGs, which are easier to flush and can accommodate larger particles, as they have larger lumens. Clogging is precipitated by attempts to pass crushed tablets and other insoluble medications through the PEJ, as well as by inspissation of the feeding solution. This tendency to clog is aggravated by inadequate postfeeding irrigation. Saline or water flushing every 4 to 6 hours is recommended even with continuous drip feedings and helps maintain patency (8,9).

Gastrointestinal bleeding is seen after the insertion of a percutaneous endoscopic jejunostomy in 15% to 30% of cases (20,23). It is difficult to attribute the bleeding directly to the PEJ device, as other etiologies, including reflux esophagitis and gastric ulceration, especially at the PEG site, may occur in these patients (20). However, these etiologies may be increased by the placement of a PEJ. Further hindering our understanding of this complication is that bleeding is often not evaluated endoscopically in these patients, especially when its magnitude does not warrant transfusion (23). Bleeding, as expected, is more likely in patients with a history of acid-peptic disease. Kaplan et al. (23) found a positive peptic ulcer disease history in all 7 of his 23 patients who bled, compared to only one patient of the remaining 16 (p <.0001). Linscheer and Murthy (28) have demonstrated an increase in gastric pH during feeding by PEG, but not PEJ. This is presumably due to the direct buffering of gastric acid by the PEG feeding, as well as to the acid secretory response to protein infusion into the proximal small bowel. They also found that gastric pH was maintained above 3.5 in 89% of patients receiving a continuous enteral infusion of cimetidine along with tube feedings via a PEG and in 69% receiving it via a PEJ. The different response between the PEG and PEJ groups was not explained. Mean serum cimetidine and gastrin levels were not significantly different in the two groups. The use of H2-blockers for bleeding prophylaxis is attractive in PEJ patients, as up to 30% of these patients manifest gastrointestinal bleeding (23). Since the avoidance of intravenous devices is a frequent goal in patients requiring long-term enteral feeding, the continuous enteral route offers an appealing alternative. Whether continuous enteral infusion would be of bene-

fit for stress ulcer prophylaxis in seriously ill patients is unknown (29).

Miscellaneous causes of PEJ malfunction may result from material breakdown or poor placement technique (8,19–21,23). Kinking of the PEJ within the small bowel or knot formation at its midpoint may occur in up to 10% of patients (8,23). Material breakdown usually results from poor maintenance technique and/or prolonged placement. Leakage occurs at the PEG–PEJ junction in 11% to 30%, cracking of the feeding port in 10%, tube rupture due to vigorous irrigation in 5%, and fracture of the mercury tip in 5% (19,20).

Overall, the mean functional life of a PEJ is 2 months (19,30,31), while PEGs frequently last for 6 months or longer. A portion of this brief functional life is attributable to high early and cumulative mortality rates (31). Whether routine replacement of jejunostomy tubes should be performed is unclear; however, tube replacement after 3 months is recommended by Sandoz (personal communication).

The 30-day mortality after PEJ placement ranges from 0% to 25% (20,31), depending upon the study population and the initial indication for the procedure. These devices are often instrumental in facilitating patient discharge to home or to a nursing facility. These facts underscore the need to evaluate candidates for the placement of a PEJ carefully, as the benefits are limited in patients with projected early mortality or who are unlikely to be discharged from the hospital (31).

Treatment of the numerous complications of a PEJ consume significant resources. This has been cited as a serious limitation to the utility of a PEJ (20). There is no question that a PEJ is more difficult to place and replace, and it requires more care than a PEG. However, it should not be utilized in the routine patient who requires an enteral feeding device. We do not feel, therefore, that this is a drawback to its use.

CONCLUSIONS

PEJ placement can be optimized by its careful positioning beyond the ligament of Treitz (24), which optimally should be confirmed by routine postprocedure radiographs (21).

As with PEGs, jejunal tube life can be extended and its complications possibly reduced with education of nurses and health care personnel in tube care, especially conscientious lavage (21).

Intensive anti-reflux measures may be indicated in those patients with a history of GE reflux or who have underlying disorders of gastric emptying that predispose to the occurrence of GE reflux. Aspiration may also be decreased in patients with poor gastric emptying by the use of a jejunostomy tube with a gastric suction port. This allows for drainage of gastric secretions (24). Interestingly, the initially described method of PEJ placement included such a decompression gastrostomy (4). These modifications should allow more widespread use of PEJ. Despite a stated goal of PEJ placement being the prevention of aspiration, this remains an ongoing problem, which is not entirely prevented by any currently used form of gastrostomy or jejunostomy.

SUMMARY

Percutaneous endoscopic jejunostomy has been developed to minimize the problems associated with PEGs, including aspiration and failure of the feeding solution to advance beyond the stomach. These goals have been partly achieved, but problems that are unique to the PEJ itself have been recognized. Familiarity with proper placement technique and care of a PEJ and awareness of the potential complications should allow safer and more widespread use.

REFERENCES

1. Ciocon JO, Silverstone FA, Graver M, et al. Tube feeding in elderly patients. Indications, benefits, and complications. *Arch Intern Med* 1988;148:429–433.
2. Cogen R, Weinryb J. Aspiration pneumonia in nursing home patients fed via gastrostomy tubes. *Am J Gastroenterol* 1989; 84:1509–1512.
3. Hassett JM, Sunby C, Flint LM. No elimination of aspiration pneumonia in neurologically disabled patients with feeding gastrostomy. *Surg Gynecol Obstet* 1988;167:383–389.
4. Burtch GD, Shatney CH. Feeding gastrostomy. Assistant or assassin? *Am Surg* 1985;51:204–207.
5. Ponsky JL, Aszodi A. Percutaneous endoscopic jejunostomy. *Am J Gastroenterol* 1984;79:113–116.
6. Shike M, Wallach C, Bloch A, et al. Combined gastric drainage and jejunal feeding through a percutaneous endoscopic stoma. *Gastrointest Endosc* 1990;36:290–292.
7. Weaver DW, Wiencek RG, Bouwman DL, et al. Gastrojejunostomy: is it helpful for patients with pancreatic cancer? *Surgery* 1987;102:608–613.
8. Gottfried EB, Plumser AB. Endoscopic gastrojejunostomy: a technique to establish small bowel feeding without laparotomy. *Gastrointest Endosc* 1984;30:355–357.
9. Lewis BS, Mauer K, Bush A. The rapid placement of jejunal feeding tubes: the Seldinger technique applied to the gut. *Gastrointest Endosc* 1990;36:139–141.
10. De Legge MH, Duckworth PF, Craig RM, et al. Percutaneous
11. Duckworth PF, Kirby DF, McHenry L. Percutaneous endoscopic gastrojejunostomy made easy: a simplified endoscopic technique. *Gastrointest Endosc* 1991;37:241.
12. MacFadyen BV, Catalano MF, Raijman I, Ghobrial R. Percutaneous endoscopic gastrostomy with jejunal extension: a new technique. *Am J Gastroenterol* 1992;87:725–728.
13. Parasher VK, Abramowicz CJ, Bell C, Wright A, Delledonne AM. Successful placement of percutaneous gastrojejunostomy PEG/J using steerable glidewire—a modified controlled "push" technique. *Gastrointest Endosc* 1993;39:255.
14. Shike M, Schroy P, Ritchie MA, et al. Percutaneous endoscopic jejunostomy in cancer patients with previous gastric resection. *Gastrointest Endosc* 1987;33:372–374.
15. Ponsky JL, Gauderer MWL. Percutaneous endoscopic gastrostomy: a nonoperative technique for feeding gastrostomy. *Gastrointest Endosc* 1981;27:9–11.
16. Shike M, Wallach C, Likier H. Direct percutaneous endoscopic jejunostomies. *Gastrointest Endosc* 1991;37:62–65.
17. Shike M, Wallach C, Gerdes H, et al. Skin-level gastrostomies and jejunostomies for long-term enteral feeding. *J Parenter Enteral Nutr* 1989;13:648–650.
18. Gauderer MWL, Picha GJ, Izont RJ Jr. The gastrostomy "Button"—a simple, skin-level, nonrefluxing device for long-term enteral feedings. *J Pediatr Surg* 1984;19:803–805.
19. Wolfsen HC, Kozarek RA, Ball TJ, et al. Tube dysfunction following percutaneous endoscopic gastrostomy and jejunostomy. *Gastrointest Endosc* 1990;36:261–263.
20. DiSario JA, Foutch PG, Sanowski RA. Poor results with percutaneous endoscopic jejunostomy. *Gastrointest Endosc* 1990;36:257–260.
21. Henderson JM, Gilinsky NH, Strodel WE. Percutaneous endoscopic jejunostomy: indications and complications in 36 patients. *Gastrointest Endosc* 1991;37:241.
22. Kadakia SC, Sullivan HO, Starnes E. Percutaneous endoscopic gastrostomy and the incidence of aspiration in 79 patients. *Am J Surg* 1992;164:114–118.
23. Kaplan DS, Murthy UK, Linscheer WG. Percutaneous endoscopic jejunostomy: long-term follow-up of 23 patients. *Gastrointest Endosc* 1989;35:403–406.
24. Lewis BS. Perform PEJ, not PED. *Gastrointest Endosc* 1990;36:311–313.
25. Cogen R, Weinryb J, Pomerantz C, Fenstemacher P. Complications of jejunostomy tube feeding in nursing facility patients. *Am J Gastroenterol* 1991;86:1610–1613.
26. Ginsberg GG, Fleischer DE, Lipman TO. Endoscopic clip-assisted placement of jejunal feeding tubes. *Gastrointest Endosc* 1993;39:251.
27. Kutcher WW, Cohen LB, Leonhardt C, Ehrlich LE. Impaired gastric emptying following percutaneous endoscopic gastrostomy (PEG). *Gastroenterology* 1989;96:A686.
28. Linscheer WG, Murthy UK. Continuous monitoring of gastric pH for evaluation of the effectiveness of cimetidine when infused simultaneously with gastric or jejunal tube feeding. *Gastrointest Endosc* 1988;34:212.
29. Wolfe MM. H$_2$ antagonists by continuous infusion: IV or IG? [Comment on ref. 12]. *Gastroenterology* 1991;101:1448–1449.
30. Murthy UK, Kaplan D, Linscheer WG. Dysutility of endoscopic feeding tubes [letter]. *Gastrointest Endosc* 1991;37:208.
31. Wolfsen HC, Kozarek RA, Ball TJ, et al. Long-term survival in patients undergoing percutaneous endoscopic gastrostomy and jejunostomy. *Am J Gastroenterol* 1990;85:1120–1122.

Advanced Therapeutic Endoscopy, 2nd Ed.,
edited by J. S. Barkin and C. A. O'Phelan.
Raven Press, Ltd., New York © 1994.

CHAPTER 20A

Enteroscopy

Push-Type Enteroscopy

David Bernstein and Jamie S. Barkin

Push enteroscopy is a technique in which the endoscope is passed under direct vision into the small bowel in a manner similar to that used in upper endoscopy. It was initially performed with a colonoscope (either adult or pediatric) and was limited to visualizing the small intestinal mucosa up to 60 cm beyond the ligament of Treitz. This technique has increased in popularity with the development of longer, more flexible enteroscopes that can reach much farther beyond the ligament of Treitz than conventional colonoscopes.

The standard adult and pediatric colonoscopes are easily accessible to most endoscopists. Their peroral use has been shown to be safe and effective in evaluating the mucosa 50 to 60 cm beyond the ligament of Treitz (1,2). The procedure can be performed easily in 1 hour or less by an endoscopist and allows both diagnostic and therapeutic access to the small bowel by the biopsy channel of the colonoscope. Several investigators have used a colonoscope or pediatric colonoscope to perform push enteroscopy. Parker and Agayoff (3) evaluated the proximal jejunum with an Olympus CF-LB2 colonoscope in 13 patients referred for small bowel biopsy. Celiac sprue was diagnosed in three, eosinophilic gastritis in one, jejunal neurofibroma in one, radiation enteritis in one, malabsorption secondary to Imuran in one, and nonspecific enteritis in one. Five patients had normal small bowel biopsies. Messer et al. (4) used a peroral colonoscope passed to at least 45 cm beyond the pylorus to evaluate 52

consecutive patients with gastrointestinal bleeding of obscure origin. Upper gastrointestinal and small bowel series, barium enema, upper endoscopy, colonoscopy, and Meckel's scan had failed to reveal a bleeding source, and they identified potential bleeding sites in 38% (20 patients). Hashimi et al. (5) found an ulcerated jejunal leiomyoma 15 cm beyond the ligament of Treitz using a peroral Olympus PCF pediatric colonoscope in a patient with unexplained gastrointestinal bleeding. Foutch et al. (6) evaluated 39 patients with gastrointestinal bleeding of obscure origin with either a CF10L or CV10L Olympus colonoscope passed 35 to 60 cm beyond the ligament of Treitz and identified a bleeding source in 38% of the patients.

New enteroscopes are being developed to allow greater visualization of the small bowel. Several important factors, including length of small bowel traversed beyond the ligament of Treitz, adequacy of tip deflection at maximum insertion of the enteroscope, adequacy of visualization of small bowel mucosa, and patient tolerance of the procedure must be considered when evaluating new enteroscopes.

We have shown that proximal jejunal enteroscopy with biopsy utilizing an SIF 10 (Olympus Corp., New Hyde Park, NY), 165 cm, fully deflectional enteroscope was a safe and effective means of visualizing the proximal jejunum and obtaining biopsies in an outpatient setting (7). One problem seen in the early use of longer enteroscopes was looping in the stomach, causing patient discomfort, and limiting the distal, effective length of the enteroscope. This insertion problem resulted from the duodenum being embedded in the retroperitoneum, thereby making transmission of a forward, propelling force difficult, causing loop formation in the stomach. Shimizu et al. (8) designed a

D. Bernstein: Division of Gastroenterology, University of Miami School of Medicine Jackson Memorial Hospital, Miami, Florida 33136.

J. S. Barkin: Division of Gastroenterology, Mount Sinai Medical Center, Miami Beach, Florida 33140.

technique in which a stiffening tube is placed beyond the duodenojejunal junction, allowing forward transmission of the enteroscope with minimal patient discomfort. They used an SIF-10L enteroscope (Olympus Corp.) with a working length of 2,175 cm and full deflection capabilities. The examination required two technicians, one to control the scope angles and one to push and pull the scope. The patient was initially placed in the left lateral decubitus position and given conscious sedation with an opioid derivative and an antispasmodic. The stiffening tube was lubricated and backloaded onto the proximal end of the enteroscope, which was passed to the duodenojejunal junction and maximally flexed to allow fixation. The enteroscope was then straightened under fluoroscopic guidance and the stiffening tube passed into the descending duodenum. It was then passed to its maximum length in the jejunum and maximally flexed to again allow fixation and straightening under fluoroscopy. The stiffening tube was advanced beyond the duodenojejunal junction to prevent loop formation in the horizontal portion of the duodenum. The enteroscope was again passed to its maximal working length. This allowed visualization of the mucosa 60 to 126 cm beyond the ligament of Treitz without any adverse effects. This technique has become accepted practice in push enteroscopy using the newer generation of longer enteroscopes.

We examined 37 patients with the SIF-10L enteroscope, equipped with a stiffening tube, for (a) evaluation of obscure gastrointestinal bleeding—28 patients, (b) evaluation after abnormal small bowel follow through—8 patients, and (c) access for endoscopic cholangiography in 1 patient with a Roux-en-Y biliary diversion (9,10). Intubation beyond the ligament of Treitz averaged 94 cm, with a range of 20 to 150 cm. A bleeding source was identified in 21 of the 28 patients (75%). In 5 of the 8 patients (63%) with abnormal small bowel follow through, barium examinations revealed pathological findings distal to the ligament of Treitz on enteroscopy.

Zuccaro et al. (11) evaluated 54 patients with gastrointestinal bleeding of obscure origin using a SIF-10.5 (Olympus Corp.) enteroscope with a working length of 2,175 cm and full tip deflection, fitted with a stiffening tube. The range of visualization beyond the ligament of Treitz was 40 to 90 cm; bleeding sites were identified in 15 patients (28%). We evaluated the SIF-10.5L enteroscope with a stiffening tube in 13 patients with gastrointestinal bleeding of obscure origin and in 4 patients with abnormal small bowel contrast examinations (12). The range of insertion of the enteroscope beyond the ligament of Treitz was 45 to 150 cm, with an average of 100 cm. This study did not distinguish the pathological diagnosis found in each group of patients studied, but did find small bowel pathology in 10 of 17 patients (59%).

We evaluated the SIF-3000 enteroscope (Olympus Corp.) fitted with a stiffening tube with a working length of 2,675 cm and full tip deflection in 42 patients with gastrointestinal bleeding of obscure origin (13). The length of scope insertion beyond the ligament of Treitz ranged from 50 to 160 cm, with a mean of 113 cm. Bleeding sites were identified in 67% of the patients; 12 (29%) were identified distal to the ligament of Treitz and 16 (38%) were identified proximal to the ligament of Treitz.

All of the enteroscopes described above are fiberoptic enteroscopes converted to video with an adapter. Recently, newer true videoenteroscopes are being evaluated. Dykman and Killian (14) evaluated a VSB-P2900 enteroscope (Pentax Precision Instrument Corp., Orangeburg, NY) with a working length of 2,500 cm., tip deflection of 120° in all four directions, and a working channel of 2.8 mm in a patient with obscure gastrointestinal bleeding. An arteriovenous malformation (AVM) in the midjejunum was identified and treated with electrocautery.

INTRAOPERATIVE ENTEROSCOPY

Intraoperative enteroscopy with a push enteroscope is considered to be the most effective method of evaluating the entire small bowel (15). This technique has been performed with a colonoscope, pediatric colonoscope, and enteroscope. During this procedure, the endoscopist passes the instrument beyond the ligament of Treitz and the surgeon telescopes the small bowel in an accordion fashion to permit visualization. The overhead lights are dimmed as the bowel is examined. Advancement of the enteroscope is always performed under direct vision because artifacts mimicking lesions may occur with scope trauma. Lesions that are detected are marked by the surgeon with a suture. The distal ileum is usually clamped during the procedure to prevent colonic distention secondary to air insufflation (16). The major indication for this procedure is gastrointestinal bleeding of obscure origin (16,17). Bowden et al. (18) report a yield of 75% in eight patients evaluated for obscure bleeding. Lewis et al. (19) compared intraoperative enteroscopy with sonde-type enteroscopy and found no difference in the diagnostic yield, with each procedure having a 77% diagnostic yield. Intraoperative enteroscopy has been used to treat patients with Peutz-Jeghers disease (20) by performing endoscopic polypectomy on small polyps within the small bowel. This technique has also been used to guide a surgeon through dense small bowel adhesions (16).

Disadvantages of intraoperative enteroscopy include the necessity for laparotomy, prolonged postoperative ileus secondary to excessive small bowel trauma (21), and the inability to interpret mucosal abnormalities secondary to scope trauma, upon withdrawal.

Indications

Enteroscopy is indicated in the following clinical settings: (a) gastrointestinal bleeding of obscure origin (3,4,10,11), (b) malabsorption (3,22), (c) confirmation and diagnosis of radiographic abnormalities (5), (d) combined enteroscopic and enteroclysis examination of the small bowel (23), (e) polypectomy (24), and, (f) access to the common bile duct in a patient with a Roux-en-Y gastrojejunostomy (10). In addition, magnifying enterocolonoscopes have been used to evaluate subtle morphological changes in the villi in inflammatory and malabsorptive disorders of the small bowel (25).

GASTROINTESTINAL BLEEDING

Enteroscopy is indicated for evaluating gastrointestinal bleeding of obscure origin when routine workup, including standard endoscopy and colonoscopy, does not reveal the bleeding source. Push-enteroscopy routinely visualizes the proximal jejunum and newer enteroscopes allow for visualization of the midjejunum. In addition to diagnostic capabilities by using biopsy forceps, push enteroscopes have the capacity to permit endoscopic treatment of bleeding lesions by applying heater probe or Bicap. Several studies have found AVMs to be the most common lesion causing bleeding of obscure origin. Foutch et al. (6) identified AVMs in 12 of 16 patients in whom enteroscopy determined a bleeding site. Eleven of the 12 (92%) were successfully treated with bipolar cautery and the twelfth patient was sent for surgical resection, with more than 30 AVMs identified in the jejunum. Zuccaro et al. (11) identified AVMs in 11 of 15 patients in whom a bleeding source was identified, all of whom were successfully treated with bipolar coagulation. We identified AVMs in 13 of 23 patients evaluated for gastrointestinal bleeding (10). Seven had AVMs distal to the ligament of Treitz and six had AVMs proximal to the ligament of Treitz. They were all treated with bipolar cautery. Lewis and Waye (26) evaluated 60 patients with gastrointestinal bleeding of obscure origin and identified a bleeding source in 20. Sixteen of the 20 (80%) were found to have AMVs as the source of bleeding.

Mass lesions such as jejunal neurofibroma (3,11), jejunal leiomyoma (1,4,5), jejunal carcinoma (4,11), lipoma (4), angiosarcoma (11), lymphangioma (4), hemangioma (10), metastatic lung carcinoma (1), and metastatic melanoma (4) have been identified on enteroscopy as causes of gastrointestinal bleeding. Non-mass lesions including radiation enteritis (3), aorto-en-teric fistula (6), and ulcer disease (6,10) have been found to be the source of gastrointestinal bleeding on enteroscopy.

Push enteroscopy is indicated in the workup of obscure gastrointestinal bleeding in the presence of a normal or equivocal results of small bowel barium study or angiogram. Arteriovenous malformations will not be seen on contrast examination as well as angiography. Zuccaro et al. (11) identified three mass lesions during push enteroscopy that were not seen on small bowel contrast or on mesenteric arteriography during push enteroscopy. Foutch et al. (1) diagnosed an ulcerated jejunal leiomyoma on enteroscopy performed secondary to gastrointestinal bleeding of obscure origin in a patient who had an equivocal selective mesenteric artery angiogram.

It is important to note that not all obscure gastrointestinal bleeding originates in the small intestine. In a retrospective study, Koren and Foroozan (27) evaluated 131 patients with obscure gastrointestinal bleeding and identified colonic angiodysplasia in 52 (40%) patients. This was the most common abnormality. We evaluated gastrointestinal bleeding of obscure origin with a push enteroscope (10) and found that 57% of the bleeding sources identified were within the reach of a standard endoscope. Another study using push enteroscopy before sonde-type enteroscopy, found bleeding sites within reach of a standard endoscope in 37% of patients (2).

MALABSORPTION

Small bowel biopsy is essential for the diagnosis of causes of malabsorption. The biopsy specimens obtained by push enteroscopy have been shown to be adequate in 76% to 100% of cases (2,28,29). We recommend that only one specimen be obtained with each passage of the biopsy forceps to minimize crush artifact and multiple areas be biopsied. Parker and Agayoff (3) used push enteroscopy to evaluate six patients with malabsorption. They made a diagnosis in four of the six patients (67%); three had celiac sprue, and the other had malabsorption secondary to Imuran.

ABNORMAL SMALL BOWEL RADIOGRAPHY CONFIRMATION

Small bowel lesions beyond the ligament of Treitz have traditionally been treated either empirically or through surgery because of the inability to evaluate these lesions by endoscopy. Small bowel enteroscopy has enabled visualization and biopsy of lesions as far as 160 cm distal to the ligament of Treitz (10). Therefore, an abnormality found on small bowel radiography, thought to be within reach of an enteroscope, should be evaluated by means of a push enteroscope. Hashimi et al. (5) report a bleeding lesion identified in the proximal jejunum by selective superior mesenteric angiography that enteroscopy revealed as an ulcerated leiomyoma.

COMBINED ENTEROSCOPY AND ENTEROCLYSIS

Enteroclysis or small bowel enema is a radiographic contrast study of the small bowel that necessitates intubation of the duodenum or jejunum before instillation of barium. It may be a useful technique in patients evaluated for gastrointestinal bleeding of obscure origin and in whom results of push enteroscopy are negative (23). Enteroclysis is uncomfortable as it requires the blind passage of a tube into the duodenum. Barkin et al. have described a combined method of enteroscopy followed by enteroclysis in patients evaluated for bleeding. Enteroscopy is initially performed and if the results are negative, enteroclysis is performed afterward. Enteroclysis is facilitated by the passage of a guidewire through the enteroscope into the distal duodenum or proximal jejunum. The enteroscope is then removed over the guidewire leaving the guidewire in the small bowel. An enteroclysis catheter is then passed over the guidewire into the small bowel with minimal discomfort to the patient (23,30).

ROUX-EN-Y GASTROJEJUNOSTOMY

We used a push enteroscope to obtain access to the common bile duct for a cholangiogram in a patient with a Roux-en-Y gastrojejunostomy. The cholangiogram revealed that the patient had rejected his liver transplant (10).

Complications

The same risks that are associated with standard upper endoscopy are also associated with push enteroscopy. These risks include medication reactions, bleeding, perforation, and aspiration. The morbidity from push enteroscopy appears to be low with few reported complications. Of 86 patients who we evaluated with push enteroscopy in two separate studies, three had complications (10,13). One patient developed a Mallory-Weiss tear after endoscopy, a second had an episode of pancreatitis thought to be secondary to trauma to the ampulla of Vater, and the third developed a pharyngoesophageal tear.

The incidence of complications in push enteroscopy is currently unknown. Further use of this technique is required to determine its safety profile.

CONCLUSION

The push enteroscopy technique is evolving at a rapid pace. Current technology enables approximately 50% of small bowel mucosa to be visualized. This enables endoscopic applications of therapeutic modalities to be applied to a greater amount of small bowel than ever before. However, push enteroscopy cannot be used to adequately visualize the entire small bowel. Newer, longer enteroscopes are continuing to be developed for evaluating the small bowel. It is hoped that with this advance in technology, the limitation of visualizing the small bowel mucosa will soon be overcome.

REFERENCES

1. Foutch PG, Sanowski MD, Kelly S. Enteroscopy: a method for detection of small bowel tumors. *Am J Gastroenterol* 1985;80: 887–890.
2. Lewis BS, Waye JD. Small bowel enteroscopy in 1988: pros and cons. *Am J Gastroenterol* 1988;83:799–802.
3. Parker HW, Agayoff JD. Enteroscopy and small bowel biopsy utilizing a peroral colonoscope. *Gastrointest Endosc* 1983;29: 139–140.
4. Messer J, Romeu J, Waye JD, et al. The value of jejunostomy in unexplained gastrointestinal bleeding. *Gastrointest Endosc* 1984;30:151(abst).
5. Hashimi MA, Sorokin JJ, Levine SM. Jejunal leiomyoma: an endoscopic diagnosis. *Gastrointest Endosc* 1985;31:81–83.
6. Foutch PG, Sawyer R, Sanowski RA. Push-enteroscopy for diagnosis of patients with gastrointestinal bleeding of obscure origin. *Gastrointest Endosc* 1990;36:337–341.
7. Barkin JS, Phillips RS, Goldberg RI. Proximal jejunal enteroscopy utilizing an SIF-10, 165 cm per oral endoscope; a routine outpatient procedure. *Gastrointest Endosc* 1988;34:202 (abst).
8. Shimizu S, Tada M, Kawai K. Development of a new insertion technique in push-type enteroscopy. *Am J Gastroenterol* 1987; 82:844–847.
9. Barkin JS, Reiner DK, Lewis BS, et al. Diagnostic and therapeutic jejunostomy with the SIF-10L enteroscope: long is really better. *Gastrointest Endosc* 1990;36:214(abst).
10. Barkin JS, Lewis BS, Reiner DK, et al. Diagnostic and therapeutic jejunostomy with the SIF-10L enteroscope: long is really better. *Gastrointest Endosc* 1992;38:55–58.
11. Zuccaro G, Barthel JS, Sivak MV. Use of a 165 cm push enteroscope in the evaluation of GI bleeding of unknown etiology. *Gastrointest Endosc* 1991;37:274(abst).
12. Barkin JS, Reiner DK. Diagnostic and therapeutic jejunoscopy with the SIF-10.5L, new enteroscope. *Am J Gastroenterol* 1992; 87:1311 (abst).
13. Barkin JS. Third generation push-type small bowel enteroscope utilizing an overtube. *Gastrointest Endosc* 1994;(in press).
14. Dykman DD, Killian SE. Initial experience with the Pentax VSB-P2900 enteroscope. *Am J Gastroenterol* 1993;88:570–573.
15. Waye, JD. Small bowel endoscopy. *Endoscopy* 1992;24:68–72.
16. Bowden TA. Endoscopy of the small intestine. *Surg Clin North Am* 1989;69:1237–1247.
17. Loffeld RJLF, Aalders GJ, Baeten CGMI. Recurrent gastrointestinal bleeding due to angiodysplasias in the small bowel. *Digestion* 1992;51:60–64.
18. Bowden TA, Hooks V, Mansberger A. Intraoperative gastrointestinal bleeding. *South Med J* 1979;72:1532–1534.
19. Lewis BS, Wenger JS, Waye JD. Small bowel enteroscopy and intraoperative enteroscopy for obscure gastrointestinal bleeding. *Am J Gastroenterol* 1991;86:171–174.
20. Barkin JS, Schonfeld W, Thomsen S, et al. Enteroscopy and small bowel biopsy—an improved technique for the diagnosis of small bowel disease. *Gastrointest Endosc* 1985;31:215–217.

21. Frank M, Brandt L, Boley S. Iatrogenic submucosal hemorrhage: a pitfall of intraoperative enteroscopy. *Am J Gastroenterol* 1981;75:209–210.
22. Mathus-Vliegan E, Tytgat G. Intraoperative enteroscopy: technique, indications and results. *Gastrointest Endosc* 1986;32:381–384.
23. Cohen ME, Barkin JS. Enteroscopy and enteroclysis; the combined procedure. *Am J Gastroenterol* 1989;84:1413–1415.
24. Gilbert DA, Buelow RG, Chung RSK, et al. Status evaluation: enteroscopy. *Gastrointest Endosc* 1991;37:673–677.
25. Tada M, Misaki F, Kawai K. Endoscopic observation of villi magnifying enterocolonoscopes. *Gastrointest Endosc* 1982;28:17–19.
26. Lewis BS, Waye JD. Chronic gastrointestinal bleeding of obscure origin: role of small bowel enteroscopy. *Gastroenterology* 1988;94:1117–1120.
27. Koren E, Foroozan P. Endoscopic biopsies of normal gastroduodenal mucosa. *Gastrointest Endosc* 1974;21:51–54.
28. Brocchi E, Corazza GR, Caletti G, et al. Endoscopic demonstration of loss of duodenal folds in the diagnosis of celiac disease. *N Engl J Med* 1988;319:741–744.
29. Scott BB, Jenkins D. Endoscopic small intestine biopsy. *Gastrointest Endosc* 1981;27:162–167.
30. McGovern R, Barkin JS. Enteroscopy and enteroclysis: an improved method for combined procedure. *Gastrointest Radiol* 1990;15:327–328.

Advanced Therapeutic Endoscopy, 2nd Ed.,
edited by J. S. Barkin and C. A. O'Phelan.
Raven Press, Ltd., New York © 1994.

CHAPTER **20B**

Enteroscopy

Sonde Enteroscopy

Blair S. Lewis

Sonde enteroscopy, also termed small bowel enteroscopy or long tube enteroscopy, can endoscopically examine the entire small intestine without the need for laparotomy. Sonde instruments rely on peristalsis to carry them into the small bowel. The endoscopic examination is performed during withdrawal.

Development of sonde enteroscopy has spanned nearly 13 years (1). Prototype sonde small intestinal fiberscope (SSIF) I thru IV had narrow fields of vision (60°) and a large diameter (11 mm). Initially, a metal hood was placed at the instrument tip and used to induce distal passage. Subsequent prototypes have utilized a balloon at the tip that is inflated upon placement in the small bowel. Early enteroscopes were fitted with magnifying lenses to evaluate villi shape and have been used in the diagnosis of tuberculosis and malabsorption states (2). Attempts to introduce tip deflection capability in the fifth prototype made the instrument too stiff for distal intubation (3,4). Oral passage, which was required with these thick instruments, was associated with patient salivation, gagging, and considerable discomfort (5). A thin, flexible, transnasal enteroscope was developed in 1986 with a tip diameter of 5 mm and a length of 2,560 mm (6). The instrument's forward angle of view was initially 90°, but was subsequently increased to 120°. This instrument, in contrast to a push enteroscope, had no biopsy or therapeutic capability and no tip deflection. An attempt to add biopsy capability to this instrument in the tenth prototype was successful, but targeting the biopsy remains a problem since there is no tip deflection (7). Present standard sonde enteroscopes, SIF-SW (small intestinal fiber-

scope—sonde, wide) do not have this biopsy channel, but remain transnasally passed with a fish-eye lens. Video technology has also been applied to sonde enteroscopy. Dabezies et al. (8) have reported on a video sonde enteroscope used in seven patients. The instrument's tip measures 11 mm, due to the presence of the video chip, necessitating oral passage. The instrument does not use a balloon and depth of intubation is limited.

The lack of tip deflection in the sonde enteroscopes leads to limitations in the endoscopic view. Visualization is rarely total even when total small bowel intubation is achieved. Abdominal palpation along with inflation and deflation of the tip balloon are the only way to control the intraluminal view. Lewis and Waye (9) estimated that approximately 50% to 70% of small bowel mucosa is observed during a standard examination. Intubation usually does not reach the ileocecal valve. The ileum is reached in 75% of examinations, with 10% reaching the ileocecal valve. Total intubation is not achieved in all cases secondary to adhesions, endoscope malfunction (such as balloon rupture), or presence of an obstructing lesion.

The original technique to position a sonde enteroscope within the jejunum was to pass the instrument transnasally, have the patient lie on the right side, and follow the patient with sequential fluoroscopy. A technique to rapidly place the small bowel enteroscope into the jejunum was developed to shorten the examination time (8). In this rapid technique, a push enteroscope, passed orally, grasps a suture affixed to the small bowel enteroscope's tip while both instruments lie within the stomach. The push instrument is advanced into the small bowel, pulling the sonde enteroscope along. Once within the jejunum the sonde instrument's

B. S. Lewis: Department of Gastroenterology, Mount Sinai School of Medicine, New York, New York 10028.

balloon is inflated, anchoring it in place as the push enteroscope is removed. The advantage of this technique is that it permits total to near-total small bowel intubation within 8 hours and thus allows the procedure to be performed on an ambulatory basis. The original technique averaged 24 hours. With the newer technique, procedure times range from 6 to 8 hours. Withdrawal times range from 45 to 60 minutes. With present standard transnasal sonde enteroscopes, the new technique of placement has become generally accepted. Still, some centers use orally passed enteroscopes that are either allowed to pass naturally through the pylorus or are passed over a previously positioned guidewire.

Sonde enteroscopy appears quite safe and no serious complications have been described. In their report of 60 patients undergoing enteroscopy, Lewis and Waye (9) reported two cases of epistaxis associated with use of the transnasal enteroscope. Lewis (10) has also recently reported enteroscopically induced trauma within the small bowel associated with "notching," which may mimic NSAID ulcers.

Presently, the major indication for sonde enteroscopy is the evaluation of the patient with obscure gastrointestinal bleeding. These are patients with either melena or occult blood loss often requiring transfusion whose site of blood loss is not diagnosed despite colonoscopy, upper endoscopy, and small bowel series. Initially, Lewis reported results of the technique in 60 patients with obscure gastrointestinal bleeding. In this report, a small bowel site of blood loss was detected in 33% (11). A more recent report by the same group detailed results in 504 patients (10). In patients with obscure GI bleeding, combined push and sonde enteroscopy documented findings in 42% of patients (12). Vascular ectasias constituted 80% of the findings and small bowel tumors accounted for 10%. Several of the tumors discovered occurred in patients after a false-negative enteroclysis (13). Similar experience has been reported by Barthel et al. (14) with a yield of 27.8% in 18 patients. Gostout et al. (15) reported a yield of 26% in 35 patients. An orally passed enteroscope was used along with a team approach to enhance patient care and shorten physician time. Van Gossum et al. (16) reported a yield of 29% in 17 patients. The sonde enteroscope has also been used to evaluate obscure bleeding in 15 patients receiving nonsteroidal anti-inflammatory drugs showing a high incidence of small bowel ulceration (17). Other indications for sonde enteroscopy have included abdominal pain, diarrhea, intestinal obstruction, determination of Crohn's disease extent, and evaluation of an abnormal x-ray of the small bowel. Lewis and Mauer (18), in a report on 32 patients, found little benefit from enteroscopy in nonbleeding indications.

Despite numerous advances in sonde enteroscopy, some physicians doubt its clinical usefulness (19). It has been stated that the development of sonde enteroscopy was unnecessary and most likely too expensive (20). It is clear, however, that the deeper one looks into the small bowel, the more one sees. Lewis (10) has compared the yields of push and sonde enteroscopy. In the report of 504 examinations using both techniques, push enteroscopy made diagnoses in 19% of patients with obscure bleeding. The addition of sonde enteroscopy yielded an additional 28%. Of 191 patients with small bowel angiodysplasia, 47% had lesions found within reach of a pediatric colonoscope, while 65% had lesions within the distal small bowel. Of 16 small bowel tumors, 69% were diagnosed at push enteroscopy while 31% were discovered with the sonde instrument.

Lewis et al. (21) compared sonde with intraoperative enteroscopy in 23 patients. Intraoperative and sonde enteroscopic findings of angiodysplasias matched exactly in number and location in 77% of cases. Preoperative sonde enteroscopy missed angiodysplasias in three patients, one in an area of traversed bowel and two in areas of the small bowel not reached by the sonde enteroscope. Intraoperative enteroscopy missed an angiodysplasia in one patient. This patient rebled acutely postoperatively and required repeat intraoperative enteroscopy.

UNUSUAL METHODS OF ENTEROSCOPY

There are other endoscopic techniques that have been used to evaluate the entire small intestine without surgery. The rope-way method of enteroscopy is the oldest method to totally intubate the small intestine (22,23). This technique involves having a patient swallow a guide string and allowing it to pass through the rectum. The string is then exchanged for a somewhat stiffer Teflon tube over which an endoscope is passed. A complete endoscopic examination can be obtained with this method. The instruments are fully therapeutic including cauterization and polypectomy. Unfortunately, the examination is painful due to tightening of the guide tube and often requires general anesthesia. Due to patient discomfort, length of time necessary for string passage, and development of better tolerated techniques, the rope-way method has largely been abandoned in the United States. Video rope-way enteroscopes have been developed with the same limitations of the nonvideo versions (24).

Endostomy involves creating enterocutaneous fistulae that can then allow a thin endoscope to intubate the small bowel (25). Frimberger et al. (25) reported this technique in one patient. The fistulae were created using standard Ponsky gastrostomy techniques in the jejunum and in the cecum. After the tracts matured in 8 to 10 days, thin (4 mm diameter) prototype endoscopes were inserted through the jejunostomy and cecostomy to evaluate the intestine. This technique must still be considered experimental.

REFERENCES

1. Tada M, Kawai K. Small bowel endoscopy. *Scand J Gastroenterol* 1984;19(suppl 102):39–52.
2. Tada M, Misaki F, Kawai K. Endoscopic observation of villi with magnifying enterocolonoscopes. *Gastrointest Endosc* 1982; 28:17–19.
3. Tada M, Akasaka Y, Misaki F, et al. Clinical evaluation of a sonde-type small intestinal fiberscope. *Endoscopy* 1977;9:33–38.
4. Tada M, Misaki F, Kawai K. Pediatric enteroscopy with a sonde-type small intestinal fiberscope (SSIF VI). *Gastrointest Endosc* 1983;29:44–47.
5. Lewis B, Waye J. A comparison of 2 sonde-type small bowel enteroscopes in 100 patients: the SSIF VII and the SSIF VI KAI. *Gastroenterology* 1988;94:A261.
6. Tada M, Shimizu S, Kawai K. A new transnasal sonde-type fiberscope (SSIF VII) as a pan-enteroscope. *Endoscopy* 1986; 18:121–124.
7. Tada M, Shimizu S, Kawai K. Small bowel endoscopy with a new transnasal sonde-type fiberscope (SSIF-Type 10). *Endoscopy* 1992;24:631(abst).
8. Dabezies M, Fisher R, Krevsky B. Video small bowel enteroscopy: early experience with a prototype instrument. *Gastrointest Endosc* 1991;37:60–62.
9. Lewis B, Waye J. Total small bowel enteroscopy. *Gastrointest Endosc* 1987;33:435–438.
10. Lewis B. Small bowel enteroscopy. *Lancet* 1991;337:1093–1094.
11. Lewis B, Waye J. Gastrointestinal bleeding of obscure origin: the role of small bowel enteroscopy. *Gastroenterology* 1988;94: 1117–1120.
12. Lewis B, Waye J. Small bowel enteroscopy for obscure GI bleeding. *Gastrointest Endosc* 1991;37:277.
13. Lewis B, Kornbluth A, Waye J. Small bowel tumors: the yield of enteroscopy. *Gut* 1991;32:763–765.
14. Barthel J, Vargo J, Sivak M. Assisted passive enteroscopy and gastrointestinal tract bleeding of obscure origin. *Gastrointest Endosc* 1990;36:222.
15. Gostout C, Schroeder K, Burton D. Small bowel enteroscopy: an early experience in gastrointestinal bleeding of unknown origin. *Gastrointest Endosc* 1991;37:5–8.
16. Van Gossum A, Adler M, Cremer M. Chronic gastrointestinal bleeding of obscure origin: role of small bowel enteroscopy. *Endoscopy* 1992;24:631(abst).
17. Morris A, Madhok R, Sturrock R, Capell, MacKenzie J. Enteroscopic diagnosis of small bowel ulceration in patients receiving non-steroidal anti-inflammatory drugs. *Lancet* 1991;337:520.
18. Lewis B, Mauer K. Sonde enteroscopy in patients without bleeding: are there other indications for enteroscopy? *Gastrointest Endosc* 1993.
19. Morrissey J. Small intestinal fiberscope (editorial). *Gastrointest Endosc* 1973;20:76.
20. Ament M. A large investment for small intestinal endoscopy (editorial). *Gastrointest Endosc* 1983;29:59–60.
21. Lewis B, Wenger J, Waye J. Intraoperative enteroscopy versus small bowel enteroscopy in patients with obscure GI bleeding. *Am J Gastroenterol* 1991;86:171–174.
22. Deyhle P, Jenny S, Fumagalli J. Endoscopy of the whole small intestine. *Endoscopy* 1972;4:155–157.
23. Classen M, Fruhmergen P, Koch H. Peroral enteroscopy of the small and large intestine. *Endoscopy* 1972;4:157–162.
24. Sato N, Tamegai Y, Yamakawa T, Hiratsuka H. Clinical applications of the small intestinal videoendoscope. *Endoscopy* 1992; 24:631(abst).
25. Frimberger E, Hagenmuller, Classen M. Endostomy: a new approach to small-bowel endoscopy. *Endoscopy* 1989;21:86–88.

Advanced Therapeutic Endoscopy, 2nd Ed.,
edited by J. S. Barkin and C. A. O'Phelan.
Raven Press, Ltd., New York © 1994.

CHAPTER 21

Management of Severe Lower Gastrointestinal Bleeding

Dennis M. Jensen and Gustavo A. Machicado

Lower gastrointestinal (LGI) bleeding in adult patients usually is self-limited rather than severe and ongoing (1). For the self-limited bleeding in ambulatory adults, internal hemorrhoids, colonic polyps, colonic cancer, and colitis are often diagnosed with elective evaluation. While self-limited LGI bleeding accounts for more than 85% of patients whom we see as gastroenterologists, approximately 15% have severe, ongoing hematochezia. These patients require hospitalization and urgent evaluation (1).

The diagnostic and therapeutic approach to the patient with severe LGI bleeding has not been well standardized due to the differences in availability of certain tests or techniques, the experience and training of the physician, and the presentation of the patient. Nevertheless, resuscitation of these patients should be early, vigorous, and in an intensive care unit. Different techniques such as angiography, scintigraphy, and emergency colonoscopy have been used to determine the site and the nature of the bleeding lesion. Angiography, colonoscopy, and surgery can also be used for emergency treatment. Over the past 10 years, videoendoscopy has dramatically improved the images and the ability of assistants to be active participants in the procedure. This is very helpful to the endoscopist who has now become an endoscopic "surgeon" and can treat many lesions of the GI tract that were previously only surgically approachable.

In this chapter on severe LGI bleeding, our purposes are (a) to review the tests available for diagnosis and treatment, (b) to present our approach to diagnosis and

treatment (1), and (c) to compare the results for diagnosis and treatment of emergency visceral angiography, colonoscopy, and scintigraphy.

METHODS

Radiologic Studies

Barium Enema

There is no role for emergency barium enema (BE) in a patient with severe hematochezia. BEs are rarely diagnostic and never therapeutic in such patients. Also, barium in the colon precludes emergency colonoscopy or visceral angiography until the barium clears. This may take several days.

CT Scan or MRI

In our experience, abdominal computed tomography (CT) or magnetic resonance imaging (MRI) may be helpful for diagnosis of an aortoviscus fistula in a patient presenting with severe hematochezia. Previous arteriosclerotic vascular disease or abdominal aneurysm surgery would direct one to these tests in highly selected cases. Most patients with severe hematochezia do not require such diagnostic testing.

Angiography

When the rate of arterial bleeding is 0.5 cc/min or more, selective visceral angiography may be positive. Angiography can be used for diagnosis and treatment of colonic, small bowel, or UGI lesions. The diagnostic

D. M. Jensen and G. A. Machicado: Department of Medicine, Division of Gastroenterology, University of California–Los Angeles, Center for the Health Sciences, Center for Ulcer Research and Education, Los Angeles, California 90024-1684.

yield varies with patient selection, timing of the procedure, and skill of the angiographers. Yields range from 12% to 69% (1). Besides extravasation of contrast into the lumen, abnormal vessels consistent with tumors or arteriovenous malformations may be diagnosed (2). With selective catheterization, different techniques have been used to control GI bleeding including vasopressin infusion, autologous clots, metal coils, absorbable gelatin (Gelfoam), and tissue glues (3). Bowel-related complications of angiography and these treatments may be serious, such as bowel ischemia or infarction. Other complications of angiography are hematomas, arterial embolization, and renal failure (from the IV contrast). In many institutions, emergency visceral angiography is used to complement emergency colonoscopy.

Scintigraphy

The threshold rate of bleeding for localization with radioisotope scanning is 0.1 cc/min or more. Two different types of scintigrams are available: (a) sulfur colloid with technetium and (b) autologous red blood cells (RBCs) tagged with technetium. The sulfur colloid is rapidly cleared from the circulation after IV injection but will extravasate into the gut lumen during active bleeding. Repeat IV injection may be performed. The tagged RBCs stay in the vascular space for about 24 hours. Gamma camera scans early (at 1 or 4 hours) are often useful for localization of severe active bleeding. As an example, among 23 patients with ongoing hematochezia, 78% were reported to have positive RBC scans (4). For 11 of the patients who had emergency surgery, the bleeding site was confirmed in 82% (9 patients). Delayed RBC scans at 12 or 24 hours may detect intermittent GI bleeding. Recently, 29 patients with severe hematochezia had RBC scans and 41% were reported to be positive (5). In many institutions scintigraphy has replaced emergency visceral angiography as an adjunct to colonoscopy, because of its higher yield, lower morbidity, and lower cost (1,4).

Scintigraphy has a significant rate of incorrect localization and we recommend caution in surgery on the basis of a positive RBC scan alone. Hunter and Pezim (6) reported an incorrect localization of the bleeding site with RBC scans in 13 of 52 patients (25%) with positive scans. Of these, 7 (13%) UGI bleeds were erroneously localized to the lower GI tract. This large localization error is possible since the positive area on a RBC scan depends on the time of bleeding, gut transit time, and the time of scanning. Moreover, of 19 patients who underwent surgery based solely on a positive scan, 8 underwent the wrong operation, for a surgical error rate of 42%.

Emergency Surgery

In most institutions, emergency surgery for diagnosis or treatment of severe LGI bleeding is reserved for patients with one of the following: (a) hypotension or shock, despite resuscitative efforts; (b) continued bleeding with transfusion of six or more units of blood and no diagnosis by emergency colonoscopy, angiography, or scintigraphy; (c) a specific segmental diagnosis such as diverticulosis, cancer, or extensive angiomata made by colonoscopy, but bleeding persists; (d) recurrent or continued slower bleeding with 6 or more units of blood transfused when a specific diagnosis has been made by other techniques (1,7,8). Emergency surgery has a higher mortality than elective surgery and the mortality has been reported to vary with transfusion requirement.

In a recent surgical series by Bender et al. (8) 49 patients with total abdominal colectomies for severe LGI bleeding had a mortality of 27%. Mortality for elective surgery, performed after the bleeding stopped was 7%. The surgical mortality increased from 8% (1 of 13 patients) for those patients transfused less than 10 U RBCs to 45% (9 of 20 pts) for patients transfused 10 or more units RBCs. In our experience (1), when segmental resection could be performed during emergency surgery because the lesion had been localized by emergency colonoscopy, mortality was lower than when more extensive resection was required.

Distinguishing Different Bleeding Rate

It is important to characterize the rate of bleeding and the clinical status of the patient before selecting a particular diagnostic approach. A massively bleeding patient should have ongoing resuscitation and surgical intervention as urgently as possible to control the bleeding and prevent exsanguination. By massive LGI bleeding we mean bleeding at such a rate that the patient remains in shock and cannot be stabilized with transfusions, fluids, and ICU care. This presentation is very uncommon for LGI bleeding sites, in our experience. Such patients usually cannot wait for diagnostic studies such as angiography or colonoscopy. Emergency surgery should be undertaken in the most expeditious manner. Intraoperative colonoscopy, upper endoscopy, or enteroscopy (small bowel endoscopy) may be considered to find the bleeding lesion, if it is not obvious at laparotomy (9).

The most common presentation is when the patient has hematochezia (bright red blood or darker stools) and then stops bleeding spontaneously (1). These patients can be evaluated electively since they stabilize easily after admission. Bleeding internal hemorrhoids, the most common diagnosis responsible for intermittent bleeding in ambulatory adults, must be excluded by anoscopic examination. If anoscopy (and possibly flexible sigmoidoscopy) is negative for a rectal lesion, a colonoscopy within 24 hours of presentation is recommended for hospitalized patients to detect stigmata of recent hemorrhage. For outpatients with a small amount of bright red blood (BRB) and no anemia, anoscopy and elective colonoscopy are recommended. Except for diagnosing of bleeding internal hemorrhoids or rectal lesions, we do not consider anoscopy and flexible sigmoidoscopy with air contrast barium enema as adequate for diagnosis of serious bleeding lesions in the colon for patients more than 40 years of age. Cancers, polyps, and angiomata cannot be excluded when these tests are negative.

The patient with severe hematochezia that persists or recurs and does not stop spontaneously is the one who presents the diagnostic management dilemma. This is the subgroup in which we pursue a vigorous diagnostic and therapeutic approach.

Our Approach

General Measures

Our first approach to patients with severe hematochezia is to start resuscitative measures early in the ICU to stabilize the patient. These patients also have consultation by a general or GI surgeon who follows the patient during hospitalization. Initially, an orogastric or nasogastric (NG) tube is placed to determine whether signs of UGI bleeding (coffee grounds, blood, or clots) are evident. In the face of ongoing hematochezia, anemia, and hypotension, a patient with an UGI source of hematochezia usually has these NG aspirate signs of bleeding. If bile without blood returns from the NG tube in this clinical setting, a lesion proximal to the ligament of Treitz is very unlikely as the source of severe hematochezia. Patients with signs of UGI hemorrhage require emergency panendoscopy prior to consideration for colonoscopy. This will exclude UGI lesions or permit endoscopic hemostasis. Based upon our results (1), we also recommend enemas to clear blood and stool from the distal colon, and a flexible sigmoidoscopy with turnaround in the rectum and anoscopy with a slotted anoscope to exclude rectosigmoid sources of severe hematochezia, prior to preparation for emergency colonoscopy.

If the panendoscopy and flexible sigmoidoscopy are negative, we recommend cleansing the colon with an oral purge followed by emergency colonoscopy in the ICU when the colon is clear of stool, blood, and clots. Should the colonoscopy and the upper endoscopy not be diagnostic, then we proceed with scintigraphy and angiography. For those patients who present with less

severe LGI bleeding or who stop bleeding, colonoscopy within 24 hours of presentation is also the initial diagnostic and therapeutic procedure of choice.

Emergency Endoscopy and Colonoscopy

We evaluated 100 consecutive patients who presented with persistent lower GI bleeding, requiring hospitalization for resuscitation. During stabilization with IV fluids and blood transfusions, the orogastric tube was placed and sigmoidoscopy performed in the ICU. The colon was then prepared for colonoscopy by using a polyethylene-sulfate purge (10) orally or via nasogastric tube. Metoclopramide (10 mg IV before and q 3–4 hours) facilitated gastric emptying and reduced nausea. The purge solution was administered 1 liter every 30 to 45 min over 3 to 5 hours, until the rectal effluent was clear of stool and clots. Usually, no more than 5 to 8 liters of solution were necessary to achieve this goal. Patients received blood products for correction of anemia and coagulopathies and were continually monitored in an ICU. Once the colon was clear of clots and stool, colonoscopy was performed at the bedside safely and effectively.

These patients were usually older, with a mean age of 77 years, and two-thirds were males. The majority (90%) had other medical or surgical conditions. During emergency colonoscopy, the diagnosis of a bleeding site was based upon (a) active bleeding from the lesion, (b) stigmata of recent hemorrhage such as a visible vessel or adherent clot resistant to washing with an endoscopic catheter, or (c) blood in the area and clean lesion without other lesions to explain the blood in that bowel segment.

RESULTS

General

Colonoscopy yielded a diagnosis in 74% of patients (Fig. 1). Panendoscopy revealed a UGI source in 11% (often a duodenal ulcer or angiomata), presumed small bowel bleeding (when the panendoscopy and colonoscopy were negative, yet fresh blood or clots were coming through the ileocecal valve) accounted for 9%, and no site was found in 6%. In these elderly patients, diverticulosis was a common incidental finding (not the bleeding site), seen in more than 70% of patients. Figure 2 shows the colonic diagnoses. The most common colonic lesions responsible for persistent bleeding in our series were angiomata usually of the right colon (30% of total and 41% of all colonic lesions). Diverticuli accounted for the next most common bleeding site (23% of the colonic bleeding sites). Colonic polyps or cancers (15% colonic sites), focal colitis (12%), lesions

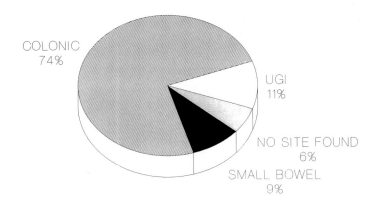

FIG. 1. Final diagnosis by the CURE Hemostasis Group of 100 patients hospitalized for severe hematochezia.

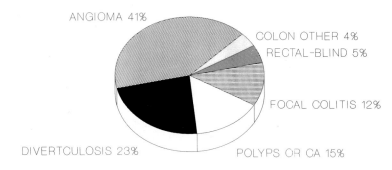

FIG. 2. Colonic diagnoses for the 100 patients who had severe hematochezia.

in the blind part of the rectum (5%), and other colonic sources (4%) were responsible for bleeding in smaller groups of patients.

Treatment

The majority (64%) of these patients required some form of intervention for control of hemorrhage. Angiographic embolization was the treatment in 1 (1%) of our patients. Surgery was the treatment in 24% of patients. Hemostasis via colonoscopy controlled the bleeding in 39% of patients. (See Figs. 3 and 4 for an example for angioma coagulation.) Therapeutic colonoscopy was performed with bipolar coagulation (BICAP or Gold Probe), heater probe, polypectomy snares, or lasers [argon or neodymium-yttrium-aluminum garnet (Nd: YAG)].

Method for Colonic Coagulation

Because of the thin wall of the colon, particularly in the cecum, caution and particular attention to detail are recommended while coagulating lesions anywhere in the colon. The bleeding site must be identified and well visualized prior to treatment via colonoscopy. Irrigation and suctioning should be used gently to avoid mucosal trauma, which can masquerade as angiomata. Distention of the bowel during treatment should be avoided since it thins out the bowel wall and makes

transmural coagulation more likely. Apply the contact probes with little pressure and low power to achieve adequate coagulation. Larger probes (3.7 mm diameter) have better coagulation characteristics and are preferred over the smaller ones (2.4 mm). Argon lasers are inconvenient for ICU or emergency treatments. However, these are very effective and safe for treatment of angiomata due to their absorption characteristics (11–13). Nd:YAG laser is also effective for coagulating lesions of the colon. However, due to its deeper

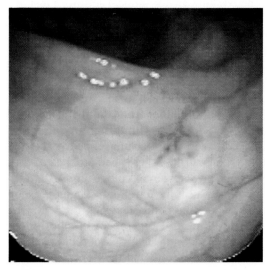

FIG. 3. Right colon angioma in a patient with severe hematochezia.

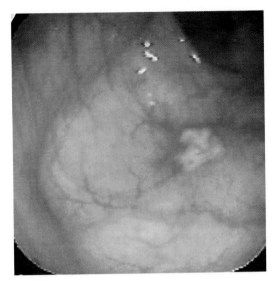

FIG. 4. After coagulation with bipolar electrocoagulation.

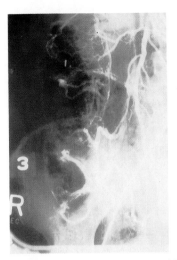

FIG. 5. Visceral angiogram of the patient with more than 100 right colon angiomata on colonoscopy. The angiogram revealed six different tufts consistent with angiomata.

coagulation, there is a higher incidence of complications such as delayed bleeding, postcoagulation syndrome, and perforation after coagulation of flat colon lesions such as angiomata (14–16).

Comparison of Angiography and Colonoscopy for Diagnosis

For our initial 17 patients, both emergency colonoscopy and angiography were performed. The diagnostic yield was 82% for colonoscopy and 12% for emergency angiography. No complications occurred with colonoscopy but 9% of patients had complications of angiography. The latter included hematomas, arterial thrombosis, and renal failure due to the IV contrast. Another five patients with small bowel or UGI bleeding sites had angiography and panendoscopy. In these patients the diagnostic yield of angiography was 20% and of endoscopy 100%. The diagnostic yield per specific lesion of colonoscopy versus angiography is listed in Table 1.

TABLE 1. *Diagnostic yield of colonoscopy vs. angiography by specific lesion*

	N	Colonoscopy (%)	Angiography (%)
Angioma	5	80	20
Diverticulosis	5	75	25
Bleeding Ca or	2	100	0
polyps	3	66	0
Small bowel lesions	2	100	0
Blind rectal lesions	1	100	0
Endometriosis			
	17	82 (14/17)	12 (2/17)
Total yield			

As an indication of the sensitivity of colonoscopy for diagnosis of angiomata, we will briefly discuss the case of a 70-year-old Caucasian woman presenting with severe hematochezia and anemia. After resuscitation and purge, she had a colonoscopy, which revealed numerous (>100) angiomata of the right colon, some with oozing. The five bleeding angiomata were coagulated to control active bleeding and, due to the number of lesions, a right hemicolectomy was planned. Prior to the surgery and after further stabilization of the patient, an angiogram was performed to rule out small bowel angiomata and other proximal bleeding sites. Selective superior mesenteric artery, inferior mesenteric artery, and celiac catheterization were performed. No extravasation was noted but only six different tufts of blood vessels consistent with right colonic angiomata were seen (Fig. 5). This emphasizes the lack of sensitivity of angiography for diagnosis of colon angiomata. No small bowel lesions were found. Subsequently, the patient had an elective right hemicolectomy and has not rebled in 4 years of follow-up.

Scintigraphy—Our Current Approach

During the last half of our hematochezia study, patients whose diagnosis for ongoing or recurrent hematochezia was not made by emergency endoscopy or colonoscopy during hospitalization had technetium RBC scans. Figure 6 gives an example of a positive scan. Twenty-five of these scans were performed and four (16%) were positive at 1 or 4 hours. Patients with positive scans had emergency angiography (one patient) or colonoscopy (three patients) and a positive

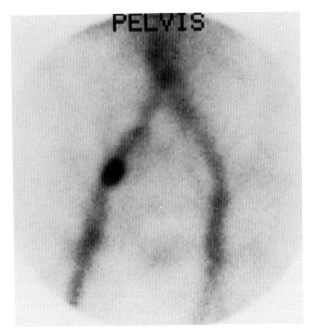

FIG. 6. Positive 1-hour technetium tagged RBC scintigram in a patient with severe hematochezia. The diagnosis of bleeding diverticulosis was confirmed by colonoscopy.

diagnosis was made in three. In comparison, another three patients (12%) had interpretations of 24-hour scans as positive, but further evaluation for a bleeding site was negative in all. Now in our institutions, patients with ongoing hematochezia and no diagnosis with panendoscopy and colonoscopy after purge undergo an emergency tagged RBC scan with 1- and 4-hour scans. If either is positive for a colonic localization, an emergency colonoscopy is repeated. If the likely location is the small bowel, small bowel push enteroscopy or an emergency angiogram is performed. Therefore, the RBC scan is used as a screening test for emergency angiography (or repeat colonoscopy) and the diagnostic yield of angiography has significantly increased.

DISCUSSION

With colonoscopy for management of severe lower GI bleeding, a specific diagnosis can often be made and treated. Even though colonoscopy is feasible in the unprepared colon, the true incidence of colonic angiomata as the source of bleeding could never be determined if one were to rely only on active bleeding to clear the stool from the colon. Angiomata and other small lesions such as polyps are obscured by overlying blood, clots, and stool (17–20). The incidence of colonic angiomata causing severe colonic bleeding is much higher (approximately 30%) than previously reported.

Confirming our results, Caos et al. (21) evaluated 35 consecutive patients who presented with acute hematochezia. The volume of sulfate purge required to clean the colon and the time required for colonoscopy to the cecum were similar to those of a comparative group of patients undergoing elective colonoscopy. The oral purge was well tolerated by all patients. A colonic bleeding site was found in 24 of 35 patients (69%). Nonbleeding colonic lesions were diagnosed in 8 patients and 3 patients had bleeding small bowel lesions. For a subgroup of 16 patients who had more severe bleeding, based upon the number of blood transfusions, 6 (38%) were bleeding from colonic angiomata, similar to our series. Endoscopic monopolar electrocoagulation was applied in 50% of patients and failed in one patient who then underwent surgery. No complications occurred from endoscopic therapy.

The next most common lesion causing severe bleeding in elderly patients is diverticuli, 17% in our study and 25% in the one by Caos et al. (21). Twenty percent of all patients with colonic diverticuli will have a bleeding episode sometime during their lifetime, and 5% of patients will bleed severely (22). Diverticuli bleed from eroded arterioles usually at the neck or the apex of the diverticulum (23). In our experience with 100 consecutive patients with severe hematochezia, 17% had diverticulosis as the bleeding site based upon active bleeding (8%; Fig. 7), a nonbleeding visible vessel (3%; Fig. 8), or an adherent clot (resistant to washing) in a single diverticulum (6%). Approximately half the diverticular bleeding sites were proximal to the splenic flexure. One-third of these patients had rebleeding or continued bleeding during hospitalization and therefore had emergency surgery with segmental resection. Previously, patients with active bleeding or other stigmata of hem-

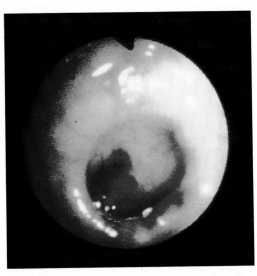

FIG. 7. A bleeding diverticulum diagnosed by emergency colonoscopy in a patient transfused 5 units RBC for severe LGI bleeding.

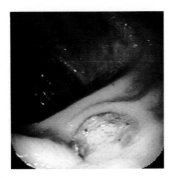

FIG. 8. A nonbleeding visible vessel on the edge of a diverticulum. The patient had recurrent LGI bleeding while hospitalized and this was the finding at emergency colonoscopy. Endoscopic coagulation was performed with a bipolar electrocoagulation probe and the patient did well.

orrhage were not treated endoscopically. However, recently we treated three patients with recurrent hematochezia during hospitalization who had a visible vessel at the edge of a diverticulum and fresh blood in the colon on emergency colonoscopy. All were treated with bipolar electrocoagulation. Techniques similar to angioma coagulation were used including low power setting, light apposition pressure, and avoidance of distention. None of the patients had rebleeding, needed more transfusions, required surgery, or had any complications of colonoscopy or coagulation (24).

Colonic cancer and polyps present more commonly with occult GI bleeding rather than severe, persistent bleeding. Benign and neoplastic polyps accounted for bleeding in 32% of cases with occult GI bleeding in one large series (25). Active severe bleeding was due to polyps or cancer in 11% and 12.5% in two other large series (1,21). Inflammatory bowel disease occasionally presents with severe lower GI bleeding. The majority of these patients do not respond to medical management and require surgical resection (26,27).

Colonic varices due to portal hypertension have been well documented to cause severe hemorrhage (28–30). Diagnosis of these lesions can be made with colonoscopy or angiography. Similar to gastroesophageal varices, bleeding colonic varices respond to portosystemic shunts (29,30), segmental colonic resections (31), or endoscopic sclerotherapy (32). Bleeding colonic varices have been reported after sclerotherapy and obliteration of esophagogastric varices (33).

Intestinal tuberculosis may cause severe colonic hemorrhage but is uncommon in the United States (34,35). With the recent influx of emigrants from Asia, one should be aware of this diagnosis as a cause of LGI bleeding. Colonic fistulization due to acute pancreatitis or pancreatic pseudocyst may cause massive colonic bleeding requiring surgical intervention (36–38). Radiation-induced rectal telangiectasias may

also be responsible for severe rectal bleeding but can be managed with endoscopic coagulation (11).

Since our first report of successful emergency colonoscopy after oral purge for severe, persistent colonic bleeding in 1981 (39), we have confirmed the feasibility and efficacy of this diagnostic procedure in the management of patients with persistent hematochezia. Other groups have also confirmed our observations that this technique is often diagnostic in the patient with acute lower GI bleeding (21,22,40,41). By evaluating these patients with initial colonoscopy and/or endoscopy, one can make a definitive diagnosis in approximately 90% of patients with ongoing hematochezia. Moreover, a large number of these patients (up to 50%) can be endoscopically treated. No further diagnostic studies are usually necessary in this circumstance and the patient can be discharged from the hospital early, after stabilization, diagnosis, and treatment.

There are no studies comparing cost-effectiveness of various approaches. However, if the patient is diagnosed and treated via endoscopy within 24 hours of admission for severe bleeding, that patient could be discharged within 48 to 72 hours of admission. This will result in significant savings in costs of hospitalization and further expensive diagnostic tests (such as angiography) or other therapy (such as surgery). In a similar manner, if colonoscopy is able to direct the surgeon to the bleeding site, a segmental resection can be accomplished rather than a subtotal colectomy. Those patients who require surgery after a specific diagnosis is made will have less morbidity, mortality, and recurrent bleeding. With a well-planned segmental resection rather than a subtotal colectomy, the patient's hospital stay will be shorter, thereby decreasing hospitalization costs.

With currently available video colonoscopes, accessories, and colonic purging during resuscitation, a well-trained colonoscopist can perform a successful colonoscopy in a patient with severe hematochezia once the colon has been cleared of stool and clots. In our opinion, this should be the management of choice. If no colonic bleeding site is found and an UGI bleed is excluded, emergency scintigrams, visceral angiography, and push enteroscopy (42) may be useful and often complementary diagnostic tests.

ACKNOWLEDGMENTS

The CURE Clinical research studies on severe lower GI bleeding in this chapter were partially funded by NIH grants AM 33273 and 17328.

REFERENCES

1. Jensen DM, Machicado GA. Diagnosis and treatment of severe hematochezia. The role of urgent colonoscopy after purge. *Gastroenterology* 1988;95:1569–1574.

2. Reuter S, Redman H, Cho K. Gastrointestinal angiography. 1986;282–338.
3. Baum S, Athanasoulis CA, Waltman AC. Angiographic diagnosis and control of large bowel bleeding. *Dis Colon Rectum* 1974; 17:447–453.
4. Bearn P, Persad R, Wilson N, et al. 99m-Technetium-labelled red blood cell scintigraphy as an alternative to angiography in the investigation of gastrointestinal bleeding: clinical experience in a district general hospital. *Ann R Coll Surg Engl* 1992;74: 192–199.
5. Ryan P, Styles CB, Chmiel R. Identification of the site of severe colon bleeding by technetium-labelled red-cell scan. *Dis Colon Rectum* 1992;35:219–222.
6. Hunter JM, Pezim ME. Limited value of technetium 99m-labelled red cell scintigraphy in localization of lower gastrointestinal bleeding. *Am J Surg* 1991;159:503–506.
7. Wright HK. Massive colonic hemorrhage. *Surg Clin North Am* 1980;60:1297–1304.
8. Bender JS, Wiencek RG, Bouwman DL. Morbidity and mortality following total abdominal colectomy for massive lower gastrointestinal bleeding. *Am Surg* 1991;57:536–541.
9. Fleckinger EG, Stanforth DC, Sinar DR, et al. Intraoperative video panendoscopy for diagnosing sites of chronic intestinal bleeding. *Am J Surg* 1989;157:137–144.
10. Davis GR, Morawski SG, Fordtran JD. Development of a lavage solution associated with minimal water and electrolyte absorption or secretion. *Gastroenterology* 1980;78:991–995.
11. Jensen DM, Machicado GA. Endoscopic diagnosis and treatment of bleeding colonic angiomas and radiation telangiectasias. Perspectives in colon and rectal surgery. 1989;2:99–113.
12. Bowers JR, Dixon JA. Argon laser photocoagulation of vascular malformation in the GI tract: short term results. *Gastrointest Endosc* 1982;28(2):126.
13. Waitman AM, Grant DZ, Chateau F. Argon laser photocoagulation treatment of patient with acute and chronic bleeding secondary to telangiectasia. *Gastrointest Endosc* 1982;28:151(abst).
14. Rutgeerts P, Van Gompal F, Geboes K, et al. Long term results of treatment of vascular malformations of the gastrointestinal tract by neodymium-YAG laser photocoagulation. *Gut* 1985;26: 586–593.
15. Johnston JH. Complications of gastrointestinal laser endoscopy. In: Jensen DM, Brunetaud JM, eds. *Medical laser endoscopy.* Netherlands: Kluwer, 1990;207–216.
16. Jensen DM. GI endoscopic hemostasis and tumor treatment—experimental results and techniques. In: Jensen DM, Brunetaud JM, eds. *Medical laser endoscopy.* Netherlands: Kluwer, 1990;45–70.
17. Forde KA. Colonoscopy in acute rectal bleeding. *Gastrointest Endoscopy* 1991;27:219–220.
18. Immordino PA. Use of colonoscopy for localization of bleeding site in severe lower gastrointestinal hemorrhage. *Conn Med* 1985;49:219–221.
19. Rex DK, Lewis BS, Waye JD. Colonoscopy and endoscopic therapy for delayed postpolypectomy hemorrhage. *Gastrointest Endoscopy* 1992;38:127–129.
20. Vellacott KD. Early endoscopy for acute lower gastrointestinal hemorrhage. *Ann R Coll Surg Engl* 1986;88:243.
21. Caos A, Benner KG, Manier J, et al. Colonoscopy after Golytely preparation in acute rectal bleeding. *J Clin Gastroenterol* 1986; 8:46–49.
22. Forde KA, Webb WA. Acute lower gastrointestinal bleeding. *Perspect Colon Rectal Surg* 1988;1:105.
23. Meyers MA, Alonso DR, Gray GF, et al. Pathogenesis of bleeding colonic diverticulosis. *Gastroenterology* 1976;71:577.
24. Savides T, Jensen DM, Machicado G, Hirabayashi K. Colonoscopic hemostasis of diverticular hemorrhage: report of three cases and of the experimental basis for treatment. *Am J Gastroenterol* 1993;in press.
25. Shinya H, Civern M, Wolf G. Colonoscopic diagnosis and management of rectal bleeding. *Surg Clin North Am* 1982;62: 897–903.
26. Robert JH, Sachar DB, Aufsis AHJ, Greenstein AJ. Management of severe hemorrhage in ulcerative colitis. *Am J Surg* 1990; 159:550–555.
27. Harvey JC, Rotstein L, Steinhardt M, et al. Massive lower gastrointestinal bleeding: an unusual complication of Crohn's disease. *Can J Surg* 1978;21:444–445.
28. Feldman J Jr, Smith VM, Warner CG. Varices of the colon. *JAMA* 1962;179:729–730.
29. Wilson SE, Stone RT, Christie JP, Passaro E Jr. Massive lower gastrointestinal bleeding from intestinal varices. *Arch Surg* 1979; 114:1158–1161.
30. Katz ALB, Shakeed A, Messer J. Colonic variceal hemorrhage: diagnosis and management. *J Clin Gastroenterol* 1985;7:67–69.
31. Orosco H, Takahashi T, Mercado MA, et al. Colorectal variceal bleeding in patients with extrahepatic portal vein thrombosis and idiopathic portal hypertension. *J Clin Gastroenterol* 1992;14: 139–143.
32. Wang M, Desigan G, Dunn D. Endoscopic sclerotherapy for bleeding rectal varices: a case report. *Am J Gastroenterol* 1985; 80:779–780.
33. Foutch PG, Sivak MV. Colonic variceal hemorrhage after endoscopic injection sclerosis of esophageal varices: a report of three cases. *Am J Gastroenterol* 1985;79:756–760.
34. Verma P, Kapur ML. Massive rectal bleeding due to intestinal tuberculosis. *Am J Gastroenterol* 1979;71:217–219.
35. Pozniak AL, Dalton-Clarke HJ, Ralphs DNL. Colonic tuberculosis presenting with massive bleeding. *Tubercle* 1985;66: 295–299.
36. Poole GV Jr, Wallenhaupt SL. Massive rectal bleeding from colonic fistula in pancreatitis. *Arch Surg* 1984;119:732–735.
37. Christensen NM, Demling R, Mathewson C Jr. Unusual manifestations of pancreatic pseudocysts and their surgical management. *Am J Surg* 1975;130:199–205.
38. Abcarian H, Eftaiha M, Kraft AR, et al. Colonic complications of acute pancreatitis. *Arch Surg* 1979;114:995–1001.
39. Jensen DM, Machicado GA. Urgent colonoscopy in patients with severe gastrointestinal bleeding. *Gastroenterology* 1981;80: 1184(abst).
40. Schrock TR. Colonoscopic diagnosis and treatment of lower gastrointestinal bleeding. *Surg Clin North Am* 1989;69:1309–1325.
41. Schuman BM. When should colonoscopy be the first study for active lower intestinal hemorrhage? *Gastrointest Endosc* 1984; 30:372–374.
42. Waye JD. Small bowel endoscopy. *Endoscopy* 1992;24:68–72.

Advanced Therapeutic Endoscopy, 2nd Ed.,
edited by J. S. Barkin and C. A. O'Phelan.
Raven Press, Ltd., New York © 1994.

CHAPTER 22

Mucosal Marking of the Colon, or India Ink Tattoo of the Colon

Jerome D. Waye

Precise location of the tip position during colonoscopy becomes important when there is a need to relocate a lesion or an area of the colon at a later time. It may be desirable to know the precise site at which a polyp was removed in piecemeal fashion so that the area can be readily identified at the next follow-up colonoscopy. Site identification becomes necessary during a wide range of surgical practices when a specific portion of the large bowel requires resection and the lesion may not be readily apparent by visual or palpatory exploration. Following endoscopic removal of a malignant adenoma, the site may heal completely in 8 weeks, and a locator mark may assist the pathologist in identifying the place where the lesion had been.

There are six methods for identifying the location of the tip of the colonoscope. Not all the methods are equally accurate, and each will be discussed with comments on their usefulness.

LENGTH OF INSTRUMENT INSERTED

Localization by measurement of centimeters of instrument introduced into the rectum is an extremely poor method for tip localization (1). During introduction of the instrument, when there are loops in the instrument, it is possible to advance an entire long colonoscope (180 cm) into the rectum and yet the tip may still be at the sigmoid/descending colon junction (2). On the other hand, it is possible, by repositioning the instrument, removing loops, and straightening, to reach the cecum in that same patient with only 60 cm of instrument inside the rectum.

J. D. Waye: Department of Medicine, Mount Sinai School of Medicine (City University of New York), and Gastrointestinal Endoscopy Unit, Mount Sinai Hospital and Lenox Hill Hospital, New York, New York 10028.

The actual number of centimeters of instrument inserted may bear no relationship to the actual tip location within the colon (3). Measurements as recorded during insertion, when loop formation is a necessary part of scope advancement maneuvers, do not reflect the true distance of intubation, since coiling of the shaft will result in spurious overestimation of the distance from the anus to a specific lesion. Measurements may be somewhat more meaningful upon withdrawal of the instrument from the cecum when the colon becomes relatively straightened out on the instrument. During scope withdrawal following total colonic intubation, the splenic flexure is usually reached at between 40 and 50 cm of instrument inserted, the upper sigmoid colon is usually encountered at approximately 30 cm upon withdrawal, and the tip is usually in the midsigmoid colon at the 25-cm mark.

Nonendoscopists frequently assume that a distance of "25 cm" on the colonoscope can be equated with a 25-cm distance on a rigid sigmoidoscope. In actuality, however, the two measurements are vastly different, with the 25 cm rigid sigmoidoscope only being able to reach into the most distal portion of the sigmoid colon, whereas the flexible instrument may actually traverse twice the actual length of bowel with the same 25 cm of instrument because of the ability to straighten the colon with the flexible scope. Distances on the colonoscope cannot be correlated with distances on the rigid sigmoidoscope unless measurements on the flexible instrument are recorded on the first pass into the rectum.

Although the cecum may be measured as being only 60 cm from the rectum with the instrument straight, in that same patient, if cecal position is lost and attempts are made to reenter the cecal caput, coiling in the distal colon may result in a large length of scope required to be inserted, with the result that the new measurement may be at 140 cm from the anus when the tip regains its cecal position. Parenthetically, the insertion of the full length of the colonoscope does not mean that the end of the colon has been reached.

LOCALIZATION BY ANATOMIC CONFIGURATION

There are only two fixed points in the colon at which there is no question about the position of the instrument tip. One area is the rectum, characterized by a large and prominent vascular pattern, by the typical Houston folds, by the anal verge and anus upon withdrawal of the instrument, and by the typical perianal appearance upon performing a U-turn maneuver in the rectum. The other location with which there can be no argument is the ileocecal valve and intubation of the cecum (4,5). The appendiceal orifice is an easily recognized landmark, usually seen as a dimple at the conjunction of the teniae coli, lying beyond the lip of the ileocecal valve. To the neophyte, the appendiceal orifice may look like a diverticulum, but it is frequently surrounded by concentric circular rings, and the adjacent mucosa may contain several red circinate spots (visible only with the videocolonoscope) that represent lymphoid nodules. Once the small bowel has been entered, there is no doubt as to the full extent of the colonoscopic examination.

Landmarks are imprecise for exact localization of areas between the rectum and cecum. Even the most experienced colonoscopists may falter in their estimate of tip location (2,6). The large blue hue of the liver with its sharp edges as the distended colon flattens out when contacting the hepatic surface is an absolute endoscopic landmark. Unfortunately, that appearance may be seen wherever the colon and the liver come in contact, which may vary from the midline (midtransverse colon) to the right posterior flank as the instrument makes an acute angle (a sharp right turn) to enter the ascending colon. The splenic flexure is only rarely identified by the smooth indentation of the spleen, but its location is frequently surmised by the endoscopist through a variety of endoscopic signs, such as, upon withdrawal, when the tip is at 40 to 50 cm from the anus, there is a change in lumen direction between the transverse and descending colon. Also, with the patient lying in the left lateral position, after withdrawal of the instrument through the triangular transverse colon, a pool of fluid is encountered, indicating that the tip has entered the left upper colon and is at the splenic flexure. When the straightened instrument is withdrawn to the area of the upper sigmoid colon, at approximately 30 cm from the anus, multiple folds can be seen on alternating sides of the colon, indicating the areas of folding normally associated with the sigmoid

configuration. With accordion pleating of the sigmoid onto the colonoscope shaft due to repeated in and out motions with twisting and torque, even a long sigmoid may become deceptively short, and accurate siting of a lesion to the upper, mid-, or lower sigmoid may be spurious.

There are numerous anecdotal stories of physicians performing a difficult colonoscopy and finding a "cecal" lesion after struggling to intubate an extremely tortuous and long colon, only to have the surgeon perform a right hemicolectomy and not remove the lesion that was actually located in the splenic flexure, hidden from surgical palpation and fixed in its location by a multitude of adhesions. Patients may require a second laparotomy for surgical resection for a tumor missed at the first exploration where the localization was based on an endoscopic estimate. Because of the capriciousness of the colon anatomy and the absence of specific landmarks, localization of points between the cecum and rectum may not be truly accurate when based on the endoscopist's impression of the intraluminal view. Indeed, in a large tortuous sigmoid colon, it may be difficult to localize a lesion to even the mid- or upper sigmoid colon. Similarly, a lesion estimated by the endoscopist to be near the splenic flexure may be under the diaphragm, or either proximal or distal to the flexure, with precise location being impossible because of tortuosity and multiple bends in that area of the colon.

In the era when laparoscopic-assisted surgical colonic resection is becoming as well accepted as primary colonoscopy, there is even greater urgency to have precise lesion location, since the laparoscopist does not have the capability of palpating the colon between the fingers at exploratory laparotomy. For the laparoscopist, it is of great importance to have an easily visible marker that can be seen through the telescopic lens of the laparoscope. It is not acceptable to state that "a lesion is in the transverse colon" since a more specific localization is needed to avoid repeated surgery for missed tumors.

MUCOSAL CLIP

Clips may be placed on the mucosa at any location to assist in radiographic identification of the marked segment. However, clips tend to fall off at an average of approximately 10 days (7), with some falling off earlier and some maintaining their attachment for longer intervals. Although it has been suggested that clips may be a helpful marker for surgical localization, it has been found that the clip devices are too small to be palpated easily. In addition, the surgeon cannot be assured that a palpable clip has not been detached and is at some distance from the original placement during endoscopy. If, indeed, a surgeon palpates a clip in the sigmoid colon and resects that segment, it is possible that the clip actually had been placed at a location near the splenic flexure, became detached, and migrated distally prior to surgery.

Employment of clips requires a large-channel colonoscope with a 3.7-mm channel (8). Currently, this is not the standard, and clips are not readily available for lesion localization with any of the standard-sized colonoscopic instrumentation channels.

An endoscopically placed clip at the site of a lesion may be useful when an abdominal x-ray can be obtained shortly after fastening a clip to the mucosa. Utilizing such a clip, it was found (7) that when the endoscopist was not sure whether the cecum had been reached, in 20% of cases the impression of the endoscopist was wrong, and the cecum had not been entered. In 63.6% of cases (7 of 11), the clinical impression of the anatomic site of a small lesion was inaccurate when compared to a flat film of the abdomen taken shortly after clip application. This further demonstrates the inability to place reliance on the anatomic location of lesions using landmarks as reference points.

IMAGING TECHNIQUES—RADIOGRAPHIC AND MAGNETIC

For years, the barium enema was the standard for the surgical localization of lesions. Surgeons would post a barium enema on the viewbox in the operating room in order to be sure that the location of the lesion could be identified. The barium enema is still a method for localizing the location of polyps or cancers (3), but small lesions may not be easily identified on the barium enema x-ray examination. If a malignant polyp were endoscopically resected, it may be extremely difficult to then try to locate the area where the polyp was removed, since only a small puckering may be present (3,9) or the site may be completely healed within 3 weeks. Most colonoscopists stopped requiring preendoscopic barium enemas about 10 years ago when it became evident that a "road map" of the colon was not necessary for the successful performance of colonoscopy. A normal-appearing large bowel on a barium enema x-ray examination provides no clue on whether the subsequent colonoscopy would be easy or difficult. The lack of correlation between the configuration of the colon as seen on the x-ray examination, and the degree of difficulty with colonic intubation during colonoscopy raised the question as to whether a barium study was worthwhile as a routine prerequisite for colonoscopy.

It has become evident that colonoscopy discovers more neoplasms than does a barium study (10) and that small polyps can readily be missed on the x-ray exami-

nation. The era of "primary colonoscopy," an endoscopic examination of the large bowel as a first-step diagnostic procedure, began with the realization that colonoscopy can visualize more colon neoplasms than the barium enema can, while providing simultaneously the capability of resecting adenomas or obtaining tissue for histologic analysis. For that reason, most patients who have rectal bleeding, anemia, or a positive fecal occult blood test, have a primary colonoscopy without a preceding barium enema. It is possible to take an x-ray or to use fluoroscopy with the colonoscope tip at the lesion in order to provide some imaging method for subsequent surgical localization (11). However, with the shortening and straightening of the bowel during colonoscopy, such a method may not give an accurate representation of the location of the lesion when the colonoscope has been removed and the bowel returns to its normal anatomic configuration.

New methods of inductive sensing with a low-intensity magnetic field may aid in the moment-to-moment localization of the tip of the fiberoptic colonoscope as it progresses through the colon. The magnetic forces are attracted to sensors within the sheath of the colonoscope (or to sensors on a wand-like device inserted into the biopsy channel). Two different techniques have been developed in England (12,13), and will soon be ready for clinical trials. These methods have replaced such devices as metal detectors for localization of the instrument tip (14). Unlike a fluoroscopic image, which demonstrates both the scope and air in the colon as a contrast media, the electromagnetic field method only shows the colonoscope itself, but is capable of a three-dimensional format.

INTRAOPERATIVE ENDOSCOPY

It is possible to localize the site of a tumor, or a resected polypectomy site, by performing intraoperative colonoscopy (15–17). Except for the dedicated surgical colonoscopist, this technique has been avoided by most endoscopists because of the burden of having to perform an endoscopic examination in the operating room with all the constraints of moving into the operative theater, positioning of the patient, handling the scope, and trying to use maneuvers such as torque and straightening techniques with the abdomen open. The amount of air insufflated to perform luminal visualization can create problems with surgical techniques once the endoscopist has completed the necessary localization. Because the site of a polypectomy may heal within 3 weeks, there is a possibility that a polypectomy site may not be seen during an intraoperative endoscopy.

The most common indication for intraoperative colonoscopy is to identify the site of a previously resected colonic lesion. Some authors (18) suggest that the use of intraoperative colonoscopy results in a "decrease in operation time," but the question arises as to whether the decrease is in relation to multiple colotomies (very time-consuming) or to previous marking of the site prior to the exploratory operation (requiring no operative time). The surgeon would not have to wait for the intraoperative endoscopy to be performed if a site were marked prior to the operative procedure.

DYE INJECTION

The ideal method for lesion localization is to have an easily identifiable marker that will immediately draw the attention of the surgeon or endoscopist (6). This can be achieved with injection of dye solutions. An experimental study (19) demonstrated that, of eight different dyes injected into the colon wall in experimental animals, only two persisted for more than 24 hours. These were indocyanine green and India ink. The indocyanine green was visible up to 7 days after injection, and it is known that India ink is a permanent marker that lasts for the life of the patient. Other dyes such as methylene blue, indigo carmine, toluidine blue, lymphazurine, hematoxylin, and eosin all were absorbed within 24 hours, leaving no residual stain at the injection site. Indocyanine green is approved by the Food and Drug Administration (FDA) for human use, but India ink has not been so approved. Indocyanine green is not associated with any significant tissue reaction and is relatively nontoxic (19). It provides excellent staining of the serosal surface and draining lymphatics for up to 7 days following its injection.

Clinical experience with indocyanine green tattoo in 12 patients (20) demonstrated that the dye was easily visualized on the serosal surface of the colon at surgery within 36 hours following injection.

Most experience with dye injection technique has been accumulated with India ink as a permanent marker (21,22). The stain lasts for at least 10 years (23) with no diminution in intensity at that duration. A permanent marker may be worthwhile for several reasons. A lesion requiring surgery may be injected and, for clinical reasons, surgery may be postponed for several weeks, at which time a vital dye such as indocyanine green will have been absorbed, leaving the operating surgeon with no visible evidence of its having been injected. Sometimes it is desirable to mark the site of a resected polyp for subsequent endoscopic localization when it is anticipated that the area will be difficult to find on a follow-up examination, especially when the lesion is located around a fold or behind a haustral septum. During a repeat colonoscopy at a later time (3 to 6 months) to assess the completeness of polypectomy, if only a small remnant of tissue remains, it

could be easily overlooked when the endoscopist must scan an entire section of the colon. A stain with a permanent marker such as India ink will draw immediate attention to the site, enabling a more accurate and complete assessment. For the surgeon, a locator stain will aid immeasurably the efforts to seek and resect an area of the bowel containing the site of the lesion. When the lesion is relatively small, such as a previously endoscopically resected malignant polyp that requires surgical resection, the site may not be evident from the serosal surface and may not even be palpable. If the lesion to be resected is in a redundant sigmoid colon or near the splenic flexure, it may be impossible to locate by either visual means or by palpation. Occasionally, even large lesions may not be palpable by the surgeon if they are soft and compressible (16). As previously mentioned, visible marking must be used for precise surgical intervention for laparoscopic-assisted colon resections.

There have been reported complications with India ink injection. The complications may be related to the wide variety of organic and inorganic compounds contained in the ink solution, such as carriers, stabilizers, binders, and fungicides (24). It has been conjectured that autoclaving the various additives to the carbon particles and water could result in additional substances capable of eliciting an inflammatory or allergic response. In one reported case, endoscopic tattooing at a polypectomy site was performed 18 hours prior to surgery, using India ink diluted 1:10 with sterile water and autoclaved. Two 0.5-ml mucosal injections were made proximal and distal to the polypectomy site using a sclerotherapy needle. Following resection, pathologic examination revealed an abscess extending through the muscularis mucosa. The consideration was that a chemical irritant could have caused the abscess or that enteric bacteria were inoculated with the injection needle. Indeed, in an experimental study on endoscopic tattooing of the dog colon, two of eight injected dyes, India ink and hematoxylin, resulted in an adverse tissue reaction. The India ink injection produced a significant inflammatory infiltrate as well as microhemorrhage and thrombosis, while hematoxylin resulted in mucosal ulceration (25).

Another report of adverse complications in humans detailed two cases in which a total of 2.0 ml of autoclaved India ink was injected following an equal volume dilution with sterile saline. In one patient, histologic examination revealed fibroblastic proliferation in an area of abundant black pigment, while the other case demonstrated, in addition to chronic inflammatory cell infiltration associated with ink injection, fat necrosis both in the serosal surface adjacent to a tumor and within the pericolic fat. In this latter case, the India ink had diffused extensively into the sigmoid colon and its mesentery and into loops of small bowel that were adherent to the sigmoid colon. Neither of these two patients had any clinical symptoms (26).

Most authors who have reported on the use on India ink have not noted any significant sequelae. A recent pathology investigation (23) of resected specimens demonstrated that two of ten patients who had India ink injected between 7 and 45 days prior to surgery revealed acute inflammation at the injection site. Both of the patients demonstrating an inflammatory response had surgery within 7 days of India ink injection. Five of ten had submucosal fibrosis, which correlated with deeper levels of India ink deposit. One additional case had focal fibrosis confined to the serosal surface. In these patients, the India ink was used in dilutions of 1:10 or 1:100, but the concentration of ink did not appear to be a factor in the degree of the fibrotic response. The extent of the reactive inflammatory response was deemed by the pathologist to be minimal in all cases.

Because of the possibility that congeners are responsible for the tissue reaction to India ink, it has been suggested that a pure charcoal suspension may be utilized effectively for marking the colon (24). Six patients injected with a 5% weight/volume suspension of micronized carbon particles (2–5 μm in diameter) had no adverse reaction (27), although surgery was not subsequently performed in any of these patients.

It is possible that the toxic properties of India ink may be partially ameliorated by marked dilution of the ink. It has been described that ink diluted to 1:100 with saline produces as dark a spectral photometric pattern as undiluted India ink (28), and in clinical tests the mark made by 1:100 diluted India ink is readily visible by the endoscopist and by the operating surgeon. A small volume injection may increase the safety of the procedure (29,30).

METHOD FOR INDIA INK INJECTION

Diluted India ink in a volume per volume ratio of 1:100 with sterile saline results in a concentration of ink that is readily visible by both the endoscopist and the operating surgeon (23). Therefore, greater concentrations need not be employed.

To further decrease the possibility of an inflammatory response from ink injection, it may be worthwhile to ensure the absence of any contaminating bacteria in the India ink. This can effectively be accomplished by autoclaving the dilute solution of India ink, or by passing it through a 0.22-μm Millipore filter, which prevents bacterial passage. This type of filter is readily available at any hospital, since this is the filter size that is used to prevent bacterial contamination of total parenteral nutrition (TPN) solutions. Passage of dilute India ink through this filter results in clogging of the filter in about 10% of instances. When the filter clogs, only a few milliliters of solution may be pushed through the filter, and then with greater force only a clear liquid effluent may be obtained, since all of the ink particles become trapped within the filter, permitting only water to pass through. The clogging of the filter with large particles of carbon can be effectively eliminated by using two filters in tandem; a 0.4-μm Millipore filter may be attached directly to the 10-ml syringe containing the dilute India ink solution. The 0.4-μm filter may then be directly connected to a 0.22-μm Millipore filter that is, in turn, attached to the hub of the sclerotherapy needle. Using this technique, it is possible to easily inject several cc's of India ink solution into the mucosa as necessary, while being assured that bacterial sterility is guaranteed.

A standard sclerotherapy needle is utilized, but it should be long enough to be inserted through the entire length of a colonoscope, and stiff enough so that it will not crinkle up as it is being forced through the biopsy port when the tip of the instrument is deep in the colon and the colonoscope shaft has several convolutions and loops. Ideally, the needle should enter the mucosa at an angle to permit injections into the submucosa, rather than to have the needle pierce the bowel wall. The edges of intrahaustral folds should be targeted. If during an injection a submucosal bleb is not immediately seen, the needle should be pulled back slightly, since the needle tip may have penetrated the full thickness of the wall and the ink may be squirting into the peritoneal cavity. An intracavity injection is not a clinical problem (9,20), but it can scatter dark pigment around the abdominal cavity, which may be somewhat disconcerting for the surgeon.

Since the colonoscopist cannot know which portion of the bowel is the superior aspect, multiple injections should be made circumferentially in the wall around a lesion to prevent a single injection site from being located in a "sanctuary" site, hidden from the eyes of the surgeon as the abdomen is opened with the patient lying supine (31). Each injection should be of sufficient volume to raise a bluish bleb within the mucosa at the injection site. The injection volume may vary from 0.1 to 0.5 ml. If injections are made a few centimeters from the lesion, the surgeon should be told whether the injections are proximal or distal to the site. With the 1:100 dilution of India ink, endoscopic visualization is still possible should some of the ink spill into the lumen, whereas with the more concentrated solutions, the endoscopic picture becomes totally black when ink covers the bowel walls (9).

Most endoscopists who use India ink to mark colonic lesions do not prescribe antibiotics prior to its use, although it has been suggested that prophylactic antibiotics be given before injections of indocyanine green (20).

The India ink is indeed a permanent marker, with

endoscopic visualization of the tattoo site being possible in every case on follow-up examination without diminution in color up to an interval of 10.5 years following initial injection (23).

The brand of India ink does not seem to be important, but a water-soluble India ink is preferred to "permanent" India ink. Carbon-particle India ink must be used rather than permanent black fountain pen–type ink. The fountain pen–type of permanent ink is highly alkaline, and injection of that into the colon wall has been reported (anecdotally) to cause necrosis of the colon wall. To assure that the ink contains carbon particles, a drop of India ink may be placed on a glass slide, and with tilting the slide, tiny dots of carbon may be seen to flow down the slide within the border of the fluid.

The use of sterile, diluted India ink is a safe and effective method for marking lesions through the colonoscope. The technique is rapid, safe, and provides an easily visible permanent marker for subsequent endoscopic localization, or for the surgeon during exploratory laparotomy. For laparoscopic-assisted colectomies, endoscopic tattooing is an essential preoperative maneuver. There are only two dyes that are useful in the preoperative marking of the colon lesions, and these are indocyanine green and India ink. For long-term identification of a polypectomy site, India ink is the only dye that has been shown to result in a permanent mucosal and serosal stain.

REFERENCES

1. Dunaway MT, Webb WR, Rodning CB. Intraluminal measurement of distance in the colorectal region employing rigid and flexible endoscopes. *Surg Endosc* 1988;2:81–83.
2. Waye JD. Colonoscopy without fluoroscopy (editorial). *Gastrointest Endosc* 1990;36:72–73.
3. Frager DH, Frager JD, Wolf EL, Beneventano TC. Problems in the colonoscopic localization of tumors: continued value of the barium enema. *Gastrointest Radiol* 1987;12:343–346.
4. Waye JD, Atchison MAE, Talbott MC, Lewis BS. Transillumination of light in the right lower quadrant during total colonoscopy (letter to editor). *Gastrointest Endosc* 1988;34:69.
5. Waye JD, Bashkoff E. Total colonoscopy: is it always possible? *Gastrointest Endosc* 1991;37:152–154.
6. Hilliard G, Ramming K, Thompson J Jr, Passaro E Jr. The elusive colonic malignancy. A need for definitive preoperative localization. *Am Surg* 1990;56:742–744.
7. Tabibian N, Michaletz PA, Schwartz JT, et al. Use of endoscopically placed clip can avoid diagnostic errors in colonoscopy. *Gastrointest Endosc* 1988;34:262–264.
8. Hachisu T, Miyazaki S, Hamaguchi K. Endoscopic clip-marking of lesions using the newly developed HX-3L clip. *Surg Endosc* 1989;3:142–147.
9. Shatz BA, Thavorides V. Colonic tattoo for follow-up of endoscopic sessile polypectomy. *Gastrointest Endosc* 1991;37:59–60.
10. Irvine EJ, O'Connor J, Frost RA, Shorvon P, Somers S, Stevenson GW, Hunt RH. Prospective comparison of double contrast barium enema plus flexible sigmoidoscopy v colonoscopy in rectal bleeding: barium enema v colonoscopy in rectal bleeding. *Gut* 1988;29:1188–1193.
11. Cirocco WC, Rusin LC. Documenting the use of fluoroscopy during colonoscopic examination: a prospective study. *Surg Endosc* 1991;5:200–203.
12. Bladen JS, Anderson AP, Bell GD, Rameh B, Evans B, Heatley DJ. Non-radiological technique for three-dimensional imaging of endoscopes. *Lancet* 1993;341:719–722.
13. Williams C, Guy C, Gillies D, Saunders B. Electronic three-dimensional imaging of intestinal endoscopy. *Lancet* 1993;341:724–725.
14. Leicester RJ, Williams CB. Use of metal detector for localisation during fibresigmoidoscopy or limited colonoscopy. *Lancet* 1981;2:232–233.
15. Forde KA, Cohen JL. Intraoperative colonoscopy. *Ann Surg* 1988;207:231–233.
16. Richter RM, Littman L, Levowitz BS. Intraoperative fiberoptic colonoscopy. Localization of nonpalpable colonic lesions. *Arch Surg* 1973;106:228.
17. Sakanoue Y, Nakao K, Shoji Y, Yanagi H, Kusunoki M, Utsunomiya J. Intraoperative colonoscopy. *Surg Endosc* 1993;7:84–87.
18. Kuramoto S, Thara O, Sakai S, Tsuchiya T, Oohara T. Intraoperative colonoscopy in the detection of nonpalpable colonic lesions—how to identify the affected bowel segment. *Surg Endosc* 1988;2:76–80.
19. Hammond DC, Lane FR, Welk RA, Madura MJ, Borreson DK, Passinault WJ. Endoscopic tattooing of the colon: an experimental study. *Am Surg* 1989;55:457–461.
20. Hammond DC, Lane FR, Mackeigan JM, Passinault WJ. Endoscopic tattooing of the colon: clinical experience. *Am Surg* 1993;59:205–210.
21. Ponsky JL, King JF. Endoscopic marking of colon lesions. *Gastrointest Endosc* 1975;22:42–43.
22. Cohen LB, Waye JD. Colonoscopic polypectomy of polyps with adenocarcinoma: when is it curative? In: Barkin JS, ed. *Difficult decisions in digestive diseases.* Chicago: Year Book Medical Publishers, 1989;528–535.
23. Novak JS, Waye JD, Harpaz N. India ink tattoo of the colon: clinical and pathological follow-up. Submitted for publication, 1993.
24. Lightdale CJ. India ink colonic tattoo—blots on the record (editorial). *Gastrointest Endosc* 1991;37:71.
25. Park SI, Genta RS, Romeo DP, Weesner RE. Colonic abscess and focal peritonitis secondary to India ink tattooing of the colon. *Gastrointest Endosc* 1991;37:68–71.
26. Coman E, Brandt LJ, Brenner S, Frank M, Sablay B, Bennett B. Fat necrosis and inflammatory pseudotumor due to endoscopic tattooing of the colon with India ink. *Gastrointest Endosc* 1991;37:65–68.
27. Naveau S, Bonhomme L, Preaux N, Chaput JC. A pure charcoal suspension for colonoscopic tattoo. *Gastrointest Endosc* 1991;37:624–625.
28. Salomon P, Berner J, Waye JD. Sterilization of India ink for endoscopic tattoo. Submitted for publication.
29. Poulard JB, Shatz B, Kodner I. Preoperative tattooing of polypectomy site. *Endoscopy* 1985;17:84–85.
30. Shatz BA. Small volume India ink injections (letter to the editor). *Gastrointest Endosc* 1991;37:649–650.
31. Hyman N, Waye JD. Endoscopic four quadrant tattoo for the identification of colonic lesions at surgery. *Gastrointest Endosc* 1991;37:56–58.

Advanced Therapeutic Endoscopy, 2nd Ed.,
edited by J. S. Barkin and C. A. O'Phelan.
Raven Press, Ltd., New York © 1994.

CHAPTER 23

Managing Large Colonic Polyps

Mark Schiele and David Lieberman

It is likely that most colon cancers arise from adenomatous polyps. Several studies have demonstrated that larger polyps with villous histology are more likely to be cancerous. The risk of cancer in polyps steadily increases with size of the polyp. The risk of cancer in a polyp 1.0 to 1.9 cm in size is 8% to 15%, in a 2.0 to 2.9 cm polyp 14% to 22%, and in a 3.0 cm or larger polyp 21% to 33% (1). Large benign adenomas (>1.0 cm) also have a high risk of developing cancer if left untreated—a risk of 1% per year (2).

In the precolonoscopy era, patients found to have large polyps on barium studies required partial colectomy for removal of what were often benign but high-risk lesions. In the colonoscopy era, we now routinely detect large polyps during the colon examination and need to make decisions about the appropriate method for removal. Endoscopic polypectomy is suitable for most small polyps (less than 1 cm) and pedunculated polyps. Large sessile polyps and pedunculated polyps with broad-based stalks often pose a difficult dilemma for the endoscopist. This chapter discusses the decision-making required for endoscopic management of large colonic polyps. We focus on patient preparation, the decision to treat the patient endoscopically or surgically, and finally, endoscopic techniques.

PATIENT PREPARATION

Polypectomy is greatly facilitated by a good bowel preparation. Multiple regimens are available and commonly include polyethylene glycol solutions, phospho-

rus-containing purgatives, magnesium citrate, and various other preparations. Mannitol has become obsolete as a purgative secondary to concerns of gas explosion during electrocautery (3). The other listed preparations are generally effective, tolerated, and reduce bacterial counts sufficiently to greatly reduce the likelihood of gas explosion. There are various reports of electrolyte and fluid imbalance as a result of these laxatives, although clinically significant problems are unusual.

Persons undergoing diagnostic colonoscopy should prepare for possible therapeutic procedures by stopping any anticoagulants or antiplatelet drugs prior to study. Aspirin inhibits platelet aggregation and usually should be stopped 1 week prior to study. If the patient is receiving heparin, it should be discontinued several hours before the procedure. Patients on coumadin may be instructed to hold their coumadin dose several days prior, until the prothrombin time normalizes. Depending on the procedure performed, the patient may then start back on the coumadin as an outpatient. Nonsteroidal anti-inflammatory drugs can cause platelet dysfunction also, and strong consideration should be made to stop these drugs prior to colonoscopy. The recognition of anticoagulant or antiplatelet drug use by the patient is especially critical when polypectomy of a large polyp is planned.

Proper use of sedatives may greatly facilitate endoscopic procedures. Not all patients will require sedation, but when necessary, "conscious sedation" is perhaps the safest approach. Ideally, a patient will be able to respond to painful stimuli, be able to change position, and remain calm during the examination. The most useful medicines are benzodiazepines and opiates. Benzodiazepines such as diazepam and midazolam are particularly useful because of their relaxing and amnestic effects. These are administered by slow intravenous infusion. If untoward effects such as respiratory depression occurs with these agents, flumazenil

M. Schiele: Division of Gastroenterology, Oregon Health Sciences University, Portland, Oregon 97201.

D. Lieberman: Department of Medicine, Oregon Health Sciences University and Department of Gastroenterology, Veterans Administration Medical Center, Portland, Oregon 97207.

has proven useful as a benzodiazepine antagonist and works rapidly. An opiate analgesic may be most useful for colonoscopy because of their analgesic effect. In addition, opiates such as Demerol often provide a euphoric effect. Naloxone can be given to antagonize the narcotic effect of respiratory suppression if needed. Sedatives such as droperidol and other neuroleptics may have a limited role in patient sedation. Routine usage of these latter drugs is not recommended because of their long duration of action and the absence of an antagonist drug.

POLYPECTOMY OR COLECTOMY?

Upon encountering a colonic polyp, the endoscopist will be faced with the decision to attempt either endoscopic or surgical resection. If the polyp is endoscopically inaccessible or the patient expresses unwillingness to undergo attempt at this form of resection, then surgery should be offered.

Obviously malignant sessile polyps are best managed surgically. These may appear as irregular, waxy, friable, ulcerated, or multilobulated neoplasms (4). Endoscopic resection of these neoplasms would not likely be curative. Pedunculated neoplasms of the same appearance may be relatively easier to remove; however, the probability of complete removal is not high because of stalk invasion by tumor. Thus, consideration should be given to initial surgical resection.

The decision regarding less obviously malignant polyps is more difficult. Some endoscopists will biopsy large, benign-appearing polyps and let the histology assist in their decision to resect endoscopically or surgically. A cancerous section of the polyp may be missed, though, and the false-negative rate has been noted to be unacceptably high in some series (5). Furthermore, a biopsy may reveal carcinoma, but after complete histologic examination the carcinoma may be noninvasive, resulting in unnecessary surgical resection. To avoid confusion, some authors feel biopsies are not helpful, and the policy of attempting complete excision of all but the malignant-appearing polyp, if accessible, seems prudent.

One factor to consider is whether the polyps are too large to resect. Pedunculated polyps have an inherent advantage due to the presence of a narrow stalk; thus, these polyps can usually be snared, even up to 5 to 8 cm in size. The polyp head may have to be trimmed piecemeal to allow placement of the snare around the polyp. Large sessile polyps may be amenable to endoscopic removal as well, given the popularity of the piecemeal polypectomy approach as outlined below. Given this approach, 75% of all polyps greater than 3.0 cm were resectable through the colonoscope in one series (6). It must be kept in mind that the risk of hem-

orrhage is greater in larger size polyps. In one series of 1,795 polypectomies, all of the major hemorrhages occurred in polyps greater than 2.0 cm in size (7). In another study of 1,485 polypectomies, 12 of 14 major hemorrhages occurred while resecting polyps greater than 1 cm (8).

Polyps that are best suited for surgical resection include large, flat, "carpet-like" polyps several centimeters in size (9). Also, polyps whose base extends over two haustral folds may be difficult to endoscopically resect due to inaccessibility. Although techniques such as BICAP probe, laser ablation, or fulguration with monopolar biopsy forceps have been described for these situations, if the patient is a good surgical candidate, this would provide more definitive and secure therapy.

Occasionally the endoscopist encounters a patient who is not a surgical candidate yet has a polyp that is large or suspicious for carcinoma. In the poor surgical candidate or those refusing surgery, standard polypectomy techniques should be tried. Laser ablation can be combined with polypectomy in such cases and is discussed below.

INACCESSIBLE AND POORLY POSITIONED POLYPS

Successful endoscopic resection of a polyp requires proper access and positioning prior to polypectomy. There are several reasons that a polyp may be inaccessible. If the patient has a particularly tortuous colon, it may not be possible to reach a polyp. In experienced hands this is seldom the case. Other causes for inaccessibility include significant diverticular disease, polyps wrapped around a bend in the colon, and polyps located deep between folds.

Polypectomy in patients with diverticular disease may be challenging if the involved segment is narrowed and thickened. Standard colonoscopes may be too large and inflexible to maneuver in a narrowed diverticular segment. The use of small caliber endoscopes in these cases may allow easier passage and manipulation of snares (10). This greater flexibility of the tip may assist in removing polyps in the rectum, where polyps can hide behind the valves. In addition, the use of mini-snares has been advocated in tight positions (9). These mini-snares open to 2.0 to 2.5 cm in length and 1.3 to 1.5 cm in width. This is distinctly smaller than the conventional snare, which is 6.2 cm when fully extended with a diameter of 3 cm. The use of the larger snares may lead to bending of the wire when opened in a narrow segment.

Management of polyps that wrap around a fold is problematic. Waye (9) has advocated piecemeal resection of these polyps by first removing the proximal portion. Scarring after the polypectomy may flatten out the distal site and allow for subsequent resection at a later date. If the lesion does not contain invasive malignancy or meet the criteria for surgical polypectomy, the remaining polyp should be removed in 3 to 6 months (9).

Polyps that are tucked between folds or just behind folds can be difficult to find and remove. Overinsufflation may impair accessibility, thus, aspiration to decompress the colon may help. Repositioning the patient and/or the endoscope may make a polyp more accessible. Ideally, the colonoscope should be manipulated such that the polyp is in the five o'clock position. This allows the best visualization since the wire snare emerges into the visual field at the five o'clock position. Care must be taken to not apply too much torque to the scope, particularly when working in the proximal colon, because of the risk of perforation. This is especially true when a loop is formed in the colon.

If a polyp is seen during intubation of the colon and is in good position for resection, the polyp should be removed at that time. This is especially true for polyps that are less than 1 cm and may not be easily seen upon withdrawal. It is safe to proceed past a fresh polypectomy site and complete the colonoscopy (11). This approach may require withdrawing the colonoscope to retrieve the polyp and then reinserting it. This is generally much easier than the initial intubation. In contrast, if a large polyp is encountered, one may wish to complete the colonoscopy first because of the possibility that a carcinoma may be found more proximally that would require surgical resection. The endoscopist and patient may be saved significant time and some risk.

POLYPECTOMY EQUIPMENT

The endoscopist should be thoroughly familiar with the polypectomy equipment available in the endoscopy unit. The essential components include an electrosurgical unit, wire snares, hot biopsy forceps, injection needles, and retrieval devices.

The most widely used energy source for polypectomy is continuous, pure coagulation current. The electrosurgical unit may have options for either cutting current, coagulation current, or a blend of both. Coagulation current heat will help seal blood vessels during polypectomy, and it is for this reason that it is advocated. The experience by Macrae et al. (7) was that after switching from blended to pure coagulation current at low settings, typically 15 to 25 W, the incidence of hemorrhage after polypectomy fell considerably. In a more recent comparison of blended or pure coagulation current in 1,485 snare polypectomies, there were no significant differences in the number of bleeding events (8). A difference did occur in the timing of the

hemorrhage in that blended current caused immediate hemorrhage (up to 12 hours), while pure coagulation current resulted in delayed hemorrhage (2 to 7 days) (8). Although it may be preferable to have an immediate complication while the patient may be under observation rather than at home, the use of pure coagulation current still is favored by most endoscopists.

Monopolar electrocoagulation is the most popular technique. A ground plate is applied to the patient that receives current that is sent from the snare through the body's tissues. Bipolar current may have some advantages but is less widely used. Data from animal gastric pseudopolypectomy have shown that bipolar snare requires less energy and damaged significantly less underlying mucosa compared with a monopolar snare (12). This may prove to decrease perforation and the colon coagulation syndrome, and clinical trials seem warranted to investigate this possibility.

There are a wide variety of snares available. A large snare extends as much as 6 cm or so and widens to 3 cm. The smaller snare will extend about 3 cm and opens to 1 cm. Newer mini-snares are available in sizes 1.3 by 2.0 cm (oval) or 1.5 cm by 2.5 cm (hexagonal). It makes little difference as to whether the loop has an oval or hexagonal shape. Each snare has an insulated plastic handle and a slide bar mechanism to open and close the snare. It is essential that the tip of the snare be retractable 1 to 2 cm into the sheath. Sufficient guillotine force may not be generated unless this condition is met, since the plastic sheath may compress when performing endoscopy.

STANDARD POLYPECTOMY TECHNIQUE

Proper positioning is the first step in assuring successful polypectomy. As mentioned above, the five o'clock position is preferred. Also, to facilitate full loop opening, it will help to have a straight or tubular view of the colon. Smaller snares are useful if the polyp is at an angulation, thus allowing full opening of the snare. In a patient with an actively peristaltic colon, it often helps to give glucagon, 0.5 mg to 1 mg. In patients who are anxious and restless, it may help to increase the sedation, especially if there are multiple, difficult polypectomies to be done.

Pedunculated polyps are snared over the head portion and the wire gently tightened around the stalk. Sessile polyps may also be snared in this manner, with creation of a pseudostalk by lifting the base away from the mucosa. The maximum diameter of the base should be 2.0 to 2.5 cm if attempting a single transection. This may result in a base sized 1.0 to 1.5 cm in diameter once the snare is tightened (13).

The snare should be opened slowly so as to avoid laceration or perforation of the bowel wall. By maneuvering the colonoscope shaft and controls, the snare is placed over the head of the polyp. Prior to loop closure, the insulated sheath of the snare should be positioned very near the stalk at the intended transection site. The ideal site of transection for a pedunculated polyp is just below the polyp head, allowing some portion of the stalk to be sent for histological analysis. If the transection is too low on the pedicle, there is a risk of significant mucosal burn or even perforation. The ideal site for closure on a sessile polyp is at the junction of the polyp base and the colonic wall, after tenting the polyp into the lumen.

After determining the optimal site of transection, the loop is then slowly closed with attention paid to the mark on the handle indicating the point of loop closure. It is critical to avoid tightening the snare too much because of a risk of premature transection and bleeding due to lack of cautery application. With larger, firm polyps the point of loop closure may be felt as some resistance, but with softer, fleshy polyps there may be some doubt as to when the loop is fully closed. This is when it is helpful to have a notion of the expected amount of tissue to be snared, so the distance from the mark on the snare indicating the loop closure point can be compared. If there is a discrepancy, normal mucosa may be inadvertently snared. The snare may then be reopened slightly, and the endoscope shifted slightly to allow the normal mucosa to slide out. At this point, it may help to move the snared polyp to and fro and assess if the bowel wall moves along with the polyp. If it does then inadvertent snaring of normal mucosa is a possibility. If the snared polyp moves but not the bowel wall, the safe polypectomy may be performed.

When it is determined that it is safe to proceed, current is applied. After evidence of thermal delivery, such as the presence of a white coagulum, the snare is slowly closed in concert with short bursts of coagulating current. The transected polyp will lie close to the transection site and may then be retrieved. As discussed earlier, polyps of size 8 mm or less may be suctioned through the colonoscope channel if a suction trap apparatus is available. For larger polyps, suction may be applied directly to the polyp and the scope withdrawn. The larger polyp may also be retrieved with the wire snare, basket, or three-pronged grasper. Close attention should be paid to the polypectomy site and an assessment for bleeding and the completeness of polypectomy.

ENDOSCOPIC RESECTION OF LARGE POLYPS

Large colonic polyps pose a particular challenge to endoscopists. Most authors define ''large'' colonic polyps as those greater than or equal to 3.0 cm (5). This distinction is made since the incidence of malignancy increases with polyps as they approach and exceed this size (1). These polyps are uncommon, ranging in frequency from 4.1% to 7.5% of all polyps, based on reports of consecutive polypectomies (1). Large polyps raise questions regarding technical ability to resect endoscopically, malignancy assessment, and surveillance issues.

All the previous suggestions concerning routine polypectomy apply to resecting large, sessile polyps. Proper preparation, timing, and positioning in addition to experience and sound judgment are required. Sessile polyps with bases greater than 2.0 to 2.5 cm should be removed by the piecemeal technique. This technique also applies to polyps that are awkwardly positioned around folds in the colon or polyps with heads too large to allow snare passage.

To start the piecemeal polypectomy, the snare should be placed around a portion of the polyp. Whether this be the center of the polyp or the edge is not critical, but if possible the edge is the preferred starting point (Fig. 1). The least number of snare placements is ideal, so a preset attack plan is worthwhile. When starting at the edge, the tip of the snare should be placed at the polyp margin while the snare is fitted around a portion of the polyp. At this point the wire will be buried in the polyp and difficult to see. As the snared section of the polyp is tented toward the lumen, the snare may be jiggled to and fro to check for normal mucosa entrapment as described above. Occasionally, the portion of the polyp snared is so large as to touch the surrounding wall of the colon, thus, there is a risk of current leakage from this portion causing both decreased current through the cutting wire and burn of the colonic wall. By moving the polyp to and fro during current delivery, the tendency to burn the normal mucosa will be less.

If the conditions appear safe, current is then applied along with snare wire closure. It is prudent to allow coagulation current to be applied for 3 to 4 seconds prior to wire retraction. The usual white coagulum may not be visualized because of the buried wire. The wire snare is then closed slowly until transection of this portion of the polyp. Instead of immediately retrieving this polyp fragment, it is best to proceed with the next piecemeal resection.

Proceeding in this way, another piece of the polyp is removed until the base is cleared of polyp. Total removal of the polyp may not be possible during the first session, thus a follow-up examination may be needed for complete resection. On examination of the polyp base after the initial resection, it may appear that residual tissue is present. This may actually be the case, but edema and swelling can give this appearance as well. The surface of the polypectomy site may be further treated with current by a hot biopsy forceps

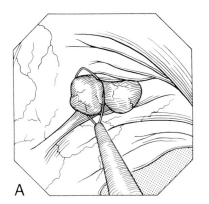 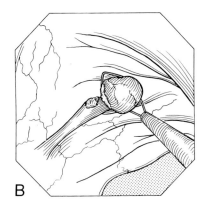 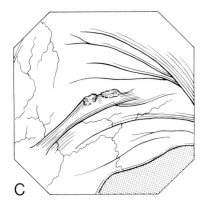

FIG. 1. Piecemeal resection of a bi-lobed, 2-cm polyp.

laid tangentially (9). Reexamination in 3 to 6 months is recommended after piecemeal polypectomy.

MUCOSAL INJECTION OF POLYPS

The most serious bleeding complications of polypectomy appear to be associated with the snare removal of sessile polyps larger than 2 cm and broad-based pedunculated polyps. Macrae et al. (7) found that the risk of postpolypectomy bleeding was closely related to the diameter of the stalk in the pedunculated polyp. In fact, they point out that the diameter of the stalk was of more importance than the size of its head in predicting the likelihood of bleeding (7). These authors suggested attempting to snare the polyp stalk at the narrowest point near the polyp head and then replacing the snare lower down the stalk and applying strangulation to the stalk if bleeding occurs. Over the past 2 years at our center we have been using 1-cc injections of epinephrine 1:10,000 via a sclerotherapy needle prior to removal of broad-based pedunculated polyps. Our hypothesis is that such broad stalks may contain large blood vessels to feed the polyp and the use of a constricting agent injected mucosally may reduce the risk of immediate bleeding. These patients may still be at risk for late bleeding complications several days after polypectomy and should be followed appropriately. We typically ask patients to avoid the use of aspirin and nonsteroidal anti-inflammatory drugs for 1 to 2 weeks after such a major polypectomy. The mucosal injection of epinephrine has not been well studied in this setting and further investigation is needed to validate the benefits of this prepolypectomy intervention.

There has been increasing interest in the removal of flat colon polyps with small snares. Some investigators have suggested that a submucosal injection of saline prior to the attempted polypectomy may elevate the mucosa away from the serosal surface and make snare removal of such lesions a safer procedure. This approach is currently under investigation and follow-up data on the adequacy of polyp removal by this technique are still needed.

LASER ABLATION OF POLYPS

Surgical treatment is usually recommended for patients with polyps that cannot be completely removed with endoscopic polypectomy. However, in patients who are poor surgical candidates due to underlying medical problems, other approaches have been considered. Tumor ablation with lasers has been used for palliation of rectosigmoid cancers. Brunetaud et al. (14) reported good palliative results in patients with rectal sigmoid cancers who were not candidates for curative resection. The extent of circumferential involvement of the bowel wall was the primary prognostic factor influencing overall success in survival for 12 months. Application of this technology for treatment of benign lesions of the colon has now been reported. These series include patients with lesions unsuitable for polypectomy or with incomplete polypectomy. In addition, these series include patients who are poor surgical candidates or who refuse surgery.

Mathus-Vliegen and Tytgat (15) presented follow-up data with a mean duration of over 3 years on 196 patients with adenomas that were treated by neodymium: yttrium-aluminum garnet (Nd:YAG) laser. Ablation of tumor depended on the extent of the lesion. Ablation was achieved in only 34 of 61 (56%) of patients with extensive lesions defined as greater than 4 cm or involving two-thirds of the circumference. Ablation was accomplished in 71 of 78 patients with intermediate lesions (1–4 cm) and in 41 of 44 patients with small lesions (less than 1 cm). This approach is not without significant complications including symptomatic stenoses in 7% and minor complications in 36%. Malignancy was discovered in 9% of patients, many of whom subsequently went to surgery (16).

Brunetaud et al. (14) reported total tumor destruction by laser in 81% of the evaluated patients but had less success in larger, more extensive lesions. Subsequent cancer was found in 8.9% of their patients. Patrice et al. (16) reported a 17.9% cancer rate in polyps undergoing laser ablation. These results underline a major concern about laser photoablation of adenomas; that is, the risk of undetected cancer. Thus, this technique currently seems most appropriate for patients who are not surgical candidates.

These studies suggest that laser ablation of large polyps is an option but has definite limitations and should not be the treatment of choice. Laser therapy is less likely to achieve complete tumor ablation if the lesions are large and circumferential and such patients are more likely to have complications including stenosis from multiple treatments. For patients with smaller lesions the risk of fatal complications of surgery need to be balanced against the risk of undetected carcinoma.

COMPLICATIONS FROM POLYPECTOMY

As with any procedure, polypectomy has a defined set of possible complications. The most significant complications are those involving hemorrhage and perforation. Removal of large polyps is associated with increased risk to the patient.

Hemorrhagic Complications

The incidence of postpolypectomy hemorrhage is about 2% (7,8,13,17). Major hemorrhage requiring transfusion has a lower incidence, which is 0.4% to 0.9% (8). As mentioned above, Macrae et al. (7) found that significant hemorrhage occurred more frequently in pedunculated polyps with large stalks and sessile polyps larger than 2 cm. Using pooled data from four series, in polyps generally greater than 3.0 cm, hemorrhage occurred in 5% of the resections (6). Some episodes of bleeding may be prevented. One avoidable cause is closure of the wire snare prior to applying coagulation current. This shears blood vessels before they are coagulated. Likewise, closing the snare too quickly will give the same result. Occasionally, a patient may have an unrecognized bleeding disorder as the cause.

There are two recognized patterns of postpolypectomy hemorrhage. The first is immediate hemorrhage, or that occurring within 12 to 24 hours after polypectomy. The second is a delayed hemorrhage, which occurs from 1 to 14 days after polypectomy. Several techniques can be used to endoscopically control the bleeding. Shinya and Wolff (18) described using a solution of 5 ml 1:10,000 epinephrine mixed with 50 ml iced saline to irrigate a bleeding site. The discrete site of bleeding may then undergo application of more coagulating current if necessary. A recent report by Rex et al. (19) has shown that prompt repeat colonoscopy for delayed postpolypectomy hemorrhage is effective and safe. In nine consecutive cases, they used colonoscopy to identify the bleeding site and various combinations of injection therapy, electrocautery, and thermal treatment to halt hemorrhage. A variety of pharmacologic agents have been used by various endoscopists and include pure ethanol, hypertonic saline-epinephrine mixture, or sclerosants. Whereas epinephrine solutions act by constriction of blood vessels, pure ethanol injection leads to necrosis of blood vessels and thrombosis of vessels. A clear benefit of any specific solution in lower tract bleeding has not been demonstrated.

For immediate bleeding after polypectomy, the remnant stalk of a pedunculated polyp may be grabbed with the snare and held for 5 to 10 minutes. Further current may be applied but risks causing snare entrapment in the pedicle. Another technique to control immediate bleeding is to use a sclerotherapy needle and inject a 1:10,000 epinephrine solution around the bleeding site (13). If the above measures fail, angiography and transcatheter infusion of vasopressin remains an option for the patient who continues to bleed (20). For those patients who are candidates, surgical resection remains an option.

Risk of Perforation

The risk of perforation from colonoscopic polypectomy is about 0.1% to 0.3%. Large polyps do not appear to increase the risk, although sessile polyps are slightly more hazardous to resect compared with pedunculated polyps (5). There is a continuum of complications related to coagulation burn extending from a colon coagulation syndrome to frank perforation. Pain during the procedure indicates a transmural burn or perforation, but these events may also initially be silent. The colon coagulation syndrome refers to patients that develop lower quadrant abdominal pain, fever, and leukocytosis. If there is no indication of perforation or diffuse peritonitis, these patients may be managed conservatively with bowel rest and consideration of antibiotics administration. Once frank perforation is detected, surgery should be expedited. Delayed symptoms may be noted and may indicate extension of burn injury to the serosa, even possibly resulting in delayed perforation.

THE HISTOLOGY OF LARGE COLORECTAL POLYPS

Interpreting the histology of large colonic polyps may be difficult, especially those removed piecemeal. Polyps are considered to show evidence of invasive carcinoma if they have malignant cells extending below the muscularis mucosa, presence of malignancy at the margin of a completely resected polyp, malignant cells invading the lymphatics or venous system, or a histology showing a poorly differentiated carcinoma (21). If these criteria are adhered to strictly, the incidence of recurrent malignancy would be rare (5).

Large polyps removed piecemeal pose an occasional problem for the pathologist. Determining the margin of resection and proper orientation was reported to be a problem in 18% of piecemeal polypectomies done by Nivatvongs et al. (22). However, in this series no foci of invasive carcinoma was missed. Every attempt should be made to facilitate recovery of the entire polyp for pathologic examination.

If a large polyp is adequately examined and completely removed colonoscopically, and if it fulfills the criteria to exclude the above evidence for invasive malignancy, then colectomy and lymph node excision for staging may not be warranted, although this remains to be firmly established in the literature (5).

CONCLUSIONS

Advances in colonoscopy and polypectomy technique now permit endoscopists to remove most polypoid lesions from the colon. Large polyps present special challenges, which have been detailed in this chapter. When dealing with large sessile polyps, the endoscopist must weigh the risk that the lesion contains unsuspected invasive carcinoma against the risk of surgical resection. Sessile lesions greater than 4 cm are more likely to harbor cancer and are less likely to be completely ablated with endoscopic techniques, including piecemeal resection and laser photoablation. Most of these patients should undergo surgical resection if they are acceptable surgical candidates. Local recurrence of adenomas after endoscopic removal of large polyps is common and mandates that such patients have surveillance examinations after the initial polypectomy. Since recurrence may well be due to incomplete removal of adenomas during the baseline study, we suggest early (3–6 months) follow-up for all patients undergoing piecemeal resection of large sessile polyps.

It is hoped that future studies will determine the benefits of using mucosal injection of epinephrine in large stalks to prevent hemorrhage, submucosal saline injection for resection of flat polyps, mini-snares, and use of bipolar versus monopolar current for snares. On the horizon are new methods for assessing whether all adenomatous tissue has been resected using autofluorescence spectroscopy or computer-enhanced magnified colonoscopic images. Endoscopic ultrasound may be able to provide information about the depth of involvement with neoplastic tissue. Refinement of polyp abla-

tion methods is under study with determination of the most appropriate laser technique and new application of photodynamic therapy. Perhaps the real key to dealing with large polyps is their prevention. It is hoped that future colon cancer screening strategies will allow us to target sensitive screening tests like colonoscopy for high-risk individuals and prevent the development of large polyps and cancer.

REFERENCES

1. Shinya H, Wolff WI. Morphology, anatomic distribution and cancer potential of colonic polyps: an analysis of 7000 polyps endoscopically removed. *Ann Surg* 1979;190:679–683.
2. Stryker SJ, Wolff BG, Culp LE, Libbe SD, Ilsrup DM, MacCarthy RZ. Natural history of untreated colonic polyps. *Gastroenterology* 1987;93:1009–1013.
3. Bigard MA, Gaucher P, Lassalle C. Fatal gas explosion during colonoscopic polypectomy. *Gastroenterology* 1979;77:1307–1310.
4. Shinya H. *Colonoscopy: diagnosis and treatment of colonic disorders*. New York: Igaka-Shoin, 1982.
5. Gyorffy EJ, Amontree JS, Fenoglio-Preiser CM, Gogel HK, Blessing LD. Large colorectal polyps: colonoscopy, pathology, and management. *Am J Gastroenterol* 1989;84:898–905.
6. Bedogni G, Bertoni G, Ricci E, Conigliaro R, Pedrazzoli C, Rossi G, Meinero M, et al. Colonoscopic excision of large and giant colorectal polyps: technical implications and results over eight years. *Dis Colon Rectum* 1986;29:831–835.
7. Macrae FA, Tan KG, Williams CB. Towards safer colonoscopy: a report of 5000 diagnostic or therapeutic colonoscopies. *Gut* 1983;24:376–383.
8. Van Gossum A, Cozzoli A, Adler M, Taton G, Cremer M. Colonoscopic snare polypectomy: analysis of 1485 resections comparing two types of current. *Gastrointest Endosc* 1992;38:472–475.
9. Waye JD. Approach to the difficult polyp. In: Barkin J, Cesar A, O'Phelan, eds. *Advanced therapeutic endoscopy*. New York: Raven Press, 1990;105–113.
10. Rogers BHG. The use of small caliber endoscopes in selected cases increases the success rate of colonoscopy. *Gastrointest Endosc* 1989;35:352.
11. Waye JD. Techniques of polypectomy: hot biopsy forceps and snare polypectomy. *Am J Gastroenterol* 1987;82:615–618.
12. Tucker RD, Platz CE, Sievert CE, Vennes JA, Silvis SE. *In vivo* evaluation of monopolar versus bipolar electrosurgical polypectomy snares. *Am J Gastroenterol* 1990;85:1386–1390.
13. Waye JD. Gastrointestinal polypectomy. In: Geenen JE, Fleisher DE, Waye JD. eds. *Techniques in therapeutic endoscopy*. 2nd ed. Philadelphia: JB Lippincott, 1992.
14. Brunetaud JM, Mosquet L, Houcke M, et al. Villous adenoma of the rectum: results of endoscopic treatment with argon and neodynium:YAG lasers. *Gastroenterology* 1985;89:832–837.
15. Mathus-Vliegen EM, Tytgat GN. The potential and limitations of laser photoablation of colorectal adenomas. *Gastrointest Endosc* 1991;37:9–17.
16. Patrice T, Jutel P, Lavignolle A, Taupignon A, Cloarec D, le Bodic L. Adenoma laser therapy. *Dig Dis Sci* 1987;32:109–110.
17. Gilbert DA, Hallstrom AP, Shaneyfelt SL, et al. The national ASGE colonoscopy survey—complications of colonoscopy. *Gastrointest Endosc* 1984;30:156.
18. Shinya H, Wolff WI. Colonoscopic polypectomy: technique and safety. *Hosp Pract* 1975;10:71–78.
19. Rex DK, Lewis BS, Waye JD. Colonoscopy and endoscopic therapy for delayed post-polypectomy hemorrhage. *Gastrointest Endosc* 1992;38:127–129.
20. Sanchez F, Rogerg M, Vujic I, Chuang V. Transcatheter control of post-polypectomy hemorrhage. *Gastrointest Radiol* 1986;11:254–256.
21. Morson BC. The polyp-cancer sequence in the large bowel. *Proc R Soc Med* 1974;67:451–457.
22. Nivatvongs S, Snover DC, Fang DT. Piecemeal snare excision of large sessile colon and rectal polyps: is it adequate? *Gastrointest Endosc* 1984;30:18–20.

Advanced Therapeutic Endoscopy, 2nd Ed.,
edited by J. S. Barkin and C. A. O'Phelan.
Raven Press, Ltd., New York © 1994.

CHAPTER 24

Endoscopic Management of Acute Colonic Pseudo-obstruction

David T. Walden and Norman E. Marcon

Acute colonic pseudo-obstruction (ACPO), also known as Ogilvie's syndrome, is a form of colonic ileus characterized by dilation of the colon without evidence of mechanical obstruction (1). It is generally a condition of hospitalized patients and carries a significant morbidity and mortality, primarily resulting from cecal perforation, if not recognized and managed appropriately (2).

The etiology of ACPO is not precisely known, but imbalance of autonomic innervation to the colon (specifically, parasympathetic denervation) resulting in cessation of motility has been postulated as the cause. Gas may then accumulate as a result of aerophagia and bacterial overgrowth, thereby leading to distention. As distention progresses, splitting of the tenia coli occurs with compromise of serosal arterial flow, resulting in ischemia and subsequent ulceration, necrosis, and perforation (3).

ACPO usually occurs as a consequence of severe medical or surgical disease. In a large review, ACPO was associated with recent surgery in 49% of patients and with medical conditions in 45%. ACPO may occur at any age, but is most common in the sixth decade. A male preponderance of 1.5–4.0:1 has been reported (4–6). Conditions and factors associated with ACPO are outlined in Table 1.

DIAGNOSIS

The most common presenting complaint is marked abdominal distention, which occurs in virtually all patients (7). Distention usually progresses gradually over

D. T. Walden and N. E. Marcon: Division of Gastroenterology, The Wellesley Hospital, Toronto, Ontario M4Y 1J3, Canada.

2 to 3 days, but may be more acute in some cases. Mild-to-moderate abdominal pain is a frequent complaint, reported in 83% of patients with ACPO in one large review (6). Nausea and vomiting occur in 50% to 80% of cases (6,8). Dyspnea may result from distention in some patients (9). A reduction in stool volume is common, but some patients continue to pass flatus and liquid stool.

On examination, the abdomen is distended and tympanitic, but is generally soft. Bowel sounds are present in most patients. Abdominal tenderness was seen in 64% of patients with viable bowel and in 87% of patients with ischemia or perforation in one series (6). Low-grade fever is commonly seen. Gastric aspiration yields small volumes of nonfeculent fluid (10).

There are no specific laboratory findings useful in the diagnosis of ACPO. A mild leukocytosis of 12,000 to 15,000/mm^3 with left shift is often seen. Marked leukocytosis may indicate ischemia or perforation, occurring in nearly all patients with these complications (6). Serum electrolyte disturbances usually reflect the underlying disease process (11).

Flat and upright roentegenography of the abdomen is the most important diagnostic study in cases of suspected ACPO. The most common finding is a dilated, gas-filled proximal colon, usually without air-fluid levels (Fig. 1) (10,12). An abrupt "cutoff" is frequently noted between the dilated and nondilated segments at the hepatic (18%) or splenic (56%) flexures or in the descending or sigmoid colon (27%) (6,13). The mucosal pattern and haustral markings are usually preserved in ACPO in contrast to toxic megacolon complicating severe inflammatory bowel disease where mucosal edema (thumbprinting) may be seen (14). Coexisting small bowel dilation is not unusual (6). Upright films should be reviewed for evidence of free air, but this is

223

TABLE 1. *Causes of acute colonic pseudo-obstruction*

General
  Myocardial infarction
  Congestive heart failure
  Renal failure
  Respiratory failure
  Pancreatitis
  Systemic lupus erythematosus
  Metastatic carcinoma
  Idiopathic
Drugs
  Narcotics
  Phenothiazines
  Tricyclic antidepressants
  Calcium channel blockers
  Clonidine
Metabolic
  Hypokalemia
  Hyponatremia
  Hypocalcemia
  Hypothyroidism
Toxic
  Alcoholism
  Lead poisoning
Infectious
  Sepsis
  Pneumonia
  Meningitis
  Herpes zoster
  Tuberculous peritonitis
Neurological
  Organic brain syndrome
  Stroke
  Multiple sclerosis
  Myotonic dystrophy
  Parkinson's disease
  Guillain-Barré syndrome
Surgical
  Multiple trauma
  Burns
  Coronary bypass
  Craniotomy
  Lumbar laminectomy
  Fracture
  Hip replacement
  Nephrectomy
  Cystectomy
  Herniorrhaphy
OB/Gyn
  Vaginal delivery
  Cesarean section
  Therapeutic abortion
  Hysterectomy

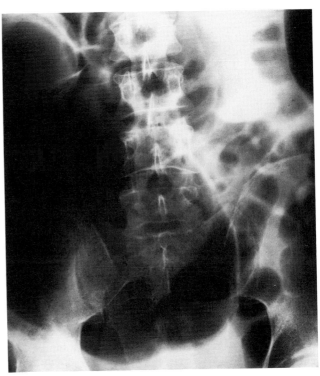

FIG. 1. Massive dilation of cecum and ascending colon.

DIFFERENTIAL DIAGNOSIS

The differential diagnosis of ACPO most importantly includes mechanical obstruction of the colon due to neoplasm, adhesions, incarcerated hernia, cecal or sigmoid volvulus, or fecal impaction. Mesenteric is-

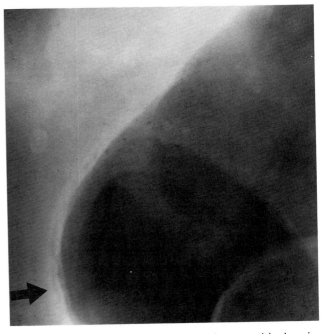

FIG. 2. Intramural air *(arrow)* indicating cecal ischemia.

absent in about half of cases of ACPO with documented perforation (3). Careful attention must be given to the walls of the dilated segments as the presence of intramural air is strongly indicative of ischemic injury (Fig. 2). Cecal diameter should be measured whenever ACPO is suspected with a value of 12 cm or greater, indicating need for aggressive management in most cases as discussed below.

chemia may produce similar findings and is encountered in many of the same clinical settings (14,15). Chronic intestinal pseudo-obstruction is characterized by a history of recurrent episodes of obstructive symptoms and is generally seen in ambulatory patients (16). Other causes of severe abdominal distention are acute gastric dilation and adynamic intestinal ileus, the former easily distinguished on x-ray and the latter characterized by absence of bowel sounds along with evidence of concurrent small bowel dilation on x-ray.

MANAGEMENT

The goal of management of ACPO is prevention of colonic perforation and its morbid sequelae while attempts are made to improve the precipitating condition. Factors associated with increased mortality include advanced age, cecal diameter greater than 14 cm, duration of distention greater than 7 days, presence of ischemia or perforation, and need for surgical therapy (6). Management strategies have been divided into three levels (17), which are discussed below. Level 1 measures are supportive and emphasize removal of exacerbating factors and treatment of the underlying disease process. Level 2 measures include colonoscopic and radiologic decompression techniques. Level 3 involves surgical therapy. A rigid sequential management program is not implied as level 1 measures are used in all patients, but not to the exclusion of more aggressive decompression whenever clinically indicated. To select the appropriate initial therapy, there must be assessment of cecal diameter and exclusion of mechanical obstruction.

Cecal Diameter and Perforation Risk

According to the law of Laplace, the pressure required to stretch the wall of a hollow viscus decreases in inverse proportion to its diameter. Thus, the cecum would be predicted to be at highest risk for pressure-related injury as it is the segment of greatest diameter in the colon. Kozarek and Sanowski (18) have shown using human cadavers that the pressure necessary to induce colonic perforation is indeed lowest in the cecum.

Cecal perforation has been reported as a complication in approximately 15% of ACPO cases and carries a mortality of 43% to 75%, largely due to severe underlying disease (3,19,20). Cecal diameter is an imperfect indicator of impending perforation and must be considered in the overall clinical context. Normal cecal diameter is 3.5 to 8.5 cm (11); a diameter ≥9 cm is cause for concern and indicates a need for serial follow-up with abdominal x-rays at 12- to 24-hour intervals. Cecal perforation did not occur in any case of ACPO where

the diameter was ≤12 cm in a large review, whereas ischemia or perforation was seen in 23% of patients with cecal diameter over 14 cm (6). Also, there have been reports of patients with cecal diameters of up to 25 cm in whom perforation did not occur (21). Moreover, unrecognized perforation may result in cecal decompression, giving a false sense of security if cecal diameter is considered as an isolated parameter.

Given the absence of strong correlation between cecal diameter and risk of perforation, arbitrary thresholds have been selected by various authors ranging from 9 to 14 cm, above which aggressive management is indicated (7,11). We generally elect a period of conservative management in stable patients presenting with a cecal diameter of 12 cm or less and proceed to early decompression in cases where the initial cecal diameter is greater than 12 cm or where there is clinical deterioration. Clinical assessment of noncommunicative or unresponsive patients in the intensive care unit may be difficult and underscores the need for regular abdominal examination and x-ray assessment every 12 to 24 hours during the initial stages of management.

Of note, in a series of 24 cancer patients with ACPO presenting with cecal diameters ranging from 9 to 18 cm managed conservatively without colonoscopic or surgical decompression, spontaneous improvement occurred in 96% in a mean of 3 days with no perforations and no ACPO-related deaths (22). This observation suggests that there may be a subset of cancer patients with ACPO that is more likely to respond to conservative management and tolerates distention with fewer complications. However, perforation is well-described in cancer patients with ACPO and there is no reliable method of predicting which patients might be managed conservatively and which should undergo decompression. Given that these patients are debilitated and are especially intolerant of perforation, we do not modify our management approach simply because the patient has cancer and will proceed to decompression as necessary following the criteria outlined below.

Exclusion of Mechanical Obstruction

Mechanical obstruction must be excluded in all cases of suspected ACPO, either by contrast enema or colonoscopy. Patients in whom conservative management (see below) is initially elected should undergo water soluble contrast enema with an agent such as diatrizoate (Gastrografin). Barium should be avoided as it may interfere with visualization in the event that colonoscopy is required and may result in peritoneal soilage if an unexpected perforation is present. Once contrast has reached the dilated segment without demonstrable evidence of obstruction, the examination should be terminated in order to prevent increased distention. Contrast enema may be of therapeutic value in the case of sigmoid volvulus in which reduction may occur. Also, the osmotic character of these agents may promote emptying of the distal bowel in patients with ACPO. Colonoscopy may be carried out safely in the unprepared bowel in this setting and has the advantage of allowing both diagnosis and therapy with a single procedure. It is our practice to forgo contrast enema in cases where early colonoscopic decompression is anticipated. However, contrast enema is mandatory in cases where the dilated segment is not successfully reached with colonoscopy. Neither contrast enema nor colonoscopy should be attempted in patients with peritoneal irritation or evidence of perforation (23).

INITIAL THERAPY

The focus of level 1 management of ACPO is supportive care and removal of exacerbating factors, measures appropriate for all patients. Mechanical obstruction should be excluded at this point as outlined above. Patients are kept NPO and a nasogastric tube is placed to low intermittent suction to reduce the accumulation of swallowed air. Fluids are given as necessary and electrolyte abnormalities are corrected. Drugs such as narcotic analgesics, clonidine, phenothiazines, and anticholinergics should be discontinued. Oral laxatives are not indicated. Gentle tap water enemas may be given to eliminate formed stool from the rectum. Rectal tube placement is seldom helpful and should be avoided except in the few cases in which dilation extends to the sigmoid colon, as there is a risk of perforation (6). Patients should be rolled from side to side and into the prone position to promote movement of gas through the colon as in the management of toxic megacolon (24).

There have been cases reports of successful treatment of ACPO with prokinetic agents. An elderly woman with ACPO complicating congestive heart failure and pneumonia responded rapidly to cisapride 10 mg IV given every 4 hours with a marked decrease in cecal diameter (25). Another patient was treated with erythromycin (a motilin agonist) 250 mg IV every 8 hours for 3 days with resolution of colonic dilation (26). Neither patient experienced recurrence. These agents are safe in the absence of mechanical obstruction and may prove to be useful adjuncts in the treatment of ACPO. Metoclopramide is not useful in this setting. Epidural anesthesia was used in a small series of ACPO patients with some success in reducing distention (27).

NONOPERATIVE DECOMPRESSION

The success of conservative measures is variable, ranging from 32% to 96% with a recurrence rate of approximately 30% (11,17,22,28). Patients must be followed closely with abdominal films every 12 to 24 hours and should undergo prompt decompression if cecal diameter remains above 12 cm for more than 24 hours, if dilation progresses, or if there is clinical deterioration.

Colonoscopic decompression (CD) is the most important of the level 2 measures, with radiologic decompression and endoscopic cecostomy rarely indicated. Since its description in 1977 (29), CD has become the preferred technique, allowing effective decompression with minimal complications in most cases of ACPO and reducing the need for surgery. Subsequent refinements involving placement of transanal decompression tubes have increased the initial success rate and have limited recurrences.

Technique of Colonoscopic Decompression

Bowel preparation is contraindicated in ACPO and is unnecessary in most cases as the stool is usually liquid and does not interfere with insertion. A tap water enema may be administered 30 minutes before CD if formed stool is present in the rectum. CD may be performed without sedation in most cases. Fluoroscopy is strongly recommended to confirm the depth of insertion and to maintain wire position when a decompression tube is to be placed; however, successful CD may be performed at the bedside in patients too ill to transport.

A large channel colonoscope is preferred for decompression, but is not essential. The colonoscope is inserted and cautiously advanced above the air-fluid interface using minimal air insufflation and appropriate suction. Frequent irrigation is often required in the rectum and sigmoid. Formed stool is generally confined to the rectum if present. Need for the "slide-by" maneuver should be minimized through the use of fluoroscopy to identify the correct direction for advancement. Despite lack of preparation, it has been our experience that insertion usually proceeds in a timely manner and is not significantly more difficult than colonoscopy in the prepared bowel. However, there are cases in which the presence of large quantities of formed stool renders the procedure considerably more labor-intensive, demanding patience and persistence on the part of the endoscopist. Effective decompression generally requires that the tip of the colonoscope be advanced proximal to the hepatic flexure (17). When this area is reached, the underlying mucosa should be carefully assessed. The findings of mucosal duskiness or ulceration are indicative of ischemic injury (Fig. 3) and should preclude further advancement, although decompression should be carried out before termination of the procedure. In the absence of these findings, in-

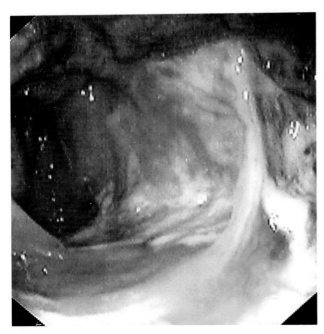

FIG. 3. Endoscopic appearance of cecal ischemia. Note mucosal erythema and ulceration.

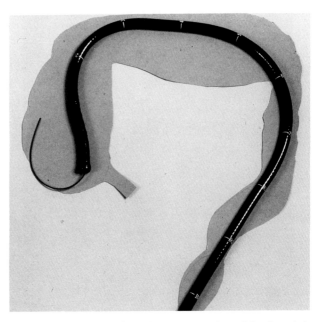

FIG. 4. Colonoscopic placement of guidewire into cecum.

sertion to the cecum should be completed with special attention paid to examination of the antimesenteric aspect of the anterior colonic wall, which is at highest risk for ischemic injury (30). The presence of ischemic mucosal changes is an indication for prompt surgical therapy, as most patients are seriously ill and are poorly tolerant of perforation.

Decompression is accomplished by slowly withdrawing the colonoscope with suctioning of both air and liquid stool until collapse of the lumen is achieved. Frequent irrigation may be required during this portion of the procedure. This method allows effective decompression in approximately 80% to 89% of cases (4,6), but recurrence has been a major problem with rates of 44% to 58% reported (28,31).

To increase the success of decompression and to avoid recurrent episodes of dilation and need for further procedures, techniques of colonoscopic tube placement have been developed. The earliest of these involved use of a modified 16 French Baker jejunostomy tube. A loop of suture in the tip of the tube was grasped by biopsy forceps and used to carry the tube to the ascending colon (32). While providing satisfactory decompression, the disadvantages of this technique include the inability to irrigate and suction without employing a double-channel colonoscope and the risk of displacing the tube upon endoscope withdrawal.

We have had success with a Seldinger technique (31,33) in which a 480-cm 0.035-inch guidewire is advanced through a colonoscope positioned in the cecum or ascending colon until a coil is noted under fluoros-

copy (Fig. 4). The colonoscope is then withdrawn over the wire with initial decompression carried out by thorough suctioning. The position of the wire tip is monitored throughout endoscope withdrawal using fluoroscopy. A Salem sump tube of at least 140 cm in length or an enteroclysis tube modified with extra side holes cut near the tip is then lubricated and advanced over the wire under fluoroscopic guidance (Fig. 5). Insertion usually proceeds easily, but looping may be noted. Should this occur, advancement may be facilitated by

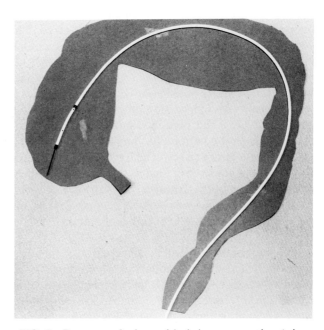

FIG. 5. Passage of wire-guided decompression tube.

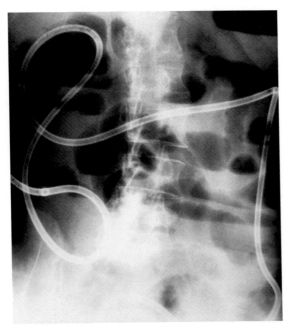

FIG. 6. Decompression tube positioned in cecum.

withdrawing the tube a short distance and reinserting with axial rotation while withdrawing a short length of wire from the cecal coil. In the situation where added wire stiffness may be required to aid tube passage, a 6 French biliary stent placement catheter may be inserted over the wire as far as the right colon prior to decompression tube insertion.

Following placement, the wire is removed, and the tube is secured to the inner thigh and connected to low intermittent suction. The tube should be irrigated with 100 cc of water every 2 hours to prevent clogging. Efficacy of decompression should be confirmed by abdominal films shortly after tube placement (Fig. 6) and then on a daily basis until the condition has resolved. The decompression tube is left in place while the precipitating condition is treated. Resolution of ACPO generally occurs within 3 to 6 days, but may occasionally require longer (17). We have noted no adverse effect in patients with transanal decompression tubes in place for in excess of 1 week. The tube may be removed once the patient's general condition has improved and abdominal distention has been resolved for 24 hours, but often will pass spontaneously under these circumstances once colonic motility resumes. Failure of a properly positioned tube to provide ongoing decompression suggests tube migration or clogging and may necessitate repeat CD.

As an alternative bedside technique for decompression tube placement in patients in whom fluoroscopy is not practical, a 10 French nasobiliary tube may be placed directly through the colonoscope into the dilated segment without the need for wire guidance. While this method may provide some added benefit

over CD alone, clogging may limit its effectiveness. Use of a large-caliber fenestrated overtube is an alternative technique that may reduce the likelihood of clogging (34).

Colonoscopic decompression tube placement is technically easy, does not significantly prolong procedure time, and is effective in both initial decompression and prevention of recurrence. In a retrospective comparison of 9 ACPO patients who underwent CD alone with 11 patients who underwent colonoscopic decompression with enteroclysis tube placement by a wire-guided technique (CDT), there were no recurrences in the CDT group versus a 44% recurrence rate in the CD group (31). We now utilize tube placement as initial management in all cases of ACPO requiring colonoscopic decompression.

Complications

Considering the frequency of severe concurrent illness and the lack of bowel preparation, complications of CD are surprisingly rare. In a thorough review of published series, the overall complication rate of CD was 2.9% with a mortality rate of 1.0% (4). Complications included respiratory arrest in a burned patient, hypotension (35), and a non-fatal cecal perforation (36). The only death occurred in a patient who developed a sigmoid perforation 8 days after CD (37).

Percutaneous Endoscopic Cecostomy (PEC)

Endoscopic techniques may be used to provide percutaneous decompression when repeated attempts at CD are unsuccessful (38,39). Ponsky et al. (39) have described cecostomy using a method similar to that employed for percutaneous endoscopic gastrostomy, which resulted in satisfactory decompression through a large caliber tube in two cases. This technique should be considered in the rare instance of cecal dilation refractory to CD. PEC requires passage of the colonoscope to the cecum. If this is possible, failure of CD with tube placement to provide satisfactory decompression is highly unusual and should always be attempted first. PEC is not a substitute for surgical therapy in cases where ischemic injury has occurred.

Radiologic Decompression

Successful cecal decompression has been reported using a technique of computed tomography (CT)-directed percutaneous puncture via the retroperitoneal approach (40). This technique may be of value when CD is not available and in patients who are unable to tolerate further endoscopic or surgical procedures.

SURGERY

Tube cecostomy is the preferred operative decompression technique in ACPO and may be performed under local anesthesia in critically ill patients (41), but carries a mortality of 12% to 30% (6). Laparoscopic cecostomy in ACPO has recently been described (42). Laparotomy with resection of the involved segments is indicated in cases where ischemic injury or perforation has occurred and is associated with a mortality rate of 36% to 44%, largely the result of severe concurrent illness (6).

SUMMARY

The key to successful management of ACPO is early recognition and prevention of perforation through exclusion of mechanical obstruction, identification and elimination of precipitating factors, and judicious use of decompression techniques as indicated by clinical status and cecal diameter. Colonoscopic decompression tube placement is safe and effective and should be the initial procedure whenever decompression is indicated. Endoscopic and radiologic cecostomy may be helpful in rare instances. Surgery is seldom required except in cases of ischemic injury or perforation.

REFERENCES

1. Ogilvie H. Large-intestine colic due to sympathetic deprivation. *Br Med J* 1948;2:671–673.
2. Dorudi S, Berry AR, Kettlewell MGW. Acute colonic pseudo-obstruction. *Br J Surg* 1992;79:99–103.
3. Gierson ED, Storm FK, Shaw W, Coyne SK. Caecal rupture due to colonic ileus. *Br J Surg* 1975;62:383–386.
4. Gosche JR, Sharpe JN, Larson GM. Colonoscopic decompression for pseudo-obstruction of the colon. *Am Surg* 1989;55:111–115.
5. Norton L, Young D, Scribner R. Management of pseudo-obstruction of the colon. *Surg Gynecol Obstet* 1974;138:595–598.
6. Vanek VW, Al-Salti M. Acute pseudo-obstruction of the colon (Ogilvie's syndrome). *Dis Colon Rectum* 1986;29:203–210.
7. Geelhoed GW. Colonic pseudo-obstruction in surgical patients. *Am J Surg* 1985;149:258–265.
8. Apostolakis E, Thiel R, Bircks W. Acute pseudo-obstruction of the colon (Ogilvie's syndrome) following open heart surgery. *Thorac Cardiovasc Surg* 1990;38:371–373.
9. Wojtalik RS, Lindenauer SM, Kahn SS. Perforation of the colon associated with adynamic ileus. *Am J Surg* 1973;125:601–606.
10. Choo Y-C. Ileus of the colon with cecal dilatation and perforation. *Obstet Gynecol* 1979;54:241–245.
11. Bachulis BL, Smith PE. Pseudoobstruction of the colon. *Am J Surg* 1978;136:66–72.
12. Adams JT. Adynamic ileus of the colon. An indication for cecostomy. *Arch Surg* 1974;109:503–507.
13. Freilich HS, Chopra S, Gilliam JI. Acute colonic pseudo-obstruction or Ogilvie's syndrome. *J Clin Gastroenterol* 1986;8:457–460.
14. Bryk D, Soong KY. Colonic ileus and its differential roentgen diagnosis. *Am J Roentgenol* 1967;101:329–337.
15. Feldman RA, Karl RC. Diagnosis and treatment of Ogilvie's syndrome after lumbar spinal surgery. *J Neurosurg* 1992;76:1012–1016.
16. Faulk DL, Anuras S, Christensen J. Chronic intestinal pseudo-obstruction. *Gastroenterology* 1978;74:922–931.
17. Fausel CS, Goff JS. Nonoperative management of acute idiopathic colonic pseudo-obstruction (Ogilvie's syndrome). *West J Med* 1985;143:50–54.
18. Kozarek RA, Sanowski RA. Use of pressure release valve to prevent colonic injury during colonoscopy. *Gastrointest Endosc* 1980;26:139–142.
19. Lowman RM, Davis L. An evaluation of cecal size in impending perforation of the cecum. *Surg Gynecol Obstet* 1956;103:711–718.
20. Nanni G, Garbini A, Luchetti P, Nanni G, Ronconi P, Castagneto M. Ogilvie's syndrome (acute colonic pseudo-obstruction). *Dis Colon Rectum* 1982;25:157–166.
21. Baker DA, Morin ME, Tan A, Sue HK. Colonic ileus. Indication for prompt decompression. *JAMA* 1979;241:2633–2634.
22. Sloyer AF, Panella VS, Demas BE, Shike M, Lightdale CJ, Winawer SJ, Kurtz RC. Ogilvie's syndrome. Successful management without colonoscopy. *Dig Dis Sci* 1988;33:1391–1396.
23. Nakhgevany KB. Colonoscopic decompression of the colon in patients with Ogilvie's syndrome. *Am J Surg* 1984;148:317–320.
24. Present DH, Wolfson D, Gelernt IM, Rubin PH, Bauer J, Chapman ML. Medical decompression of toxic megacolon by "rolling." *J Clin Gastroenterol* 1988;10:485–490.
25. MacColl C, MacCannell KL, Baylis B, Lee SS. Treatment of acute colonic pseudoobstruction (Ogilvie's syndrome) with cisapride. *Gastroenterology* 1990;98:773–776.
26. Bonacini M, Smith OJ, Pritchard T. Erythromycin as therapy for acute colonic pseudo-obstruction (Ogilvie's syndrome). *J Clin Gastroenterol* 1991;13:475–476.
27. Lee JT, Taylor BM, Singleton BC. Epidural anesthesia for acute pseudo-obstruction of the colon (Ogilvie's syndrome). *Dis Colon Rectum* 1988;31:686–691.
28. Nano D, Prindiville T, Pauly M, Chow H, Ross K, Trudeau W. Colonoscopic therapy of acute pseudoobstruction of the colon. *Am J Gastroenterol* 1987;82:145–148.
29. Kukora JS, Dent TL. Colonoscopic decompression of massive nonobstructive cecal dilation. *Arch Surg* 1977;112:512–517.
30. Spira IA, Wolff WI. Gangrene and spontaneous perforation of the cecum as a complication of pseudo-obstruction of the colon. *Dis Colon Rectum* 1976;19:557–562.
31. Harig JM, Fumo DE, Loo FD, Parker HJ, Soergel KH, Helm JF, Hogan WJ. Treatment of nontoxic megacolon during colonoscopy: tube placement versus simple decompression. *Gastrointest Endosc* 1988;34:23–27.
32. Bernton E, Myers R, Reyna T. Pseudo-obstruction of the colon. *Curr Surg* 1983;40:30–31.
33. Messmer JM, Wolper JC, Loewe CJ. Endoscopic-assisted tube placement for decompression of acute colonic pseudo-obstruction. *Endoscopy* 1984;16:135–136.
34. Burke G, Shellito PC. Treatment of recurrent colonic pseudo-obstruction by endoscopic placement of a fenestrated overtube. *Dis Colon Rectum* 1987;30:615–619.
35. Starling JR. Treatment of nontoxic megacolon by colonoscopy. *Surgery* 1983;94:677–682.
36. Strodel WE, Nostrant TT, Eckhauser FE, Dent TL. Therapeutic and diagnostic colonoscopy in non-obstructive colonic dilatation. *Ann Surg* 1983;197:416–421.
37. Bode WE Beart RW Jr, Spencer RJ, Culp CE, Wolff BG, Taylor BM. Colonoscopic decompression for acute pseudoobstruction of the colon (Ogilvie's syndrome). *Am J Surg* 1984;147:243–245.
38. Ganc AJ, Faria Netto AJ, Morrell AC, Plapler H, Ardengh JC. Transcolonoscopic extraperitoneal cecostomy. A new therapeutic and technical proposal. *Endoscopy* 1988;20:309–312.
39. Ponsky JL, Aszodi A, Perse D. Percutaneous endoscopic cecostomy: a new approach to nonobstructive colonic dilation. *Gastrointest Endosc* 1986;32:108–111.
40. Crass JR, Simmons RL, Frick MP, Maile CW. Percutaneous decompression of the colon using CT guidance in Ogilvie syndrome. *AJR* 1985;144:475–476.
41. Groff W. Colonoscopic decompression and intubation of the cecum for Ogilvie's syndrome. *Dis Colon Rectum* 1983;26:503–506.
42. Duh QY, Way LW. Diagnostic laparoscopy and laparoscopic cecostomy for colonic pseudo-obstruction. *Dis Colon Rectum* 1993;36:65–70.

Advanced Therapeutic Endoscopy, 2nd Ed.,
edited by J. S. Barkin and C. A. O'Phelan.
Raven Press, Ltd., New York © 1994.

CHAPTER 25

Endoscopic Management of Colonic Strictures: Technology and Follow-Up

David Bernstein and Howard D. Manten

Colonic stricture is not an uncommon problem encountered by gastroenterologists and surgeons, and recent advances in colonoscopic capabilities have shifted its initial therapy from the surgical arena to the gastrointestinal endoscopy suite. Colonoscopy has allowed access to strictures previously inaccessible to rigid sigmoidoscopy, has improved the ability to diagnose the etiology of colonic strictures, and has enabled endoscopic therapy of colonic strictures to be performed safely and effectively.

The diagnosis of colonic stricture is usually made after symptoms of obstruction or partial obstruction are described and either a barium or Gastrografin contrast enema reveals the presence of colonic narrowing. Asymptomatic colonic strictures are occasionally seen on routine contrast enemas. However, spasm may mimic the appearance of strictures on radiologic contrast examination. Therefore, all strictures seen on contrast examination must be confirmed by colonoscopy. Bernard et al. (1) found that single contrast enema established the diagnosis in 38% of colonic strictures and that colonoscopy following single contrast enema increased the diagnostic accuracy to 81%. We therefore recommend that all radiologic colonic strictures be confirmed by colonoscopy and that all strictures be biopsied at colonoscopy to rule out the presence of neoplasm.

It is imperative that a stricture be evaluated prior to therapy. Forde and Treat (2) reported that an adult colonoscope of standard diameter and stiffness was unable to traverse 54% of colonic strictures seen on contrast exam. Kozarek et al. (3) used an Olympus XQ-10 pediatric upper endoscope with a 9.8 mm diameter

and 102 cm length (Olympus Corp., New Hyde Park, NY) to successfully traverse 27 of 31 (87%) colonic strictures or fixed sigmoid loops that could not be traversed with a standard Olympus CF-1T-10L colonoscope with a 13.7 mm diameter and 168 cm length. Bat and Williams (4) utilized a PCF 10 pediatric colonoscope with a diameter of 11.3 cm (Olympus) to pass through 13 strictures that could not be passed with an adult colonoscope. The use of smaller-diameter endoscopes has improved the ability to traverse colonic strictures. However, this does not mean that smaller-diameter instruments such as pediatric colonoscopes should be the instrument of choice. Although the increased flexibility and smaller diameter allow for passage through the stricture, they do not always allow for complete evaluation of the remaining colon, as Kozarek et al. were able to reach the cecum only 60% of the time using a smaller pediatric endoscope (Olympus XQ-10). We therefore advocate the initial use of an adult colonoscope in the evaluation of colonic stricture. If an adult colonoscope is unsuccessful in passing the stricture, a pediatric colonoscope is the logical next choice to continue the evaluation. In our experience, we have utilized a pediatric upper endoscope to examine the colon in patients with strictures unable to be traversed with a pediatric colonoscope and have been able to reach the cecum in the majority of cases (5).

The addition of brush cytology and biopsy of the stricture will increase the diagnostic yield of colonoscopy and should be performed when the stricture is seen through the colonoscope. Mortensen et al. (6), in a report on the evaluation of 29 benign and 55 malignant strictures, found that biopsy alone was correct in 68% of patients, cytological brushing alone was correct in 81% of cases, and a combination of biopsy and brushing gave a diagnostic yield of 88%. Benvenuti et al. (7)

D. Bernstein and H. D. Manten: Division of Gastroenterology, University of Miami School of Medicine/Jackson Memorial Hospital, Miami, Florida 33101.

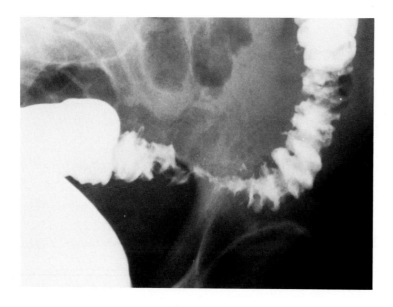

FIG. 1. Colonic stricture on barium enema (*arrows*).

reported a 100% diagnostic yield utilizing both brush cytology and biopsy in evaluating malignant colorectal stricture.

The most common site of stricture is the sigmoid colon (70–77%) followed by the descending colon (15%), with the remainder of the sites scattered throughout the colon and ileocolonic anastomoses (1,2).

DILATATION OF COLONIC STRICTURES

The initial evaluation of a colonic stricture should determine whether or not it is benign or malignant (Figs. 1 and 2). Once this is determined, a decision

must be reached on treatment of the stricture. Endoscopic therapy should be reserved for symptomatic strictures whose benefit of treatment outweighs the risks of the procedure. Several different techniques of dilatation are available to the colonoscopist and are listed in Table 1. Regardless of the technique used in dilation, the colon should be adequately prepped prior to the examination. We recommend an oral colon preparation utilizing 4 liters of a polyethylene glycol solution (e.g., Golytely, Nulytely) the day prior to examination and a gentle tap water enema on the morning of the procedure in patients with partial colonic obstruction secondary to stricture. In patients with complete obstruction, we do not recommend the above regimen but instead prep the colon with two tap water enemas (5).

Prior to dilation, informed consent with careful explanation of the risk of perforation and bleeding must be obtained from the patient. The patient should be

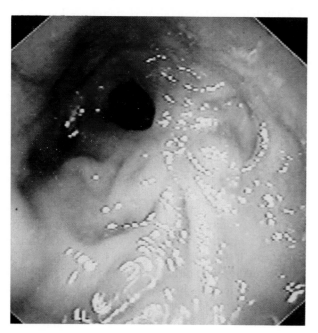

FIG. 2. Anastomotic stricture of the colon.

TABLE 1. *Techniques of colonic stricture dilatation*

Balloon dilatation
  Transendoscopic dilatation
    Through the scope
    Over a wire
  Nontransendoscopic dilatation over a wire
  Combined
Rigid dilatation
  Foley catheter dilatation
  Modified Lister urethral dilatation
  Modified Stark dilatation
  Progressive sigmoidoscopes of increasing diameter
  Hollow-core dilatation
    Savary dilatation
    Eder-Puestow dilatation
    Maloney dilatation
Electrocautery incision
Laser ablation

made aware that the dilation process may require several sessions and that surgical treatment may be required in the event dilation fails as well as for complications of the procedure.

After the dilation is complete, the patient should be observed for several hours and the vital signs should be monitored. A Hypaque enema should be performed to confirm dilation and to ensure no perforation has occurred. The patient may be discharged on a regular diet with careful instruction regarding symptoms of bleeding and perforation. The physician should contact the patient the following day to be sure no untoward effects of the procedure have occurred.

Balloon Dilation

The first description of the clinically successful use of hydrostatic balloon dilation catheters was reported by Gruntzig and Hopff (8) in 1974 in treating atheromatous lesions of the iliac, femoral, and popliteal vessels. Since this original description, balloon dilation catheters have been used to dilate stenotic lesions in the cardiovascular and urological systems (9). London et al. (10) were the first to apply balloon dilation to the gastrointestinal tract in 1980 in treating esophageal strictures. Subsequently, balloon catheter dilation has been applied to the upper gastrointestinal tract, the biliary tree, and the colon (11,12). In 1983, Ball et al. (13) dilated ischemic strictures in colons of infants with balloon catheters (13). Brower and Freeman (14) in 1984 were the first to utilize balloon catheter dilation in the adult colon. In our study, we reported eight of ten patients with rectosigmoid strictures who were successfully treated with balloon dilation (5).

Balloon dilation catheters offer several advantages over conventional rigid dilation techniques. Balloon dilation allows for direct visualization and affords the endoscopist greater control over the procedure. The flexibility of balloon catheters makes them ideally suited for tortuous segments of the gastrointestinal tract such as the sigmoid colon, and these catheters are able to be passed through tight strictures. On inflation, the balloon exerts a radial pressure on the stricture as opposed to the longitudinal and shearing forces of conventional rigid dilating methods. The radial pressure is transmitted equally throughout the segment and, in theory, should decrease the risk of perforation. The balloons are constructed of an inelastic polymer and can only be inflated to a preset maximum diameter. Excess pressure will not lead to overinflation but will result in the ripping of the balloon. The procedure is well tolerated and may be done in an outpatient facility under conscious sedation. This technique appears to be effective and relatively safe, although it is not without risk.

Balloons are available in a variety of lengths and diameters. The decision regarding the type of balloon to use is dictated by the etiology, length, and diameter of the stricture. Wire-guided and balloon dilators can be passed directly or transendoscopically.

Multiple studies have reported successful technical dilatation of colonic strictures with balloon catheters. Successful balloon dilation is defined as the ability to easily pass the endoscope through the stricture immediately following the dilation (15). A national survey of hydrostatic balloon dilation of colonic strictures reported a technical success rate of 79% with 56% achieving immediate symptomatic relief and 75% of those patients reporting symptomatic relief for greater than 3 months. The subset of patients with anastomotic strictures reported an 86% technical success rate with 73% achieving immediate symptomatic relief and 86% of those patients reporting relief for greater than 3 months (16). Balloon size appears to be important in symptomatic relief. Balloons of size 21 to 40 French had a 50% success rate as defined symptomatically, while balloons greater than 51 French had a 90% improvement in symptoms (16).

Balloon dilation may not be completely successful after a single session and multiple dilations are sometimes required to adequately relieve symptoms. We recommend starting with a small caliber stricture and bringing the patient back for repeat dilation every 2 to 4 weeks until symptoms abate.

Transendoscopic Balloon Dilation

Transendoscopic balloon dilation is commonly used in colonic stricture. These balloons are excellent for stricture therapy as they are passed through a standard endoscopic biopsy channel and can be introduced into the stricture under direct vision. Fluoroscopy is not required to perform transendoscopic balloon dilation (15,17). Despite these studies showing successful transendoscopic balloon dilation, we recommend the use of fluoroscopy in all colonic dilation.

Standard equipment for transendoscopic balloon dilation includes (a) balloons of various length and diameter (Fig. 3), (b) a pressure gauge to monitor pressure, (c) an inflation device, and (d) silicone spray or liquid.

Standard transendoscopic balloons vary in diameter and length and have different maximum inflatable pressures. Transendoscopic balloons vary in diameter from 4 to 25 mm. Balloon length ranges from 2 to 8 cm, with the length of the radiopaque guidewire either 180 or 210 cm. The maximum recommended pressures in pounds per square inch (PSI) is dependent on balloon size and should not be exceeded. These maximum pressures are found on the balloon packaging and on the balloon hub. All through-the-scope (TTS) balloons

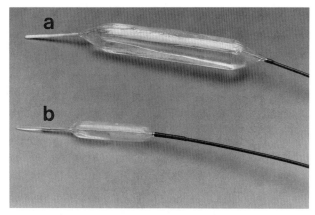

FIG. 3. Balloon dilators. **a:** Through-the-scope balloon (Microvasive). **b:** Bard balloons.

(Microvasive) will fit through a standard 2.8-mm endoscopic biopsy channel except the 20 mm and 25 mm TTS balloons, which require a 3.7-mm biopsy channel. TTS balloons have a built-in guidewire or stiffener that enables transendoscopic passage. Hobbs transendoscopic balloon dilators are placed over a guidewire and fit through a standard 2.8-mm endoscopic biopsy channel. We prefer to use longer transendoscopic balloons (6–8 cm) as shorter balloons tend to slip out of a stricture during inflation.

Inflation of the balloon may be obtained with a syringe, a screw-type inflation syringe (Medi-tech), a Rigiflator inflation-deflation gun (Microvasive), or newer digital inflation devices (Fig. 4). Mechanical inflation devices are very useful in dilation since they help decrease the incidence of overinflation and allow for a more uniform pressure throughout the dilation period.

The technique of transendoscopic balloon dilation is as follows. First, the balloon is inflated prior to insertion into the colonoscope to evaluate for leaks. The colonoscope is then passed to the stricture and, if possible, through the stricture. The colonoscope is withdrawn 1 to 2 cm distal to the stricture. The balloon catheter is well lubricated with silicone and passed into the endoscopic biopsy channel and into the stricture under direct vision. The balloon is positioned in the center of the stricture, inflated to the recommended inflation pressure, and maintained in position for 60 seconds. If the procedure is performed under fluoroscopy, the balloon waist is positioned in the center of the stricture and the balloon is inflated with either air or a contrast material diluted with saline or water. Effacement of the waist signifies stricture dilation (Fig. 5). The balloon is then deflated and repositioned, and the sequence of inflation repeated two to three times. We believe fluoroscopy is immensely valuable in transendoscopic balloon dilation as it allows for better visu-

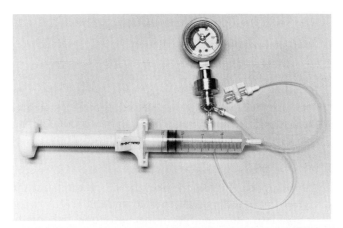

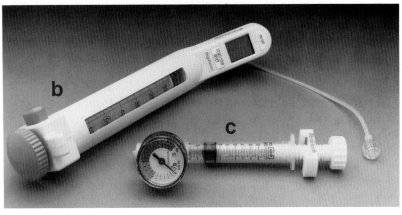

FIG. 4. Balloon inflation devices. **a:** Rigiflator (Microvasive). **b:** Digiflator (Microvasive). **c:** Screw type inflation balloon (Medi-tech).

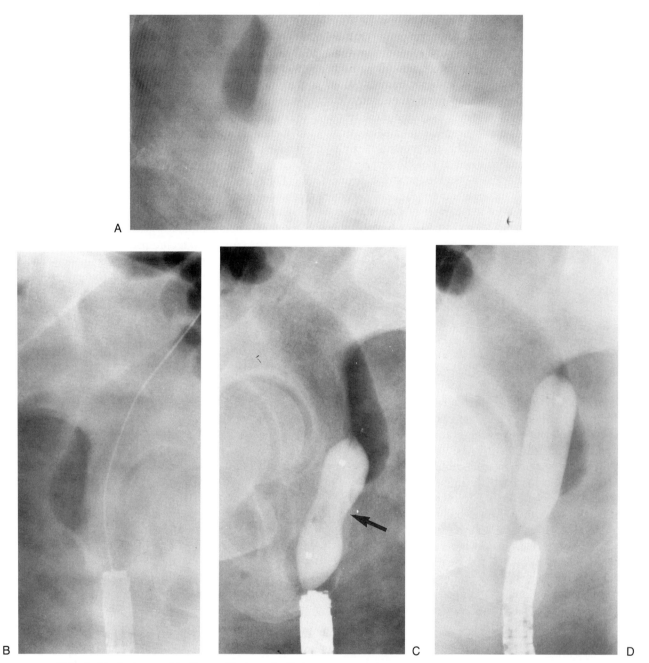

FIG. 5. Technique of balloon dilation. **A:** Colonoscope at level of stricture. **B:** Guidewire above stricture. **C:** Balloon catheter with waistband. **D:** Balloon catheter with flattening of waistband.

alization of the dilation and aids in positioning the waist of the balloon into the center of the stricture. Once dilation has been accomplished, the transendoscopic balloon should be removed from the colonoscope. The balloon is deflated by applying negative pressure to the catheter by withdrawing on a 60-cc syringe. Negative pressure should be maintained while withdrawing the balloon in order to decrease the resistance in the biopsy channel and facilitate catheter removal.

New transendoscopic balloons are currently under development that will have variable diameters, so that a single balloon can be inflated to multiple diameters by varying the inflation pressure. For example, a balloon inflated to 20 PSI will have a diameter of 12 mm and the same balloon inflated to 40 PSI will have a diameter of 18 mm. The efficacy of these balloons is currently being evaluated in clinical trials.

Nontransendoscopic Wire-Guided Balloon Dilation

Gruntzig balloon dilation is frequently used in the dilation of vascular strictures. This technique of passing a balloon over a previously placed guidewire under fluoroscopy has been adapted for use in many other organs including the colon. Wire-guided balloon dilation of the colon has been described with and without the use of an endoscope (18,19). We recommend that regardless of the technique employed, the guidewire be positioned under fluoroscopy secondary to the technical difficulties of diverticula, angulation, and haustral folds inherent in the colon. The procedure of wire-guided balloon dilation utilizing a colonoscope is as follows. The colonoscope is passed to the stricture and a guidewire is passed through the endoscopic biopsy channel and through the stricture. It is important to position the guidewire at least 5 to 10 cm beyond the stricture to avoid retraction of the guidewire from the stenotic area while the balloon is positioned (20,21). Once the guidewire is in position, the endoscope is withdrawn while the proper position of the wire is maintained by fluoroscopy. If there is any question regarding the position of the wire, an endoscopic retrograde cholangiopancreatography (ERCP) catheter may be exchanged over the guidewire and water-soluble contrast injected to confirm the position of the catheter. After confirmation of the position, the guidewire is reintroduced and the catheter removed. The wire-guided balloon should be inflated prior to introduction into the colonoscope to evaluate for leakage. The balloon is then lubricated with silicone and fed over the guidewire under fluoroscopic guidance into the stricture. The balloon is partially inflated and positioned such that the waist of the balloon is noted in the central portion of the stricture. Newer balloons are premarked with two radiopaque markers in the center of the balloon to facilitate balloon positioning. The balloon is then inflated and deflated as with the TTS balloons. Effacement of the waist signifies stricture dilation (22,23). The maximum inflation pressure (PSI) is noted on the balloon package and catheter hub and varies depending upon balloon size. After dilation, the colonoscope is passed to the stricture to evaluate the success of the procedure.

Wire-guided balloons are available in diameters of 4 to 40 mm (Microvasive, Medi-tech, Bard) and are able to be passed over a 0.038-inch guidewire. The balloons vary in length from 2 to 8 cm and the catheter lengths vary from 95 to 180 cm. Inflation devices are similar to those used in transendoscopic balloons.

Wire-guided balloon dilation of rectal and colonic strictures has been reported without the use of a colonoscope (24–26). Under fluorosocpic guidance, a J-shaped guidewire within a catheter is passed to the area of the stricture. The guidewire is removed from the catheter and water-soluble contrast material is injected through the catheter to outline the stricture. The J-shaped guidewire is then passed through the catheter and advanced at least 20 cm proximal to the stricture

(25). The catheter is removed and a wire-guided balloon is advanced under fluoroscopy into the stricture. The balloon is partially inflated and the waist is positioned in the center of the stricture. Dilation is performed as in transendoscopic balloon dilation. This technique has been described solely in rectal and low-lying anastomotic strictures. We feel it is effective in these situations but its use is limited in more proximal lesions secondary to difficulty in passing a guidewire through the entire colon without endoscopic guidance.

Dilation of a colonic stricture distal to an ostomy is a special circumstance in which wire-guided balloon dilation has been utilized (27,28). This combined technique has been employed with up to a 96% success rate (27). The combined technique requires an endoscope to be passed into the rectum and up to the level of the stricture and a second endoscope to be passed through the colostomy and down to the stricture. A guidewire is then passed through the stricture from below and grasped with a snare and removed via the ostomy. An over-the-wire balloon dilation catheter is passed into the stricture under fluoroscopic guidance and inflated (Fig. 6). This technique allows for an endoscope to be passed to the stricture for direct visualization of the dilation. Bedogni et al. (27) modified this technique by introducing a pediatric fiberscope with a Miller-Abbott balloon attached into the stricture after his initial dilation with a wire-guided balloon dilation catheter. This enabled the stricture to be dilated to 2 to 3 cm under retrograde view of the endoscope.

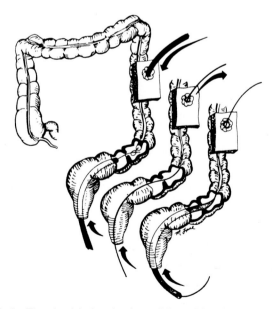

FIG. 6. The double intubation of "combined technique." Two endoscopes in place with guidewire transfer from operator at rectal limb to operator at ostomy end. After both endoscopes are withdrawn, wire-guided balloons or hollow-core dilators (Savary-Gilliard type) may be passed over the wire to dilate the stricture.

Rigid Dilation Techniques

Several techniques have been employed in the dilation of rectal and colonic strictures utilizing rigid dilation devices (29–32). Hegars metal dilators (31), Foley catheters (32), modified Lister urethral dilators (31), modified Stark dilators (30) and sigmoidoscopes of increasing diameter (33) have been useful in the dilation of strictures in the upper rectum and lower sigmoid colon but are limited to these distal structures by their length. Hollow-core rigid dilators such as Savary-Gilliard, Eder-Puestow, and Maloney mercury dilators may be employed to dilate colonic strictures but these dilators must be used either under direct vision or over a guidewire with fluoroscopic guidance (34). As in the esophagus, these strictures should be dilated slowly and progressively with a maximum of three dilators passed at each session. The combined technique for dilation of a stricture distal to an ostomy has been employed utilizing Savary-Gilliard over the wire dilators (27) and Eder-Puestow over the wire metal olives (35). The technique is identical to the combined procedure described using over-the-wire balloon dilators. As with Savary-Gilliard and Eder-Puestow dilation in the colon and esophagus, generally a maximum of three dilators should be passed sequentially at each dilation session. After each dilation session, a colonoscope should be inserted in an attempt to traverse the stricture.

Electrocautery Dilation

Electrocautery has been used to treat strictures of the esophagus (21) and duodenum (36) and in the treatment of achalasia (37), in addition to its use in the treatment of sphincter of Oddi obstruction. Colonic stricture following the use of an end-to-end anastomosis (EEA) stapler device appears to be responsive to treatment with electrocautery using a standard or a needle-knife papillotome (38,39). The EEA stapler inverts the intestinal border and therefore the stenosis presents as a diaphragm-like narrowing. The procedure is performed by introducing the papillotome through the biopsy channel of the endoscope to reach the level of the stricture. The papillotomy knife is then passed be-

yond the stenotic diaphragm and the stenotic ring is cut utilizing a blended current in two, three, or four points along its circumference (Fig. 7). The length and depth of each cut must be determined by the operator in order to avoid injury to normal colonic mucosa. After the incisions are made, the colonoscope should be passed through the stricture to further dilate the area. Accordi et al. (38) successfully treated 11 patients in this fashion and had excellent results after 1 year without any reported complications. This technique may be combined with transendoscopic balloon dilation either to facilitate sphincterotome placement or for further dilation after initial cutting with electrocautery.

Laser Therapy

Laser therapy has proven to be effective in the gastrointestinal tract in the palliative treatment of malignant tumors, in the preventive management of recurrent villous adenomas, and in achieving hemostasis (40,41). Multiple studies have found neodymium:yttrium-aluminum garnet (Nd:YAG) laser ablation to be effective in the recanalization of malignant strictures of the colon and rectum (42–47). Nd:YAG laser has been successfully used in the treatment of benign anastomotic strictures, Crohn's strictures, and radiation strictures (40,41,48). An international survey of the treatment of benign stenoses of the colon and rectum with laser showed a 95% and 100% success rate, respectively, in relieving obstruction and obtaining long-term symptom relief (49). As many as 30 treatments per stricture were required to obtain these results. Chen et al. (50) successfully applied Nd:YAG laser therapy to treat a colonic stricture caused by an EEA stapler device.

To perform laser ablation, the laser fiber is passed through the biopsy channel of the endoscope, positioned within 10 mm of the target, and laser energy is applied. Vaporization of the tissue to a depth of 1 to 2 mm into the wall is necessary. The step-by-step photocoagulation is performed beginning with the part of the stricture closest to the tip of the endoscope. Mechanical dilation may be performed after laser ablation to increase the diameter of the stricture. This proce-

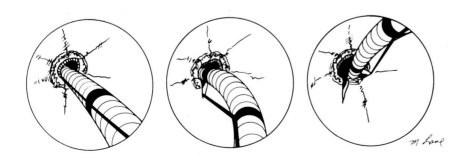

FIG. 7. Electrocautery dilation of an anastomotic stricture. A standard papillotome is inserted through the endoscope into the stricture; then, under direct vision, small incisions are made in each quadrant.

dure has allowed passage of the colonoscope in all reported cases after a single dilation.

Complications of Dilation

There are currently no studies that fully evaluate the complication rates of the dilatation of colonic strictures. An overall complication rate of 7.8% was found in balloon dilation of colonic strictures in the American Society of Gastrointestinal Endoscopy (ASGE) survey of hydrostatic balloon dilation (16). Three perforations (4.7%) and two episodes of bleeding (3.1%) were reported in the 64 patients undergoing colonic balloon dilation. These rates are higher than the respective perforation and bleeding rates after routine colonoscopy. These complications may be lessened by following some basic precautions. On insertion of the colonoscope, prolonged "slide-by" should be avoided as a fixed loop may produce more bowing and increase the risk of perforation. Overinsufflation should be avoided as air may accumulate proximal to the stricture and cause severe pain and discomfort. In addition, overzealous manipulation should be avoided as it may increase the risks of perforation and bleeding especially in colons that have fixed loops secondary to surgical adhesions or previous peritoneal inflammation.

ETIOLOGY OF COLONIC STRICTURES

Many etiologies have been associated with colonic stricture formation (Table 2). Diverticular disease with associated muscular hypertrophy is the most common

TABLE 2. *Etiology of colonic stricture*

Most common
 Diverticulosis
 Postsurgical anastomosis
 Inflammatory bowel disease
 Malignancy
Less common
 Postradiation stenosis
 Ischemia
  Necrotizing enterocolitis
  Vasculitis
 Infection
  Amoebiasis
  Actinomycosis
  Schistosomiasis
  Tuberculosis
  Lymphogranuloma venereum
 Endometriosis
 Extrinsic compression
  Pancreatitis
  Carcinomatosis
 Blunt abdominal trauma
 Foreign body perforation
 Essential mixed cryoglobulinemia

cause of colonic narrowing (51); however, few cases of endoscopic treatment of these narrowed segments are reported in the literature. Balloon dilatation was reported to be technically accomplished in the ASGE survey in five cases of diverticular narrowing with relief of symptoms for greater than 3 months seen in only 67%. One dilation was complicated by severe bleeding (16). It is unclear why such a void in the literature exists, but it suggests that either few patients with diverticular narrowing become symptomatic or few endoscopists are willing to dilate diverticular narrowing.

Anastomotic Stricture

Anastomotic strictures are the most common colonic strictures to undergo colonoscopic therapy. Stenosis of a colonic anastomosis has been shown to occur in 1% to 4.2% of all postsurgical patients (24,35,52) and are most common following low anterior rectal resection. These may result from perianastomotic inflammation, ischemia, recurrent tumor, or recurrent inflammatory bowel disease (53). Most of these strictures dilate spontaneously during the first postoperative year (54); those that remain symptomatic must be treated. Treatment traditionally has been surgical but several recent studies have shown efficacy in colonoscopic treatment. The ASGE national survey reports 86% long-term symptom relief with colonoscopic dilation of these strictures (16). Fregonese et al. (55) treated 16 patients with anastomotic strictures with balloon dilation and found a 100% success rate at 28.9 months. Several studies have shown success rates of greater than 90% in treating anastomotic strictures colonoscopically (22,28,54,56). Accordi et al. (38) reported success in eight patients with anastomotic strictures following EEA stapling treated with a papillotomy knife to cut the narrowing. A single patient in this series required repeat dilatation at 1 year.

Inflammatory Bowel Disease

Inflammatory bowel disease (ulcerative colitis and Crohn's disease) can cause strictures in the active phase of the disease due to mucosal and submucosal inflammation or in the chronic phase as a result of fibrosis. Colonoscopic treatment of strictures has been shown to be effective in active disease (57) as well as in stricture secondary to fibrosis. Bloomberg et al. (17) dilated 27 patients with stricture secondary to Crohn's disease and showed complete resolution of symptoms in 18 patients, improved symptoms in 5, and no improvement in 4 patients. The mean follow-up was 19 months and all patients, including the group with no long-term benefits, showed some relief immediately postdilation. Breysem et al. (15) successfully dilated

16 patients with Crohn's strictures and had immediate symptomatic relief in 14 patients and long-term improvement in 9 patients. Williams and Palmer (58) successfully dilated five of seven patients with Crohn's strictures and achieved long-term symptomatic improvement in all five cases. Brower (59) and Kirtley et al. (60) have reported successful treatment of terminal ileal strictures secondary to Crohn's using balloon dilation. Malignant colorectal strictures have been reported to occur in Crohn's disease in as many as 6% of strictures (61). Therefore, it is essential to biopsy all colonic strictures in Crohn's patients as malignant strictures should be treated with surgery. Interestingly, Yamazaki et al. (61) reported a high false-negative rate in the biopsy of malignant Crohn's strictures. Overall, it appears that colonoscopic dilation of benign strictures secondary to Crohn's disease is very useful and may help delay or prevent further surgical intervention. We reported eight colonic Crohn's strictures treated successfully with transendoscopic balloon dilatation utilizing either through-the-scope balloon dilators (Microvasive) or 20 mm (Hobbs) balloon catheter placed over a guidewire (20).

Postirradiation Stricture

Irradiation delivered to tumors in the pelvis may lead to the development of strictures in the rectum and the small bowel. Strictures in the anorectal area have been treated with manual dilation; however, strictures more proximal in the rectum and colon have traditionally been treated surgically (62). There have been several reports of colonoscopic treatment of radiation strictures. Ricci et al. (28) reported two cases of postirradiation sigmoid strictures treated successfully with wire-guided Savary dilation requiring three sessions each. Graham et al. (63,64) reported two cases of postirradiation strictures treated with TTS balloon dilation, and reported success in a stricture of 4 cm length and failure in a stricture of 7 cm. The role of colonoscopic treatment of postirradiation strictures remains undefined and therefore further evaluation of this treatment should be undertaken.

Ischemic Stricture

Ischemic stricture formation is the most common long-term complication of necrotizing enterocolitis, occurring in 3% to 36% of infants who recover from this disorder (13,65). Balloon dilation techniques have replaced surgical treatment of focal and nonobstructive strictures, thus reserving surgical treatment for radiographically diffuse and obstructive strictures. Ball et al. (13) reported dilation of five infants with nine focal intestinal strictures. Eight of the nine strictures were

located in the defunctionalized colon distal to an enterostomy. One perforation at the level of the splenic flexure occurred secondary to a technical error in guidewire placement. Successful treatment of the remaining strictures allowed closure of the enterostomy without a formal laparotomy.

Malignant Stricture

Malignant strictures of the colon cannot be definitively treated with dilation, and surgery must be performed whenever possible. Dilatation to relieve obstruction should be reserved for nonsurgical candidates as it provides only temporary relief. The ASGE survey on balloon dilation (16) in colon cancer reports a 60% immediate symptomatic relief rate and a 25% rate of symptomatic relief at 3 months. A 20% complication rate was seen in this group. We have used a technique of dilating malignant strictures combining balloon dilation and laser. In our technique, the stricture is dilated with a balloon to allow scope passage. After the scope is passed proximal to the stricture, the laser probe is placed through the biopsy channel and applied to the stricture upon withdrawal.

Miscellaneous Causes of Stricture

Trauma of many etiologies including blunt abdominal trauma and surgical trauma have been reported to cause colonic stricture (66). Pancreatitis may lead to the development of marked transverse colonic edema and inflammation secondary to its proximity to the colon, and to stricture formation (67). Carcinoma from adjoining organs may compress the bowel leading to narrowing. Endometriosis (68) and pneumatosis coli (51) may also lead to colonic narrowing. There are currently no reported cases of colonoscopic therapy for strictures secondary to these conditions. Infectious diseases such as amoebiasis, tuberculosis, schistosomiasis, actinomycosis, and lymphogranuloma venereum can lead to stricture formation (51). Collagen vascular disease and essential mixed cryoglobulinemia have also been reported to lead to colonic stricture (69).

REFERENCES

1. Bernard D, Morgan S, Tasse D. Colonoscopic assessment of radiological strictures of the colon. *Can J Surg* 1986;29:239–242.
2. Forde KA, Treat MR. Colonoscopy in the evaluation of strictures. *Dis Colon Rectum* 1985;28:699–701.
3. Kozarek RA, Botoman VA, Patterson DJ. Prospective evaluation of small caliber upper endoscope for colonoscopy after unsuccessful standard examination. *Gastrointest Endosc* 1989;35:333–335.

4. Bat L, Williams CB. Usefulness of pediatric colonoscopes in adult colonoscopy. *Gastrointest Endosc* 1989;35:329–332.

5. Manten HD, Zara J, Raskin JB, et al. Balloon dilatation of rectosigmoid strictures: transendoscopic approach. *Gastrointest Endosc* 1986;32:162–164.

6. Mortensen NJ, Eltringham WK, Mountford RA, et al. Direct vision brush cytology with colonoscopy: an aid to the accurate diagnosis of colonic strictures. *Br J Surg* 1984;71:930–932.

7. Benvenuti GA, Prollo JC, Kirsner JB, et al. Direct vision brushing cytology in the diagnosis of colo-rectal malignancy. *Acta Cytol* 1974;18:477–481.

8. Gruntzig AR, Hopff H. Perkutane rekanalisation chrnescher arterieller verschlusse mit einem neuen dilatation-katheter. *Dtsche Med Wochenschr* 1974;99:2502–2505.

9. Musher DR, Boyd A. Esophagocolonic stricture with proximal fistulae treated by balloon dilation. *Am J Gastroenterol* 1988;83:445–447.

10. London RL, Trotman BW, DiMarino AJ, et al. Dilatation of severe esophageal strictures by inflatable balloon catheters. *Gastroenterology* 1980;80:173–175.

11. Siegel JH, Yatto RP. Hydrostatic balloon catheters: a new dimension of therapeutic endoscopy. *Endoscopy* 1984;16:231–236.

12. Whitworth PW, Richardson RL, Larsen GM. Balloon dilatation of anastomotic strictures. *Arch Surg* 1988;123:759–762.

13. Ball WS, Kosloske AM, Jewell PF, et al. Balloon catheter dilatation of focal intestinal strictures following necrotizing enterocolitis. *J Pediatr Surg* 1985;20:637–639.

14. Brower RA, Freeman LD. Balloon catheter dilation of a rectal stricture. *Gastrointest Endosc* 1984;30:95–97.

15. Breysem Y, Janssens JF, Vantrappen G, et al. Endoscopic balloon dilation of colonic and ileo-colonic Crohn's strictures: long term results. *Gastrointest Endosc* 1992;38:142–147.

16. Kozarek RA. Hydrostatic balloon dilation of gastrointestinal stenoses: a national survey. *Gastrointest Endosc* 1986;32:15–20.

17. Bloomberg B, Rolny P, Jarnerot G. Endoscopic treatment of anastomotic strictures in Crohn's disease. *Endoscopy* 1991;23:195–198.

18. McClean GK, Cooper GS, Hartz WH, et al. Radiologically guided balloon dilation of gastrointestinal strictures: part 1. *Radiology* 1987;165:35–40.

19. McClean GK, Cooper GS, Hartz WH, et al. Radiologically guided balloon dilation of gastrointestinal strictures: part 2. *Radiology* 1987;165:41–43.

20. Manten HD, Goldberg RI, Roger AI, et al. Transendoscopic balloon dilatation of Crohn's strictures in the gastrointestinal tract. In: Rachmilewitz D, ed. *Inflammatory bowel 1990*. The Netherlands: Kluwer, 1990;32.

21. Raskin JB, Manten HD, Harary A, et al. Transendoscopic electrosurgical incision of lower esophageal rings: a new treatment modality. *Gastrointest Endosc* 1985;31:391–393.

22. Aston NO, Owen WJ, Irving JD. Endoscopic balloon dilatation of colonic anastomotic strictures. *Br J Surg* 1989;76:780–782.

23. Grundy A, Page JE. Treatment of colonic anastomotic strictures with 'thru the scope' balloon dilators. *J R Soc Med* 1991;84:569.

24. Banerjee AK, Walters TK, Wilkins R, et al. Wire guided balloon coloplasty—a new treatment for colorectal strictures. *J R Soc Med* 1991;84:136–139.

25. DeLange EE, Shaffer HA. Rectal strictures: treatment with fluoroscopically guided balloon dilation. *Radiology* 1991;178:475–479.

26. Dobson HM, Robertson DA. Balloon catheter dilatation of an ileocolic stricture. *Clin Radiol* 1988;39:202–204.

27. Bedogni G, Ricci E, Pedrazzoli C, et al. Endoscopic dilation of anastomotic colonic stenosis by different techniques: an alternative to surgery. *Gastrointest Endosc* 1987;33:21–23.

28. Ricci E, Conigliaro R, Maria GM, et al. Endoscopic management of colonic stenoses. *Endosc Rev* 1989;6:9–25.

29. Dencker H, Johansson JI, Norryd C, et al. Dilator for treatment of strictures in the upper part of the rectum and the sigmoid. *Dis Colon Rectum* 1973;16:550–552.

30. Duce AM, Badia de Yebenes A, Garces G, et al. Instrument for dilatation of stenotic colorectal anastomosis. *Dis Colon Rectum* 1990;33:160–161.

31. Hood K, Lewis A. Dilator for rectal strictures. *Br J Surg* 1986;73:633.

32. Mazier WP. A technic for the management of low colonic anastomotic stricture. *Dis Colon Rectum* 1973;13:113–116.

33. Bacon HE. *Anus, rectum, sigmoid colon: diagnosis and treatment*, 3rd ed. Philadelphia: JB Lippincott, 1963;1127.

34. Dooley MC, Levison SL. Postoperative sigmoid colonic strictures—a new guided dilation technique. *Gastrointest Endosc* 1983;29:229–230.

35. Thies E, Lange V, Miersch WD. Peranal dilatation of a postsurgical colonic stenosis by means of a flexible endoscope. *Endoscopy* 1983;15:327–328.

36. Venu RP, Geenen JE, Hogan WJ, et al. Endoscopic electrosurgical treatment for strictures of the gastrointestinal tract. *Gastrointest Endosc* 1984;30:97–100.

37. Ortega JA, Madureri V, Perez L. Endoscopic myotomy in the treatment of achalasia. *Gastrointest Endosc* 1980;26:8–10.

38. Accordi F, Sogno O, Carniato S, et al. Endoscopic treatment of stenosis following stapler anastomosis. *Dis Colon Rectum* 1987;30:647–649.

39. Neufeld DM, Shemesh EI, Kodner IJ, et al. Endoscopic management of anastomotic colon strictures with electrocautery and balloon dilation. *Gastrointest Endosc* 1987;33:24–26.

40. Sander R, Poesl H. Nd:YAG laser treatment of non-neoplastic GI stenoses. *Gastrointest Endosc* 1986;32:170(abst).

41. Sander R, Poesl H, Spuhler A. Management of non-neoplastic stenosis of the GI tract: a further indication for Nd:YAG laser application. *Endoscopy* 1984;16:149–151.

42. Brunetaud JM, Maunoury V, Ducrotte P, et al. Palliative treatment of rectosigmoid carcinoma by laser endoscopic photoablation. *Gastroenterology* 1987;92:663–668.

43. Buchi KN. Endoscopic laser surgery in the colon and rectum. *Dis Colon Rectum* 1988;31:739–745.

44. Daneker GW, Carlson GW, Hohn DC, et al. Endoscopic laser recanalization is effective for prevention and treatment of obstruction in sigmoid and rectal cancer. *Arch Surg* 1991;126:1348–1352.

45. Eckhauser ML. Laser therapy of colorectal carcinoma. In: Schwesinger WH, Hunter JG, eds. *Surgical clinics of North America: lasers in general surgery*. Philadelphia: WB Saunders, 1992;597–607.

46. Kiefhaber P, Kiefhaber K, Huber F. Pre-operative neodymium: YAG laser treatment of obstructive colon cancer. *Endoscopy* 1986;18(suppl 1):44–46.

47. Mathus-Vliegen EMH, Tytgat GNJ. Laser ablation and palliation in colorectal malignancy: results of a multicenter inquiry. *Gastrointest Endosc* 1986;32:393–396.

48. Sasako M, Iwasaki Y, Takami M, et al. Endoscopic laser treatment for the post-operative anastomotic stricture of the digestive tract. *Gastrointest Endosc* 1982;24:2028(abst).

49. Loffler A, Dienst C, Velasco SB. International survey of laser therapy in benign gastrointestinal tumors and stenoses. *Endoscopy* 1986;18(suppl 1):52–62.

50. Chen PC, Wu CS, Chang-Chien CS, et al. YAG laser endoscopic treatment of an esophageal and sigmoid stricture after end-to-end anastomosis stapling. *Gastrointest Endosc* 1984;30:258–260.

51. Williams CB. Diverticular disease and strictures. In: Hunt RH, Waye JD, eds. *Colonoscopy—techniques, clinical practice and colour atlas*. London: Chapman and Hill, 1981;363–381.

52. Barrozo AO, Azizi E, Jordan G. Repeated balloon dilation of a severe colonic stricture. *Gastrointest Endosc* 1987;33:320–322.

53. Dinneen MD, Motson RW. Treatment of colonic anastomotic strictures with 'through the scope' balloon dilators. *J R Soc Med* 1991;84:264–266.

54. Skreden K, Wiig JN, Myrvold HE. Balloon dilation of rectal strictures. *Acta Chir Scand* 1987;153:615–617.

55. Fregonese D, Di Falco G, Di Toma F. Balloon dilatation of anastomotic intestinal stenosis: long term results. *Endoscopy* 1990;22:249–253.

56. Pietropaolo V, Masoni L, Ferrara M, et al. Endoscopic dilation of colonic postoperative strictures. *Surg Endosc* 1990;4:26–30.

57. Linares L, Moriera LF, Andrews H, et al. Natural history and treatment of anorectal strictures complicating Crohn's disease. *Br J Surg* 1988;75:653–655.

58. Williams AJ, Palmer KR. Endoscopic balloon dilatation as a therapeutic option in the management of intestinal strictures resulting from Crohn's disease. *Br J Surg* 1991;78:453–454.

59. Brower RA. Hydrostatic balloon dilation of a terminal ileal stricture secondary to Crohn's disease. *Gastrointest Endosc* 1986; 32:38–40.

60. Kirtley DW, Willis M, Thomas E. Balloon dilation of recurrent terminal ileal Crohn's disease. *Gastrointest Endosc* 1987;33: 399–400.

61. Yamazaki Y, Ribiero MB, Sachar DB, et al. Malignant colorectal strictures in Crohn's disease. *Am J Gastroenterol* 1991; 86:882–885.

62. Ernest DL, Trier JS. Radiation enteritis and colitis. In: Sleisenger MH, Fordtran JS, eds. *Gastrointestinal disease*, 4th ed. Philadelphia: WB Saunders, 1989;1339–1382.

63. Graham DY. Evaluation of the effectiveness of through the scope balloons as dilators of benign and malignant gastrointestinal strictures. *Gastrointest Endosc* 1987;33:432–435.

64. Graham DY, Tababian N, Schwartz JT, et al. Balloon dilatation of gastrointestinal strictures: thru the scope. *Gastrointest Endosc* 1986;32:151(abst).

65. Renfrew DL, Smith WL, Pringle KC. Pre anal balloon dilatation of a post-necrotizing enterocolitis stricture of the sigmoid colon. *Pediatr Radiol* 1986;16:320–231.

66. Davidson BR, Everson NW. Colonic stricture secondary to blunt abdominal trauma—report of a case and review of the literature. *Postgrad J Med* 1987;63:911–913.

67. Mann NS. Colonic involvement in pancreatitis. *Am J Gastroenterol* 1980;73:357–362.

68. Pillay SP, Hardie IR. Intestinal complications of endometriosis. *Br J Surg* 1980;67:677–679.

69. Ferrari BT, Ray JE, Robertson HD, et al. Colonic manifestations of collagen vascular disease. *Dis Colon Rectum* 1980;23: 473–477.

Advanced Therapeutic Endoscopy, 2nd Ed.,
edited by J. S. Barkin and C. A. O'Phelan.
Raven Press, Ltd., New York © 1994.

CHAPTER 26

Treatment of Hemorrhoidal Disease with Endoscopic Injection Sclerotherapy

John D. Mellinger and Jeffrey L. Ponsky

Hemorrhoidal disease is estimated to affect more than half of Americans over age 50 (1), and is the most frequent cause of anorectal bleeding overall (2). Despite significant progress in recent years adding to our understanding of the anatomy (3) and physiology (4) of hemorrhoidal pathology, the plethora of symptoms attributed to hemorrhoids remain frequent presenting complaints in clinical practice. Many patients so affected undergo endoscopic evaluation to exclude less benign sources of hematochezia or other anorectal symptomatology prior to definitive therapy.

The treatment of hemorrhoids historically has included simple measures such as dietary therapy, surgical hemorrhoidectomy, and a variety of nonoperative therapies including injection sclerotherapy and rubber band ligation. The latter therapies have enjoyed considerable popularity because of their potential to induce submucosal fixation and resulting ablation of hemorrhoidal tissues in an office setting. In more recent years, infrared photocoagulation, direct current, bipolar or monopolar electrocoagulation, heater probe coaptive coagulation, laser coagulation, and cryodestruction have all been touted as acceptable means of achieving a similar effect (2,5–8). Despite this proliferation of new methodologies and the utility of flexible endoscopy in evaluating anorectal bleeding, only laser therapy had been previously described as a flexible endoscopic technique (9). Due to equipment and cost implications, as well as reports of complicating stric-

ture formation (10), endoscopic laser therapy for hemorrhoidal disease has not proved to be a widely applicable treatment method.

Injection sclerotherapy is the oldest and most widely applied nonoperative technique for hemorrhoidal disease. Initially popularized in the late nineteenth century by practitioners often labeled as charlatans (5,11), injection sclerotherapy has been very widely applied in Europe, where its economy, efficacy, and relative safety have been well attested (12–14). Success rates in the 85% range for relief of bleeding and minor prolapse have been documented in very large series (15). Even in centers favoring rubber band ligation as another traditional nonoperative therapy, injection techniques have been recognized for their ability to facilitate more rapid and equally durable results, with less associated patient discomfort (14). Moreover, in comparative studies of injection sclerotherapy and newer techniques such as infrared photocoagulation, the former has been found to be equally efficacious, to require fewer treatment sessions, and to be less costly from an equipment standpoint (6).

Despite the above, injection sclerotherapy has not achieved widespread popularity in this country. Dissatisfaction on the part of patients and some physicians with anoscopic techniques, along with well-documented instances of allergic reaction to a variety of available sclerosants (2,4,16,17), appear to have been important factors in this regard.

In 1989, we began a clinical trial of endoscopic injection sclerotherapy using 23.4% saline solution in the nonoperative treatment of symptomatic hemorrhoids (18). This concept was developed from several observations. First, as described above, anoscopic injection treatment of hemorrhoids is well attested historically. Second, the recent popularity of endoscopic injection

J. D. Mellinger: Department of Surgery, United States Air Force Medical Center, Wright-Patterson AFB; and Department of Surgery, Wright State University, Dayton, Ohio 45401.

J. L. Ponsky: Department of Surgery, Mount Sinai Medical Center; and Department of Surgery, Case Western Reserve University, Cleveland, Ohio 44106.

techniques in the treatment of esophageal varices, bleeding peptic disease, and postpolypectomy colonic bleeding has made the materials and technique of endoscopic injection both accessible and familiar to most gastrointestinal specialists. Third, flexible endoscopy is usually performed in the evaluation of anorectal symptoms and is well tolerated by patients. The advent of videoendoscopy has afforded magnified views of the distal rectum not achieved by earlier methods of exposure and inspection, creating the potential for more precise and better-monitored therapies. Finally, recent reports on the use of 23.4% saline as a nonallergenic sclerosant in the treatment of vascular blemishes and telangiectasias (16,19) suggested the potential utility of this agent as a low-morbidity alternative to previous sclerosing agents.

TECHNIQUE

Endoscopic hemorrhoidal sclerotherapy is performed from a retroflexed position in the rectal vault at the completion of a standard flexible sigmoidoscopic or colonoscopic examination. This position allows optimal visualization of the distal rectum and upper anal canal. The retroflexed position is achieved by first positioning the tip of the endoscope in the inflated midrectum. The tip of the endoscope is then deflected upward while the insertion tube is simultaneously advanced and torqued in a counterclockwise direction. Coordination of these two synchronous maneuvers consistently allows a retroflexed position to be attained in a smooth and comfortable fashion (Fig. 1). Just prior to retroflexion, a standard endoscopic injection catheter

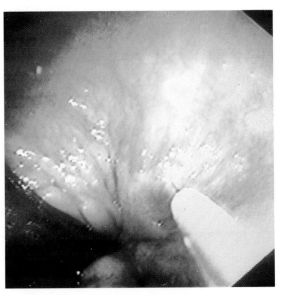

FIG. 2. The sclerotherapy needle is introduced beneath the mucosa of the hemorrhoidal column just proximal to the dentate line.

(Flexitip Sclerotherapy Needle with 5-mm, 25-gauge retractable needle, Bard Interventional Products, Tewksbury, MA) is passed through the endoscope's working channel to the tip of the instrument. This helps to avoid difficulty with catheter passage and maneuvering in the acutely angled, retroflexed position. Once in this position, the distal rectum and anal canal are carefully inspected, using manipulation of the insertion tube and fine deflection of the control knobs in a braked position. Care is required to avoid excessive torquing or looping of the endoscope during these maneuvers, which will otherwise make subsequent fine catheter manipulations difficult. Overdistention of the rectum in this position may efface hemorrhoidal complexes and obscure their precise location and proximal extent. Other distal anorectal pathology is carefully searched for prior to commencing treatment.

Following the diagnostic examination, the injection catheter is advanced, the needle extended, and the catheter preflushed with 23.4% saline solution (LyphoMed, Rosemont, IL). Hemorrhoidal columns are injected near their proximal extent (Fig. 2). After initial needle placement through the mucosa, gentle lifting of the needle and endoscope tip into the lumen can help confirm an appropriate submucosal placement. Following needle placement, a very small volume of sclerosant is first injected to ensure the site does not retain somatic innervation, which is not uncommon in the 1- to 2-cm transition zone immediately proximal to the dentate line. If no somatic (i.e., focal, sharp) pain is noted with initial limited injection, the treatment proceeds. Appropriate submucosal injection is further confirmed at this point by ease of injection and recogni-

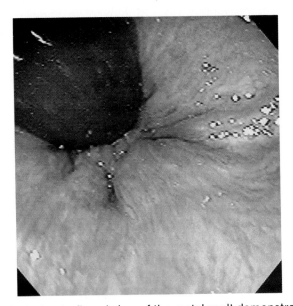

FIG. 1. A retroflexed view of the rectal vault demonstrating grade I internal hemorrhoids.

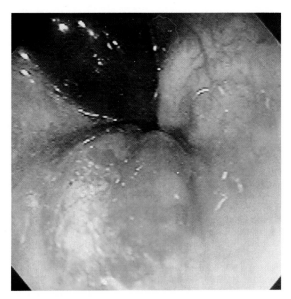

FIG. 3. After injection, a submucosal wheal will be noted at the area of the hemorrhoid. This indicates that the sclerosant has diffused in the submucosal plane.

tion of dissemination of the sclerosant in the submucosal plane (Fig. 3). Deep needle placement is manifested by failure of such a submucosal wheal to develop on initial injection. Superficial needle placement may be heralded at this point by raising a relatively confined, unusually pale and focal wheal, suggesting intramucosal injection. Once appropriate needle placement is so confirmed, 1 to 2 ml of 23.4% saline are injected at that site. In patients with several columns or near circumferential disease, three or four injections are placed so as to allow a circumferential submucosal wheal to be produced. Instances of postinjection bleeding are treated by simple observation or, in rare instances, by further injection at the bleeding site.

At the completion of injection, the needle and catheter are retracted, the endoscope returned to an antegrade viewing position, and air is suctioned from the rectum prior to endoscope withdrawal. Mild nonnarcotic analgesics and sitz baths are provided for postprocedural discomfort when necessary, although most patients have not required them.

RESULTS

Endoscopic retrograde hemorrhoidal sclerotherapy, similar to its anoscopic forebear, has had its greatest efficacy in patients with symptomatic grade I (bleeding only) or II (bleeding and spontaneously reducing prolapse) hemorrhoids. In this group, approximately 90% of patients have been very satisfied with both the method and results of therapy. While the success profile is not quite as high, the technique can often be

used effectively in grade III (prolapse requiring manual reduction) disease as well. Treatment is generally reserved for patients who have failed to have adequate symptom control on dietary fiber supplements or other conventional therapies. The technique has not and should not be utilized in settings of isolated external hemorrhoidal disease, other active nonhemorrhoidal anorectal pathology, or in the face of acute thrombosis. This technique has been used in several patients who have failed to have adequate symptom control following other therapies such as rubber band ligation or surgical hemorrhoidectomy. Acceptable outcomes and high patient satisfaction have also been noted in this setting, where a method that does not further ablate rectal mucosal surface area offers some theoretical advantages. Endoscopic sclerotherapy has also been used successfully in patients with minor degrees of nonhemorrhoidal rectal mucosal prolapse.

Recurrent bleeding has been noted in 10% to 15% of patients 3 or more months after initial therapy. Repeat injections of persistent hemorrhoidal tissue distal to the previous injection sites has been effective in obtaining more lasting symptom relief in some such cases. In other instances, the degree of recurrent symptoms has been mild enough that patients have not desired further intervention.

No serious complications have been noted with this technique, including no infectious complications, acute thromboses, anal fistulae, delayed hemorrhage, or stricture formation. No untoward reactions to the sclerosant itself have been encountered. One patient experienced acute rectal mucosal prolapse immediately after treatment, which was easily reduced and did not recur. Two patients early in our experience had persistent anorectal discomfort for 1 to 2 weeks after therapy, which was aggravated by prolonged standing or sitting. Anoscopic evaluation in this setting failed to disclose any specific etiology for these symptoms, although sphincter spasm perhaps related to injection in close proximity to somatically innervated epithelium was suspected.

DISCUSSION

With the proliferation of comparably effective nonoperative submucosal fixation techniques for hemorrhoidal treatment, determination of optimal therapy for a given patient has become increasingly complex. Fortunately, many patients experience spontaneous improvement in symptoms (20), or present with advanced disease that dictates more aggressive therapy such as surgical hemorrhoidectomy. For the remainder of patients with moderate hemorrhoidal symptoms not responsive to dietary therapy, the technique herein described appears to offer several potential advantages.

First, by utilizing an injection methodology, endoscopic retrograde hemorrhoidal sclerotherapy is derived from a well-attested historical context of efficacy and safety. Injection therapy uses techniques familiar to most contemporary therapeutic endoscopists, and relies on economical materials available in any endoscopy suite. By relying on an endoscopic methodology, this method allows magnified visualization of the distal rectum unparalleled by the predominant transanal techniques otherwise available, facilitating precise therapy with continuous visual monitoring during treatment. In addition, the endoscopic method allows simultaneous diagnostic evaluation and therapy, and achieves a high patient acceptance rate typical of many current endoscopic techniques. Finally, by avoiding ablation of rectal mucosal tissue, this technique may be particularly safe in controlling recurrent symptoms after more aggressive or ablative therapies such as banding or surgical hemorrhoidectomy.

Further evaluation of this technique, including comparative evaluations with other methods of hemorrhoidal therapy, is indicated. For the present, patients with bleeding secondary to grade I or II hemorrhoids appear to be excellent candidates for the approach described. In this setting, one can anticipate a high success rate and patient satisfaction profile, with minimal treatment morbidity.

REFERENCES

1. Hass PA, Hass GP, Schmultz S, et al. The prevalence of hemorrhoids. *Dis Colon Rectum* 1983;26:435–439.
2. Smith LE. Hemorrhoids: a review of current techniques and management. *Gastroenterol Clin North Am* 1987;16:79–91.
3. Thomson WHF. The nature of haemorrhoids. *Br J Surg* 1975; 62:542–552.
4. Burkitt DP, Graham-Stewart CW. Haemorrhoids—postulated pathogenesis and proposed prevention. *Postgrad Med J* 1975; 51:631–636.
5. Faulconer HJ. Hemorrhoids: alternative treatments. *J Ky Med Assoc* 1988;86:617–620.
6. Ferguson EF. Alternatives in the treatment of hemorrhoidal disease. *South Med J* 1988;81:606–610.
7. Pearl RK, Abcarian H. Nonoperative therapy of hemorrhoids. *Infect Surg* 1989;8:411–417.
8. Zinberg SS, Stern DH, Furman DS, Wittles JM. A personal experience in comparing three nonoperative techniques for treating internal hemorrhoids. *Am J Gastroenterol* 1989;84:488–492.
9. Yu JC, Eddy HG Jr. Laser: a new modality for hemorrhoids. *Am J Gastroenterol Colon Rectum Surg* 1985;1:9–10.
10. Schrock TR, Guthrie JF, Shub HA, Smith LE, Stern HS. Lasers in colon and rectal surgery. *Perspect Colon Rectum Surg* 1989; 2:55–69.
11. Andrews E. The treatment of hemorrhoids by injection. *Med Rec* 1879;15:451.
12. Goligher JC. *Surgery of the anus, rectum and colon*, 4th ed. London: Balliere Tindall, 1980.
13. Graham-Stewart CW. Injection treatment of hemorrhoids. *Br Med J* 1962;1:213–216.
14. Sim AJW, Murie JA, Mackenzie I. Comparison of rubber band ligation and sclerosant injection for first and second degree hemorrhoids: a prospective clinical trial. *Acta Chir Scand* 1981; 147:717–720.
15. Kilbourne NJ. Internal hemorrhoids: comparative value of treatment by operative and by injection methods. *Ann Surg* 1934;99: 600–608.
16. Bodian EL. Techniques of sclerotherapy for subacute venous blemishes. *J Dermatol Surg Oncol* 1985;11:696–704.
17. Schneider KW. Anaphylactic shock after hemorrhoidal sclerosing with quinine. *Coloproctology* 1980;4:255–256.
18. Ponsky JL, Mellinger JD, Simon IB. Endoscopic retrograde hemorrhoidal sclerotherapy using 23.4% saline: a preliminary report. *Gastrointest Endosc* 1991;37:155–158.
19. Lupo MLP. Sclerotherapy: review of results and complications in 200 patients. *J Dermatol Surg Oncol* 1989;15:214–219.
20. Senapati A, Nicholls RJ. A randomized trial to compare the results of injection sclerotherapy with a bulk laxative in the treatment of bleeding hemorrhoids. *Int J Colorect Dis* 1988;3: 124–126.

Advanced Therapeutic Endoscopy, 2nd Ed.,
edited by J. S. Barkin and C. A. O'Phelan.
Raven Press, Ltd., New York © 1994.

CHAPTER 27

Is Hot Biopsy Appropriate for Treatment of Diminutive Colon Polyps?

Shailesh C. Kadakia and Fred H. Goldner

The term *polyp* is derived from the Greek word *polypus*, meaning many-footed, although most colon polyps have a single stalked or sessile base (foot) and a rounded head with possibly many lobes (arms). Colon polyps are defined as mucosal protuberances into the lumen of the colon (1), and are divided into two broad categories of nonneoplastic and neoplastic polyps. Nonneoplastic polyps include mucosal excrescences, hamartomatous polyps, inflammatory polyps, and hyperplastic polyps. Neoplastic polyps of the colon include adenomas (tubular, tubulovillous, and villous) and carcinomas. Polyps may vary in size from a few millimeters to several centimeters in size. Diminutive polyps are generally defined as sessile polyps of 5 mm or less by most endoscopists (2–6). Rarely, it has been defined as a sessile polyp of 8 mm or smaller in size (7) but this is not widely accepted.

It is now generally accepted that colorectal cancer arises from a previously benign neoplastic polyp (8). Colorectal carcinoma is the second most common cause of cancer death in the United States with 151,000 new cases and 61,300 deaths estimated in 1989 (9). It is the second most common cause of cancer death (after lung cancer–related death) in men and the third most common cause of cancer death (after lung and breast cancer–related death) in women (9). Natural history studies of untreated colonic polyps have revealed that the cumulative risk of diagnosis of colon cancer

at the polyp site at 5, 10, and 20 years was 2.5%, 8%, and 24%, respectively (10). Much indirect evidence suggests an adenoma-carcinoma sequence, but it is difficult to predict development of colonic carcinoma in any one individual with an adenoma except in patients with familial polyposis coli and Gardner's syndrome. The adenoma-carcinoma sequence suggests that untreated adenomas become carcinomas over time (11). This fact has been substantiated by a number of important observations, including (a) adenomatous origin of minute adenocarcinomas, (b) morphologic association between adenomas and invasive carcinomas, (c) high incidence of colon cancer in untreated patients with familial adenomatosis polyposis, (d) similarities between adenomas and carcinomas at the molecular level, (e) epidemiology of colonic adenomas and carcinomas, and (f) the natural history of adenomas. In addition, proctosigmoidoscopy and removal of rectosigmoid polyps has been shown to reduce the incidence and mortality rate of subsequent rectosigmoid cancer (12–14). It is, therefore, important to detect colonic adenomas and remove them prior to their developing into carcinoma. This strategy may result in decreased mortality from colon cancer.

The American Cancer Society and the National Cancer Institute have recommended the screening of average-risk asymptomatic patients over the age of 50 years for the development of colon cancer with annual fecal occult blood testing and flexible sigmoidoscopy every 3 to 5 years after the initial negative flexible sigmoidoscopy. For these reasons and widespread availability of fiberoptic flexible endoscopes, interest in colorectal polyps has increased considerably. Neoplastic polyps, such as adenomas, are of great interest due to their malignant potential. The incidence of carcinoma in diminutive polyps ranges from 0% to 0.1% (2–4,15). In

S. C. Kadakia: Department of Medicine, University of Texas Health Science Center at San Antonio, San Antonio, Texas 78234-6200; and Gastroenterology Service, Department of Gastrointestinal Endoscopy, Brooke Army Medical Center, Fort Sam Houston, Texas 78234-6265.

F. H. Goldner: Department of Medicine, University of Texas Health Science Center at San Antonio, San Antonio, Texas 78234-6200; and Department of Medicine, Brooke Army Medical Center, Fort Sam Houston, Texas 78234-6265.

general, all polypoid lesions greater than 5 mm in diameter should be removed. The decision to perform colonoscopy for removing polyps of 5 mm or less should be individualized based on patient's age, past history, family history, and the presence of other diseases (16). Unfortunately, the effects of removing all colon polyps in a population on the subsequent development of colon cancer is not definitely known despite the widespread availability of colonoscopy. Whether eradication of diminutive adenomas reduces the subsequent incidence of colorectal cancer has not been well proven. Although a variety of techniques such as cold biopsy (6), bipolar probe coagulation (BICAP probe) (6), snare polypectomy (17), and laser ablation have been used in the treatment of diminutive polyps, the most common method of obliterating diminutive mucosal polyps of the colon is by the monopolar hot biopsy forceps technique (16). However, the question remains: Is hot biopsy forceps appropriate for treatment of diminutive colon polyps?

EPIDEMIOLOGY OF DIMINUTIVE POLYPS

The older literature has suggested a high prevalence of hyperplastic polyps among diminutive polyps (5,18,19). However, numerous recent studies utilizing endoscopy have reported a preponderance of adenomas among diminutive colon polyps. Granqvist et al. (2) found that 37% of 300 polyps were adenomas. Waye et al. (15) in their experience found 61% of 1,046 polyps to be neoplastic. Tedesco et al. (3) reported 49% incidence of neoplastic polyps in a series of 329 polyps of less than 5 mm. Feczko et al. (4), in a series of 62 polyps of less than 5 mm found 47 (76%) to be of neoplastic variety. Even an autopsy study has shown that 60% of adenomatous polyps are less than 5 mm in diameter (20). The reasons for this diversity of low prevalence of adenomas in older studies and a significantly higher prevalence in recent studies are many and include the specimens obtained only from the rectum, rectosigmoid, or resected portion of the colon at surgery in the older reports (5,18,19). If one examines the colonoscopic data, most small colon polyps are in fact found in the rectosigmoid colon (15). In addition, some studies have examined the polyps removed at rigid proctoscopy instead of at colonoscopy (20). The histopathologic examination of diminutive polyps is mandatory to confirm their neoplastic nature since the accuracy of visual determination is poor (21).

TECHNICAL ASPECTS

Electrosurgical Generators

Any solid-state electrosurgical unit consisting of a high frequency current generator with two electrodes is suitable for hot biopsy forceps technique (21,22). These units provide coagulation current (interrupted power output), cutting current (continuous power output), or a combination of both forms resulting in "blended current." Coagulation current causes desiccation and coagulation of the tissue without cutting. Cutting current results in rapid tissue heating and vaporization resulting in incision of the tissue without coagulation. In using electrocautery it is important to become familiar with one specific brand, whichever one the operator finds simple and easy to use, since the current delivery varies among various brands or even within the same brand. Many modern units are combined monopolar-bipolar generators, but are more expensive than standard monopolar generators.

Monopolar Hot Biopsy Forceps

The monopolar hot biopsy forceps was used initially by Williams (23) in 1973. This biopsy forceps is electrically insulated, which permits current to flow through its entire length. The current applied to the grasped tissue passes through the patient to the ground plate and back to the generator. Small hot biopsy forceps, with a cup diameter of 2.3 mm when closed and a length of 7 mm when open, as well as large hot biopsy forceps with a cup diameter of 3.2 mm when closed and a length of 8 mm when open, are available for clinical use.

Endoscopic Technique Using Monopolar Hot Biopsy Forceps

Pure coagulation current should be used in all cases. Williams (24) recommends a current of 15 to 20 W for 1 to 2 seconds. The polyp is grasped with the forceps and tented away from the wall toward the colon lumen. This tenting will allow the current density and temperature rise to be highest in the narrow tented segment. However, if the forceps touches the opposite wall, current flow and density may be highest at the point of wall contact with an increased risk of transmural injury. With application of the current, heat is generated at the base of the polyp, which is endoscopically visible as whitening of the mucosa. When this whitened zone is about 1 to 2 mm in size, coagulation should be stopped to minimize further tissue injury (7,21,24). The tissue entrapped in the jaws of the forceps is unaffected by the heat and is available for accurate histologic evaluation. The degree of tissue injury is dependent upon many factors, including tissue resistance, current output, and electrical contact. The technique of polypectomy utilizing monopolar hot biopsy forceps may be complicated by certain factors. For example, it may be difficult to avoid contact with the adjacent normal mucosa due to tangential orientation of the grasped polyp with resultant coagulation at the polyp site as well as at the adjacent wall. Tenting may be difficult due to the location of the polyp (for example, at the splenic or hepatic flexure). The colonic wall may be thinned further by overdistention of the colon, thereby increasing the risk of transmural coagulation, deeper tissue injury, and possible colonic wall perforation.

Bipolar Hot Biopsy Forceps

Recently, the bipolar hot biopsy forceps has been used for diminutive colon polyps or normal mucosa (25). The theoretical advantage of bipolar forceps is the limited injury to the colonic wall. The use of 2.3 mm bipolar forceps in canines has shown virtual absence of transmural injury in the gastric and colonic wall 24 to 72 hours after application (25). However, the tissue within the forceps failed to provide interpretable biopsy specimens due to the thermal injury. Further studies in animals and humans are needed to show efficacy and safety of bipolar forceps. In addition, further technical advances are also necessary to improve the quality of the tissue specimen for better histopathologic diagnosis.

IS HOT BIOPSY FORCEPS TREATMENT FOR DIMINUTIVE POLYPS EFFECTIVE?

Once the decision to treat a diminutive polyp is made, monopolar hot biopsy forceps is the most commonly used device. This technique allows removal of diminutive polyps for histopathologic study while the remainder of the polyp is assumed to be obliterated by the thermal effects on the surrounding colonic tissue. However, this assumption may not be correct. In fact, two recent prospective studies examining the efficacy of hot biopsy forceps for obliteration of diminutive polyps have shown that hot biopsy forceps do not obliterate all polyps (26,27). Vanagunas et al. (26) randomized patients with diminutive polyps (defined as ≤6 mm in size) in the rectum and sigmoid colon to hot biopsy treatment with either electrocautery for 2 seconds (fixed duration) or electrocautery until visible necrosis of the polyp base was evident (variable duration). Sigmoidoscopy was performed at 4 weeks after treatment to determine the adequacy of polyp eradication. In the fixed duration cautery group, 11 of 21 polyps (52%) were eradicated, compared with 12 of 14 polyps (86%) in the variable duration cautery group. Despite the small number of patients and polyps in each group, the authors achieved a statistical significance of $p = .04$. When analyzed according to whether or not visible necrosis was achieved (some of the polyps in the fixed duration cautery group showed necrosis with 2-sec cautery), 19 of 23 polyps (83%) were eradicated when

the necrosis was evident, compared to 5 of 12 (42%) without necrosis ($p = .004$). Based on their results, diminutive polyps are eradicated endoscopically in 83% of the polyps when there is visible necrosis. The corollary is that there is a 17% failure rate of polyp eradication even with visible necrosis.

Does the endoscopically visible eradication mean that there is also histologic eradication? Does the endoscopically visible polyp at 4 weeks mean that there is still an adenoma (histologically proven) left behind? The answers to these questions are not available from this study. The authors did not rebiopsy (cold or hot) the endoscopically visible polyp to prove that the visible polyp indeed had the same histology as the original polyp.

In another prospective study, we examined the efficacy of hot biopsy forceps in patients with diminutive polyps (27). The polyps were treated with hot biopsy forceps in a standard manner using a pure coagulation current setting of 2.5 (Valley Lab SSE2L electrocautery high frequency current generator) for a period of 1 to 2 seconds until a white coagulum was visible at the base. Of the 39 total patients, 23 patients with 37 biopsy sites underwent flexible sigmoidoscopy at both 1 and 2 weeks. At 1 week, 23 had bland ulcers of 4 to 8 mm in size with a white base. The ulcers decreased in size or they disappeared in most patients at 2 weeks' follow-up. At 1 week, six polyp remnants were found and at 2 weeks five remnants were found, resulting in incomplete destruction of the polyp in 11 of the total of 62 biopsy sites (17.7%) examined. This confirms the findings of Vanagunas et al. (26), who also noted a failure rate of 17% in their group. However, in contrast to Vanagunas et al., we rebiopsied all endoscopically visible remnants using the conventional cold biopsy forceps and confirmed the histology of the remnants to be the same as original polyp in all instances. Based on these two studies, it is obvious that the colonoscopist cannot assume that the monopolar hot biopsy forceps is reliable in eradication of diminutive polyps. If the coagulation current is applied until the base of the diminutive polyp is white, the eradication rate seems to be 83% and the failure rate 17% in both series (26,27).

Recently, bipolar coagulation probe (BICAP probe) has been compared to conventional cold biopsy in evaluating the eradication of diminutive polyps (defined as 5 mm or less by the authors) by Woods et al (6). Seventy-seven polyps (mean polyp size 2.9 mm) were randomized to BICAP probe and 79 polyps (mean size 2.8 mm) to cold biopsy. Flexible sigmoidoscopy performed at 3 weeks showed residual polyp in 21% of BICAP probe–treated polyps compared to 29% of cold biopsy–treated polyps ($p > .05$). However, one has to wonder about the residual adenomatous tissue in cold biopsy–treated polyps despite the lack of endoscopically invisible remnant of polypoid tissue at the polypectomy site. Bipolar coagulation probe may be advantageous due to a lesser degree of transmural burn. However, it is not universally available and the probes are more expensive than monopolar hot biopsy forceps. In addition, one has to perform cold biopsy prior to bipolar probe treatment to obtain specimen for accurate histopathologic evaluation. The major advantages of hot biopsy forceps treatment are its simplicity, familiarity with the technique by most endoscopists, universal availability of the equipment, excellent specimen retrieval for histopathologic interpretation, and relatively low expense. Potential disadvantages may be incomplete eradication and complications from thermal injury to the colon wall.

The cold biopsy forceps is easy to use, relatively inexpensive, universally available, familiar to all endoscopists, and provides excellent specimens, but its efficacy in eradication of adenomas is unknown. Cold snare polypectomy (without electrocautery) of diminutive polyps has all advantages of cold biopsy forceps but may be somewhat overaggressive therapy for diminutive polyps, and its efficacy for eradication is also unknown. Bipolar biopsy forceps may be safer than hot biopsy forceps due to less transmural burn (similar to BICAP probe), but requires an electrosurgical generator with bipolar capacity, is relatively more expensive than monopolar forceps, has not been used in humans, provides unacceptable specimen, and its efficacy rate for eradication of diminutive polyps is also unknown. Finally, it must be emphasized that there are no trials comparing the efficacy of hot biopsy forceps with cold snare polypectomy without electrocauterization, snare cauterization, conventional cold biopsy forceps, bipolar coagulation probe, or bipolar hot biopsy forceps.

IS HOT BIOPSY FORCEPS TREATMENT FOR DIMINUTIVE POLYPS BENEFICIAL?

Although, hot biopsy forceps treatment has been recommended by some authors to remove all diminutive polyps (3,4,15,16,21,24), whether this is actually beneficial and if this constitutes the "standard of care" remains quite controversial (28). The reason for not removing the diminutive polyp is the extremely low incidence of high-grade dysplasia (formerly called carcinoma in situ) to virtual nonexistence of invasive carcinoma. Therefore, the short-term and long-term risk-to-benefit ratio as well as economic considerations may suggest that these polyps be ignored. However, most endoscopists remove diminutive polyps at the time of colonoscopy because they are unwilling to take the extremely small risk of missing the carcinoma within the polyp. Also, the growth pattern of adenomatous diminutive polyps show that 50% of diminutive polyps grow

in size, suggesting that many of the diminutive polyps will eventually require definitive treatment, particularly in younger patients. Therefore, some prefer to treat diminutive polyps at index colonoscopy rather than enter them into a surveillance program because of the uncertainties of patient compliance, the occasional findings of carcinoma in diminutive polyps, and the limited understanding of the growth pattern (29). The American Society for Gastrointestinal Endoscopy (ASGE) recommends removing or destroying all such diminutive polyps at the time of colonoscopy for any indication (16).

It is suggested that a surveillance colonoscopy be performed after removal of an adenoma. The optimal follow-up intervals have not been established. It is reasonable to perform repeat colonoscopy at a 1-year interval to detect missed synchronous polyps in patients with multiple benign polyps who appear to be greater risks for recurrent polyps (16). It is not known whether patients with a single polyp should be reexamined in 1, 2, or 3 years after initial polypectomy (16). In either case, once the colon has been cleared of any adenomas, routine follow-up every 3 to 5 years is recommended in the absence of special risk factors (16). What about the surveillance strategies in patients with only diminutive polyps that have been treated with monopolar hot biopsy forceps? There are no recommendations for surveillance colonoscopy in patients who have only a diminutive polyp(s). It is conceivable that surveillance colonoscopy may be done at longer intervals in patients with diminutive polyps. Many factors such as associated medical conditions and very old age will affect the decision regarding continued follow-up in patients with diminutive polyps.

The above-described studies (26,27) raise some important questions about whether the polyp found in the vicinity of a polyp previously treated by hot biopsy forceps indeed represents a recurrent polyp versus an incompletely eradicated initial polyp. The result of this conclusion might cause the physician to inappropriately maintain heightened concern over the propensity toward polyp recurrence in a given patient and thereby delay lengthening the interval between subsequent surveillance colonoscopy. This has obvious cost-and-risk benefit implications as has been shown recently by Ransohoff et al. (30). Utilizing cost-effectiveness analysis of colonoscopic surveillance and complications of colonoscopy, the authors determined that a program of colonoscopy every 3 years will incur 1.4% risk of colon perforation, 0.11% risk for death, and direct physician cost of $2,071 for the colonoscopy. With 100% effectiveness of colonoscopic surveillance every 3 years, one death from cancer will be prevented by 283 colonoscopies, incurring 0.6 perforation, 0.04 death, at a cost of $82,000 in a 50-year-old man with 2.5% cumulative risk of colon cancer death.

In light of current data, we feel that patients with adenomas including diminutive adenomas should undergo surveillance colonoscopy until the colon is cleared of all adenomas at which time the follow-up colonoscopies can be done every 3 to 5 years.

IS HOT BIOPSY FORCEPS TREATMENT OF DIMINUTIVE POLYPS SAFE?

The complications of colonoscopic polypectomy range from 0.8% to 4.5% depending upon the size of the polyp (31–34). Nivatvongs (31,32) in his experience with 1,555 colonoscopic polypectomies reported 19 (1.2%) complications. The polyp sizes ranged from 0.5 to 6 cm. No complications occurred when 5-mm polyps were removed and only two incidences of bleeding for polyps between 6 and 10 mm. Webb et al. (33) reported an overall complication rate of 0.8% in their experience with 1,000 colonoscopic polypectomies in 591 patients. All complications were postpolypectomy bleeding with no perforations and none requiring blood transfusions. Polyps less than 5 mm were excluded from the analysis for reasons that are not clear. In clinical practice, massive bleeding after treatment of diminutive polyps with monopolar hot biopsy forceps has been reported in isolated case reports (27,35,36). Rex et al. (37) reported a series of 29 patients with postpolypectomy bleeding, with 20 patients requiring no specific therapy and 9 requiring endoscopic treatment consisting of various combinations of injection therapy, electrocautery, or thermal injury to control bleeding. Of these 9 patients, 3 had diminutive polyps. Two patients required three units of packed cell transfusion and one required 18 units. There have been three major bleeding episodes associated with hot biopsy forceps at our institution over a 3-year period (27).

In a recent survey, Wadas and Sanowski (38) reported that 16% of respondents who used monopolar hot biopsy forceps reported complications including bleeding, perforation, and postpolypectomy coagulation syndrome. The risk of major bleeding was 0.41% and the risk of perforation was 0.05% among 13,081 monopolar hot biopsy procedures. The risk of bleeding was highest at 0.52% in the ascending colon. There were 12 cases of abdominal pain and fever and one death. In the study by Rex et al. (37), two major bleeding episodes occurred in the cecum and one in the ascending colon. Recent studies evaluating eradication of diminutive polyps by monopolar hot biopsy forceps have not described any complications but the number of patients and polyps in both studies was very small (26,27). Larger series are required to demonstrate more significant complications. The generator current settings are much lower (average 2.5) in controlled studies (27) compared to those reported in the survey (average

3.5) (38). The incidence of perforation is also more common in the right colon probably due to the relatively thin colonic wall in this segment of colon compared to the rest of the colon. Bleeding that fails to stop spontaneously after treatment of diminutive polyps with hot biopsy forceps can be controlled with a variety of therapeutic endoscopic modalities such as injection of 1 to 2 ml aliquots of 1:10,000 solution of epinephrine, intravenous vasopressin, heat probe, BICAP probe, or repeat application of monopolar hot biopsy forceps (21,37,39). All of these are probably reasonable options but controlled trials or systematic evaluation of each therapy is lacking in the literature. We use epinephrine injection combined with bipolar probe coagulation to achieve hemostasis after polypectomy.

The postpolypectomy coagulation syndrome occurring after hot biopsy treatment is characterized by abdominal pain, fever, abdominal tenderness usually at the site of polypectomy, and leukocytosis due to transmural burn to the level of visceral peritoneal reflection. There is no evidence of free peritoneal air suggesting colonic perforation. Most patients with postpolypectomy coagulation syndrome can be managed by conservative treatment consisting of nil per mouth, intravenous fluids, and intravenous antibiotics.

CONCLUSIONS AND RECOMMENDATIONS

Most diminutive polyps should be removed at the time of colonoscopy. Monopolar hot biopsy is a relatively simple and straightforward technique to apply. The major advantage of the hot biopsy forceps is simultaneous tissue biopsy and electrocoagulation of the remainder of the polyp. At present, there are no data that such treatment of diminutive polyps causes reduction in colorectal cancer. Recent studies have failed to show that hot biopsy forceps is absolutely perfect in eradicating diminutive polyps and colonoscopists can no longer assume that this method is reliable in obliterating diminutive polyps. In the presence of white coagulum at the base of the polyp at the time of current application using pure coagulation current will eradicate about 85% of the diminutive polyps. This eradication rate is only 40% in the absence of visible whitening of the base. Whether this endoscopic determination of eradication of the polyp results in actual histologic destruction of all adenoma cells is unknown.

Can modifications in technique improve efficacy? We are reluctant to recommend increasing duration or intensity of current application, as this may increase complications. We recommend a pure coagulation current of 2.5 to 3 for 1 to 2 seconds when using monopolar hot biopsy forceps. The base of the polyp should have 1 to 2 mm of whitening with this technique. The bipolar hot biopsy forceps in animal studies shows decreased transmural injury but there is no information on its use in humans. In addition, bipolar hot biopsy forceps does not provide interpretable histopathologic specimens. Until better techniques are developed, colonoscopists should probably continue to apply the present monopolar hot biopsy method, keeping in mind the shortcomings described. For the obliteration of diminutive polyps, there is a need for controlled trials comparing the efficacy and safety of monopolar hot biopsy with other techniques such as cold snare polypectomy without electrocauterization, snare electrocoagulation, conventional cold biopsy forceps removal, cold biopsy combined with thermal probe coagulation, bipolar probe coagulation alone, and bipolar hot biopsy removal.

ACKNOWLEDGMENT

The opinions and assertions herein are the private views of the authors and are not to be construed as reflecting the views of the Department of the Army or the Department of Defense.

REFERENCES

1. Boland RC, Itzkowitz SH, Kim YS. Colonic polyps and gastrointestinal polyposis syndromes. In: Sleisenger MH, Fordtran JS, eds. *Gastrointestinal disease: pathophysiology, diagnosis, management*, 4th ed, vol 2. Philadelphia: WB Saunders, 1989;1483.
2. Granqvist S, Gabrielsson N, Sundelin P. Diminutive colonic polyps, clinical significance and management. *Endoscopy* 1979;11:36–42.
3. Tedesco FR, Hendrix JC, Picken CA, Brady PG, Mills LR. Diminutive polyps: histopathology, spatial distribution and clinical significance. *Gastrointest Endosc* 1982;28:1–5.
4. Feczko PJ, Bernstein MA, Halpert RD, Ackerman LV. Small colonic polyps: a reappraisal of their significance. *Radiology* 1984;152:301–303.
5. Pagtalunana RJ, Dockerty MB, Jackman RJ, et al. The histopathology of diminutive polyps of the large intestine. *Dis Colon Rectum* 1965;120:1259–1265.
6. Woods A, Sanowski RA, Wadas DD, Manne RK. Eradication of diminutive polyps: a prospective evaluation of bipolar coagulation versus conventional biopsy removal. *Gastrointest Endosc* 1989;35:536–540.
7. Waye JD. Techniques of polypectomy: hot biopsy forceps and snare polypectomy. *Am J Gastroenterol* 1987;82:615–618.
8. Winawer SJ. Introduction to position papers from the third international symposium on colorectal cancer. *CA* 1984;34:130–133.
9. Cancer statistics. *CA* 1989;39:1–21.
10. Stryker SJ, Wolff BG, Culp CE, et al. Natural history of untreated colonic polyps. *Gastroenterology* 1987;93:1009–1013.
11. Burt RW, Samowitz WS. The adenomatous polyp and the hereditary polyposis syndromes. *Gastroenterol Clin North Am* 1988;17:657–678.
12. Gilbertsen VA. Proctosigmoidoscopy and polypectomy in reducing the incidence of rectal cancer. *Cancer* 1974;34:936–939.
13. Gilbertsen VA, Nelms JM. The prevention of invasive cancer of the rectum. *Cancer* 1978;41:1137–1139.
14. Dales LG, Friedman GD, Collen MF. Evaluating periodic multiphasic health checkups: a controlled trial. *J Chronic Dis* 1979;32:385–404.
15. Waye JD, Lewis BS, Frankel A, Geller SA. Small colon polyps. *Am J Gastroenterol* 1988;83:120–122.
16. American Society for Gastrointestinal Endoscopy. The role of colonoscopy in the management of patients with colonic polyps. *Gastrointest Endosc* 1988;34:6S–7S.
17. Tappero G, Gaia E, De Giuli P, Martini S, Gubetta L, Emanuelli G. Cold snare excision of small colorectal polyps. *Gastrointest Endosc* 1992;38:310–313.
18. Arthur JF. Structure and significance of metaplastic nodules in the rectal mucosa. *J Clin Pathol* 1968;21:735–743.
19. Lane N, Kaplan H, Pascal R. Minute adenomatous and hyperplastic polyps of the colon and rectum: divergent patterns of epithelial growth with specific associated mesenchymal changes. *Gastroenterology* 1971;60:537–555.
20. Arminski TC, McLean DW. Incidence and distribution of adenomatous polyps of the colon and rectum based on 1000 autopsy examinations. *Dis Col Rectum* 1964;7:249–261.
21. Waye JD. Endoscopic treatment of adenomas. *World J Surg* 1991;15:14–19.
22. Peleman RR, Kinzie JL, Desai TK, Ehrinpreis MN. Colonoscopic polypectomy. *Gastroenterol Clin North Am* 1988;17:851–858.
23. Williams CB. Diathermy-biopsy. A technique for the endoscopic management of small polyps. *Endoscopy* 1973;5:215–218.
24. Williams CB. The use of hot biopsy. *Endosc Rev* 1985;6:12–17.
25. Kimmey MB, Silverstein FE, Saunders DR, Haggitt RC. Endoscopic bipolar forceps: a potential treatment for the diminutive polyps. *Gastrointest Endosc* 1988;34:38–41.
26. Vanagunas A, Jacob P, Vakil N. Adequacy of "hot biopsy" for the treatment of diminutive polyps: a prospective randomized trial. *Am J Gastroenterol* 1989;84:383–385.
27. Peluso F, Goldner F. Follow-up of hot biopsy forceps treatment of diminutive colonic polyps. *Gastrointest Endosc* 1991;37:604–606.
28. Hoffmann SMJ. Response to Dr. Vanagunas [Letter]. *Am J Gastroenterol* 1989;84:1468.
29. Vanagunas A. Reply to Dr. Hoffmann. *Am J Gastroenterol* 1989;84:1468–1469.
30. Ransohoff DF, Lang CA, Kuo HS. Colonoscopic surveillance after polypectomy: considerations of cost effectiveness. *Ann Intern Med* 1991;114:177–182.
31. Nivatvongs S. Complications in colonoscopic polypectomy: lessons to learn from an experience with 1576 polyps. *Am Surg* 1988;54:61–63.
32. Nivatvongs S. Complications in colonoscopic polypectomy: an experience with 1555 polypectomies. *Dis Colon Rectum* 1986;29:825–830.
33. Webb WA, McDaniel L, Jones L. Experience with 1000 colonoscopic polypectomies. *Ann Surg* 1985;201:626–632.
34. Bedogni G, Bertoni G, Ricci E, et al. Colonoscopic excision of large and giant colorectal polyps. *Dis Colon Rectum* 1986;29:831–835.
35. Dyer WS, Quigley, Noel SM, et al. Major colonic hemorrhage following electrocoagulation (hot) biopsy of diminutive colonic polyps: relationship to colonic location and low-dose aspirin therapy. *Gastrointest Endosc* 1991;37:36–34.
36. Quigley EMM, Donovan JP, Linder J, Thompson JS, Straub PF, Paustian FF. Delayed, massive hemorrhage following electrocoagulating biopsy ("hot biopsy") of a diminutive colonic polyp. *Gastrointest Endosc* 1989;35:559–563.
37. Rex DK, Lewis BS, Waye JD. Colonoscopy and endoscopic therapy for delayed postpolypectomy hemorrhage. *Gastrointest Endosc* 1992;38:127–129.
38. Wadas DD, Sanowski RA. Complications of the hot biopsy forceps technique. *Gastrointest Endosc* 1980;3:32–37.
39. Dill JE. Vasopressin in postpolypectomy bleeding [Letter]. *Gastrointest Endosc* 1987;33:399.

Advanced Therapeutic Endoscopy, 2nd Ed.,
edited by J. S. Barkin and C. A. O'Phelan.
Raven Press, Ltd., New York © 1994.

CHAPTER 28

Indications and Techniques for Nasobiliary Stenting

John T. Cunningham

Endoscopic cannulation of the pancreatic duct (PD) and common bile duct (CBD) with retrograde injection of contrast media was first described by McCune et al. (1) in 1968. More prolonged cannulation for pancreatic juice sampling and exfoliative cytological studies were soon to follow, but these techniques were hampered by the necessity for prolonged intubation of the patient with the endoscope (2,3). The logical extension of this technique was to develop a method for continuous deep cannulation of the PD or CBD with the endoscope removed from the patient (4–6). One report included descriptions of its use to decompress malignant biliary obstruction and cholangitis (6).

With the development of plastic and metal indwelling endoprosthesis, continuous nasobiliary stenting has been used much less frequently. As the field of therapeutic endoscopy in both the pancreas and biliary tree expands, the use of continuous access stents needs to be readdressed. A list of its advantages and disadvantages are listed in Table 1.

INSERTION

The diagnostic portion of the procedure can be performed with standard diagnostic or therapeutic side-viewing duodenoscopes. Once the diagnostic portion of the procedure is completed the desired system is cannulated with a catheter or papillotome through which a long straight-tipped or J-tipped guidewire can be passed. The preferred wire is 0.035 inch in diameter, 400 to 480 cm in length, with a short soft tip. Guidewires of smaller caliber or with longer soft tips can

make deep placement of the nasobiliary stent more difficult. The stents are 5 to 7 French (Fr) in external diameter, and I prefer the 7 Fr as there are fewer problems with occlusion and aspiration is easier. The stent is slid over the guidewire by the endoscopist while the assistant applies gentle back traction on the wire so that the rate of advancement of the catheter is equal to the rate of wire extraction, producing no net change in the wire position relevant to the duct or structure being cannulated.

Cooperation and communication between the operator and the assistant are paramount to successful stent positioning. If the assistant is applying too much back traction the wire will lose its deep position or back out of the desired location. This is corrected by the operator advancing the catheter and wire together into the desired position or by holding the stent stationary and having the assistant advance the wire through the stent to the proper position. Inadequate back traction will result in bending or buckling of the wire and may create patient discomfort if advanced too far peripherally. The operator should stop advancing the stent and have the assistant pull the wire until the desired position is achieved. Once the wire and stent are in place

TABLE 1. *Advantages and disadvantages of nasobiliary stents*

Advantages
  Repeat biliopancreatic access without reendoscopy
  Stent removal without reendoscopy for temporary decompression
  Prolonged fluid sampling
Disadvantages
  Premature stent dislodgment by confused patient
  Patient acceptance and comfort
  Loss of fluid and electrolytes

J. T. Cunningham: Department of Medicine, Gastroenterology Division, Medical University of South Carolina College of Medicine, Charleston, South Carolina 29425.

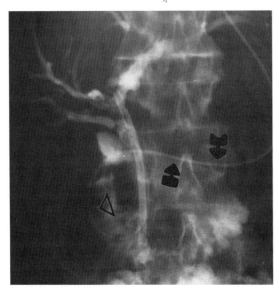

FIG. 1. Proper final position of a nasobiliary catheter with a smooth duodenal loop *(open arrow)* and natural gastric curve *(large arrows).*

the endoscope is withdrawn with constant fluoroscopic monitoring. The stent/guidewire assembly is pushed into the endoscope operating channel as the instrument is withdrawn so as to leave a loop of stent catheter in the duodenum and follow the natural sweeping curvature of the stomach (Fig. 1). Some of the catheter systems have preformed loops that will reconform when the guidewire is removed.

After the endoscope is retracted off the stent, it must be converted to a nasobiliary position (6). A nasoenteric tube is passed through the nose into the hypopharynx and pulled out through the mouth either by grasping with forceps or by digital manipulation. The stent/guidewire is passed through the end of the nasal oral tube and pulled out of the nose (Fig. 2). It is important

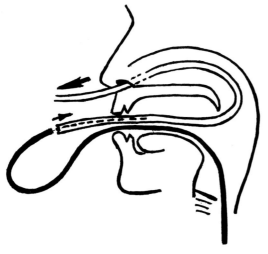

FIG. 2. Technique for conversion of the nasobiliary catheter from oral to nasal position.

to leave the guidewire in the stent during the conversion from oral to nasal intubation as it is common for the polyethylene catheter to twist or kink in the hypopharynx during conversion. The guidewire is removed and the position confirmed by contrast injection and aspirate to ensure proper function of the catheter. The tubing is fixed to the external nares and placed for gravity drainage.

MATERIALS

Most of the commercially available stents are made of 5, 6, or 7 Fr polyethylene tubing, which allows the material to be preformed into various shapes (Fig. 3). The straight stents with a distal pigtail (Fig. 3A) have a tendency for the pigtail to reform when the stent tip passes from the stiff core, to the transitional zone, onto the soft tip; therefore, it is important to have a deep cannulation with the wire so the transitional zone of the wire is above the area of desired stent placement. If unable to place the wire deeply then one of the straight-tipped stents may be more desirable (Fig. 3C).

There is usually no difference in the use of a 5 or 7 Fr in the ease of passage. The stents of larger caliber are probably better utilized in the biliary tree where the secretions are more viscous, and 5 Fr used for aspiration of pancreatic fluid. The selection of a specific shape of catheter is more arbitrary and dependent on the need for long-term cannulation and the area to be cannulated. It is difficult to reform a pigtail in a nondilated system and straight-tipped stents might be preferred. If there may be a need to reinsert guidewires or delivery systems for localized radiation at a later time, then a 7 Fr catheter with a preformed duodenal loop and straight tip (Fig. 3C) is more effective.

If the stent is not being used for continuous infusion then it should be maintained by flushing with 5 to 10 cc of sterile normal saline four times a day followed by aspiration to ensure ease of return. If the catheter is in a closed or confined space then it should be left open to gravity drainage. Should occlusion occur then more forceful flushing may clear the system, but this should be done with fluoroscopic monitoring. A long guidewire will occasionally clear a blocked stent; fluoroscopic monitoring is mandatory and is usually more successful in 7 Fr than 5 Fr systems.

CLINICAL APPLICATION

With the development of indwelling stents and their apparent greater patient acceptance, there has been much less use of prolonged nasobiliary (NB) stenting. Two issues relevant to the increasing application of pancreatobiliary endoscopy as a therapeutic modality should change the attitude toward the use of NB stents.

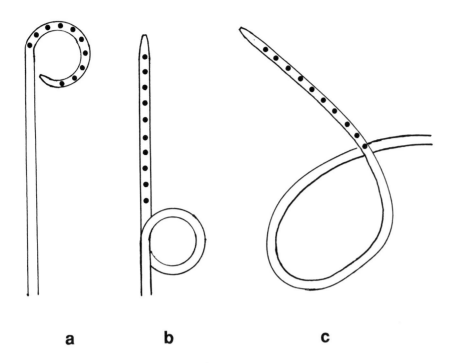

a   b   c

FIG. 3. Examples of the distal configuration of stents. **A:** Straight catheter with distal pigtail. **B:** Straight shaft with more proximal pigtail. **C:** Preformed duodenal loop with straight distal tip.

First is the increased use of endoscopic retrograde cholangiopancreatography (ERCP) as a first line in the diagnosis and therapy of acutely ill patients (7). The second is providing a safe method of decompression when the initial procedure is unsuccessful, particularly in high-risk patients where the alternative therapies carry a high morbidity or mortality (8). The potential clinical indications are listed in Table 2.

Ascending Cholangitis

Early retrospective studies of endoscopic sphincterotomy (ES) and CBD stone extraction versus surgery with CBD exploration failed to demonstrate marked benefit except in the elderly high-risk patient who underwent ES alone with gallbladder left in situ (9). Ascending cholangitis can occur when intraductal pressure exceeds 22 cm H_2O and cholangiovenous reflux occurs. Bacteremia is common when pressures exceed 30 cm H_2O (10). Two studies have indicated the benefit of endoscopic drainage over surgery in the face of ongoing cholangitis (11,12). The latter study was a prospective randomized trial in which a partial sphincterotomy with NB stent insertion with no attempt at stone extraction was the endoscopic aim. This raises an important issue as to whether some of the higher endoscopic morbidity and mortality in earlier studies was related to the sphincterotomy and stone extraction, and that our primary initial goal should be relief of the cholangitis. The placement of stents without sphincterotomy does not appear to increase the incidence of complications over those of diagnostic ERCP (13). The disadvantage to such an approach is the need for additional procedures or later surgery. Further clinical trials may better delineate who can be managed in a single procedure versus those requiring the least invasive approach and multiple procedures.

Another issue is whether any internal drainage is needed in conjunction with the external NB drain. If the goal is purely to ensure adequate drainage then the external drain should be sufficient. However, if there is doubt about being able to maintain patency or position then the addition of an internal stent in conjunction with the external should be considered.

TABLE 2. *Indications for nasobiliary stents*

Emergent decompression in severe acute cholangitis
Repeat visualization and drainage of endoscopically managed pseudocysts
Infusion of mono-octanoin or methyl tert-butyl ether
Removal of viscous biliary secretions in malignant biliary obstruction
During preoperative evaluation of malignant biliary obstruction
Delivery system for brachytherapy

Stone Therapy

Inability to extract CBD stones is still a significant problem during the initial endoscopy, though mechanical lithotriptors have diminished the incidence. Nasobiliary stents can be used to localize stones for radiographically guided extracorporeal shock wave litho-

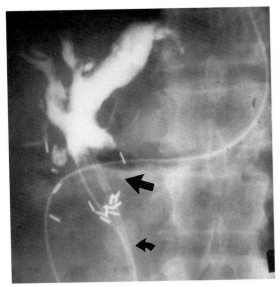

FIG. 4. Mono-octanoin infusion over large intraductal stone *(large arrow)* with a 10-Fr stent *(curved arrow)* providing decompression into the duodenum.

tripsy (14), or, if radiolucent stones are present, for perfusion of mono-octanoin (15) or methyl tert-butyl ether (16). The success rates of the two infusion methods is limited, but stone size or consistency may be altered sufficiently to allow for more effective endoscopic removal (16). Mono-octanoin is a very viscous, lipid-solubilizing monoglyceride that should be infused through a 7 Fr catheter and, due to the volumes infused, requires free flow into the duodenum. This man-

dates that an adequate papillotomy be performed or that an indwelling stent (I prefer 10 Fr) be placed (Fig. 4).

Several points relevant to infusion therapy need to be made. Mono-octanoin requires continuous infusion with the recommendation that intraductal pressure be monitored. This is not mandatory if patient symptoms are monitored and adequate flow into the duodenum has been provided. Prolonged infusion of up to 2 weeks is recommended, but if on repeat nasobiliary cholangiography there is no interval change in stone size after 3 days, then successful dissolution is unusual.

Malignant Obstruction

ERCP is often used early in the management of biliary obstruction and injection of contrast into a blocked system is associated with a significant incidence of cholangitis (17). Therefore, the endoscopist should be able to provide decompression if obstruction is encountered. Early reports used nasobiliary catheters (18), but patient preference soon had them supplanted by indwelling stents (19). Many of these patients are best managed by palliative procedures and a 7-Fr straight-tipped nasobiliary catheter can be used to deliver intraluminal radiation with less systemic side effects (20) (Fig. 5). A cholangiogram is obtained just prior to the loading of the hot guidewire to precisely localize the tumor.

Patients with indwelling stents frequently present with occlusion and cholangitis. A small number will

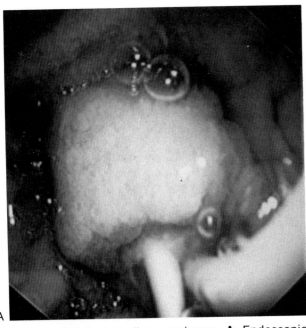

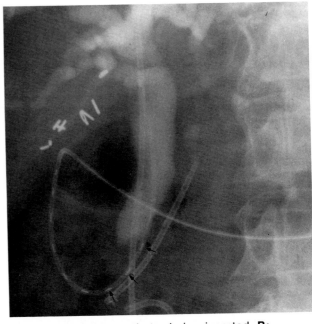

FIG. 5. Ampullary carcinoma. **A:** Endoscopic view with nasobiliary catheter being inserted. **B:** Iridium 192 bead placement *(arrows)*. Note both PD and CBD decompressed with indwelling stents.

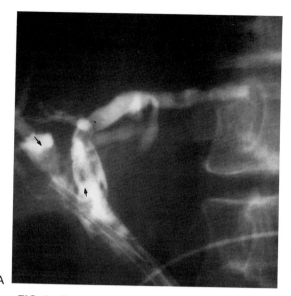
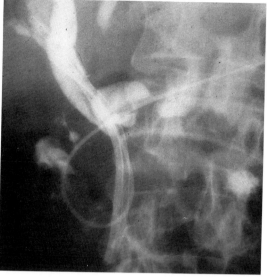

FIG. 6. Pancreatic carcinoma with **(A)** thick intrabiliary secretions (*arrows*) after endoscopic stent placement and **(B)** after lavage with normal saline and duct aspiration.

have rapid reocclusion of replacement endoprostheses. This is heralded by thick mucoid secretions in the biliary tree. We place a nasobiliary beside the newly placed Amsterdam-style stent to aspirate and flush the ducts and obtain delayed cholangiograms to ensure adequate drainage (Fig. 6).

Biliary Leaks

Biliocutaneous fistulae, cystic duct stump leaks, and CBD and common hepatic duct leaks have been managed with a variety of endoscopic methods including nasobiliary stenting (21). There is no consensus as to the preferred method of management. But many reports suggest rapid closure of most leaks when there is ablation of the duodenobiliary pressure gradient whether by stent, sphincterotomy, or a combination of the procedures. A nasobiliary stent has the advantage of facilitating revisualization of the biliary tree at intervals to assess the status of the leak, and reendoscopy is not necessary for stent removal.

Pancreatic Disease

Nasopancreatic drains have been used to bypass dominant PD strictures (22) and have been endoscopically inserted into pancreatic pseudocysts (23). The drains have the clinical advantage of facilitating revisualization of the cyst with the nasopancreatic tube. This technique offers no decided advantage over percutaneous methods and carries significant morbidity and mortality, and it should be performed only by expert endoscopists.

CONCLUSION

Nasobiliary drainage is a technique that is infrequently used in most clinical endoscopic practices. Therapeutic endoscopists should be familiar with the proper technique for insertion and have a familiarity with the various types of materials available. As the theater of therapeutic endoscopy widens, it will become a more commonly utilized and valuable tool in patient therapy.

REFERENCES

1. McCune WS, Shore PE, Moscovitz H. Endoscopic cannulation of the papilla of Vater; a preliminary report. *Ann Surg* 1968;167:752–756.
2. Hatfield ARW, Whittaker R, Gibbs DD. The collection of pancreatic fluid for cytodiagnosis using a duodenoscope. *Gut* 1974;15:305–307.
3. Robberecht P, Cremer M, Vandermeers A, Piret MCV, et al. Pancreatic secretion of total protein and of three hydrolases collected in healthy subject via duodenoscopic cannulation. *Gastroenterology* 1975;69:374–380.
4. Kurachi T. Trials of endoscopical biliary drainage [translation]. *Gastroenterol Endosc (Tokyo)* 1974;16:832.
5. Shapiro HA, Cotton PB. Leaving a balloon-tip catheter in the bile duct at duodenoscopy: a new technique for sequential collection of pure bile in man. *Lancet* 1975;2:13–15.
6. Nagai N, Toki F, Oi I, et al. Continuous endoscopic pancreatocholedochal catheterization. *Gastrointest Endosc* 1976;23:78–81.
7. Leese T, Neoptolemos JP, Baker AR, Carr-Locke DL. Management of acute cholangitis and the impact of endoscopic sphincterotomy. *Br J Surg* 1986;73:988–992.
8. Cairns SR, Dias L, Cotton PB, et al. Additional endoscopic procedures instead of urgent surgery for retained common bile duct stones. *Gut* 1989;30:535–540.
9. Neoptolemos JP, Davidson BR, Shaw DE, et al. Study of common bile duct exploration and endoscopic sphincterotomy in a consecutive series of 438 patients. *Br J Surg* 1987;74:916–921.

10. Yoshimoto H, Ikeda S, Tanaka M, Matsumoto S. Relationship of biliary pressure to cholangiovenous reflux during endoscopic retrograde balloon catheter cholangiography. *Dig Dis Sci* 1989; 34:16–20.

11. Lai ECS, Paterson IA, Tam PC, et al. Severe cholangitis: the role of emergency nasobiliary drainage. *Surgery* 1990;107: 268–272.

12. Lai ECS, Mok FPT, Tan ETS, et al. Severe cholangitis: the role of emergency nasobiliary drainage. *N Engl J Med* 1992;326: 1582–1586.

13. Wootton FT, Hoffman BJ, Cunningham JT, Marsh WH. Does endoscopic stent insertion without sphincterotomy increase the risk of pancreatitis? *Am J Gastroenterol* 1992;87:1296(abst).

14. Saurbruch T, Stern M. Fragmentation of bile duct stones by extracorporeal shock waves. *Gastroenterology* 1989;96: 146–152.

15. Palmer KR, Hoffman AR. Intraductal mono-octanoin for the direct dissolution of bile duct stones: experience in 343 patients. *Gut* 1986;27:196–202.

16. Diaz D, Bories P, Ampelas M, et al. Methyl tert-butyl ether in the endoscopic treatment of common bile duct radiolucent stones in elderly patients with nasobiliary tube. *Dig Dis Sci* 1992; 37:97–100.

17. Kiil J, Kruse A, Rokkjaer M. Endoscopic biliary drainage. *Br J Surg* 1987;74:1087–1090.

18. Laurence BH, Cotton PB. Decompression of malignant biliary obstruction by duodenoscopic intubation of the bile duct. *Br Med J* 1980;1:522–523.

19. Huibregtse K, Tytgat GN. Palliative treatment of obstructive jaundice by transpapillary introduction of large bore bile duct prosthesis. *Gut* 1982;23:371–375.

20. Levitt MD, Laurence BH, Cameron F, Klemp PFB. Transpapillary iridium-192 wire in the treatment of malignant bile duct obstruction. *Gut* 1988;29:146–152.

21. Binmoeller KF, Katon RM, Shneidman R. Endoscopic management of post operative biliary leaks: review of 77 cases and report of two cases with biloma formation. *Am J Gastroenterol* 1991;86:227–231.

22. Huibregtse K, Schneider B, Vrij AA, Tytgat GNP. Endoscopic pancreatic drainage in chronic pancreatitis. *Gastrointest Endosc* 1988;34:9–15.

23. Cremer M, Deviere J, Engelholm L. Endoscopic management of cysts and pseudocysts in chronic pancreatitis: long-term follow-up after 7 years experience. *Gastrointest Endosc* 1989;35: 1–9.

Advanced Therapeutic Endoscopy, 2nd Ed.,
edited by J. S. Barkin and C. A. O'Phelan.
Raven Press, Ltd., New York © 1994.

CHAPTER 29

Endoscopic Approach to the Gallbladder

Richard A. Kozarek

The development and widespread application of laparoscopic cholecystectomy have dramatically changed the need for endoscopic intubation of the gallbladder. Nevertheless, both percutaneous gallbladder puncture with direct cholecystoscopy and stone removal and retrograde gallbladder cannulation for drain or stent placement are occasionally required and may have future applicability if the dream of chemical cholecystectomy becomes a reality. Tables 1 and 2 define past, current, and potential future applications utilizing these techniques.

TECHNIQUES

Retrograde Cannulation of the Gallbladder

Retrograde cystic duct cannulation, using conventional guidewires and endoscopic retrograde cholangiopancreatography (ERCP) catheters, was initially described a decade ago (1). Cystic duct angulation and tortuosity, however, precluded direct gallbladder access in most instances. Since that time, there has been an explosion of endoscopic accessories to include catheters specifically designed to seat in the cystic duct, torquable guidewires, and toposcopic balloon systems. These accessories, in turn, have rapidly become superfluous with the development of hydrophilic wires (Glide wire, Microvasive, Inc., Belmont, MA; Tracer/nitinol wire, Wilson-Cook, Inc., Winston-Salem, NC), which, when introduced into the cystic duct orifice, can be doubled and readily advanced into the gallbladder (2) (Fig. 1).

Technically, guidewire cannulation can be facilitated by direct cystic duct cannulation with an ERCP cathe-

ter. Should the latter prove difficult, a change in patient or scope position is usually adequate, although use of a balloon catheter or double-lumen sphincterotome with variable inflation volumes or wire tension, respectively, will allow various approaches to the cystic duct orifice. Cystic duct manipulation itself is variably but often exquisitely painful, arousing the patient from a deep narcosis and comparable to the sensation patients experience with balloon dilation of the common bile duct. As noted above, hydrophilic wires usually double prior to their advancement into the gallbladder and particularly acute cystic duct angulation may require change in patient position or even manual abdominal pressure with the patient supine. I usually try to insert two to three loops of wire into the gallbladder proper (Fig. 2) and utilize this loop in conjunction with fixation of the external end of the wire to advance an ERCP catheter into the neck of the gallbladder to allow retrograde cholecystoscopy using a miniscope, place a naso-

TABLE 1. *Potential applications for percutaneous cholecystoscopy*

Stone extraction
Assurance of complete stone dissolution
Mucosal biopsy
Direct cystic duct occlusion in conjunction with chemical/thermal mucosal ablation

TABLE 2. *Potential applications for retrograde gallbladder cannulation*

Removal of obstructing cystic duct calculus
Placement of nasogallbladder drain
   Acute cholecystitis
   Study of gallbladder physiology
Placement of gallbladder stent
   Chronic cholecystitis
Retrograde cholecystoscopy
? Chemical cholecystectomy

R. A. Kozarek: Department of Gastroenterology, Virginia Mason Clinic; and Department of Medicine, University of Washington, Seattle, Washington 98111.

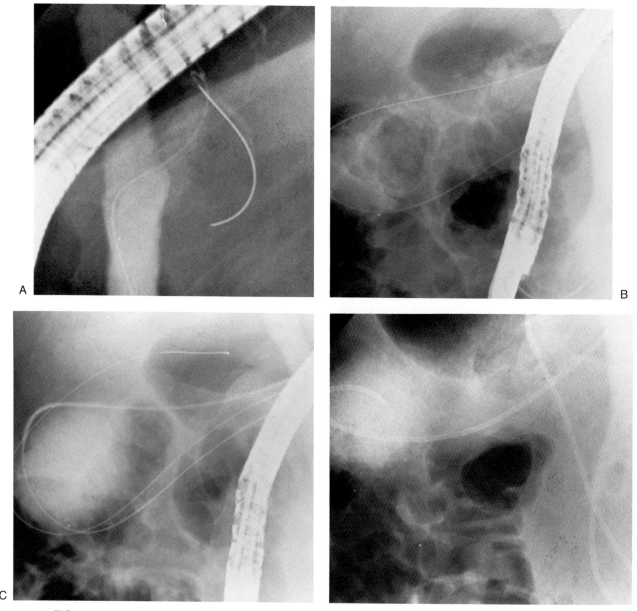

FIG. 1. Nitinol wire in the cystic duct orifice **(A)**. A diabetic patient with suppurative cholecystitis, renal transplant, severe heart failure. The guidewire is advanced to form a loop in gallbladder **(B)**. A 7-Fr catheter (*arrow*) is inserted over the guidewire and into the gallbladder **(C)**. Nasogallbladder drain **(D)**. Culture demonstrated four different gram-negative rods and enterococcus. There was rapid symptom defervescence. Laparoscopic cholecystectomy was performed 5 days later.

gallbladder drain for decompressive purposes (Figs. 1 and 2), or place a double pigtail stent from the gallbladder neck to the duodenum (Fig. 3). The former can be used in the acutely ill patient with empyema or Mirizzi's syndrome. The latter is occasionally indicated in high-risk portal hypertensive patients with recurrent cholecystitis or biliary colic. Alternatively, drains can be used to facilitate gallstone dissolution, or the guidewire itself can be used as a stent to effect cystic duct stone extraction utilizing over-the-wire extraction balloons or stone baskets.

RESULTS

In 1984, I published a prospective study successfully performing cystic duct and/or gallbladder cannulation at the time of ERCP in 37 of 50 (74%) consecutive cases (1). I also concluded that this was a technical parlor trick unless a solvent could be found that safely dissolved gallstones *in vivo*. This study antedated clinical trials utilizing either methyl tert-butyl ether (MTBE), extracorporeal shock wave lithotripsy (ESWL), or their combination.

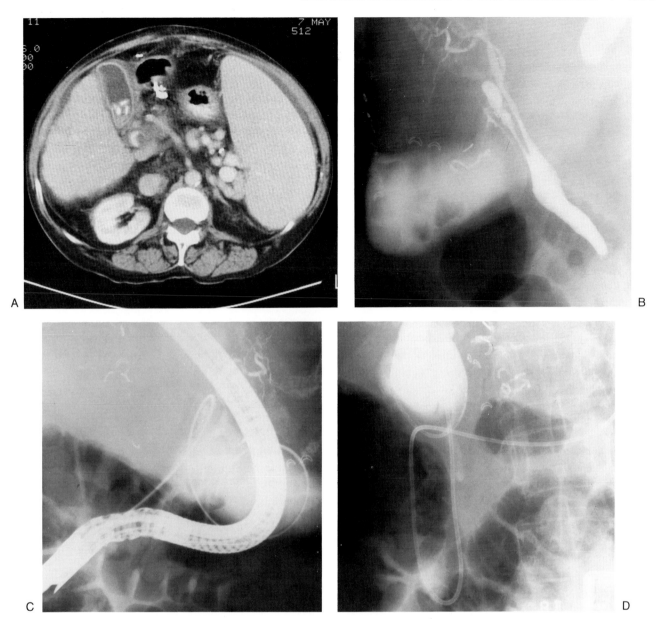

FIG. 2. Calcified gallstones in cirrhotic patient with acute cholecystitis. Note the irregular liver and large spleen **(A)**. ERCP in patient depicted in A **(B))**. A 0.035-inch guidewire is placed in gallbladder **(C)** followed by nasogallbladder drain **(D)**. The drain was ultimately exchanged for a double pigtail stent.

Since that time, a number of investigators have utilized nasogallbladder cannulation in conjunction with the above-mentioned technologies. Ponchon et al. (3) successfully cannulated the cystic duct in five patients, leaving a nasogallbladder drain in two, and they used this access to dissolve residual stone fragments with MTBE post-ESWL stone fragmentation. Maydeo et al. (4), in turn, were able to effect gallbladder cannulation in 45 of 50 patients with gallstones, 34 of whom underwent combined therapy; 60% of the latter were stone-free within 10 days. Procedure-related complications included three cases of pancreatitis, one guidewire impaction, and one cystic duct perforation. Foerster et al. (5) used nasogallbladder MTBE infusion as the sole treatment in 14 patients with gallstones, effecting litholysis in 8. Finally, Feretis et al. (6) endoscopically placed gallbladder catheters successfully in 20 of 23 patients (87%) with gallstones, including 4 patients with initial cystic duct obstruction. These authors utilized a radiopaque Teflon dilating catheter to facilitate guidewire and subsequent catheter insertion. Combining ESWL with MTBE infusion resulted in gallstone elimination in 14 of 18 (78%) patients. One patient developed mild pancreatitis and no mortality was noted.

Despite the relative safety and technical success rates noted in the series mentioned above, it appears

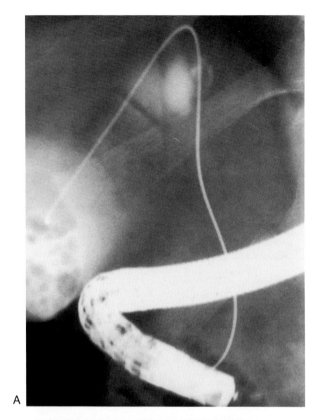

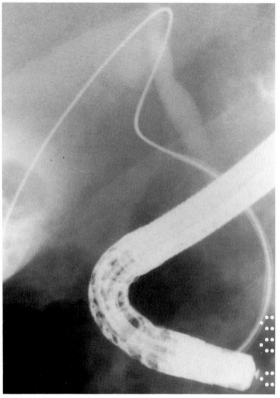

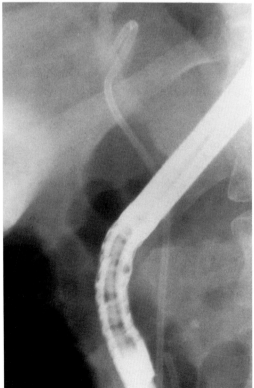

FIG. 3. Direct gallbladder cannulation with guide-wire **(A)**; note gallstones. A double pigtail stent from neck of gallbladder to duodenum **(B,C)** pre-cluded recurrent biliary colic, multiple bouts of bacterial peritonitis in a cirrhotic patient.

that there is little use for this combined technology today. Instead, I utilize nasogallbladder drains primarily to decompress an acutely inflamed gallbladder in an extremely high-risk surgical patient in an attempt to convert an urgent situation into an elective (and possibly) laparoscopic one. Other authors have utilized similar technology in the treatment of Mirizzi's syndrome, fragmenting or dissolving the impacted cystic duct stone with ESWL, electrohydraulic lithotripsy, or mono-octanoin infusion, respectively (7–9). Alternatively, in the prohibitive risk patient the drainage catheter can be exchanged for a double pigtail stent, which allows long-term gallbladder drainage by preventing stone impaction in the gallbladder neck as well as hydrops and empyema. I have had one such cholecystoduodenal stent in place for several years in a decompensated cirrhotic patient who previously had presented with recurrent biliary colic and multiple episodes of spontaneous bacterial peritonitis.

Finally, in addition to decompression, solvent infusion, and stent placement, selective gallbladder cannulation at the time of ERCP has allowed direct cholecystoscopy through the cystic duct. For instance, Foerster et al. (10) utilized a 0.5-mm miniscope in-

serted through a retrograde catheter system to successfully visualize portions of the gallbladder and cystic duct in almost 80% of attempts. Lacking tip deflection, biopsy channel, and insufflation and suction channels, the use of this instrument in the gallbladder should be considered investigational.

PERCUTANEOUS CHOLECYSTOSCOPY

The second endoscopic approach to the gallbladder requires either laparoscopic, or more commonly percutaneous, access. Popularized by Kellet et al. (11) as well as other investigators (12,13), the latter approach requires transperitoneal or transhepatic gallbladder puncture, tract maturation and dilation, and flexible or rigid endoscopic visualization of the gallbladder (Fig. 4). Such visualization has been utilized to fragment stones with mechanical or laser lithotripsy and facilitates fragment extraction (14,15). For instance, Gillams et al. (16) performed percutaneous cholecystolithotomies (PCCL) on 113 patients, utilizing local anesthesia in 10 patients and general anesthesia in the remainder. Contraindications included an intrahepatic

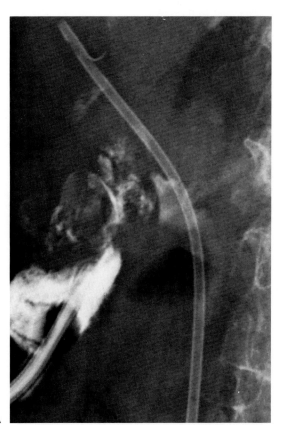
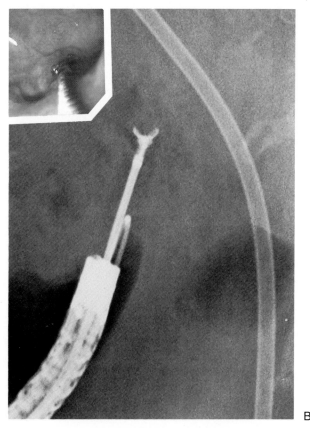

A   B

FIG. 4. Percutaneous cholecystogram demonstrating filling defects and irregular gallbladder **(A)** in a patient who presented with Mirizzi's syndrome. Note the biliary stent. Direct cholecystoscopy and biopsy **(B,** *insert***)** in the patient depicted in A. Diagnosis: chronic cholecystitis, gallbladder carcinoma.

or small, shrunken, thick-walled gallbladder. Procedure time averaged 1 hour and complete stone removal was accomplished in 88% (100/113 patients). There was a 7.6% incidence of complications, all managed conservatively. The authors concluded that PCCL is both safe and effective in clearing the gallbladder of calculi. Van Heerden et al. (17) found that 1 of 13 patients developed stone recurrence at a mean follow-up of 11 months post-PCCL.

Alternatively, percutaneous endoscopy has also been used to assure complete gallstone dissolution following MTBE infusion. For instance, Zakko et al. (18) have utilized transhepatic cholecystoscopy with a 2.2-mm miniscope, following MTBE-facilitated gallstone dissolution. No complications were noted.

Because of the risks of the percutaneous approach (bleeding, bile leak, pain) as well as the widespread utilization of laparoscopic cholecystectomy, direct cholecystoscopy will continue to be relegated to a bit part in the treatment of gallstone disease unless chemical or thermal cholecystectomy can be done easily and safely (19–21).

REFERENCES

1. Kozarek RA. Selective cannulation of the cystic duct at time of ERCP. *J Clin Gastroenterol* 1984;6:37–40.
2. McCarthy JH, Miller GL, Laurence BH. Cannulation of the biliary tree, cystic duct and gallbladder using a hydrophilic polymer-coated steerable guide wire. *Gastrointest Endosc* 1990;36:386–389.
3. Ponchon T, Beroud J, Mestes JL, Chayvialle JA. Gallbladder lithotripsy: retrograde dissolution of fragments. *Gastrointest Endosc* 1988;34:468–469.
4. Maydeo A, Nam VCH, Soehendra N. Extracorporeal shock wave lithotripsy and gallstone dissolution with MTBE via a nasovesicular catheter. *Gastrointest Endosc Clin North Am* 1991;1:167–182.
5. Foerster EC, Matek W, Domschke W. Endoscopic retrograde catheterization of the gallbladder: direct dissolution of gallstones. *Gastrointest Endosc* 1990;36:444–450.
6. Feretis ChB, Malas EG, Mansouras AJ, et al. Endoscopic transpapillary catheterization of the gallbladder followed by external shock wave lithotripsy and solvent infusion for the treatment of gallstone disease. *Gastrointest Endosc* 1992;38:19–22.
7. Martin DF, Tweedle EF, Rao PN. Endoscopic gallbladder catheterization and extracorporeal shockwave lithotripsy in the management of Mirizzi's syndrome. *Endoscopy* 1988;20:321–322.
8. Delcenserie R, Joly J-P, Dupas J-L. Endoscopic diagnosis and treatment of Mirizzi's syndrome. *J Clin Gastroenterol* 1992;15:343–346.
9. Binmoeller KF, Thonke F, Soehendra N. Endoscopic treatment of Mirizzi's syndrome. *J Clin Gastroenterol* 1993;39:532–536.
10. Foerster EC, Schneider MU, Matek W, Domschke W. Transpapillary cholecystoscopy. *Endoscopy* 1989;21:381–383.
11. Kellet MJ, Wickham JEA, Russell RCG. Percutaneous cholecystolithotomy. *Br Med J* 1988;290:433–436.
12. Picus D, Marks V, Hicks ME, et al. Percutaneous cholecystolithotomy: preliminary experience and technical considerations. *Int Radiol* 1989;173:487–491.
13. Hruby W, Stackl W, Urban M, et al. Percutaneous endoscopic cholecystolithotripsy. *Int Radiol* 1989;173:477–479.
14. Hawes RH, Kopecky KK. Percutaneous cholecystolithotripsy using the pulsed dye laser. *Gastrointest Endosc Clin North Am* 1991;1:137–148.
15. Geisinger MA. Percutaneous biliary stone extraction: radiologic and combined radiologic-endoscopic techniques. *Gastrointest Endosc Clin North Am* 1991;1:105–124.
16. Gillams A, Curtis SC, Donald J, et al. Technical considerations in 113 percutaneous cholecystolithotomies. *Radiology* 1992;183:163–166.
17. van Heerden JA, Begura JW, LeRoy AJ, Bender LE. Early experience with percutaneous cholecystolithotomy. *Mayo Clin Proc* 1991;66:1005–1009.
18. Zakko SF, Rashid S, Ramsby GR. Diagnostic percutaneous cholecystoscopy after nonsurgical treatment of gallstones. *Gastrointest Endosc Clin North Am* 1991;1:127–136.
19. Cuschieri A, Abd El Ghany AB, Holley MP. Successful chemical cholecystectomy: a laparoscopic guided technique. *Gut* 1989;30:1786–1794.
20. Becker CD, Quenville NF, Burhenne JH. Gallbladder ablation through radiologic intervention: an experimental alternative to cholecystectomy. *Radiology* 1989;171:235–240.
21. Becker CD, Iache JS, Malone DE, et al. Ablation of the cystic duct and gallbladder: clinical observations. *Radiology* 1990;176:687–690.

Advanced Therapeutic Endoscopy, 2nd Ed.,
edited by J. S. Barkin and C. A. O'Phelan.
Raven Press, Ltd., New York © 1994.

CHAPTER 30

Management of Strictures and Use of Self-Expanding Biliary Stents: Techniques and Applications

David L. Carr-Locke

CURRENT ENDOSCOPIC PRACTICE

Indications and Results

Once a decision has been made to provide palliation for malignant biliary obstruction, in the 80% or so of cases in whom this is possible without recourse to surgery, it should be achieved with minimum disturbance to the patient and with as good a quality of life as possible for the remaining weeks or months. In a consecutive personal series of over 1,000 patients referred for endoscopic retrograde cholangiopancreatography (ERCP) for the evaluation of cholestasis, the spectrum of diagnoses established was gallstones in 36%, pancreatic cancer in 22%, normal (intrahepatic cholestasis) in 14%, bile duct cancer in 8%, ampullary tumors in 7%, metastatic compression of the bile duct in 4%, dilated common bile duct (CBD) in 2% (following spontaneous stone passage), benign CBD stricture secondary to chronic pancreatitis in 2%, traumatic CBD stricture in 2%, sclerosing cholangitis in 2% and unknown in 1%. The 41% of patients suffering from a malignant cause comprised 22% pancreatic, 8% biliary, 7% ampullary, and 4% metastatic to the portal nodes. In excess of 80% were deemed incurable or unresectable on noninvasive imaging.

The placement of endoscopic endoprostheses or stents has become accepted as palliation for malignant biliary obstruction. The morbidity associated with stent insertion varies from 0% to 36% depending on

D. L. Carr-Locke: Department of Endoscopy, Brigham and Women's Hospital; and Department of Medicine, Harvard Medical School, Boston, Massachusetts 02115.

what individual centers choose to include as complications (1–13), but major morbidity is probably well under 10%. Mortality within 1 month of the procedure is 10% to 18% and median survival is about 6 months (1–3). An endoscopic approach has been shown to be superior to surgical bypass (Table 1) and percutaneous placement of endoprostheses (4,5,7,8,14).

Techniques

The endoscopic insertion of a plastic endoprosthesis across the papilla has become widely practiced over the last decade, especially since the development of 3.7 and 4.2 mm diameter channel duodenoscopes allowing the passage of 10 and 11.5 French gauge stents (Fig. 1). The methodology and range of plastic endo-

TABLE 1. *Randomized controlled trial of endoscopic versus surgical palliation in malignant biliary obstruction*

	Endoscopy		Surgery
N	101		103
Success (%)	94		91
Complications (%)	10	*	28
Procedure mortality (%)	4	*	14
30-day mortality (%)	7	*	17
Late jaundice (%)	18	*	3
Duodenal obstruction (%)	6	*	1
Hospital stay days	9	*	13
Survival weeks	22	*	26

* Statistically significant differences $p < .05$.
Data from ref. 8 and PB Cotton (*personal communication*, 1992).

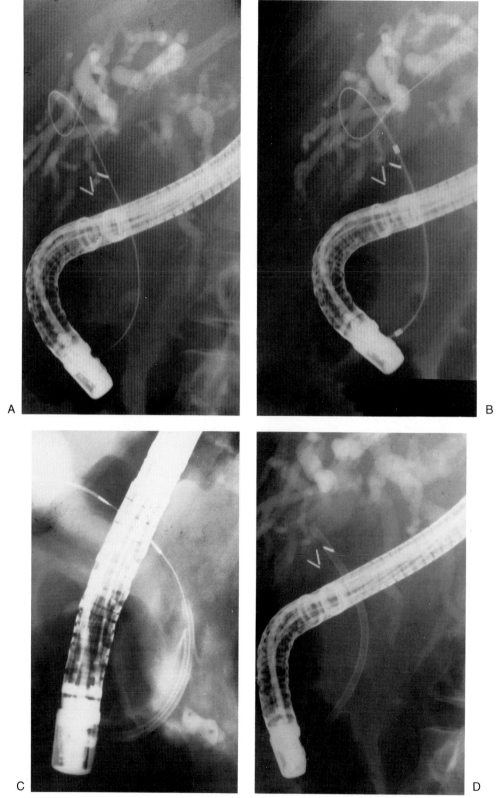

A

B

C

D

FIG. 1. Steps in plastic endoprosthesis insertion: **A:** guidewire placement, **B:** guidewire and guide catheter, **C:** 10-French stent being inserted over cytology sheath and brush, **D:** final position of stent.

TABLE 2. *Results of endoscopic palliation in malignant biliary obstruction*

	Tumor position			
	Ampullary	Low CBD	GB	Hilar
N	112	679	71	640
Success (%)	96	84–90	86	91–96
Complications (%)	8–32	10–19	14	8–60
30-day mortality (%)	1–3	10–17	13	10–33
Late jaundice (%)	36	37	25	40–68
Duodenal obstruction (%)	23	5–7.5	5	—
Survival months	9–14	4.5–6	5	2–6

Data from refs. 3, 6, 8, 9, 17.

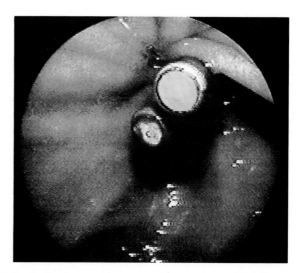

FIG. 2. Endoscopic appearance of occluded endo-prostheses.

prosthesis equipment currently available has been well standardized and there have been no major recent developments (1–9,15).

Experience with endoprosthesis insertion suggests that, in centers performing it regularly, a technical success rate of at least 85% should be expected with relief of jaundice and pruritus in 80% or more (1–11) (Table 2). Hydrophillic guidewires may speed the process and often permit access across strictures resistant to standard wires. Steerable and torque-stable wires have made some difference to selective intrahepatic cannulation. Some experts use curved catheters or a catheter with a side hole close to the tip. A sphincterotome can also be used as a deflecting device. Two wires can be placed through the channel of a stenting endoscope into both hepatic ducts in hilar lesions. Many experts do not use sphincterotomy for stent insertion unless they plan to use two stents. The "snap back" technique is useful for overcoming resistance at the papilla or strictures.

PLASTIC ENDOPROSTHESIS OCCLUSION

Stent occlusion may occur from 1 week to over 15 months after placement, with a mean of about 5 months (16–26). Patients with a clogged endoprosthesis can present with malaise, low-grade fever, or mild disturbance of liver enzymes. These symptoms and signs must be recognized, as jaundice and acute cholangitis will supervene.

Several variables may be involved, including bile flow, bile composition, bacterial contamination, and endoprosthesis characteristics such as length, shape, design, position, size, number, and material (polyethylene and other similar polymers). Attempts at manipulating all of these have been made *in vitro* (16–22) but with little progress to date in clinical practice. Ideally, the shape of the endoprosthesis should conform to the bile duct and provide anchorage to prevent migration. The double pigtail catheters initially used were soon replaced by straight stents with bends or curves and cut flaps on the upper and lower ends of the stent to prevent migration. The suggestion that absence of side holes reduces clogging has not yet been confirmed. Side holes may be necessary, especially in hilar lesions. Experimental data suggesting that leaving the tip of the stent above the papilla may prolong stent life have not been verified in clinical practice.

The maximum outside diameter of such stents is limited by the diameter of the instrument channel in the duodenoscope being used for the procedure. Initially, 7- and 8-French stents were inserted, but with the development of larger-diameter duodenoscopes the insertion of 10- to 11.5-French tubes became possible; they are now standard and perform better than smaller-diameter endoprostheses (19). Endoscopic replacement of a clogged stent is usually technically simple and replacement is associated with resolution of symptoms. Macroscopically, the material in a blocked stent resembles biliary sludge or brown pigment stones (Fig. 2) consisting mainly of calcium bilirubinate with some calcium palmitate and unidentified organic material together with bacteria (16–19) (Table 3). Endoprostheses

TABLE 3. *Composition of stent occlusion material compared to bile*

	Stent sludge (% dry weight)	Bile (% dry weight)
Bile acid	9 ± 4	56 ± 6
Cholesterol	5 ± 3	3
Lecithin	6 ± 3	20 ± 2
Bilirubin	12 ± 7	
Protein	25 ± 12	5 ± 1
Residue	20 ± 10	
Total	77 ± 20	84 ± 6

From ref. 18.

removed 2 months after insertion are usually covered with a layer of protein and bacterial remnants, and this is especially prominent around the side flaps and side holes. This bacterial "biofilm" is found consistently on surfaces of other biomedical devices connecting sterile organs with colonized organs or with the environment, such as urinary catheters, peritoneal dialysis catheters, and vascular catheters. Bacteria form biofilms by polysaccharide production, which cements the bacterial cell to the surface and mediates adhesion to sister cells. Further bacterial multiplication leads to the formation of adherent microcolonies that eventually coalesce. The polysaccharide matrix protects the bacteria from the host defense mechanisms and from toxic substances such as antibiotics, biocides, and surfactants. It is most likely that this layer is the first step in the clogging process.

Light and electron microscopic studies of blocked and functioning stents have shown that the material blocking the lumina is composed of a matrix of bacterial cells and fibrillar anionic extracellular products (16–18). Crystals of calcium bilirubinate, calcium palmitate, and cholesterol are embedded within the matrix and the bacteria are attached to the stent surface by a fibrillar matrix. Bacterial enzyme activity (β-glucuronidase and phospholipase) lead to the deposition of crystals. The use of antibiotics or antibiotic- or bacteriostatic-impregnated stents has not prevented this clogging phenomenon from occurring. The use of gallstone dissolution agents, mucolytic agents, and choleretic agents have also been ineffective in clinical practice, although encouraging *in vitro* effects have been demonstrated (20–22).

PLASTIC ENDOPROSTHESIS MANAGEMENT

The regular occurrence and predictability of plastic stent occlusion, with its serious principal complication of sepsis, militates in favor of planned removal and replacement at approximately 3- to 4-month intervals (1–4). The variability of stent survival, however, and the difficulty of predicting this in an individual patient would support the conservative approach of close clinical follow-up to anticipate early symptoms of biliary obstruction or cholangitis (23,25). Both systems are in current use in different centers, but from practical considerations, largely determined by patient referral populations and their geographical distribution, a mixed compromise is common. The cost-benefit of elective exchange has not been rigorously evaluated.

A number of techniques are available for endoprosthesis removal and replacement using a therapeutic duodenoscope:

1. Remove the stent by grasping the intraduodenal segment with a snare, biliary basket, or stent re-

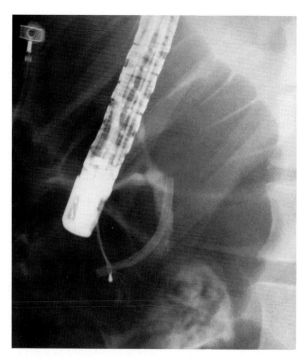

FIG. 3. Removal of occluded stent by snare extraction and removal of endoscope.

moval forceps and withdraw it with the endoscope from the patient and start again with guide catheter and guidewire (Fig. 3).
2. Remove the stent in the same way but release it in the stomach, return to the duodenum and start again, collecting the first stent from the stomach at completion of the procedure (Fig. 4).
3. Remove the stent within the endoscope by grasping it close to the tip and extract it through the channel while maintaining a cannulating position, then start again.
4. Place a guidewire alongside the first stent then extract it using method 2 and replace a new stent over the wire in the usual way.
5. Do method 4 but extract the stent within the scope and replace as in method 3.
6. Do method 5 but place the guidewire within the stent to be extracted.
7. Place a guidewire through the stent and employ the Soehendra (Fig. 5) or other stent extractor method (25,26) through the endoscope channel and place a new stent over the same wire in the usual way. The current extraction device is rather rigid and can force the stent proximally into the bile duct before it can be retrieved. Each method may be appropriate in different circumstances but, in general, methods 1 and 2 are probably used most frequently, with a growing enthusiasm for the most innovative technique of method 6.

Stent dislocation spontaneously or during attempted extraction into the bile duct may present problems of

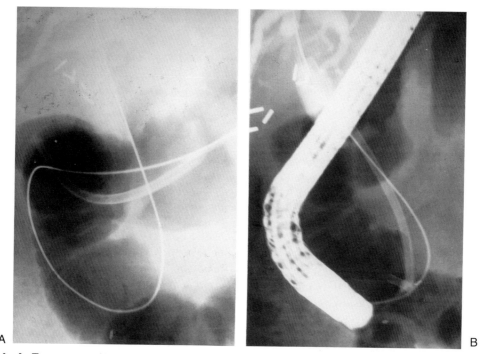

A   B

FIG. 4. A: Temporary deposit in stomach and **B:** Removal of occluded stent by snare extraction with guidewire alongside stent to maintain access.

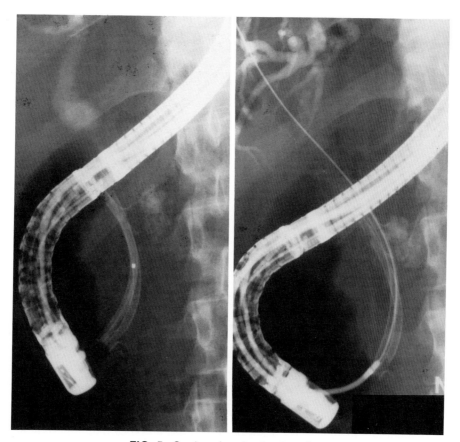

FIG. 5. Soehendra stent extraction.

retrieval but a previously placed intra-stent guidewire will allow use of the Soehendra extractor, or a basket can be used in the same way as for stone extraction. In the event of upward dislocation above a malignant stricture, balloon or catheter dilatation of the stenosis will be necessary before extraction can be attempted by snare or basket.

Inflating a balloon above the upper tip of the stent may be helpful but it is usually necessary to "go fishing" with a snare or basket. Stents that have migrated distally with impaction of the tip in the contralateral duodenal wall can be removed either by making a loop around the stent with a guidewire grasped with a snare passed alongside it or by grasping the stent with appropriate forceps.

The replaced stent should not automatically be assumed to be of the same length as that removed and the same care and attention to insertion technique should be taken as on the first occasion.

METALLIC EXPANDABLE ENDOPROSTHESES

In search of a solution to the problem of plastic stent occlusion, larger-diameter expandable metallic stents have been developed by a number of manufacturers. All types have been first deployed through the percutaneous transhepatic route (27–33) and some have not yet become available in an endoscopically usable form

in the United States, such as the Strecker and Palmaz devices.

Gianturco Z Stent

There is limited experience with the endoscopic Gianturco Z stent (Wilson-Cook), which is available as single 8-mm by 30-mm units when fully expanded (30,34,35) and can be linked end to end to cover the necessary stricture length (Fig. 6). The advantages of this device are its self-expanding nature, relative inexpensiveness, and deployment at the site of positioning of the delivery system. The disadvantages, however, have been the suboptimal delivery system, the frequent need for multiple end-to-end placements in order to cover a malignant stricture, and the theoretical and observed disadvantage that the open strutted construction may allow early occlusion by tumor ingrowth.

Strecker Stent

The Strecker stent (Microvasive, Boston Scientific Corp.) has a single tantalum thread interlocking woven meshwork construction, attains a maximum diameter of 8 mm, and is available in lengths of 4, 6, and 8 cm

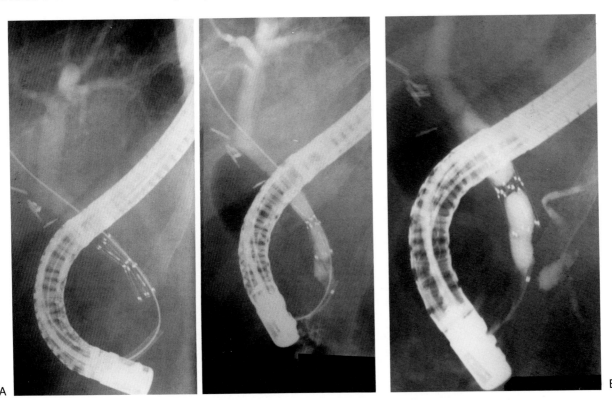

A   B

FIG. 6. A: Radiograph of Gianturco Z stent placed across mid–bile duct stricture and **B:** after tumor ingrowth has occluded stent.

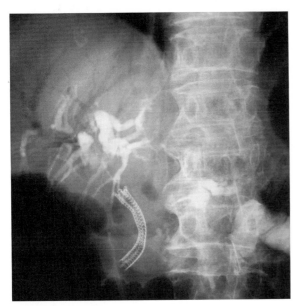

FIG. 7. Radiograph of Strecker stent across low bile duct stricture (with acknowledgment to Drs. R. Dumas and J. Delmont, Nice, France).

(Fig. 7). It requires balloon expansion at the time of placement and leads to technical failures in up to 18%, and there is no subsequent self-expansion in its original form (25,27,36). Early clinical results from nonrandomized studies are encouraging, with improved results compared with conventional plastic stents, although there is an early cholangitis rate of about 3.5% and an occlusion rate of 18% during the follow-up period. One randomized trial (27) included these devices but used the endoscopic version in common bile duct lesions and the transhepatic version for hilar lesions, compared with plastic stents inserted by the same routes. Unfortunately, all metallic stents (Strecker and Wallstent patients) were reported together, suggesting an overall improvement in palliation with less time in the hospital, a lower incidence of early cholangitis, and a lower late-occlusion rate. In Europe a self-expanding Strecker device produced from nitinol is under evaluation and the results of randomized controlled trials are awaited.

Wallstent

Most experience has been gained with the self-expanding metallic Wallstent (Schneider Stent, Inc.), which is delivered on an 8 French gauge system of 100-mm length but expands to 30 French gauge in its fully expanded form of 68-mm length (25–43) (Fig. 8). A shorter, 42-mm length has also become available for endoscopic use. The original "rolling membrane" de-

livery system, which required pressurization to separate the covering membrane from the constrained stent and shaft before attempted deployment, has been replaced by the "Unistep" system, which allows retraction of the covering membrane after internal wetting because of its inner hydrophyllic coating. The prepared system is positioned across the malignant stricture over a standard 0.035-inch guidewire and can be passed through a 3.2 mm diameter endoscope channel, although larger channels afford continued suction capabilities during deployment. Preliminary sphincterotomy or dilation of the stricture is unnecessary.

Controlled slow release of the Wallstent requires careful coordination between the endoscopist and assistant to maintain full control of the device as it expands and shortens. It is usual to leave a short length of less than 10 mm of the stent exposed in the duodenal lumen after release if the stricture to be crossed is distal, but when the stricture is more proximal the Wallstent may be deployed completely within the bile duct. Anecdotally, it is recommended that the distal end of the Wallstent should not be left immediately adjacent to the papilla in view of its tendency to straighten with time and the potential for interference with the sphincter mechanism. The stent can be repositioned during placement but only in the direction of the duodenum and before 50% deployment has taken place. Care must be exercised at initial positioning to ensure that the tip of the system is not located within a small intrahepatic duct, which will prevent expansion of the released stent and subsequent removal of the delivery catheter. This potential problem also exists when the malignant stricture is such that the stent cannot expand sufficiently to allow removal of the delivery catheter. Traction on the catheter and patience usually achieve catheter removal. In the rare event that an excessive length of Wallstent protrudes from the papilla, it is feasible to grasp the stent with a snare and extract it by withdrawing the duodenoscope. Premature deployment of the Wallstent within, or attempts to extract a Wallstent through, the endoscope channel result in severe endoscope damage and should be avoided.

Initial open studies were conducted in Europe and results have been reported (28,36–38,43) in a total of 293 patients with malignant biliary obstruction. The patient population was representative of the usual spectrum of malignant biliary lesions and technical success of implantation was high, although some failures of deployment occurred (37). Early morbidity was very low but late occlusion by tumor ingrowth or overgrowth appeared in 10% as a new problem not previously encountered with plastic stents (Fig. 9). Sludge occlusion was reported in only 2%. After the Wallstent became available for endoscopic use in the United States, a multicenter open study (Carr-Locke et al., *unpublished data*, on file at Schneider, Inc.) was undertaken to as-

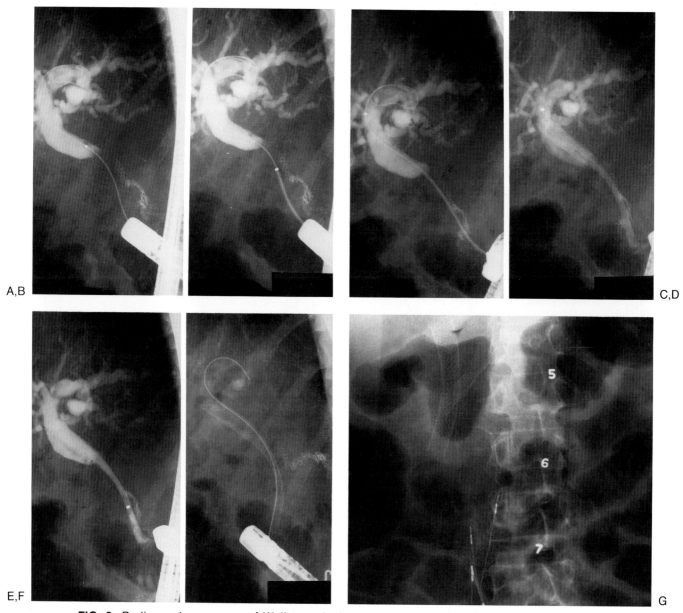

FIG. 8. Radiograph sequence of Wallstent deployment in a patient with recurrent tumor after pancreaticoduodenectomy showing **A:** initial diagnostic catheter and guidewire placement, **B:** insertion of Wallstent delivery system, **C:** position prior to deployment, **D:** immediately after deployment with delivery catheter in place, **E:** contrast injection through delivery catheter on withdrawal, **F:** guidewire placed in preparation for a second Wallstent, **G:** fully expanded Wallstent 2 weeks after insertion.

sess ease of implantation, associated complications, and long-term performance. The study involved 101 patients, 54 female and 47 male, with a mean age of 67 (range 38–100) and strictures due to pancreatic carcinoma in 33, metastatic tumors in 19, cholangiocarcinoma in 21, gallbladder carcinoma in 6, and a range of other tumors in 22. Implantation of the Wallstent was successful in all, with 78 in the common bile duct or common hepatic duct and 23 in the hilar region. Early complications (less than 30 days) included seven deaths unrelated to stent placement, and stent obstruc-

tion with mucin in one (10 days postimplant). Late complications consisted of 24 nonrelated stent deaths due to underlying disease, 9 patients with recurrent jaundice due to tumor ingrowth or overgrowth of the stent, 2 stents clogged with sludge, and 1 stent migrated. The study group concluded that the Wallstent was easy to place in bile duct and hilar strictures with acceptable early complications and good initial drainage.

The theoretical advantages that the Wallstent, with a 30 French luminal diameter compared with conven-

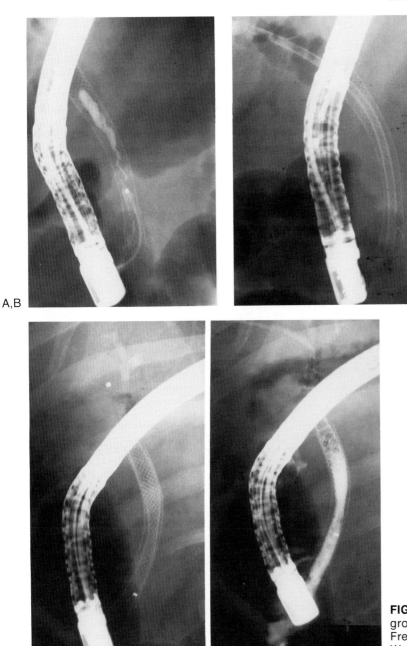

A,B

C

FIG. 9. Radiographic appearance of **A:** tumor ingrowth through Wallstent and **B:** treatment by 10 French plastic endoprosthesis or **C:** second Wallstent.

tional 10- or 11.5-French stents, would provide equal or superior initial bile drainage, prolonged stent patency, avoidance of stent exchanges, and facilitation of side-branch drainage through the open meshwork, making it a cost-effective, safe alternative for palliation of malignant bile duct obstruction, could only be decided by suitably controlled trials, and three have now been reported (29,40,41).

The Wallstent Study Group in the United States has conducted a randomized trial of the Wallstent versus conventional 10-French biliary stents to evaluate these variables (40). Of 182 patients randomized, 94 received Wallstents and 88 plastic stents with a 97% and 95% successful implantation rate, respectively. The range

of tumors was similar to the previous European and United States open studies with 47% to 51% pancreatic, 15% to 28% bile duct, 13% to 16% metastatic, and 12% to 18% others. Patients were also randomized by site of lesion, with 30% hilar and 70% bile duct in each treatment group. Early complications within 30 days included 3% occluded plastic stents, no occluded Wallstents, and 6% to 7% deaths from underlying disease. Late stent complications after 30 days were sludge occlusion of plastic stents in a further 25% and Wallstents in 5%, but tumor ingrowth or overgrowth only in the Wallstent group in 10%, making overall complication rates 16% for Wallstents and 31% for plastic stents ($p < .05$). This advantage was observed irrespective of tumor site and was more marked for patients who had received previous plastic stents where occlusion rates were three times higher. Life table analysis showed no difference in patient survival, but the mean time to stent occlusion was prolonged to 132 days for Wallstents and the probability of plastic stent occlusion was 2.8 times greater than for Wallstents. The implications of these findings are that there are significant clinical advantages of the Wallstent and, despite the higher initial expense of the device, a cost-benefit advantage resulting from the reduced need for subsequent intervention.

Of the two other prospective trials, one, from two centers in Germany and the United States (29), included 62 patients randomized to receive plastic stents in 31 and metal stents in 31 placed endoscopically or by a combined percutaneous-endoscopic approach, with Wallstents in 70% and Strecker stents in 30%. This study showed a higher patency failure rate (11% vs. 5%), a higher cholangitis rate (10% vs. 3%), longer hospitalization times (10 vs. 3 days), and higher overall treatment costs associated with plastic compared with metal stents. The other study, from Holland (41), randomized 105 patients, 49 patients to Wallstents and 56 to plastic stents, with no difference in overall survival (median 149 days) but prolonged stent patency (273 vs. 126 days, $p = .006$), lower stent occlusions and other complications (33% vs. 54%), and a 28% reduction in interventions for complications and stent occlusions for Wallstents, which the authors deduced had a significant impact on cost-effectiveness.

The problem of tumor ingrowth through the meshwork may be overcome by the development of a silicone covering (44) or the emergence of newer metallic stents that do not have an open framework (45).

The place of self-expanding metallic stents for benign biliary disease remains to be established (46–48).

ACKNOWLEDGMENT

The author wishes to acknowledge the assistance of Dr Angelo Ferrari in the preparation of the illustrations.

REFERENCES

1. Cotton PB. Endoscopic methods for relief of malignant obstructive jaundice. *World J Surg* 1984;8:854–861.
2. Huibregtse K, Katon RM, Coene PP, Tytgat GNJ. Endoscopic palliative treatment in pancreatic cancer. *Gastrointest Endosc* 1986;32:334–338.
3. Siegel JH, Snady H. The significance of endoscopically placed prostheses in the management of biliary obstruction due to carcinoma of the pancreas: results of nonoperative decompression in 277 patients. *Am J Gastroenterol* 1986;81:634–641.
4. Brandabur JJ, Kozarek RA, Ball TJ, Hofer BO, Ryan JA, Traverso LW, Freeny PC, Lewis GP. Nonoperative versus operative treatment of obstructive jaundice in pancreatic cancer: cost and survival analysis. *Am J Gastroenterol* 1988;83:1132–1139.
5. Sheperd HA, Royle G, Ross APR, Diba A, Arthur M, Colin-Jones D. Endoscopic biliary endoprosthesis in the palliation of malignant obstruction of the distal common bile duct—a randomised trial. *Br J Surg* 1988;75:1166–1168.
6. Deviere J, Baize M, DeToeuf J, Cremer M. Long term follow-up of patients with hilar malignant stricture treated by endoscopic internal biliary drainage. *Gastrointest Endosc* 1988;34:95–101.
7. Andersen JR, Sorensen SM, Kruse A, Rokkjaer M, Matzen P. Randomised trial of endoscopic endoprosthesis versus operative bypass in malignant obstructive jaundice. *Gut* 1989;30:1132–1135.
8. Dowsett JF, Russell RCG, Hatfield ARW, Cotton PB, Speer AG, Houghton J, Lennon T, Stanesby L, Macrae K, Ahern R. Malignant obstructive jaundice: what is the best management? A prospective randomised trial of surgery vs endoscopic stenting. *Gut* 1989;30:128.
9. Cullingford GL, Srinivasan R, Carr-Locke DL, Endoscopic endoprosthesis for malignant biliary obstruction. *Gut* 1989;30:A1458.
10. Mizuma Y, Ikeda E, Mukai H, Yasuda K, Nakajima M. ERBD vs PTBD in the management of inoperable malignant obstructive jaundice. *Gastroenterology* 1992;102:A323.
11. Boender J, Nix GA, Schutte HE, Lameris JS, van Blankenstein M, Dees J. Malignant common bile duct obstruction: factors influencing the success rate of endoscopic drainage. *Endoscopy* 1992;22:259–262.
12. Marsh WH, Cunningham JT. Endoscopic stent placement for obstructive jaundice secondary to metastatic malignancy. *Am J Gastroenterol* 1992;87:985–990.
13. Motte S, Deviere J, Dumonceau J-M, Serruys E, Thys J-P, Cremer M. Risk factors for septicemia following endoscopic biliary stenting. *Gastroenterology* 1991;101:1374–1381.
14. Clarke BD, Lehman GA. "Cloggology" revisited: endoscopic or surgical decompression of malignant biliary obstruction. *Am J Gastroenterol* 1990;85:1533–1534.
15. Kadakia SC, Starnes E. Comparison of 10 Fr gauge stent with 11.5 French gauge stent in patients with biliary tract diseases. *Gastrointest Endosc* 1992;38:454–459.
16. Leung JWC, Ling TKW, Kung JLS, Vallance-Owen J. The role of bacteria in the blockage of biliary stents. *Gastrointest Endosc* 1988;34:19–22.
17. Huibregtse K. *Endoscopic biliary and pancreatic drainage.* Stuttgart: Georg Thieme Verlag, 1988.
18. Speer AG, Cotton PB, Rhode J, Seddon AM, Neal CR, Holton J, Costerton JW. Biliary stent blockage with bacterial biofilm. *Ann Intern Med* 1988;108:546–553.
19. Speer AG, Cotton PB, MacRae KD. Endoscopic management of malignant biliary obstruction: stents of 10 French gauge are preferable to stents of 8 French gauge. *Gastrointest Endosc* 1988;34:412–417.
20. Coene PPLO. *Endoscopic biliary stenting: mechanisms and possible solutions of the clogging phenomenon.* MD Thesis, CIP-DATA Koninklijke Bibliotheek den Haag, 1990.
21. Sung JY, Shaffer EA, Lam K, Costerton JW. Inhibition of *E. coli* adhesion on biliary stents by bile salts with different hydrobicities. *Gastrointest Endosc* 1992;38:263.
22. Hurwich DB, Poterucha JJ, Nixon DE, Cockerill FR, Moyer TP, Thistle JL. Preventing biliary stent occlusion. *Gastrointest Endosc* 1992;38:263.
23. Johanson JF, Frakes JT. Optimal timing for stent replacement in malignant biliary strictures. *Gastrointest Endosc* 1992;38:254.
24. Cessot F, Sauterau D, Le Sidaner A, Moesch C, Berry P, Florence J, Deviois B, Pillegand B. Obstruction delay of biliary endoprostheses. *Gastroenterology* 1992;102:A304.
25. Soehendra N. A new method for exchanging biliary stents. *Endoscopy* 1990;22:271–272.
26. Mitooka H, Honsako Y, Ohno S, Miyamoto M, Aoyama N, Kasuga M. Simpler technique for replacing an obstructed biliary endoprosthesis. *Gastroenterology* 1992;102:A322.
27. Yoshioka T, Sakaguchi H, Yoshimura H, Tamada T, Ohishi H, Uchida H, Wallace S. Expandable metallic biliary endoprosth-

eses: preliminary clinical evaluation. *Radiology* 1990;177:253–257.

28. Lammer J. Biliary endoprosthesis, plastic versus metal stents. *Radiol Clin North Am* 1990;28:1211–1222.

29. Knyrim K, Wagner HJ, Starck E, Hertberg A, Pausch J, Vakil N. Metall oder Kunststoffendoprosthesen bei malignem Verschulssikterus. Ein randomisierter und prospektiver Vergleich. *Dtsch Med Wochenschr* 1992;117:847–853.

30. Kozarek RA, Ball TJ, Patterson DJ. Metallic self-expanding stent application in the upper gastrointestinal tract: caveats and concerns. *Gastrointest Endosc* 1992;38:1–6.

31. Salomonowitz EK, Antonucci F, Heer M, Stuckmann G, Egloff B, Zollikofer CL. Biliary obstruction: treatment with self-expanding metal prostheses. *J Vasc Interv Radiol* 1992;3:365–370.

32. Jackson JE, Roddie ME, Chetty N, Benjamin IS, Adam A. The management of occluded metallic self-expandable biliary endoprostheses. *Am J Roentgenol* 1991;157:291–292.

33. Nicholson DA, Chetty N, Jackson JE, Roddie ME, Adam A. Patency of side branches after peripheral placement of metallic biliary endoprostheses. *J Vasc Interv Radiol* 1992;3:127–130.

34. Shim CS, Lee MS, Kim JH, Cho SW. Endoscopic application of Gianturco-Rosch biliary Z-stent. *Endoscopy* 1992;24:436–439.

35. Kawase Y, Takemura T, Hashimoto T. Endoscopic implantation of expandable metal Z stents for malignant biliary strictures. *Gastrointest Endosc* 1993;39:65–67.

36. Neuhaus H, Hagenmuller F, Classen M. Self-expanding biliary stents, preliminary clinical experience. *Endoscopy* 1989;21:225–228.

37. Bethge N, Wagner HJ, Knyrim K, Zimmerman HB, Starck E, Pausch J, Vakil N. Technical failure of biliary metal stent deployment in a series of 116 applications. *Endoscopy* 1992;24:395–400.

38. Huibregtse K, Carr-Locke DL, Cremer M, et al. Biliary stent occlusion—a problem solved with self-expanding metal stents? *Endoscopy* 1992;24:391–394.

39. Cotton PB. Metallic mesh stents—is the expanse worth the expense? *Endoscopy* 1992;24:421–423.

40. Carr-Locke DL, Ball TJ, Connors PJ, Cotton PB, Geenen JE, Hawes RH, Jowell PS, Kozarek RA, Lehman GA, Meier PB, Ostroff JW, Shapiro HA, Silvis SE, Vennes JA. Multicenter randomized trial of Wallstent biliary endoprosthesis versus plastic stents. *Gastrointest Endosc* 1993;39:310.

41. Davids PHP, Groen AK, Rauws EAJ, Tytgat GNJ, Huibregtse K. Randomized trial of self-expanding metal stents versus polyethylene stents for distal malignant biliary obstruction. *Lancet* 1992;340:1488–1492.

42. Cremer M, Deviere J, Sugai B, Baize M. Expandable biliary metal stents for malignancies: endoscopic insertion and diathermic cleaning for tumor ingrowth. *Gastrointest Endosc* 1990;36:451–457.

43. Dertinger S, Ell C, Fleig WE, Hochberger J, Karn M, Gurza L, Hahn EG. Long-term results using self-expanding metal stents for malignant biliary obstruction. *Gastroenterology* 1992;102:A310.

44. Sievert CE, Silvis SE, Vennes JA, Abeyta B, Brennecke LH. Comparison of covered vs uncovered wire stents in the canine biliary tract. *Gastrointest Endosc* 1992;38:A262.

45. Goldin E, Wengrower D, Fich A, Safra T, Verstandig A, Globerman O, Beyar M. A new self-expandable and removable metal stent for biliary obstruction. *Gastrointest Endosc* 1992;38:A251.

46. Gillams A, Dick R, Dooley JS, Wallsten H, El-din A. Self-expandable stainless steel braided endoprosthesis for biliary strictures. *Radiology* 1990;174:137–140.

47. Costamagna G, Perri V, Mutignani M, Gabbrielli A, Crucitti F. Long-term results of endoscopic self-expanding metal stents in benign biliary strictures. *Gastroenterology* 1992;102:A309.

48. Deviere J, Cremer M, Baize M, Sugai B, Vandermeeren A. Management of common bile duct stricture due to chronic pancreatitis using metal mesh self expandable stents. *Gastrointest Endosc* 1992;38:288.

Advanced Therapeutic Endoscopy, 2nd Ed.,
edited by J. S. Barkin and C. A. O'Phelan.
Raven Press, Ltd., New York © 1994.

CHAPTER 31

The Hydrophilic Guidewire

John Baillie

Gastrointestinal endoscopists have borrowed quite a few techniques and technologies from their colleagues in interventional radiology (1–3), cardiology (4), and urology (5). Possibly the most useful of these has been the adaptation of guidewire technology for use in endoscopic retrograde cholangiopancreatography (ERCP). ERCP was largely a diagnostic modality until the evolution of duodenoscopes with large instrument channels and high-quality optics. The ability to achieve and maintain access to the biliary tree and pancreas is the key to therapeutic ERCP. Although most of the current generation of ERCP-trained endoscopists learned to use guidewires for nasobiliary drain and stent placement, guidewires are increasingly being used for non-stenting procedures. The wire-guided papillotome is a good example. Even experienced endoscopists encounter difficulty from time to time in maintaining their access to the common bile duct during sphincterotomy.

As the physics of electrocautery require that a very small length of the papillotome wire be in contact with tissue during the sphincterotomy, there is always a risk that the sphincterotome will fall out. This is a particularly unwelcome occurrence when it proves impossible to recannulate the common bile duct. The obvious solution to this problem, which was surprisingly slow in coming, was to design a papillotome through which a guidewire could be passed. The initial designs were considerably less flexible than their non-guidewire counterparts, making them cumbersome to use. However, refinement of this technology has rendered the guidewire papillotome increasingly user friendly.

One of the basic skills that the modern trainee in ERCP must master is the exchange of a variety of catheters over a guidewire. Once access to the desired duct has been achieved with a guidewire, it is a relatively simple matter to exchange the initial catheter or cannula for a variety of ERCP accessories, including dilating and retrieval balloons, wire-guided baskets, nasobiliary drains, stents, etc. The standard ERCP guidewire is 0.035 inch in diameter. Thinner guidewires are available (0.018, 0.021, and 0.025 inch) but these have the drawback of being less rigid than the 0.035-inch wire. Just the right combination of flexibility and rigidity is necessary for therapeutic ERCP work.

GUIDEWIRE DESIGN

The standard ERCP guidewire is a very useful tool but it has several disadvantages. First, it is not electrically insulated. This raises concern about its use for maintaining access during electrocautery (sphincterotomy). Even if there is no actual arcing between the sphincterotome wire and the guidewire, the proximity of the electrical elements in the sphincterotome-guidewire combination make current induction a potential risk. The second disadvantage of standard guidewires is their potential for causing injury. Significant axial forces can be transmitted through the tip of the wire, which can perforate the bile duct wall (Fig. 1) and create false tracks, especially through malignant tissue. Finally, the physical properties of the standard guidewire are often inadequate for the challenges presented by tortuous ducts and tight strictures.

To overcome these problems, considerable efforts have been made to develop soft, pliable, and electrically insulated guidewires. The hydrophilic guidewire meets these design requirements. The hydrophilic guidewire has a basic metal core, akin to those in standard guidewires, with a soft polymer plastic coating (Figs. 2 and 3). As the name suggests, this coating is hydrophilic or "water loving." When flushed with water or saline, this covering becomes soft and pliable. It is important to distinguish the hydrophilic guidewire

J. Baillie: Department of Medicine, Division of Gastroenterology, Duke University Medical Center, Durham, North Carolina 27710.

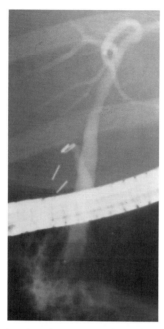

FIG. 1. Retroduodenal extravasation of contrast at ERCP following perforation caused by a standard guidewire used to assist bile duct cannulation.

from the purely Teflon-coated, woven guidewire. The physical properties of the latter are not altered by contact with liquid. As it is electrically insulated, there is no risk of electrical current leak or induction, which might cause injury to the patient or the ERCP operators. Hydrophilic coating makes the wire slippery, which has the disadvantage that it is more easily displaced than standard wires during catheter exchanges. Endoscopy nurses and assistants must take particular care when catheters are being exchanged not to pull the wire out of the desired duct. The slipperiness of the wires makes them difficult to hold in place using the elevator (bridge) of the duodenoscope. Accordingly, a high level of coordination is required between the endoscopist and his or her assistant during the procedure.

TORQUE STABILITY AND OTHER REFINEMENTS

Some of the hydrophilic guidewires that have been produced commercially are advertised as being torque-stable (6). These so-called torque-stable wires usually have an angled tip design, which allows the wire to be directed under fluoroscopic control. In practice, angled hydrophilic wires are not completely torque-stable. However, they are useful in attempting selective cannulation, for example, when access to the right or left main intrahepatic ductal system is required (Fig. 4), or when trying to negotiate a particularly tortuous stricture (Figs. 5–7) (7). Hydrophilic guidewires may be especially useful when attempting to place two or more biliary stents across a hilar stricture (Fig. 8) (8). Sometimes it is desirable to have a stiffer guidewire in place for stenting or other therapeutic manipulation. Once the desired site has been reached using a hydrophilic guidewire, this can easily be exchanged for a standard 0.035-inch metal guidewire through a catheter. The modern therapeutic ERCP endoscopist needs to be familiar with and comfortable using a variety of catheters and guidewires to achieve the best results. Early hydrophilic guidewires were difficult to visualize on fluoroscopy. More modern designs incorporate radiopaque markers (Fig. 2), which render them more easily identifiable.

CYSTIC DUCT CANNULATION

Hydrophilic guidewires have been used to negotiate the valves (of Heister) in the cystic duct for gallbladder cannulation (9). Although it is an attractive idea to attempt gallstone dissolution using solvents administered via a nasocystic drain, the vogue for this endoscopic tour de force has died with the advent of laparoscopic cholecystectomy. Laparoscopic surgery rendered this approach irrelevant. There are now few indications for endoscopic retrograde cannulation of the gallbladder.

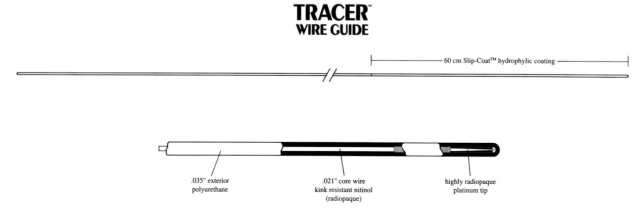

FIG. 2. TRACER hydrophilic guidewire (courtesy of Wilson-Cook Medical, Inc.).

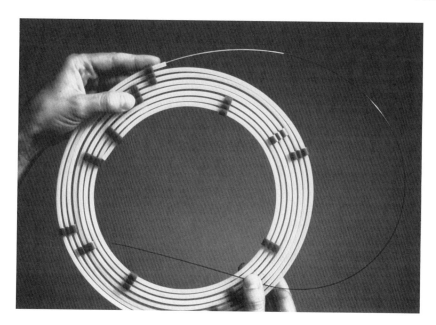

FIG. 3. Hydrophilic guidewire in its delivery sheath.

However, when this *is* necessary a hydrophilic guidewire will greatly improve the chances of success.

HYDROPHILIC GUIDEWIRES AND ELECTROCAUTERY

The widespread use of wire-guided sphincterotomes has raised concern regarding the electrical safety of these devices. Schoenfeld and colleagues (10) assessed the electrical properties of standard guidewires and

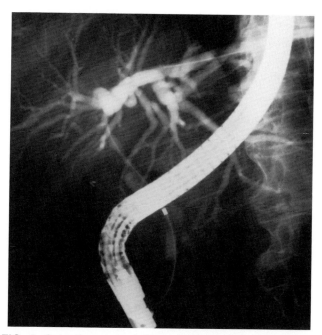

FIG. 4. Selective cannulation of left intrahepatic biliary system using a hydrophilic wire. Note the radiopaque tip for ease of visualization under fluoroscopy.

compared them to two commercially available plastic-coated alternatives. Wire-guided sphincterotomes have a septum separating the guidewire from the cutting wire (Fig. 9). Should this septum be defective, an electrical short circuit can occur. Even if the septum remains intact, loss of complete electrical insulation will allow current induction in the guidewire with potential for problems. The standard guidewire provided no electrical insulation; measured current was equivalent in both the sphincterotomy cutting wire and the guidewire. In comparison, the plastic-coated guidewires allowed no current flow, regardless of the power setting.

Johlin et al. (11) reported six electrosurgical incidents and one complication that occurred during guidewire-assisted sphincterotomy. They conducted studies on three types of guidewires: Teflon painted, Teflon sheathed, and polymer coated. Scanning electron micrography demonstrated surface imperfections in the painted Teflon guidewire coating, which create the potential for electrical short circuits between the cutting wire and guidewire (through a septal defect in a double channel catheter). Septal defects were found in 1 of 4 "factory fresh" sphincterotomes studied and 6 of 57 (11%) of those used in the clinical setting. The capacitatively coupled, induced current on the guidewires was measured at 13 to 35 mA for typical sphincterotomy settings. In contrast, the induced current on sheathed guidewires without any insulation defects was measured at < 1 mA for typical operating powers. As both short circuits and induced currents place the patient at risk for burns or perforation at the distal end of the guidewire, the authors suggest the use of Teflon-sheathed wires rather than Teflon-painted ones, if the wire is to be left in place during sphincterotomy. The

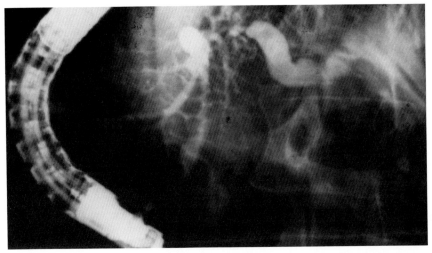

FIG. 5. Tight stricture of the pancreatic duct (later proved to be malignant).

Teflon sheath is said to offer the thickest insulation, a very low probability of surface defects, and therefore a high index of safety during electrosurgery. Teflon-sheathed guidewires are much less likely to have surface defects that would allow electrical short circuits. The painted Teflon, which should be an effective electrical insulator, covers the bulk of the guidewire, but there are many small defects in the coating that expose the underlying wire core. In contrast, Teflon-sheathed wires have a thicker insulating coat that is sealed at both ends. A typical commercially available example has a proprietary, urethane-based polymer coating over a solid nitinol wire. Another variant has an 0.035 inch exterior diameter Teflon tube annealed onto a solid, ferrous wire. Both of these so-called glidewires become slippery when moist.

Johlin et al. (11) found that approximately one in ten double-channel sphincterotomes assessed by them displayed physical evidence of electrical problems as evidenced by an inability to initiate a cut or by sparking (arcing) of the catheter tip or the guidewire introducer site. An electrical phenomenon that always occurs when using a double-channel sphincterotome and a metal-core guidewire is capacitatively coupled current. The flow of radio frequency current along the cutting wire induces a current to flow in the guidewire. Capacitively coupled currents may then flow through any exposed metal on the guidewire into the patient.

Tucker and Silvis (12) found an induced current on a Teflon-painted guidewire of 8 mA at a power setting of 50 W. A Teflon-painted guidewire with its exposed metal tip will continually subject the patient to all induced current in that guidewire. However, the induced current on the metal core components of the metal-core Teflon-sheathed guidewire would only flow into a patient if there was a fault such a break or a tear in the insulating sheath at the end that is in contact with the patient. Induced currents in the 8- to 10-mA range

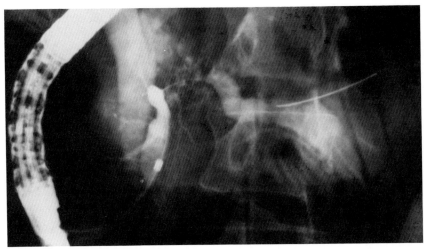

FIG. 6. Hydrophilic guidewire used to access stricture for cytology brushing and stenting.

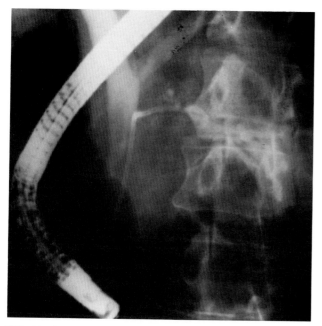

FIG. 7. A 5 French gauge polyethylene stent placed across stricture using hydrophilic guidewire.

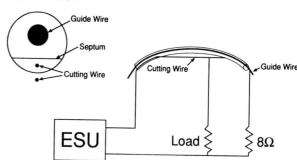

FIG. 9. Diagram of the electrical circuit used to measure the induced current on metal and insulator components of the guidewires. The sphincterotome was inside the operator channel of the endoscope, while the guidewire was inside the double channel sphincterotome. The magnified cross section was obtained at the level of the bowed sphincterotome. (From ref. 11, with permission.)

may not be clinically relevant; they are probably too small to cause tissue injury even if applied for prolonged periods. Higher values, in the 20 mA plus range, have potential to cause injury. Induced currents in a Teflon-painted guidewire are still considerably less than those present if the guidewire and the cutting wire are in a short circuit in a dual-channel sphincterotome with a septal defect. Johlin et al. calculated that transient currents in the region of 60 mA could be generated at the tip of a Teflon-painted guidewire, with potential for tissue injury.

SUMMARY

Hydrophilic guidewires have been a major addition to the armamentarium of the ERCP endoscopist. They provide a means of access through tight and irregular strictures in the biliary tree and pancreas (Figs. 5–7). A certain degree of torque stability increases the success rate for selective cannulation within the intrahepatic bile ducts (Fig. 8). Hydrophilic guidewires facilitate cystic cannulation on the rare occasions when this procedure is indicated. The hydrophilic coating provides electrical insulation, more reliably on Teflon-sheathed than painted Teflon wires. This is a significant safety feature when performing sphincterotomy with a guidewire maintaining bile duct access.

ACKNOWLEDGMENT

I am grateful to Bruce McBride, Director of Product Design, Wilson-Cook Medical, Inc., for Fig. 2, Glenn Hoskin (Wilson-Cook) and Lynne Thomas, RN (Montclair Center for Digestive Diseases) for technical assistance, and Roman Pendzich for expert secretarial assistance.

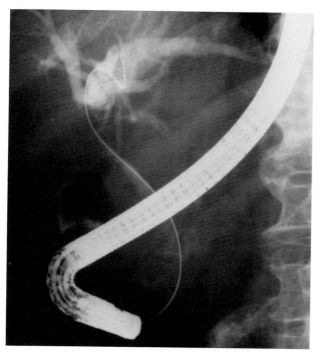

FIG. 8. Hydrophilic guidewire being used to selectively cannulate beyond a tight hilar stricture.

REFERENCES

1. Hosoki T, Hashimoto T, Masuike M, Marukawa T, Takunaga K, Kuroda C, Kozuka T. Slippery coaxial catheter system. *Radiology* 1989;171:858–859.
2. Kikuchi Y, Graves VB, Strother CM, McDermott JC, Basel SG,

Crummy AB. A new guidewire with kink-resistant core and low-friction coating. *Cardiovasc Intervent Radiol* 1989;12:107–109.

3. Mills P, Grundy A. Technical report: percutaneous treatment of a pancreatic duct fistula facilitated by a hydrophilic guidewire. *Clin Radiol* 1991;43:347–348.

4. Stamato NJ, O'Toole MF, Valquish E, Enger EL. A technique utilizing a steerable hydrophilic guidewire for permanent pacemaker implantation. *Pacing Clin Electrophysiol* 1992;15:1244–1247.

5. Swanson SK. Handling the "glidewire." *J Urol* 1991;146:1339.

6. McCarthy JH, Miller EL, Lawrence BH. Cannulation of the biliary tree, cystic duct and gallbladder using a hydrophilic polymer-coated steerable guide wire. *Gastrointest Endosc* 1990;36:386–389.

7. Venu RP, Geenen JE, Vas TC. A new guidewire technique for biliary strictures. *Gastrointest Endosc* 1991;37:553–555.

8. Hoffman BJ, Cunningham JT, Marsh WH. Multiple stent placement with a new steerable guide wire. *Gastrointest Endosc* 1990;36:595–596.

9. Miller GL, Lawrence BH, McCarthy JH. Cannulation of the cystic duct and gallbladder. *Endoscopy* 1989;21:223–224.

10. Schoenfeld PS, Jones DM, Lawson JM. Conducted current on guidewires in single lumen papillotomes. *Gastrointest Endosc* 1991;37:344–346.

11. Johlin FC, Tucker RD, Ferguson S. The effect of guidewires during electrosurgical sphincterotomy. *Gastrointest Endosc* 1992;38:536–540.

12. Tucker RD, Silvis SE. Induced current on the guide wire during sphincterotomy. *Gastrointest Endosc* 1989;35:45–47.

Advanced Therapeutic Endoscopy, 2nd Ed.,
edited by J. S. Barkin and C. A. O'Phelan.
Raven Press, Ltd., New York © 1994.

CHAPTER 32

Endoscopic Therapy of the Sump Syndrome

Seth A. Cohen and Jerome H. Siegel

The sump syndrome, an unusual but well-recognized complication of a side-to-side choledochoenterostomy, results when a stagnant pool of bile and debris collects in the bypassed, or dependent, limb of the bile duct, leading to recurrent biliary colic or cholangitis. Previously, this condition was only treated surgically (1); now, therapeutic endoscopy is the treatment of choice. In this chapter we review the syndrome and discuss its management utilizing therapeutic endoscopic technique.

THE SUMP SYNDROME

Choledochoduodenostomies are performed in 6.3% to 8.6% of patients undergoing biliary surgery for benign disease, usually in patients with a dilated common bile duct (CBD) and recurrent stones, when complete clearance of CBD stones cannot be assured, or when drainage of the distal duct is compromised (2,3). A choledochoenterostomy allows the proximal biliary tree to drain freely into the gut, leaving the distal CBD as a potential stagnant pool if transpapillary drainage is inadequate (Fig. 1). The sump syndrome represents a diverse group of signs and symptoms developing as a result of this stagnant collection of lithogenic bile, debris, calculi, and bacteria that accumulates in the defunctionalized distal CBD. Patients present with a variety of symptoms: unexplained upper abdominal pain with normal liver chemistries, biliary colic, frank cholangitis, pyogenic liver abscesses, jaundice, or recurrent pancreatitis. Reports of the incidence of this

syndrome following choledochoduodenostomy vary from 0% to 6.9% (2,4).

It had been postulated that cholangitis could only occur in patients in whom the anastomosis had stenosed (5). Endoscopic reports have demonstrated, however, that cholangitis does indeed occur in the absence of anastomotic stenosis (6,7). Several factors are thought to be important in the pathogenesis of the sump syndrome: (a) length of the excluded limb of the bile duct, (b) presence of inadequate papillary drainage ("papillary stenosis" or dysfunction of the sphincter of Oddi), (c) obstruction of the anastomosis either by stenosis or by calculi or debris, and (d) the presence of retained stones in the distal CBD after surgery (6–8).

Before the advent of therapeutic endoscopy, repair of the sump syndrome demanded an additional operation. Repeat biliary surgery carries significant morbidity and mortality depending on the overall health of the patient. Several small, retrospective comparisons of surgical versus endoscopic correction of the sump syndrome show that they are equally effective (7,9). Thus endoscopic therapy, particularly in elderly, high-risk patients, should be the first line of therapy. Surgery is available for patients in whom endoscopic therapy fails.

ENDOSCOPIC DIAGNOSIS

The endoscopic approach to the diagnosis and treatment of the sump syndrome is safe and effective. It can be tailored to the specific pathophysiologic setting of the individual patient.

Patients with symptoms following choledochoduodenostomy are best evaluated with endoscopic retrograde cholangiopancreatography (ERCP). The results of ERCP evaluation of 49 symptomatic patients after choledochoduodenostomy are listed in Table 1.

S. A. Cohen: Beth Israel Medical Center; and Department of Medicine Columbia University, St. Luke's-Roosevelt Hospital Center, New York, New York, 10028.

J. H. Siegel: Department of Medicine, Mount Sinai School of Medicine; and Department of Endoscopy, Beth Israel Medical Center, North Division, New York, New York 10028.

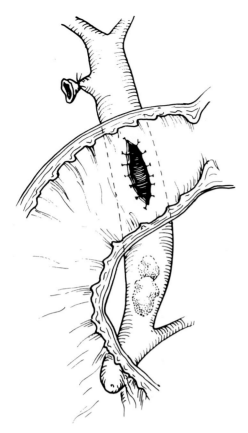

FIG. 1. An artist's representation of the sump syndrome. A lateral side-to-side choledochoduodenostomy is present, which allows free drainage of bile; several gallstones, however, are trapped in the distal limb of the common bile duct, which can lead to biliary colic and cholangitis.

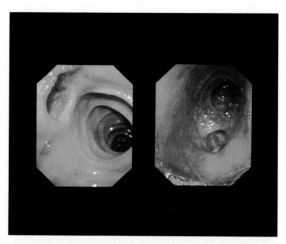

FIG. 2. Videoendoscopic photographs of a choledocho-duodenostomy. **Left:** The duodenal lumen is seen and the anastomosis is at the 10 o'clock position. **Right:** The choledochal anastomosis is viewed *en face.* Separate openings of the proximal and distal bile duct are visible.

bile duct into the jejunum, or with a GI series by watching for reflux of barium into the biliary tree.

As the duodenoscope is passed through the pylorus, during the endoscopic examination, the choledochoduodenal anastomosis should be seen on the anterior wall of the proximal duodenum (Figs. 2, 3, and 4). When the anastomosis is widely patent it can be mistaken for a duodenal diverticulum, whereas if it has stenosed to only a small orifice it can be easily overlooked by the endoscopist. Identifying this anastomosis, which may

A diagnostic ERCP performed in the setting of a previous choledochoenterostomy must identify three variables: (a) patency of the anastomosis, (b) presence of stones or debris in the bile duct, and (c) adequacy of bile drainage through the papilla. In the majority of patients, the biliary enteric anastomosis is a lateral side-to-side choledochoduodenostomy that is easily accessible with an endoscope. Despite rare reports (10), a choledochojejunostomy (CJ) anastomosis is not routinely accessible endoscopically. The CJ anastomosis can be visualized and assessed during cholangiography by observing spillage of contrast media from the

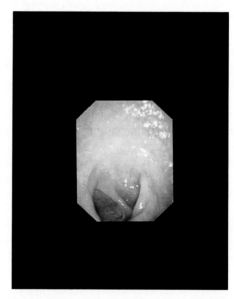

FIG. 3. Videoendoscopic photograph of a widely patent choledochoduodenal anastomosis. In the foreground is duodenal bulb, which leads directly into the distal limb of the common bile duct. The continuation of the second portion of the duodenum, which is not visible, lies at a sharp angle behind the fold at the 5 o'clock position.

TABLE 1. *Incidence of biliary pathology among 49 symptomatic patients, out of a total 173 patients, after choledochoduodenostomy*

Symptom	n	Stenosis	Choledo-chobezoar	CBD stone
Dyspepsia	26	0	0	0
Colicky pain	15	2	2	0
Cholangitis	8	8	2	8

Adapted from ref 2.

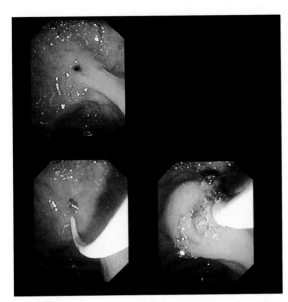

FIG. 4. Top: A stenosed choledochoduodenostomy is seen. **Bottom:** An 11.5-mm retrieval balloon is advanced through the anastomosis into the distal CBD *(left)*. Stone debris is extracted through the stoma *(right)*.

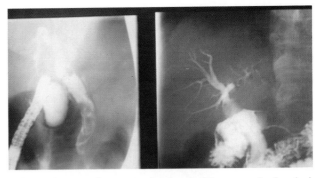

FIG. 5. Cholangiograms obtained with an occlusion balloon via the choledochoduodenostomy in a patient with the sump syndrome. **Left:** Multiple stones are seen in the distal CBD. **Right:** The intrahepatic radicles are seen with reflux of contrast media in the small bowel.

After inspection of the anastomosis, the duodenoscope is advanced down to the level of the papilla, and retrograde cholangiography is performed (Fig. 6). When the presence of a choledochoduodenostomy is inadvertently missed by the endoscopist, spillage of contrast into the proximal duodenum during cholangi-

be only a few millimeters in diameter, becomes important in patients in whom a cholangiogram via the papilla is not possible due to significant papillary stenosis.

Occlusion balloons (8.5, 11.5, and 15 mm) are useful in calibrating the diameter of the anastomosis and permit cholangiography through the stoma. Occluding the stoma with an inflated balloon prevents reflux of contrast out of the bile duct, providing a complete cholangiogram. In the absence of stones or debris, an anastomosis of 1 cm or greater provides adequate drainage and the patient should not develop symptoms. Individual openings of the proximal and distal bile duct can often be seen when the anastomosis is viewed *en face*, appearing as a saddle (Fig. 2). The natural curve of the balloon catheter and the elevator make it technically easier to obtain a cholangiogram of the proximal biliary tree since the catheter tends to enter that limb more readily. A complete cholangiogram must be performed to exclude debris or calculi. It is usually possible to flip the balloon catheter down to obtain a cholangiogram of the distal bile duct or sump to assess for filling defects and distal drainage (Fig. 5).

Because of the anastomosis, there are always air bubbles present on cholangiography, so it can be difficult to determine whether a filling defect represents a calculus or debris (Fig. 6). In this situation, if the choledochoduodenostomy is widely patent, a small-caliber forward-viewing endoscope may be passed directly through the stoma for direct, peroral, cholangioscopy, which enables the endoscopist to provide positive identification and treatment (11–13) (Figs. 7 and 8).

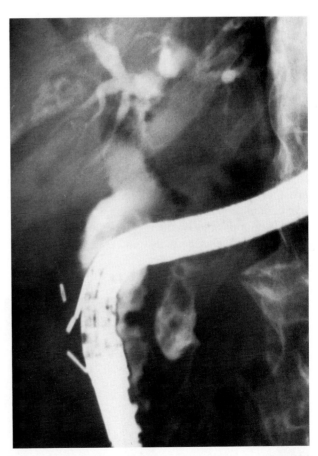

FIG. 6. A cholangiogram via the papilla in a patient with the sump syndrome. Air bubbles and stones are seen in the sump, the distal limb of the CBD. Contrast media is seen flowing out through the anastomosis into the bulb.

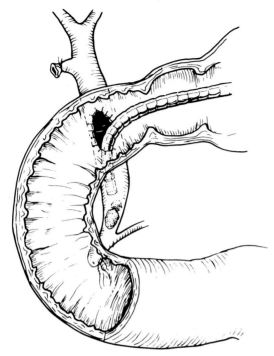

FIG. 7. An artist's representation of the technique of peroral cholangioscopy via a choledochoduodenostomy. A small-caliber, forward-viewing endoscope is advanced through the anastomosis into the distal common bile duct and identifies gallstones.

ography via the papilla makes it difficult to obtain a complete cholangiogram and may confuse the endoscopist. An important clue to the presence of an unanticipated choledochoenterostomy is pneumobilia, seen on fluoroscopy, in the absence of a sphincterotomy.

In our experience, the papilla is difficult to cannulate in a high percentage of patients with a choledochoenterostomy because of stenosis and may require selective cannulation using a guidewire. When a cholangiogram is not possible via the papilla, it must be obtained via the choledochoduodenostomy (Fig. 5), or, in cases

with a strong indication, a precut sphincterotomy is required. Occasionally, a small choledochoduodenal fistula is present and can be cannulated to access the bile duct.

A subgroup of patients who present with abdominal pain after a choledochoduodenostomy have abnormal pancreatograms. Polydorou and colleagues (7) reported 4 patients (out of a total of 17) with unexplained chronic pancreatitis associated with the sump syndrome and postulated an obstructive etiology related to the sump. We, also, have seen patients with a history of choledochoduodenostomy with unexplained recurrent pancreatitis, which is assumed to be on the basis of sphincter dysfunction.

ENDOSCOPIC THERAPY

After a diagnostic study has been completed, a decision is made as to whether mechanical biliary abnormalities explain the symptoms. Treatment should be tailored to the specific abnormality.

If the anastomosis is patent and stones or debris are present within the bile duct, extraction is required. Calculi located in the proximal biliary radicles are best removed using standard balloon or basket techniques via the choledochoduodenal anastomosis (Fig. 4). It is difficult to obtain proximal biliary cannulation via the papilla due to stenosis of the papilla and because the accessories tend to exit through the anastomosis.

Several options exist to extract stones and debris from the distal CBD. Stones can be removed through the anastomosis with a balloon or basket advanced through the endoscopic channel (12,14–15) (Fig. 9). With the anastomosis kept in view endoscopically, the balloon or basket is inserted through the anastomosis, and the stones, which are visualized on the fluoroscopy monitor, are pulled back out through the stoma. This technique is best suited for solitary stones retained after surgery. But if the stones in the sump are soft,

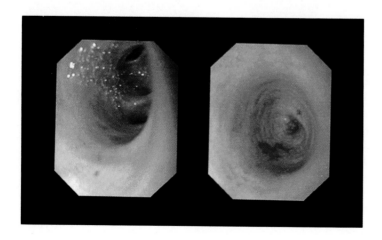

FIG. 8. Videoendoscopic photographs of peroral cholangioscopy. **Left:** The bifurcation and intrahepatic biliary radicles are seen. **Right:** The distal common bile duct is seen. No stone or debris was present.

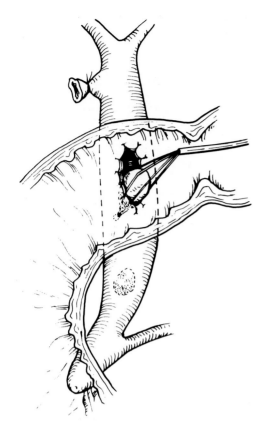

FIG. 9. A schematic representation of basket extraction of CBD stones via the choledochoduodenal anastomosis.

primary CBD stones, simple removal does not treat the underlying problem, namely a reservoir of stagnant lithogenic bile. Thus, the stones and symptoms are likely to recur (16). Definitive treatment requires establishment of adequate biliary flow to prevent stasis, which is accomplished by endoscopic sphincterotomy. One must assume, in many patients in whom a choledochoduodenostomy was performed specifically because bile drainage through the papilla was inadequate at the time of surgery (e.g., papillary stenosis, distal stricture), that bile drainage will remain compromised despite the bypass.

The technical aspects of performing endoscopic sphincterotomy and stone extraction via the papilla in patients with the sump syndrome are no different than in patients with standard anatomy (Fig. 10). However, it may require up to 3 procedures (average 1.9) in order to assure complete bile duct clearance (7). Free cannulation of the bile duct with a sphincterotome, as mentioned above, is often not possible in these patients because of papillary stenosis (17). In our experience, a precut sphincterotomy has been required with increased frequency to achieve access into the bile duct for stone clearance and drainage (12,18). Rarely, a small choledochoduodenal fistula is present on the papilla and a sphincterotome can be introduced into the

bile duct. All stones and debris should be extracted, if possible, at the time of sphincterotomy.

Stasis in the distal CBD may still occur despite performing an adequate sphincterotomy: Due to the lack of the physiologic pressure gradient, stones may recur (6). However, it is easy to remove recurrent stones and debris with balloon or basket catheters at repeat ERCP.

If there is a significant postsurgical stricture of the bile duct, endoscopic balloon dilation and long-term stent placement is indicated (19,20) (Fig. 11).

When there is a stricture of the choledochoduodenal anastomosis with inadequate drainage of the proximal biliary system associated with CBD stones or symptoms, there are three options for endoscopic treatment: (a) improving distal biliary flow through the papilla by performing a sphincterotomy, (b) dilating the stenotic anastomosis with a hydrostatic balloon, and (c) actually enlarging the stoma using a sphincterotome. As discussed, sphincterotomy in this setting does not dif-

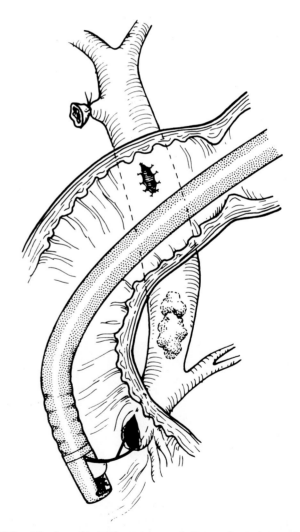

FIG. 10. A schematic representation of endoscopic sphincterotomy in a patient with the sump syndrome.

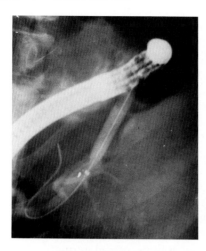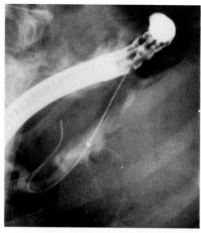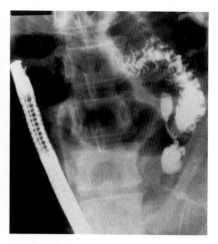

FIG. 11. **Left:** Cholangiography in a patient with stenosis of a choledochoduodenal anastomosis and stricturing of the both limbs of the bile duct. **Middle:** A guidewire and balloon are advanced through the anastomosis into the proximal bile duct. **Right:** Dilation with an 8 mm hydrostatic balloon.

fer from the standard technique. Balloon dilation of the biliary enteric anastomoses has been described by the interventional radiologists (21), but there are limited reports of this technique in the endoscopic literature (20) (Fig. 12). In our experience, balloon dilatation of the anastomosis does not lead to effective long-term results in most patients.

Blair and colleagues (17) reported a technique in which they enlarged strictured, pinhole-sized choledochoduodenal anastomoses (<1 mm) using standard diathermic sphincterotomy technique in three patients. The CBD could not be cannulated via the papilla in any patient. In two patients the anastomosis was enlarged to 1 cm, and the patients remained asymptomatic. In the third patient the anastomosis was enlarged to only 5 mm and recurrent cholestasis developed. There were no complications but all stoma had restrictured by approximately 50% on follow-up examination. This is an interesting technique that we do not perform or advocate because of the potential of life-

threatening hemorrhage. In our experience, precut papillotomy is a safer, more established technique.

A difficult therapeutic decision confronts the endoscopist when a patient presents with a convincing history of symptoms, say biliary colic or cholangitis, but a normal study is found at ERCP. Eaton and colleagues (8) reported that three of their seven patients treated with sphincterotomy improved despite the fact that they had normal studies. It is not clear whether these patients passed stones prior to cholangiography. If no stones or debris are found at ERCP, we are inclined to perform a sphincterotomy in patients who manifested objective signs, such as jaundice or significant cholangitis. These decisions must be made on an individual basis.

Patients with recurrent pancreatitis should be subclassified as recurrent acute or chronic pancreatitis on the basis of their pancreatography and clinical findings. Recurrent acute pancreatitis can be related either to debris in the sump (repeated episodes of gallstone pan-

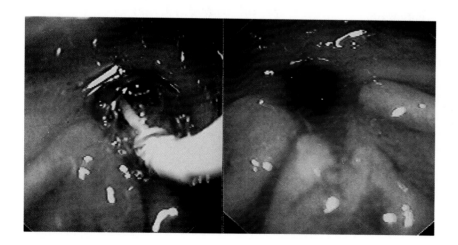

FIG. 12. Balloon dilation of a stenotic choledochoduodenal anastomosis. **Left:** A hydrostatic balloon is inflated in the anastomosis. **Right:** The stoma after dilation.

TABLE 2. *Results of series of endoscopic therapy of the sump syndrome*

Authors	Number	Anastomosis	Therapy	Outcome
Barkin et al., 1980 (14)	2	2/2 Open	Stone removal by lavage and basket extraction via the anastomosis	Asymptomatic at 18 and 60 months
Baker et al., 1985 (24)	8	3/8 Open	5 Sphincterotomy 1 Irrigation 2 Surgery	Asymptomatic 6–14 months Persistent symptoms Asymptomatic 6–14 months
Eaton et al., 1989 (8)	8	6/7 Open	7 Sphincterotomy 1 Failure	3 Asymptomatic, 3 improved, 1 surgery 14–94 months Persistent symptoms
Marbet et al., 1987 (9)	13	9/9 CD open 3/4 CJ open	8 Sphincterotomy (2 Failures) 5 Surgery	Asymptomatic 6–60 months 4 Asymptomatic, 1 persistent symptoms 1–126 months
Polydorou et al., 1989 (7)	17	10/14 CD open 1/2 CJ open	13 Sphincterotomy (2 Failures) 4 Surgery	11 Asymptomatic, persistent symptoms 6–48 months 1 Asymptomatic, 3 persistent symptoms
Siegel 1981 (6)	11	8/8 CD open 3/3 CJ open	11 Sphincterotomy	10 Asymptomatic, 1 recurrent stones 3–30 months

Adapted from ref. 7.
CD, choledochoduodenostomy; CJ, choledochojejunostomy.

creatitis) or to dysfunction of the sphincter of Oddi (8). These patients may benefit from a trial of endoscopic sphincterotomy to clear the sump and ablate the sphincter. Some patients may have chronic pancreatitis on an obstructive basis related to the sump, and a trial of sphincterotomy is warranted (7). Similarly, if a significant stricture or pancreatic stones are present, endoscopic therapy is indicated as in other patients (22,23).

RESULTS

The results of six published series of endoscopic treatment of the sump syndrome are summarized in Table 2. Technical success has varied from 78% to 100% in these retrospective reports. The few patients in whom endoscopic therapy failed were managed surgically. Two patients with coexisting sump syndrome and severe chronic pancreatitis were referred directly to pancreatoduodenectomy (7). There are no reports of any mortality and no significant morbidity occurred. Seventy-eight percent (45 out of 58) of the choledochoenterostomies were patent in this collected group of patients with the sump syndrome.

CONCLUSION

ERCP provides a safe and effective technique for the diagnosis and treatment of the sump syndrome. Endoscopic clearance of stones and debris in the sump, either distally via the transpapillary route following sphincterotomy or by direct extraction via the choledochoduodenostomy, can be achieved in most patients and is the treatment of choice for this condition. Although the sump syndrome occurs infrequently, ERCP plays a crucial role in the recognition, diagnosis, and treatment of this condition.

REFERENCES

1. McSherry CK, Fischer MG. Common bile stones and biliary-intestinal anastomoses. *Surg Gynecol Obstet* 1981;153:669–676.
2. Parrilla P, Ramirez P, Sanchez F, et al. Long-term results of choledochoduodenostomy in the treatment of choledocholithiasis: assessment of 225 cases. *Br J Surg* 1991;78:470–472.
3. Deustch AA, Nudelman I, Gutman H, et al. Choledochoduodenostomy an important surgical tool in the management of common bile duct stones. *Eur J Surg* 1991;157:531–533.
4. Delikaris PG. Choledochoduodenostomy. *Surg Ann* 1989;21:181–199.
5. Madden JL, Chun JY, Kandalaft S, et al. Choledochoduodenostomy: an unjustly maligned surgical procedure. *Am J Surg* 1970;119:45–52.
6. Siegel JH. Duodenoscopic sphincterotomy in the treatment of the "sump syndrome". *Dig Dis Sci* 1981;26:922–928.
7. Polydorou A, Dowsett JF, Vaira D, et al. Endoscopic therapy of the sump syndrome. *Endoscopy* 1989;21:126–130.
8. Eaton MC, Worthley CS, Toouli J. Treatment of postcholedochoduodenostomy symptoms. *Aust NZ J Surg* 1989;59:771–774.
9. Marbet UA, Stadler GA, Faust H, et al. Endoscopic sphincterotomy and surgical approaches in the treatment of the "sump syndrome." *Gut* 1987;28:142–145.
10. Sivak MV Jr. *Gastroenterologic endoscopy.* Philadelphia: WB Saunders, 1987.
11. Siegel JH. Biliary bezoar: the sump syndrome and choledochoenterostomy. *Endoscopy* 1982;14:238–240.
12. Siegel JH. *Endoscopic retrograde cholangiopancreatography: technique, diagnosis, and therapy.* New York: Raven Press, 1992.
13. Rösch W, Koch H. Peroral cholangioscopy in choledochoduode-

nostomy patients using the pediatric fiberscope. *Endoscopy* 1978;10:195–198.

14. Barkin JS, Silvis S, Greenwald R. Endoscopic therapy of the "sump" syndrome. *Dig Dis Sci* 1980;25:597–601.

15. Alberti-Flor JJ, Hernandez ME, Ferrer JP. Endoscopic removal of a large common bile duct stone through a choledochoduodenostomy [Letter]. *Gastrointest Endosc* 1988;34:369.

16. Polydorou AA, Chisholm EM. Management of the sump syndrome after choledochoduodenostomy [Letter]. *Gastrointest Endosc* 1989;35:355.

17. Blair AJ, Leung JWC, Cotton PB. Endoscopic treatment of stomal stenosis after choledochoduodenostomy: preliminary report. *Surgery* 1985;97:487–489.

18. Cohen SA, Kasmin FE, Resnicow KA, et al. Techniques of endoscopic sphincterotomy in a referral population. *Gastrointest Endosc* 1992;38:262 (abst).

19. Huibregtse K, Katon RM, Tytgat GNJ. Endoscopic treatment of postoperative strictures. *Endoscopy* 1986;18:133–137.

20. Siegel JH, Guelrud M. Endoscopic cholangiopancreatoplasty: hydrostatic balloon dilatation in the bile duct and pancreas. *Gastrointest Endosc* 1983;29:99–103.

21. Teplick SK, Wolferth CC, Hayes MF, et al. Balloon dilatation of benign postsurgical biliary enteric anastomotic strictures. *Gastrointest Radiol* 1982;7:307–310.

22. Kozarek RA, Ball TJ, Patterson DJ. Endoscopic approach to pancreatic duct calculi and obstructive pancreatitis. *Am J Gastroenterol* 1992;87:600–603.

23. Cremer M, Deviere J, Delhaye M, et al. Stenting in severe chronic pancreatitis: results of medium-term follow-up in seventy-six patients. *Endoscopy* 1991;23:171–176.

24. Baker AR, Neoptolemos JP, Carr-Locke DL, et al. Sump syndrome following choledochoduodenostomy and its endoscopic treatment. *Br J Surg* 1985;72:433–435.

Advanced Therapeutic Endoscopy, 2nd Ed.,
edited by J. S. Barkin and C. A. O'Phelan.
Raven Press, Ltd., New York © 1994.

CHAPTER 33

ERCP Biopsy and Cytology Techniques

Maurits J. Wiersema and Glen A. Lehman

The management of obstructing pancreaticobiliary lesions identified at endoscopic retrograde cholangio-pancreatography (ERCP) depends heavily on the clinical setting. Biliary strictures occurring after recent surgery, especially laparoscopic cholecystectomy, will generally be benign postoperative strictures. Elderly patients with obstructive jaundice and a double duct sign at ERCP will almost invariably have pancreatic cancer. Overall, many patients with obstructing ductal lesions seen at ERCP can be managed without histologic confirmation. However, histologic confirmation, if simple and inexpensive, would be ideal in nearly all such lesions.

A variety of nonoperative techniques can be used to establish a histologic diagnosis in pancreaticobiliary ductal strictures. These techniques can be classified into three categories: (a) percutaneous sampling with smaller-gauge cytology aspiration needles or larger-gauge cutting biopsy needles; (b) intraductal collection of fluids from the biliary or pancreatic duct for cytology analysis; and (c) endoluminal collection methods including brush cytology, fine needle aspiration (FNA), forceps biopsy, and stent retrieval or scrape biopsy. Of the percutaneous techniques, computed tomography (CT) and ultrasound-guided needle aspiration biopsy are two of the more common methods employed. The sensitivity of these techniques in detecting pancreatic carcinoma ranges from 70% to 95% (1–4). This yield decreases in primary tumors of the bile duct or strictures in which a mass is not well visualized (1–3). Intraductal sampling at ERCP is especially attractive in this latter group.

Although ERCP may identify pathology that is highly suggestive of malignancy, the ductogram lacks specificity. The addition of tissue sampling technique(s) to confirm the diagnosis would be advantageous. Definitively distinguishing benign from malignant pancreaticobiliary strictures may avoid additional diagnostic tests and aid in therapeutic decisions.

Several studies have been published that describe ERCP cytology and biopsy methods (5–16). Limited data are available supporting the utility of secretin-stimulated pure pancreatic juice collection and bile aspiration for assisting in the diagnosis of malignant pancreatic and biliary strictures (17–21). Unfortunately, the latter methods have limited sensitivity for malignant strictures (20–47%). Additionally, some have suggested the technique be carried out independently from ductography due to cytology artifact caused by the contrast medium (22). For these reasons, this technique will not be further discussed. Instead, we shall focus on the other available ERCP cytology and biopsy techniques and detail prior experience gained with these methods. This chapter focuses on biliary tissue sampling performed at ERCP, but pancreatic sampling is reviewed where data are available.

TECHNIQUES

Prior to attempting procurement of a tissue diagnosis, a satisfactory cholangiogram and/or pancreatogram is generally recommended. Defining the stricture zone will help in obtaining tissue from the correct site. In those cases where a complete duct cutoff is present and visualization of the stricture and/or proximal ductal system is not possible, sampling is possible only from the downstream margin. When obstructive jaundice is present, we generally recommend sphincterotomy to facilitate tissue sampling and endoprosthesis insertion. The available FNA catheters and transpapil-

M. J. Wiersema: Department of Medicine, Division of Gastroenterology/Hepatology, Indiana University School of Medicine; St. Vincent Hospitals and Health Care Center; Indiana Gastroenterology Inc., Indianapolis, Indiana 46260.

G. A. Lehman: Department of Medicine, Division of Gastroenterology/Hepatology, Indiana University School of Medicine, Indianapolis, Indiana 46202.

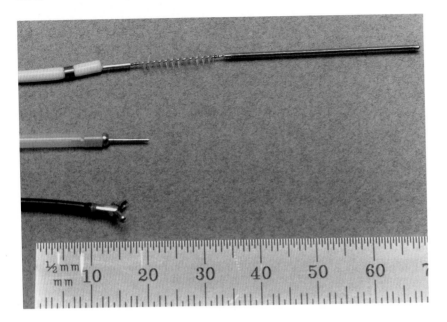

FIG. 1. The Geenen cytology brush *(top)*, Howell biliary aspiration needle *(middle)*, and a prototype malleable biopsy forceps *(bottom)* are shown. The cytology brush has a guidewire on the tip that permits maintaining access across the stricture while the sample is collected. The Howell biliary aspiration needle has several modifications that facilitate cannulation, including a metal ball tip as well as a curved distal end.

lary biopsy forceps are somewhat cumbersome for cannulation unless a sphincterotomy has been done (Fig. 1).

Brush Cytology

Several techniques are available to perform brush cytology. One method involves placement of an intraductal guidewire through the stricture. A cytology brush sheath is then advanced over the guidewire. When the cytology sheath has been advanced through the stricture as observed under fluoroscopy, the wire may be withdrawn and replaced with the brush. The brush is then extended beyond the catheter and withdrawn in a to-and-fro fashion across the area of interest (Fig. 2). The entire sheath assembly is then removed. Alternatively, the brush alone can be withdrawn, leaving the sheath within the duct or stricture. This method may result in significant cell loss while traversing the length of the catheter.

A second technique involves advancing a cytology sheath adjacent to a previously placed guidewire in a monorail fashion. The cytology sheath is prepared by punching a side hole in one wall of the tip. After the guidewire is placed across the stricture, the cytology sheath is advanced over the wire (the wire is threaded through the distal tip and then out the side hole). The sheath is then advanced through the stricture and beyond the end of the guidewire so that the sheath tip is released. A brush may then be placed through the sheath. This method has the advantage of maintaining guidewire access across the stricture zone.

A third brushing technique, which may be technically more difficult, employs direct cannulation with the cytology sheath assembly and then advancement

of the brush through the stricture under fluoroscopic guidance. This method has the advantage of not requiring a guidewire exchange; however, it will be more difficult in tight or proximal strictures. The Geenen cytology brush (Wilson-Cook, Winston-Salem, NC) has a 3-cm flexible tip that extends beyond the brush and may facilitate advancement through the stricture. Recently, a prototype model employing a hydrophilic guidewire tip has been developed and is currently undergoing evaluation.

Optimum cytology yield depends on adequate cellularity and preservation. Proper handling of cytology samples is critically important to avoid deterioration in the cellular detail. The rapid penetrating capacity of 95% ethanol makes this the fixative of choice. Although spray fixatives are available, columnar cells do not stain as well with spray fixation when compared with ethanol fixation (23).

In the reviewed studies, a variety of techniques for production of slides were employed. With brush cytology, most investigators immediately smeared the brush onto glass slides at the time of the procedure. Ryan (12) additionally placed the brush in saline to allow subsequent agitation to dislodge any remaining material. This solution was then filtered and additional slides were made. The extra yield with this technique has not been reported. Additional factors, including brush design (brush length, bristle angle), may influence sensitivity, as suggested in a recent series (24).

Fine Needle Aspiration Cytology

Recently, a ball-tipped curved catheter has been introduced (8) that facilitates procuring FNA samples

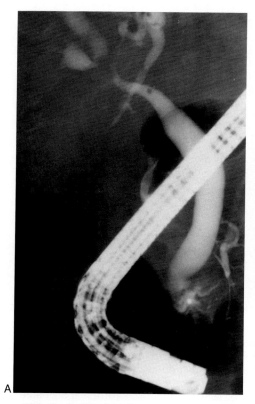

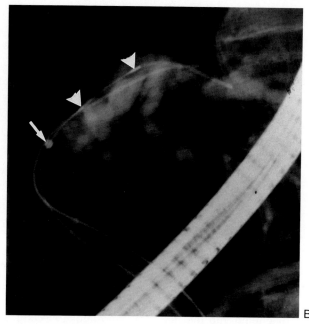

FIG. 2. A: Cholangiogram demonstrates a type III Klatskin's stricture at the hilum of the liver. There is obstruction of both the left and right intrahepatic biliary system that extends into the common hepatic duct. **B:** A guidewire has been placed across the stricture into the left intrahepatic system. The Geenen cytology brush has been advanced next to this guidewire across the stricture. The tip of the catheter is represented by the radiopaque ring *(arrow)* and the region of the brush is found between the two radiopaque lines *(arrow heads)*. The sheath will be withdrawn slightly and the brush moved within the stricture zone.

during ERCP (Howell Biliary Aspiration Needle, 22-gauge, 7-mm needle, Wilson-Cook) (Figs. 3 and 4). After cannulation, the radiopaque tip of the catheter is positioned immediately distal to the stricture. The needle is then extended into the stricture and aspirations are obtained using a 20-ml dry syringe. The needle may be gently moved back and forth within the narrowing while aspirating and then repositioned to a different site without withdrawing the assembly from the bile duct. Generally, three to five sites may be selected with release of the suction between each placement of the needle. After all aspirations have been performed, the needle is retracted and the catheter assembly is withdrawn from the endoscope. An added advantage of this method is that it can be used after deployment of an expandable metal stent (i.e., the needle is passed through the wire mesh of the stent).

After withdrawing the assembly, the contents of the needle are expressed onto glass slides and then immediately spray fixed or immersed in 95% ethanol to prevent air-drying artifact. Clearance of the aspirated material from the needle is done with forceful injection through an air-filled syringe. Flushing the needle with saline should be avoided since this may hinder cell adhesion to the glass slides. We have not routinely assessed for adequacy at the time of the aspirate; however, if this is desired, half of the slides may be processed with the Diff-Quick stain (Harleco, Gibbstown, NJ) and reviewed by an attendant cytologist or cytopathologist.

A recently described alternative method involves preparing the needle catheter with a heparin solution (100 U/ml) flushed through the entire assembly (25). The aspirate is performed and the material is then sprayed into a mucoliquefying preservative solution (Mucolex, Lerner Labs, PA). This solution is centrifuged with slides made from the cell block. In a comparative study performed by Muggia et al. (25), the yield with this new method did not appear to differ significantly from the technique of making direct smears (72% with Mucolex versus 71% with direct smears). A major advantage arises from the enhanced efficiency and reduced need for needle handling. Additional studies are needed to confirm these findings.

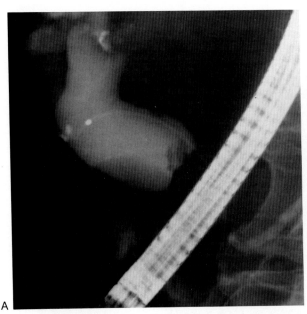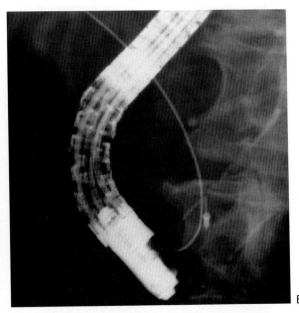

FIG. 3. A: Cholangiogram reveals obstruction of the distal duct with significant dilatation of the common bile duct proximal to the region of narrowing. A catheter with a radiopaque tip has been successfully advanced through the region of narrowing. The pancreatogram revealed ductal obstruction suggesting pancreatic carcinoma (not shown). **B:** A guidewire has been advanced through the stricture, and the Howell biliary aspiration needle is seen protruding from the sheath, extending into the region of the tumor. The endoscopist will advance and retract the needle within the stricture by 3- to 5-mm increments while suction is applied to the proximal end of the catheter assembly. Suction may be released and the needle repositioned to obtain additional material.

Transpapillary Forceps Biopsy

Forceps biopsies of pancreaticobiliary strictures may be performed with standard biopsy forceps (most commonly requiring a papillotomy to achieve cannulation) or malleable biopsy forceps, which may be curved to assist with cannulation (Olympus America, Inc., Lake Success, NY) (Fig. 5). Under fluoroscopic control, the biopsy forceps are advanced to the lesion (preferably within the stricture zone). Samples may be procured in a similar fashion as with standard endoscopic techniques; however, due to the action of the elevator and the degree of bending with the biopsy forceps, the endoscopist should ensure that the instrument is opening and closing by observing the fluoroscopy image. The optimal configuration of the jaws of the forceps needs further evaluation, and wire-guided forceps are currently under development. Specimens are preserved in buffered formalin.

Stent Retrieval and Scrape Biopsy

The replacement of previously placed stents provides an opportunity to establish a histologic diagnosis. Typically, after stent removal, adherent material is removed and placed in formalin. The stent is then washed with normal saline, which is then centrifuged and the button processed into smears. An alternative but similar technique involves a scrape biopsy where a modified dilator with plastic barbs is passed through the stricture (26). The Prince of Wales Hospital group has reported its results with both techniques and found a sensitivity of 79% (11 of 14) with stent retrieval and 60% (9 of 15) with scrape biopsy (performed percutaneously) when evaluating malignant biliary strictures (26,27). The major disadvantage with stent retrieval is the delay in diagnosis until the time of repeat ERCP for stent exchange. The scrape biopsy method, however, appears promising, and additional evaluation employing sampling via ERCP is needed.

SPECIAL TECHNIQUES

Once access across a biliary stricture has been achieved, the endoscopist may be reluctant to sacrifice it to obtain histologic material if eventual endoprosthesis placement is planned. This reluctance is most pronounced when initial traversal of the stricture was challenging. We have occasionally found that regaining access across a stricture after these tissue collection techniques have been performed may be especially difficult (perhaps secondary to edema from instrumentation). One method to alleviate this problem is to leave a guidewire in place while performing the cytology and

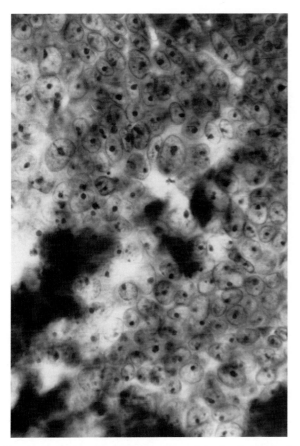

FIG. 4. Fine needle aspirate material obtained during ERCP (Fig. 3) showing malignant cells from a pancreatic adenocarcinoma. Cells show nuclear size variation with marked crowding and prominent nucleoli. Darkly stained amorphous material represents necrotic debris. Papanicolaou stain, ×400.

biopsies. Passing the FNA catheter and forceps alongside the 0.035-inch guidewire is possible in the larger-channel ERCP endoscopes. Another device that the endoscopist may find useful is a 10 to 11.5 French diameter overtube. This may be passed to the distal margin of the biliary stricture with the proximal end of the overtube protruding from the biopsy channel. This permits rapid procurement of multiple specimens without requiring repeated cannulations. Kinking of the overtube at the 180° turn in the duodenum at times may limit passage of the instruments.

TISSUE SAMPLING YIELD

Pancreatic Carcinoma

Table 1 summarizes the diagnostic yield from eight series when samples were obtained from the bile duct. Despite the presence of obstructive jaundice, overall sensitivity was generally modest at best: brush 23%, FNA 32%, and forceps biopsy 32%. A single series by

Osnes et al. (10) reported brushings from within the pancreatic duct. Twenty-one of 29 patients with pancreatic carcinoma were detected. This very high yield needs confirmation.

A component of the overall low sensitivity with transbiliary sampling methods in the diagnosis of pancreatic (and metastatic) carcinoma is secondary to the extrinsic nature of the tumor. The mass may cause compression of the bile duct without necessarily invading the lumen. Additionally, the desmoplastic tissue response accompanying pancreatic carcinoma may in part cause the ductal narrowing and would not yield malignant material with these sampling techniques. Therefore, series reporting their results from a patient group with more advanced disease may have improved sensitivity if transmural invasion of the bile duct is present. Some reports have suggested that endoscopic FNA biopsy may overcome these difficulties. In the series reported by Howell et al. (8) in which biliary samples were taken (Table 1), of 19 patients with pancreatic adenocarcinoma, none had positive brush cytology and 10 (53%) had positive FNA. The authors suggested the low brush yield in their series may be representative of a group of patients with earlier malignancies. The difficulty of any technique in procuring a diagnosis in pancreatic carcinoma is highlighted by a yield of only 77% by open surgical needle biopsy in a recent series (3).

Additional problems arise in interpretation of specimens with atypical or suspicious cells. In these cases, the cytopathologist will be unable to clearly define whether the atypia is truly secondary to an underlying malignant process or related to regional inflammation. Alternatively, this may reflect the aggressiveness, confidence, or experience of the cytopathologist. With our own series, in all cases where atypical cells suggestive of malignancy were identified on one or more collection methods, the patient was found to have a malignant lesion based on clinical follow-up or surgery (16). Similar results have been found by others (5–15). Overall, inclusion of atypia as a positive cancer diagnosis will improve the diagnostic sensitivity of all techniques by 10% to 30%. Perhaps further testing with flow cytometry may be useful in providing a more definitive diagnosis in these cases. Problems with false-positive results have not been reported in the studies reviewed (68 patients with benign strictures) (5–16); however, most series have not included a large number of patients with inflammatory processes such as primary sclerosing cholangitis or chronic pancreatitis in whom reactive changes may result in more difficult cytology interpretation.

The wide range of sensitivity among various studies with these tissue sampling techniques may in part arise from (a) different instruments used in sample procurement, (b) collection of tissue from the bile duct versus

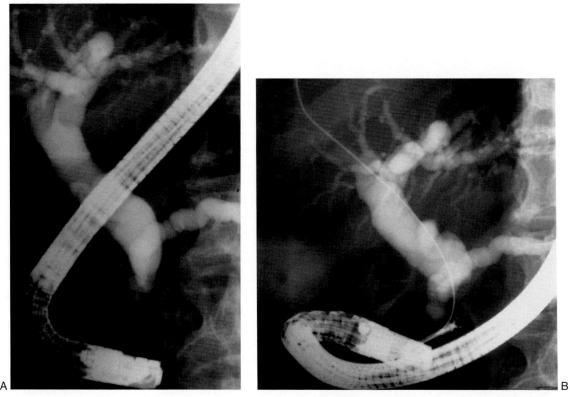

FIG. 5. A double duct sign is seen on the initial cholangiogram and pancreatogram. **A:** The common bile duct and main pancreatic duct are dilated in their proximal segments. **B:** A guidewire has been advanced through the common bile duct narrowing. The biopsy forceps has been advanced alongside the wire into the region of the narrowing, and both cups can be seen to be in the open position. Multiple tissue samples were obtained and demonstrated a pancreatic adenocarcinoma.

TABLE 1. *Sensitivity of endoscopic biliary tissue sampling techniques in patients with malignant strictures*

Series[a]	Pancreatic adenocarcinoma				Cholangiocarcinoma				Metastatic cancer			
	n	Brush	FNA	BX	n	Brush	FNA	BX	n	Brush	FNA	BX
Aabakken et al. (5)	7	–	–	1 (14.3%)	3	–	–	2 (67%)	0	–	–	–
Foutch et al. (7)	5	3 (60%)[b]	–	–	6	6 (100%)	–	–	9	2 (22%)	–	–
Howell et al. (8)	19	0 (0%)	10 (53%)	–	5	2 (40%)	4 (80%)	–	1	0 (0%)	1 (100%)	–
Rustgi et al. (11)	0	–	–	–	4	2 (50%)	–	4 (100%)	1	9 (0%)	–	0 (0%)
Ryan (12)	10	3 (30%)	–	–	9	4 (44%)	–	–	9	3 (33%)	–	–
Scudera et al. (13)	10	5 (50%)	–	–	2	2 (100%)	–	–	2	0 (0%)	–	–
Venu et al. (15)	5	3 (60%)	–	–	25	20 (80%)	–	–	12	8 (67%)	–	–
Wiersema et al. (16)	15	1 (7%)	1 (7%)	6 (40%)	13	2 (15%)	3 (23%)	5 (38%)	5	0 (0%)	2 (40%)	1 (20%)
Total	–	15/64 (23%)	11/34 (32%)	7/22 (32%)	–	38/64 (59%)	7/18 (39%)	11/20 (55%)	–	13/39 (33%)	3/6 (50%)	1/6 (17%)

[a] All studies report a specificity of 100%. Specimens with atypia only are considered negative for malignancy in this table.
[b] Number indicates patients with malignancy detected.
FNA, transpapillary fine needle aspiration; BX, forceps biopsies.
Parentheses indicate percent of samples positive for malignancy.

TABLE 2. *Sensitivity of endoscopic biliary tissue sampling techniques in patients with malignant biliary strictures and negative brush cytology*[a]

Sampling method	Pancreas carcinoma	Cholangiocarcinoma	Metastases	All cancers
FNA	7% (1/14)	9% (1/11)	40% (2/5)	13% (4/30)
BX	36% (5/14)	36% (4/11)	20% (1/5)	30% (9/30)
FNA + BX	43% (6/14)	36% (4/11)	60% (3/5)	43% (13/30)

[a] Taken from the series by Wiersema et al. (16). Specimens with atypia only are considered negative for malignancy in this table.
FNA, transpapillary fine needle aspiration; BX, forceps biopsies; FNA + BX, combined yield.

pancreatic duct, (c) the small numbers of patients in several series, and (d) the primary tumor site. In those studies where 10 or more patients with pancreatic carcinoma were evaluated, the greatest sensitivity (21 of 29, 72%) occurred in the Osnes et al. (10) series where brush cytology was obtained exclusively from the main pancreatic duct. This is tempered by 11 technical failures when brushing of the stricture zone was not possible. In the other series, the bile duct was the predominant biopsy site. As shown with the series from Howell et al. (8) and Wiersema et al. (16), the guidewire-tipped brush had inferior sensitivity (0% and 7%) when compared with the standard brush (Mill-Rose Laboratories, Mentor, OH) used in Ryan's (12) series (6 of 20, 30%). Of these 20 patients in Ryan's series, the sensitivity of sampling from the common bile duct was equal to that from the main pancreatic duct (3 of 10 for each). The higher yield in Ryan's series may in part arise from the different brush, but perhaps also from the processing of the sample. Specifically, after directly smearing material from the brush onto glass slides, the brush and sheath were placed in a saline solution and then processed using a Vortex agitator to dislodge any cellular material from the brush. This solution was then applied to a Millipore filter system (Millipore Filter Company, Bedford, MA) to retrieve the remaining cells, from which additional slides were made. A description of the added yield provided by these extra measures is not provided; however, in the two other series by Howell et al. (8) and Wiersema et al. (16), only direct smears were examined.

Currently, there is no apparent single best method for diagnosing pancreatic carcinoma at ERCP. Additional studies evaluating the utility of intraductal forceps and fine needle aspirates from the pancreatic duct are awaited. Overall, employment of multiple tissue sampling techniques in the same patient appears to offer the highest yield (Table 2) (16).

Cholangiocarcinoma

The intraluminal nature of cholangiocarcinoma has allowed greater sensitivity in establishing a diagnosis with brush, FNA, or forceps biopsies. Table 1 shows

that overall yields are brush 59%, FNA 39%, and forceps biopsy 55%. Employing a specially modified brush, Venu et al. (15) achieved a sensitivity of 80%. This is greater than our own experience (15%) and that of Ryan (12) (44%). A comparison of brush with FNA in Howell's series demonstrated a trend for greater sensitivity with FNA when compared to brush (80% vs. 40%, n = 5). We prospectively compared brush, FNA, and biopsy yields in cholangiocarcinoma. The forceps biopsy alone yield (38%) was superior to brush (15%) or FNA alone (23%), and the addition of brush and/or FNA to biopsy resulted in only an 8% improvement in yield (16).

Metastatic Carcinoma

Biliary strictures secondary to metastatic disease appear to be equally well evaluated with brush or FNA. The series from Venu et al. (15) demonstrated a sensitivity of 67% with brush, whereas our own was 0%. With FNA alone, our yield was 40%. Overall, there have not been adequate published data to reach conclusions in reference to these lesions.

Ampullary Carcinoma

The ability to endoscopically visualize the ampulla would suggest that direct forceps biopsy is the best technique for establishing a tissue diagnosis. Our experience in seven patients with ampullary adenocarcinoma undergoing triple sampling yielded a sensitivity of 71% with forceps biopsy, versus 29% for brush and 43% for FNA (16).

Miscellaneous Tumors

Data are currently too limited to determine if less common lesions such as islet cell tumors, carcinoid tumors, or cystadenocarcinomas can be accurately diagnosed by ERCP methods.

SELECTION OF TECHNIQUES

Optimally, a single sampling method that is technically easy to perform could routinely be used at ERCP to procure a tissue diagnosis. To definitively identify the best test would require a prospective evaluation of multiple sampling methods applied to the biliary and/ or pancreatic ducts where appropriate. Unfortunately, this information is unavailable. When a suspicious stricture has been identified at ERCP, the endoscopist must decide whether tissue sampling will assist in patient management. Brush cytology is simplest but offers reasonable yield only in cholangiocarcinoma. This may be enhanced with the addition of FNA and/or forceps biopsy. A trend exists for the combination of techniques to provide greater sensitivity than any single method. Fortunately, these techniques have been associated with only rare cases of mild pancreatitis or minimal bleeding, and serious complications have not been reported. Although the incidence of complications may be slightly increased with these tissue collection methods, the additional diagnostic information obtained may preclude other invasive studies and their associated morbidity and cost.

SUMMARY

Tissue sampling for pancreaticobiliary malignancy continues to evolve with improved methods. Currently, multiple sampling methods offer greater diagnostic yield than any method alone.

REFERENCES

1. Lees MR, Hall-Craggs MA, Manhire A. Five years' experience of fine-needle aspiration biopsy: 454 consecutive cases. *Clin Radiol* 1985;36:517–520.
2. Thlin L, Blind BJ, Angstrom T. Fine needle aspiration biopsy of pancreatic masses. *Acta Chir Scand* 1990;156:91–94.
3. Parsons L, Palmer C. How accurate is fine-needle biopsy in malignant neoplasia of the pancreas? *Arch Surg* 1989;124:681–683.
4. Welch TJ, Sheedy PF, Johnson CD, Johnson CM, Stephens DH. CT-guided biopsy: prospective analysis of 1,000 procedures. *Radiology* 1989;171:493–496.
5. Aabakken L, Karesen R, Serck-Hanssen A, Osnes M. Transpapillary biopsies and brush cytology from the common bile duct. *Endoscopy* 1986;18:49–51.
6. Foutch PG, Harlan JR, Kerr D, Sanowski RA. Wire-guided brush cytology: a new endoscopic method for diagnosis of bile duct cancer. *Gastrointest Endosc* 1989;35(3):243–247.
7. Foutch PG, Kerr DM, Harlan JR, Manne RK, Kummet TD, Sanowski RA. Endoscopic retrograde wire-guided brush cytol-
ogy for diagnosis of patients with malignant obstruction of the bile duct. *Am J Gastroenterol* 1990;85(7):791–795.
8. Howell DA, Beveridge RP, Bosco J, Jones M. Endoscopic needle aspiration biopsy at ERCP in the diagnosis of biliary strictures. *Gastrointest Endosc* 1992;38(5):531–535.
9. Osnes M, Serck-Hanssen A, Myren J. Endoscopic retrograde brush cytology (ERBC) of the biliary and pancreatic ducts. *Scand J Gastroenterol* 1975;10:829–831.
10. Osnes M, Serck-Hanssen A, Kristensen O, Swensen T, Aune S, Myren J. Endoscopic retrograde brush cytology in patients with primary and secondary malignancies of the pancreas. *Gut* 1979;20:279–284.
11. Rustgi AK, Kelsey PB, Guelrud M, Saini S, Schapiro RH. Malignant tumors of the bile ducts: diagnosis by biopsy during endoscopic cannulation. *Gastrointest Endosc* 1989;35(3):248–251.
12. Ryan ME. Cytologic brushings of ductal lesions during ERCP. *Gastroinetest Endosc* 1991;37(2):139–142.
13. Scudera PL, Koizumi J, Jacobson IM. Brush cytology evaluation of lesions encountered during ERCP. *Gastrointest Endosc* 1990;36(3):281–284.
14. Seifert E, Urakami Y, Elster K. Duodenoscopic guided biopsy of the biliary and pancreatic duct. *Endoscopy* 1977;9:154–161.
15. Venu RP, Geenen JE, Kini M, Hogan WJ, Payne M, Johnson GK, Schmalz MJ. Endoscopic retrograde brush cytology: a new technique. *Gastroenterology* 1990;99:1475–1479.
16. Wiersema MJ, Lehman GA, Sherman S, Hawes RH, Earle DT. Endoscopic brush cytology, fine needle aspiration, and forceps biopsy in the evaluation of malignant biliary strictures. *Gastrointest Endosc* 1993;39:336.
17. Roberts-Thomson IC, Hobbs JB. Cytodiagnosis of pancreatic and biliary cancer by endoscopic duct aspiration. *Med J Aust* 1979;1:370–372.
18. Muro A, Mueller PR, Ferrucci JT, Taft PD. Bile cytology: a routine addition to percutaneous biliary drainage. *Radiology* 1983;149:846–847.
19. Harell GS, Anderson MF, Berry PF. Cytologic bile examination in the diagnosis of biliary duct neoplastic strictures. *Am J Roentgenol* 1981;137:1123–1126.
20. Hatfield ARW, Whitaker R, Gibbs DD. The collection of pancreatic fluid for cytodiagnosis using a duodenoscope. *Gut* 1974;15:305–307.
21. Davidson B, Varsamidakis N, Dooley J, Deery A, Rick R, Kurzawinski T, Hobbs K. Value of exfoliative cytology for investigating bile duct strictures. *Gut* 1992;33:1408–1411.
22. Kozu T, Oi I, Takemoto T. In: *Proceedings of the Second European Congress*. Paris: Congress of Digestive Endoscopy, 1972.
23. Naib ZM. *Exfoliative cytology*. Boston: Little, Brown, 1985.
24. Camp R, Rutkowski MA, Atkinson K, Niedzwick L, Vakil N. A prospective, randomized, blinded trial of cytological yield with disposable cytology brushes in upper gastrointestinal tract lesions. *Am J Gastroenterol* 1992;87(10):1439–1442.
25. Muggia RA, Bosco JJ, Jones MA, Howell DA. Improved cytologic technique for endoscopic needle aspiration (ENA). *Gastrointest Endosc* 1993;39(2):318A.
26. Yip CKY, Leung JWC, Chan MKM, Metreweli C. Scrape biopsy of malignant biliary stricture through percutaneous transhepatic biliary drainage tracts. *Am J Roentgenol* 1989;152:529–530.
27. Leung JWC, Sung JY, Chung SCS, Chan KM. Endoscopic scraping biopsy of malignant biliary strictures. *Gastrointest Endosc* 1989;35(1):65–66.

Advanced Therapeutic Endoscopy, 2nd Ed.,
edited by J. S. Barkin and C. A. O'Phelan.
Raven Press, Ltd., New York © 1994.

CHAPTER 34

Technique for Retrieval of Migrated Biliary and Pancreatic Stents

Kenneth F. Binmoeller and Nib Soehendra

Migration is a relatively rare complication following endoscopic placement of plastic biliary and pancreatic stents, reported to occur in 5% to 7% of cases (1). Retrieving a dislodged stent can be extremely frustrating and may require repeated attempts using different devices (Fig. 1). This chapter describes some of the instruments and techniques that have been used to retrieve migrated stents.

CAUSES OF MIGRATION

A number of factors may contribute to the migration of stents. Stent design is an important consideration. Two basic stent shapes are widely used: pigtail and straight stents. With pigtail stents, anchorage is provided by the pigtail, which may be at one or both ends of the stent (single or double pigtail). Straight stents have side flaps for anchorage, which are cut out of the wall of the stent. There are no comparative trials establishing the superiority of one stent design to the other in terms of migration rates, but it is our experience that pigtail stents provide superior anchorage. Straight stents, however, have been shown to provide a superior drainage effect, and are therefore generally preferred over pigtail stents (2,3).

The size of the sphincterotomy is another factor that may contribute to migration. Some authors perform stent insertion without a prior sphincterotomy, which should theoretically provide better stent anchorage at the papilla. However, stent insertion and exchange are more difficult. If a sphincterotomy is performed, this should be small and not exceed 0.5 mm in length.

K. F. Binmoeller and N. Soehendra: Department of Endoscopic Surgery, University Hospital Eppendorf, Hamburg, Germany.

Stent length is a consideration that may not directly influence the risk of migration, but may have bearing on whether migration becomes clinically significant. Minor shifts in the position of a stent should be allowed for when assessing the desired length of a stent. The distal stent end should project 1 to 2 cm into the duodenum and the proximal end should extend at least 2 cm above the upper border of the stricture.

DISTAL MIGRATION

Distal migration of the stent into the intestinal tract may be complete or partial. A completely migrated prosthesis will usually pass spontaneously with the stool. Serious complications resulting from intestinal stent migration have not been reported. Partially dislodged stents may compromise drainage either due to inadequate bridging of the stricture or obstruction of end flow because of impingement on the duodenal wall. Wall injury may also occur, causing pain and in some cases even perforation (4). The partially dislodged stent is usually easy to retrieve since the intraduodenal end can be grasped under vision with a grasping forceps (rat tooth forceps, Wilson-Cook Medical, Inc., Winston-Salem NC) snare, or basket.

PROXIMAL MIGRATION

In contrast to distal migration, a proximally migrated stent must be retrieved "blindly." Fluoroscopic control provides some orientation, but this is limited to one plane. Frequent repositioning of the patient to obtain different imaging planes will improve the orientation. A trial-and-error approach is necessary and requires a coordinated effort between the endoscopist, endos-

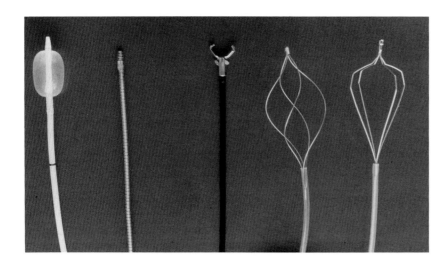

FIG. 1. Accessories available for stent retrieval. *Left to right:* Balloon catheter, stent retriever, rat tooth grasping forceps, spiral basket, Dormia basket.

copy assistant, and radiologist. The proximally migrated stent can be accessed either directly by inserting a retrieval instrument into the duct, or over the guidewire after inserting a guidewire through the migrated stent.

Direct Retrieval

The prerequisite for direct retrieval is that the stent be accessible, i.e., the instrument can be passed through the papilla and the stricture. Passing a rigid instrument through a stricture may, however, risk perforation.

The stent can be captured at the distal end using a grasping forceps, polypectomy snare, or basket. Our preference is to capture the stent with the rat tooth forceps (Fig. 2). The size of the forceps selected depends upon the caliber of the stent. The closed instru-

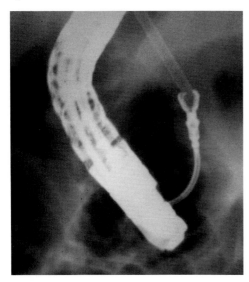

FIG. 2. Endoscopic retrograde cholangiopancreatography (ERCP) showing retrieval of a proximally migrated biliary stent with the rat tooth forceps.

ment is positioned at the distal end of the stent, opened, and then maneuvered to engage the stent. Capturing the distal side flap may be adequate to pull the stent into the duodenum.

If the distal end of the stent impinges against the ductal wall, retrieval at the proximal end can be attempted. The closed basket or snare is advanced above the stent, opened, and then withdrawn while attempting to engage the stent (Fig. 3). The balloon catheter may also be used to retrieve a stent by inflating the balloon either alongside or above the stent (Fig. 4).

The retrieval of stents in the relatively narrower pancreatic duct is usually more difficult than in the bile duct. Accordingly, miniaturized instruments have been developed (Wilson-Cook mini basket and mini snare, Wilson-Cook Medical, Inc.) for pancreatic stent removal.

Over-the-Guidewire Removal

Over-the-guidewire stent retrieval can be performed with the Soehendra stent retriever (Wilson-Cook Medical, Inc.) or the balloon catheter, both of which accommodate a guidewire. This technique allows removal of the stent through the biopsy channel of the endoscope while leaving the guidewire in place. The major advantage is that access across the stricture is not lost, thus avoiding the need to recannulate the stricture after stent removal.

Insertion of a guidewire through the lumen of the stent is the first step. A guiding catheter with a slightly curved and tapered tip (Soehendra Universal catheter, Wilson-Cook Medical, Inc.) is used to position the guidewire (400 cm long Teflon-coated stainless steel wire) at the distal end of the stent. The stent lumen is then cannulated with the guidewire. If the stent is unfavorably oriented, the hydrophilic guidewire (Terumo Glidewire, Terumo GmbH, Frankfurt, Germany;

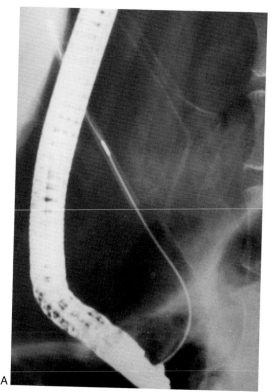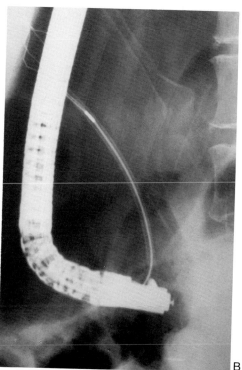

FIG. 3. ERCP showing retrieval of a proximally migrated biliary stent with the Dormia basket. **A:** Basket passed above the stent. **B:** The basket is opened and withdrawn toward the duodenum, thereby engaging the proximal end of the stent for retrieval.

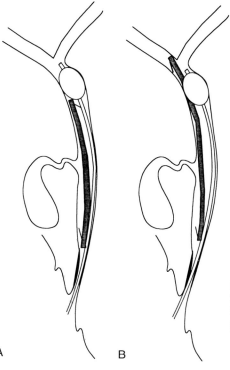

FIG. 4. Retrieval of a proximally migrated biliary stent with the balloon catheter. **A:** Balloon advanced above the stent to engage the proximal stent end. **B:** Inflation of the balloon alongside the stent. Deep migration of the stent prevented advancement of the balloon catheter above the stent.

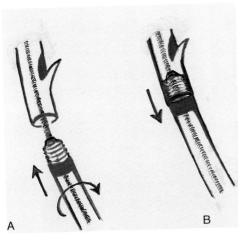

FIG. 5. Technique of over-the-guidewire stent removal using the Soehendra stent retriever. **A:** The retriever is directed toward the distal end of the stent over a previously inserted guidewire. The tip is screwed into the stent by rotating the entire device along its axis in a clockwise direction. **B:** After attaching itself to the stent, the retriever is withdrawn. The guidewire is left in place for insertion of a new stent.

Tracer Wire, Wilson-Cook Medical, Inc.) may aid access to the stent lumen. This unique guidewire is available with a straight or angled tip and is steerable using torque control. Once the stent is cannulated, the guidewire is advanced through the length of the stent and the guiding catheter is removed.

The Soehendra stent retriever consists of a flexible metal spiral sheath with a threaded tip (5). The tip is screwed into the distal end of the stent by rotating the device in a clockwise direction. Once the retriever is attached to the stent, the stent can be withdrawn through the biopsy channel of the endoscope while leaving the guidewire in place (Figs. 5 and 6).

Several technical points regarding the use of the Soehendra stent retriever should be emphasized. The device comes in different sizes to accommodate stents of different caliber (5, 7, 8.5, 10, and 11.5 Fr); hence, the caliber of the stent to be removed must be correctly identified. The inserted guidewire should be free of kinks, since these will impede smooth advancement of the retriever device. To engage the tip of the device in the stent, it is necessary to align the retriever in the axis of the stent. Engagement is facilitated by having

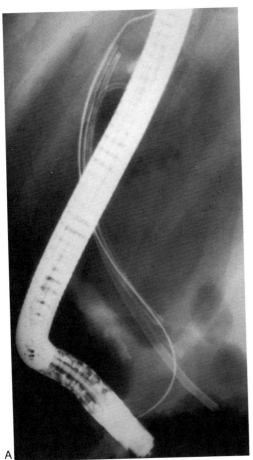
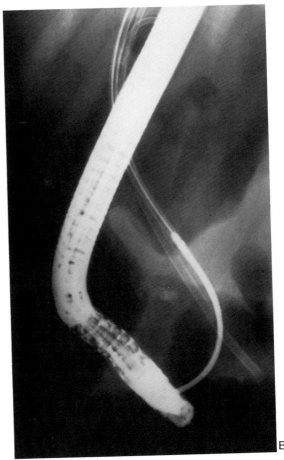

FIG. 6. ERCP radiographs showing selective removal of a proximally migrated stent with the Soehendra stent retriever in the setting of multiple biliary stent placement. **A:** A guidewire has been passed through the migrated stent **B:** Stent engaged by the retriever for withdrawal.

the endoscopy assistant maintain traction on the guide-wire while the endoscopist pushes the retriever tip into the stent.

When removing the stent with the stent retriever, close fluoroscopic monitoring is warranted to ensure that the guidewire is not removed along with the stent. Usually the guidewire will need to be advanced into the duct as the stent is withdrawn. At the point that the stent is released from the papilla, the guidewire has a tendency to catapult out of the duct. Advancing the guidewire at this stage may cause a bow to develop and dislodge the wire. Keeping the tip of the duodenoscope positioned as close to the papilla as possible will help stabilize the stent and guidewire. The elevator should be fully lowered and the control knobs unlocked to allow easy passage of the stent into the biopsy channel.

The method for retrieving a stent with the balloon catheter over a guidewire is analogous to that described for the stent retriever. Traction on the stent is produced by either inflating the balloon inside or above the stent (6).

ALTERNATIVE MANAGEMENT

If a stent cannot be removed endoscopically, one alternative is to insert a second stent. This may be reasonable in the patient with a limited life-expectancy or of high surgical risk. A guidewire is first passed through the stricture followed by stent placement in the standard fashion.

Proximal migration of biliary stents may be removable by the percutaneous route. This approach warrants particular consideration in the patient with a bifurca-tion stricture accompanied by proximal stent migration into the hepatic ducts.

CONCLUSION

A large variety of instruments and methods are available today to endoscopically retrieve the migrated biliary or pancreatic stent. The approach of choice will depend primarily upon the given duct anatomy. Direct retrieval using a grasping forceps, polypectomy snare, basket, or balloon is generally preferred if this can be performed safely. The over-the-wire method using the Soehendra stent retriever or the balloon catheter is technically more complex, but has the advantages that the migrated stent can be retrieved without having to remove the endoscope and a new stent can be inserted without having to recannulate the stricture.

REFERENCES

1. Johanson JF, Schmalz MJ, Geenen JE. Incidence and risk factors for biliary and pancreatic stent migration. *Gastrointest Endosc* 1992;38:341–346.
2. Leung WJC, Del Favero G, Cotton PB. Endoscopic biliary prosthesis: a comparison of materials. *Gastrointest Endosc* 1985;31: 93–95.
3. Rey JF, Maupetit P, Greff M. Experimental study of biliary endo-prosthesis efficiency. *Endoscopy* 1985;17:145–148.
4. Siegel J, Veerappan A. Endoscopic management of pancreatic disorders: potential risks of pancreatic prostheses. *Endoscopy* 1991;23:177–180.
5. Soehendra N, Maydeo A, Eckmann B, Brückner M, Nam V Ch, Grimm H. A new technique for replacing an obstructed biliary endoprothesis. *Endoscopy* 1992;22:271–272.
6. Martin DF. Wire guided balloon assisted endoscopic biliary stent exchange. *Gut* 1991;32:1562–1564.

Advanced Therapeutic Endoscopy, 2nd Ed.,
edited by J. S. Barkin and C. A. O'Phelan.
Raven Press, Ltd., New York © 1994.

CHAPTER 35

Precut Papillotomy

K. Huibregtse, I. Waxman, and V. K. Parasher

Since the description of endoscopic retrograde cholangiopancreatography (ERCP) in 1968 (1) and subsequent development of endoscopic sphincterotomy in 1973 (2), the use of these modalities is deeply entrenched in the nonsurgical management of a variety of pancreatobiliary disorders. Despite the continued and explosive growth in accessories used to perform such procedures endoscopic sphincterotomy is still not successful in 5% to 10% of cases. This is most commonly attributed to a failed "free cannulation" of the common bile duct (CBD). This failure may be due to acute angulation of the distal common bile duct or to an altered anatomy of the papilla caused by a tumor, an impacted stone, a congenital anomaly, a periampullary diverticulum or a Billroth II gastrojejunostomy. When this occurs special techniques are needed to gain entry into the common bile duct (3–5). These techniques are addressed in this chapter.

Precut papillotomy is the most frequently employed "special technique" to gain access into the CBD when the usual conventional methods fail. These conventional methods consist of using a tapered tip catheter, a ball-tipped cannula with a glidewire, and a double lumen papillotome with or without a glidewire (Cotton cannulatome, Wilson-Cook Medical, Inc.). Failure of CBD cannulation by standard techniques does not necessarily mean that one should proceed to more aggressive methods to obtain access to the CBD. The more aggressive the method, the greater the risks involved. When CBD cannulation fails by conventional methods, one should reconsider the indication for bile duct cannulation. Alternative methods to obtain direct cholangiography, such as percutaneous cholangiography, should be considered. A second attempt a few days later or perhaps a referral to a center with more experience and expertise should be considered before proceeding to precut papillotomy. Precut papillotomy should be performed only in patients who will most likely require therapeutic intervention for stone disease or biliary drainage. Furthermore, this technique should be used only by experienced endoscopists who have complete control over all movements of catheter and endoscope. The objective of precutting is to unroof the papilla and to make a cut in the upper part of the muscular sphincter so as to gain entry into the distal CBD. The precut papillotomy is performed either with a precut papillotome or a needle knife.

PRECUT PAPILLOTOMY WITH A PRECUT PAPILLOTOME

This papillotome is a standard papillotome without the leading piece of catheter beyond the wire (Fig. 1) (3). The tip of this papillotome is placed into the orifice of the papilla, and the wire is slightly tightened. The wire must be moved upward in the direction of the CBD while applying a combination of cutting and coagulation current. It is important not to burn too many times at the same spot since this will create edema, which occludes the pancreatic orifice and thereby increases the risk of acute pancreatitis. Furthermore, edema may make eventual cannulation more difficult. A cut of more than 5 mm should deroof the papilla and once this is achieved cannulation of the common bile duct may become possible. It is recommended that one proceed with the regular papillotomy after a precut papillotomy so as to avoid late stricturing of the papilla. The difficulty in using a precut papillotome is the inability to always orient the wire in the 11 o'clock position. One may have to bend the tip of the papillotome or use a different papillotome before obtaining a satisfactory position of the wire in order to proceed with

K. Huibregtse, I. Waxman, V. K. Parasher: Department of Gastroenterology and Hepatology, Academic Medical Center, University of Amsterdam, 1105 AZ Amsterdam, The Netherlands.

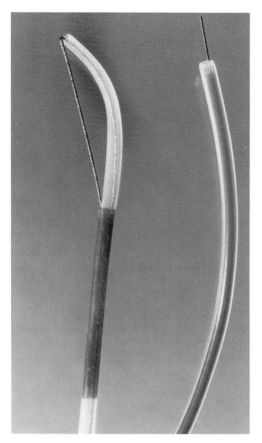

FIG. 1. Precut papillotome and needle knife papillotome.

the cut. This difficulty in controlling the direction and depth of the cut with the precut papillotome is the reason that some endoscopists prefer to use the needle knife for unroofing the papilla.

PRECUT PAPILLOTOMY WITH A NEEDLE KNIFE

A needle knife consists of a 0.2, mm diameter straight wire that can be extended 5 mm from the tip of the cannula (Wilson-Cook Medical, Inc.) (Fig. 1). The wire is retractable into the cannula. Needle knives are available whereby contrast can be injected in order to define the duct. Furthermore, the knife with the inner catheter can be removed from the outer sheath to allow guidewire insertion. The electrosurgical current setting is a conventional blended current (75% cutting and 25% coagulation), which is also employed during a standard sphincterotomy. The effect of applying electrical current to tissue via an electrosurgical device depends not only on the characteristics of the electrical current but also on other factors, such as the diameter of the wire, the length of the wire exposed to the tissue, and the pressure of the wire on the tissue. More coagulation effect is obtained with a thicker wire, which is more

exposed, and with more pressure of the wire on the tissue. The creation of edema at the site of the orifice should be avoided, because that may increase the risk of subsequent acute pancreatitis.

Before insertion of the needle knife, one should check to see if the needle protrudes from the catheter properly. Additionally, it is also important to remember that the length of the exposed wire may vary depending on the amount of bending of the plastic sheath. It is therefore advisable to check the length of the exposed wire with the plastic sheath uncoiled outside the endoscope and to carefully review the length of the exposed wire endoscopically.

Before one begins actual cutting with the knife, one should make several sham movements to determine how to direct the knife in the desired direction. These movements can be achieved by various combinations of the following 12 single movements: the catheter can be directed by (a) elevating or (b) releasing the bridge, by moving the tip of the endoscope (c) up or (d) down, (e) right or (f) left with the control knobs, turning the endoscope handle (g) clockwise or (h) counterclockwise, (i) withdrawal or (j) advancement of the endoscope, and finally (k) insertion or (l) withdrawal of the catheter. Once the optimal direction of the cut is found the wire is extended 5 mm from the tip of the catheter and inserted in the papillary orifice. The incision is made in the 11 o'clock position, which is the usual position of the bile duct (Figs. 2 and 3). The proper orientation of the cut is achieved by first creating pressure on the roof of the papilla and then continuing the cut using a combination of the above-described movements. It is essential to move the knife while applying current to avoid excessive coagulation. The papilla and sphincter should be cut layer by layer and in small increments.

The sphincter is a circular muscle that will spread open when it is incised. A precut in the correct orientation and of sufficient depth will result in a nicely "spreading open" effect of the precut wound. If the cut is made too superficial or at the right or left side of the sphincter, the wound will not spread open. A superficial cut therefore should be made slightly deeper in order to determine if the cut is in or alongside the sphincter muscle. Beginners especially tend to make the cut too much to the left alongside the sphincter. In this scenario the sphincter may sometimes be seen as bulging tissue at the right wall of the initial incision uncovered from mucosa. A cut slightly more to the right of the muscular sphincter will then result in the desired "spreading open" effect. Once this effect is seen, one may further proceed with stepwise dissection of the fibers of the muscle. As long as retraction of the muscle fibers and further spreading of the sphincter is observed one may continue with the cut, because this means that still only the upper part of the muscle has

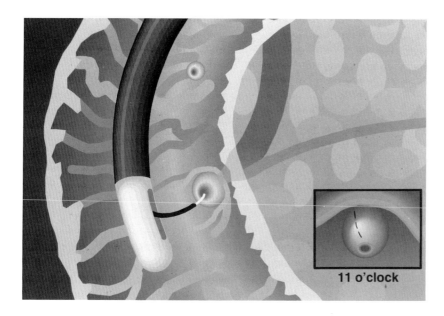

11 o'clock

FIG. 2. Schematic drawing of desired direction of precut incision.

been incised. One should never make a deeper incision when the above-described effect is no longer seen.

The incision should never be extended beyond the angle that is formed by the papillary complex and the duodenal wall. Cannulation attempts should be made following a 5 to 7 mm long incision by gently probing the papillotomy wound with a blunt ball-tip catheter. Contrast should only be injected when free cannulation is achieved. Contrast injection with the catheter stuck between the mucosa and the sphincter or in the sphincter muscle will result in edematous dissected tissue with an increased risk of false routes and failure of the procedure. The cut should be extended and made deeper when free cannulation fails, always taking into account the above-described fundamentals. The opening to the common bile duct may sometimes be seen

as a little red spot representing protruded bile duct mucosa or a yellow spot with bile flow. Most frequently, however, the opening is not clearly seen and one should continue probing with the catheter at the expected position for some time.

In the majority of cases the orifice of the CBD is located somewhere along the incision, usually at its superiormost aspect. Occasionally, one repeatedly cannulates the pancreatic duct. The bile duct should then be found at the same spot by moving the catheter more to the left and more parallel to the duodenal wall. A slightly deeper or proximal incision to the left starting at the opening to the pancreatic duct should be made. Repeat attempts for cannulation and repeat incisions should be done in an incremental fashion.

Bleeding infrequently obscures the papillotomy

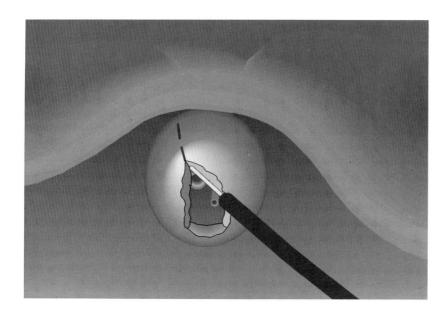

FIG. 3. The preferential position of the openings of the pancreatic duct and common bile duct following precut incision.

wound. Most bleeding stops spontaneously after a few seconds and the procedure can be continued. One should discontinue the procedure and reattempt it a few days later when continuous oozing occurs or when free cannulation fails after substantial extension of the precut. It is amazing how easy cannulation is achieved in most patients a few days later, when bleeding has stopped and edema has subsided. During a delayed attempt it is important to first inspect the papillotomy wound for an indication of the opening of the bile duct before probing with the catheter, since this may provoke bleeding again.

DIFFERENT NEEDLE KNIFE TECHNIQUES

Needle knife papillotomy was first described in bulging papilla. This technique is now referred to as infundibulotomy. An opening is made proximal to the orifice, in or just proximal to the bulging papilla. A sphincterotome may then be inserted antegrade and the bridge of tissue between the papillary orifice and the puncture site may be cut. Alternatively, a guidewire may be inserted via the puncture site through the papillary orifice. A standard sphincterotome can then be inserted over the guidewire in the CBD. This technique can only be used in the case of large bulging papillae (6).

Sherman et al. (14) described a slightly different technique of needle knife papillotomy. In many candidates for precut papillotomy repeated cannulation of the pancreas is easy, but cannulation of the CBD fails. In these patients they advise protecting the pancreas by insertion of a pancreatic stent prior to opening the CBD with the needle knife. The pancreatic stent is then removed a few days after successful bile duct cannula-

tion. No data are available to show that acute pancreatitis is prevented by this protective technique.

Papillotomy of the minor papilla is preferentially performed over a stent, which has been inserted in the dorsal pancreatic duct. The stent is then removed 5 to 7 days later. Biliary sphincterotomy in patients after Billroth II gastrojejunostomy is technically difficult. Therefore, several techniques with different sphincterotomes have been described. Using the needle knife, papillotomy can be performed, by first inserting a 7 Fr stent into the bile duct (Fig. 4). The sphincterotomy is then performed by making a cut over the stent with the needle knife. Preferentially, one should start at the orifice by placing the knife in the orifice with the elevator bridge up and then moving the knife downward by releasing the elevator bridge. This is a very difficult maneuver; one may also start the incision a few millimeters from the orifice, then moving the knife upward by closing the elevator bridge. In small increments the sphincter can be opened over the stent, which indicates the desired direction and the depth of the incision. The needle knife has also been used to create gastrocystostomies and for opening choledochal cysts (8) and duodenal duplication cysts (9,10). Leung et al. (11) used needle knife in precutting 20 patients with impacted CBD stones. In this setting the needle knife papillotomy is very safe since the impacted stone prevents the knife from penetrating deep in the tissue. The stone pops out following a short superficial cut.

RESULTS

In most published series precut papillotomy is performed in less than 10% of therapeutic biliary endoscopies. Overall success rate is over 90%; however,

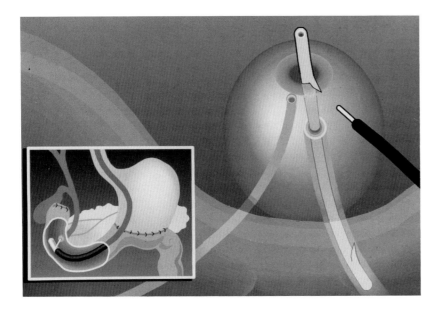

FIG. 4. Schematic drawing of a sphincterotomy over a stent in Billroth II anatomy.

TABLE 1. *Success rate of common bile duct cannulation following precut papillotomy*

Author (reference)	Overall success rate (%)	Success at first attempt (%)	Success at second attempt (%)
Huibregtse et al. (4)	91	54	37
Leung et al. (11)	95	60	35
Tweedle and Martin (7)	96	63	33
Shakoor et al. (12)	85	72	13
Dowsett et al. (13)	77	33	44
Katuscak et al. (14)	92	55	37

two attempts may be required to enhance the cumulative success rate (Table 1). The complications of precutting with the needle knife are similar to those of standard sphincterotomy (15), i.e., perforation, hemorrhage, and pancreatitis. Table 2 summarizes complication rates of several studies comparing sphincterotomy with precut papillotomy. We published our results in 190 consecutive failed biliary cannulations (4). The precut technique allowed biliary access in 171 (90%). The overall complication rate was 2.3%. Bleeding occurred in 1.6% (three cases) and pancreatitis in 1% (two cases). No perforation occurred.

Similar results were found in the series of Dowsett et al. (13). They performed the needle knife papillotomy in 96 of 748 therapeutic procedures. In 74 patients (77%) biliary access was achieved with needle knife papillotomy. Free CBD cannulation was possible immediately post–needle knife papillotomy in 34 of 74 patients. The remaining 40 patients were cannulated 2 to 5 days later. The 78% cannulation success was enhanced to 96.2% by the use of the precutting technique. The overall complication rate was 5.2%. There was an additional 2% mortality.

Contrary to this experience other groups have reported higher incidence of complications in patients undergoing precut papillotomy (7,10–12). Leung et al. (11) report a rate of 20%, while Frank et al. (16) report a rate of 16%. Shakoor et al. (12) report their experience with 1,367 patients who underwent endoscopic sphincterotomy; 1,267 (93%) were cannulated easily and underwent endoscopic sphincterotomy. Free can-

nulation was not achieved in 100 patients (53 patients from this group underwent needle knife papillotomy). In the remaining 47 patients a combined percutaneous endoscopic approach was successfully employed. Of the 53 patients that underwent needle knife papillotomy, 85% had successful cannulation. The complication rate, however, was higher (11%) than the complication rate following standard endoscopic sphincterotomy (6%). Incomplete papillotomy by performance of only a precut has a theoretical higher risk of later papillotomy stenosis. This complication, however, has yet not been described.

CONCLUSION

Precut papillotomy by needle knife or precut papillotome are important techniques to gain access into the CBD, especially when conventional measures have failed. This procedure carries an additional but acceptable risk. It is an important tool in the armamentarium of a skilled therapeutic endoscopist.

REFERENCES

1. McCune WS, Shorb PE, Moscovitz H. Endoscopic cannulation of the ampulla of Vater: a preliminary report. *Ann Surg* 1968; 167:753–756.
2. Classen M, Demling L. Steinextraktion aus dem Gallengang endoskopisch möglich. *Med Trib* 1973;27:1–5.
3. Siegel JH. Precut papillotomy: a method to improve success of ERCP and papillotomy. *Endoscopy* 1980;12:130–133.
4. Huibregtse K, Katon RM, Tytgat GNJ. Precut papillotomy via the needle knife papillotome: a safe and effective technique. *Gastrointest Endosc* 1986;32:403–405.
5. Siegel JH, Ben-Zvi JS, Pullano W. The needle knife: a valuable tool in diagnostic and therapeutic ERCP. *Gastrointest Endosc* 1989;35:499–503.
6. Osnes M, Kahr T. Endoscopic choledochoduodenostomy for choledocholithiasis through choledochoduodenal fistula. *Endoscopy* 1977;9:162–165.
7. Tweedle DEF, Martin DF. Needle knife precut papillotomy for sphincterotomy and cholangiography. *Gut* 1989;30: A1460–A1461.
8. Siegel JH, Harding GT, Chateau F. Endoscopic incision of choledochal cysts (choledochocele). *Endoscopy* 1981;13: 200–202.
9. Al Triaf I, Khan MH. Endoscopic drainage of a duodenal duplication cyst. *Gastrointest Endosc* 1992;38:64–65.
10. Johanson JF, Geenen JE, Hogan WJ, Huibregtse K. Endoscopic

TABLE 2. *Needle knife papillotomy: use and complications*

Authors (reference)	Frequency of use (%)	Complications EST (%)	Mortality EST (%)	Complications precut (%)	Mortality precut (%)
Huibregtse et al. (4)	19.2	2.1	0	2.6	0
Leung et al. (11)	3.9	N.A.	N.A.	20.0	0
Frank et al. (16)	9.7	9.0	0	16.0	1
Tweedle and Martin (7)	5.0	7.0	0	12.5	0
Shakoor et al. (12)	3.8	6.0	0.1	11.0	0
Sherman et al. (17)	15.4	7.0	0	6.2	0

therapy of a duodenal duplication cyst. *Gastrointest Endosc* 1992;38:60–64.

11. Leung JWC, Banez VP, Chung SCS. Pre-cut needle knife papillotomy for impacted common bile duct stone at the ampulla. *Am J Gastroenterol* 1990;85:991–993.

12. Shakoor T, Hogan WJ, Geenen JE. Needle knife papillotomy—efficacy and risks. *Gastrointest Endosc* 1992;38:251.

13. Dowsett JF, Polydorou AA, Vaira D, Anna'D LM, Ashraf M, Crocker J, Salmon PR, Russell RCG, Hatfield ARW. Needle knife papillotomy: how safe and how effective? *Gut* 1990;31:905–908.

14. Katuscak I, Horakova M, Frlicka P, Straka V, Macko J. Needle knife papillotomy: a necessary tool [Letter]. *Gastrointest Endosc* 1991;37:495.

15. Cotton PB, Lehman G, Vennes J, et al. Endoscopic sphincterotomy complications and their management: an attempt at consensus. *Gastrointest Endosc* 1991;37:383–393.

16. Frank V, Booth MCL, Doerr RJ, Khalafi RS, Luchette FA, Flint LM. Surgical management of complications of endoscopic sphincterotomy with precut papillotomy. *Am J Surg* 1990;159:132–136.

17. Sherman S, Ruffolo TA, Hawes RH, Lehman GA. Complications of endoscopic sphincterotomy. *Gastroenterology* 1991;101:1068–1075.

Advanced Therapeutic Endoscopy, 2nd Ed.,
edited by J. S. Barkin and C. A. O'Phelan.
Raven Press, Ltd., New York © 1994.

CHAPTER 36

Combined Procedure for Evaluation and Therapy in the Biliary Tree

Henning Schwacha and Friedrich Hagenmüller

Endoscopic retrograde cholangiography (ERC) and percutaneous transhepatic cholangiography (PTC) have the highest sensitivity and specificity for evaluating biliary tract diseases. These procedures allow the exact diagnosis of biliary tract diseases in most cases. PTC is practical even when anatomical variations of the papilla of Vater or postoperative alterations of the upper gastrointestinal tract make it endoscopically impossible to reach the papilla. For some patients in this group, neither ERC nor PTC alone is able to establish an adequate treatment. In these patients a combined percutaneous transhepatic access and an endoscopic procedure may help to find a correct treatment for biliary tract diseases. This combined procedure (CP) technically consists of simultaneous endoscopic and percutaneous procedures and has also been referred to as the "rendezvous maneuver."

TECHNIQUE

The percutaneous transhepatic approach is carried out either in a one-step manner during the same session or after a more-than-one-step procedure. The biliocutaneous fistula is established to be used as a channel for the combined percutaneous axis. Establishing a biliocutaneous fistula results from a step-by-step dilatation of the cutaneobiliary tract. This is accomplished by inserting a catheter of increasing diameter at 1- to 2-day intervals. The diameter of the biliocutaneous fistula differs from 7 to 20 Fr, depending on the therapeutic procedure planned. The combined procedure is usually performed using a guidewire, which is inserted through either the biliocutaneous tract or the PTC. The guidewire is then passed through the stricture, into the duodenum, and then into the stomach (Fig. 1). Even in patients with anatomic variations or postoperative alterations of the upper gastrointestinal tract (e.g. Billroth II resection, Roux-en-Y limb), the guidewire can be pushed deeply into either the duodenum or the jejunum in the direction of the stomach, so that it can be grasped endoscopically using either a Dormia basket or a snare (Fig. 2). Then the guidewire is drawn out

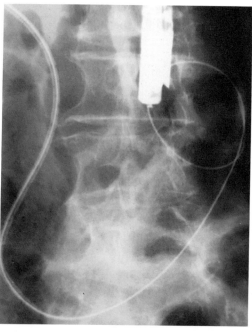

FIG. 1. Patient with impacted bile duct stones and postgastrectomy anatomy (case 1). The guidewire is inserted percutaneously and transhepatically into the duodenum and stomach.

H. Schwacha and F. Hagenmüller: Department of Medicine I, Allgemeines Krankenhauss, D-22763 Hamburg, Germany.

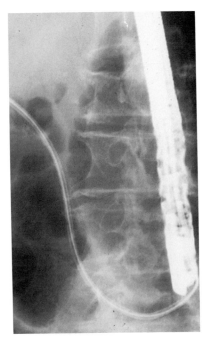

FIG. 2. The guidewire has been grasped with the endoscope.

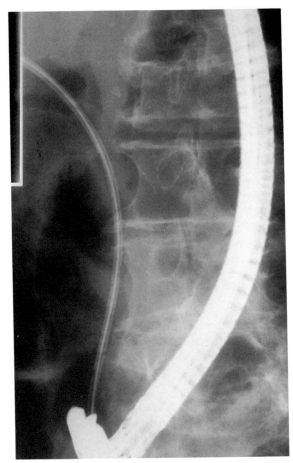

FIG. 3. The endoscope is drawn to the papilla over the wire.

perorally and used thereafter to bring the endoscope to the papilla, under fluoroscopic view (Fig. 3). A double-length wire is necessary, because the whole length of the endoscope has to be pushed over the wire, outside the patient. In some cases it is necessary to use an endoscope with an orthograde lens system (e.g., gastroscope, colonoscope) to locate the papilla of Vater, instead of a duodenoscope (1). During the combined procedure the cooperation of three experienced medical and paramedical personnel is required to perform the pull and push maneuver.

When using the combined technique for stent insertion, it is essential that the bile duct is punctured as peripherally as possible, to ensure that when the stent passes the stricture the end lies totally intraductally and not partially embedded within the liver parenchyma (2,3). In cases of central puncture, the end of the shortest stent should be placed just proximal to the stricture. Checking two planes with fluoroscopy may help to reduce the risk of incorrect stent positioning.

RESULTS

We performed 1,470 endoscopic retrograde cholangiopancreatographies (ERCPs) and 348 PTC(D) during the period 1990 to 1992. Only 11 patients (7 males, 4 females) underwent CP because of ERCP and PTC failure. Four patients had jaundice, which was found to be secondary to benign obstructions (Table 1). Common bile duct stones were found in three of these patients, one of which (case 1) underwent Billroth opera-

tion so that the papilla of Vater could not be reached endoscopically. The other two patients with bile duct stones did not have postoperative alterations of the upper gastrointestinal tract, but either a large peripapillary diverticula or an impacted dormia basket prevented an exclusive endoscopic procedure for stone extraction. All patients with common bile duct stones could be treated with a combined procedure (Fig. 4).

One patient (case 4) had undergone a cholecystectomy because of cholelithiasis and had a postsurgical complication due to an accidental ligature of the common bile duct (CBD), resulting in complete duct occlusion (Fig. 5) and a hepaticoduodenal fistula (Fig. 6). A CP allowed the fistula to be identified and dilated; a long-term drainage was performed. Seven patients (five males, two females) underwent CP due to malignant cause of jaundice (Table 2). In two of these seven patients (cases 5 and 6), endoscopic insertion of the papilla was not possible because of tumor growth in the region of the papilla of Vater. The patients were treated with CP by percutaneously inserting the metal stent into the tumor stenosis under endoscopic view, to enable appropriate positioning. One other patient

TABLE 1. *CP in benign diseases of the biliary tract*

Case no.	Age, sex	Diagnosis	Anatomy	Reason for CP	Therapeutic procedure
1	86, male	CBD, stones	Billroth II gastrectomy	Papilla of Vater not accessible	EPT and stone extraction
2	80, male	CBD, stones, biliary pancreatitis	Duodenal diverticula	EPT failure	EPT and stone extraction
3	66, female	CBD, stones	Existing biliocutaneous fistula	Dormia basket impaction	Percutaneous transhepatic electrohydraulic lithotripsy and stone extraction
4	80, female	Postsurgical occlusion of the CBD	Accidental ligature of the CBD, hepaticoduodenal fistula	Complete duct obstruction	Identification, dilatation, and drainage of the fistula

CBD, common bile duct; EPT, endoscopic papillotomy.

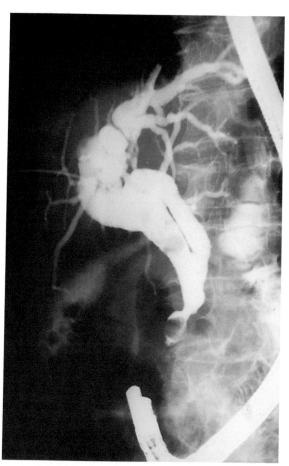

FIG. 4. Patient with common bile duct stones (case 1), Billroth II gastrectomy. Combined procedure for stone extraction.

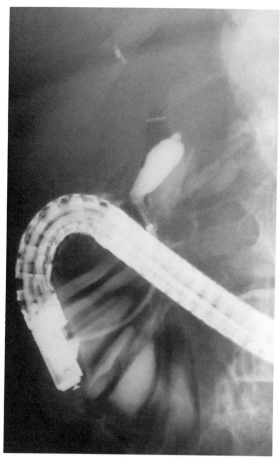

FIG. 5. Complete occlusion of the common bile duct after laparoscopic cholecystectomy and ERC (case 4).

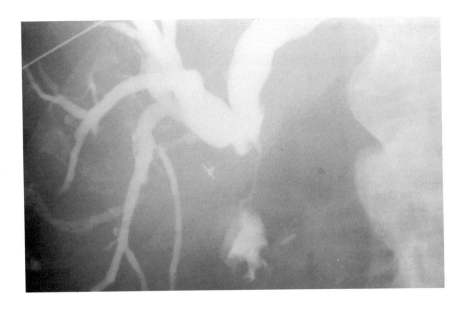

FIG. 6. Spontaneous hepaticoduodenal fistula after CBD ligature (case 4).

(case 7) had pancreatic cancer and another (case 8) had a Klatskin tumor. We used CP to insert plastic stents due to endoscopically impassable stenosis of the CBD versus liver hilus. One patient (case 9) suffered from a metastatic liver hilus stenosis that involved both hepatic ducts. Neither endoscopic nor transhepatic passage to the stenosis of the left hepatic duct was possible, so too was CP. The patient was discharged after drainage of the right hepatic duct. In one patient (case 10) a combined procedure was attempted to remove an occluded Strecker stent from the liver hilus (Fig. 7), but this also failed. A percutaneous drainage of the right hepatic duct was inserted. Another patient (case 11) had surgical implantation of a plastic stent during construction of Billroth II occluded anastomosis. Unfortunately, the stent could not be removed by CP and

TABLE 2. *CP in malignant diseases of the biliary tract*

Case no.	Age, sex	Diagnosis	Anatomy	Reason for CP	Therapeutic procedure
5	71, male	Carcinoid of papilla of Vater	Invisible orifice of papilla of Vater	Failure of cannulation of the papilla of Vater	Metal stent, percutaneous-endoscopic positioning
6	69, male	Gastric cancer	Total gastrectomy; tumor of the papilla of Vater	Failure of cannulation of the papilla of Vater	Metal stent, percutaneous-endoscopic positioning
7	67, male	Pancreatic cancer	Bile duct stenosis	Impassable stenosis	Plastic stent, percutaneous-endoscopic positioning
8	52, male	Bile duct cancer (Klatskin type III)	Liver hilus stenosis	Impassable stenosis	Plastic stent, percutaneous-endoscopic positioning
9	57, female	Breast cancer	Metastic liver hilus stenosis	Failure of cannulation of the left hepatic duct	Failure of cannulation of the left hepatic duct; percutaneous internal drainage of the right hepatic duct
10	47, female	Bile duct cancer (Klatskin type III)	Liver hilus stenosis; occluded Strecker stent	Endoscopic and percutaneous failure of stent removal	Failure of stent removal; percutaneous internal drainage of the right hepatic duct
11	63, male	Gastric cancer	Billroth II gastrectomy; occluded plastic stent after surgical implantation	Endoscopic and percutaneous failure of stent removal	Failure of stent removal; percutaneous internal drainage of the right hepatic duct

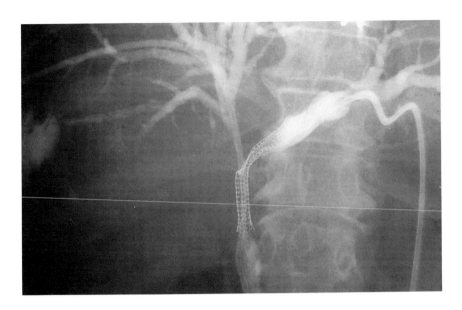

FIG. 7. Occluded Strecker stent in the hilus, not extractable by combined procedure (case 10).

a percutaneous internal drainage of the right hepatic duct was inserted. In summary, the success rate of the combined procedure in our patients was 73%.

ASSESSMENT

CP is a maneuver that is seldom used and accounts for less than 1% of all ERCPs and about 3% of all PTC examinations. However, other authors have reported a higher percentages of CP (4). In our opinion, because CP is a large-scale maneuver, it should only be done if single or sequential endoscopic or percutaneous accesses have failed. CP should only be done in patients for whom there is a reasonable expectation of worthwhile improvement in the quality of life.

INDICATIONS FOR COMBINED PROCEDURES IN BENIGN DISEASES OF THE BILIARY TREE

Endoscopic sphincterotomy can be performed successfully in up to 95% of patients. CP is indicated in patients with anatomical variations, e.g., diverticula of the duodenum, or postoperative alterations of the upper gastrointestinal tract, e.g., Billroth II resection or Roux-en-Y limb when the papilla of Vater cannot be reached endoscopically, or when intubation of the ostium of the papilla fails. In these patients, sphincterotomy can be done over a percutaneous transhepatic inserted guidewire, which is endoscopically grasped and perorally drawn out, using the combined maneuver. The success rate of the sphincterotomy rises to 99% (2).

More than 95% of patients who have choledocholithiasis can be treated successfully by endoscopy or percutaneous transhepatic sphincterotomy and stone removal or fragmentation (5). When the percutaneous route is used for treating bile duct stones, sphincterotomy may not be necessary if dilatation of the papilla of Vater is sufficient, as it allows passage of small duct stones or large stones that have been treated by electrohydraulic lithotripsy.

Few patients have large stones of the CBD that are not amenable to endoscopic or percutaneous transhepatic extraction. These patients can undergo a combined procedure for stone fragmentation and extraction, after sphincterotomy, particularly if the repeated duct stones have caused recurrent biliary pancreatitis and if CBD impaction of gallbladder stones can be expected. Precondition for all these patients is that the papilla of Vater cannot be reached endoscopically and that the patients are inoperable due to concomitant diseases and old age.

Another indication for CP in benign diseases of the biliary tract is mapping of the bilioduodenal anatomy, e.g., fistula between bile duct and duodenum, and reestablishing biliary tract continuity after iatrogenic common bile duct ligation (6). A rare indication for a CP is treatment of benign postoperative bile duct strictures by introducing stents by CP (2).

INDICATIONS FOR CP IN MALIGNANT DISEASES OF THE BILIARY TREE

Endoscopic insertion of plastic stents is successful in up to 90% of malignant, lower CBD strictures, and in up to 70% of hilar stenosis (7). In patients who cannot be treated endoscopically due to postoperative variation, tumor invasion of the papilla of Vater, and/or tightness or angulation of the stricture, or where the percutaneous approach alone is insufficient, the CP offers a chance for placing an endoprosthesis into the biliary tract (4,8–14). Even in postoperative variations, it is possible to place the endoprosthesis either endoscopically or percutaneously, due to the stability of the inserted guidewire using the CP. The overall success rate of stenting increases to 98% (low stricture) and 94% (hilar strictures) by using the combined procedure. CP is limited if a tight stenosis does not allow passage of a percutaneously inserted guidewire through the stricture into the duodenum.

The increasing application of self-expanding and expandable metal stents for treating malignant bile duct strictures make it possible to insert larger-caliber endoprostheses (15). CP allows accurate positioning of percutaneous transhepatic insertion of metal stents as the endoscopic view, especially if the region of the papilla of Vater is altered due to tumor growth. Metal stents that prominently protrude from the ampulla may result in erosions of the contralateral duodenal or jejunal wall, which may progress to perforation or ulceration. These complications could be avoided by using the combined percutaneous transhepatic and endoscopic procedure. CP fails for extraction of either ingrown metal stents or plastic stents, which are embedded in the liver parenchyma because they cannot be grasped, as shown in our two cases.

In conclusion, CP offers one more nonsurgical management option in the following constellations of findings:

1. Multiple, large CBD stones in cases where endoscopic and percutaneous stone removal have failed.
2. CBD stones with recurrent or persistent biliary pancreatitis after failure of endoscopic and percutaneous stone removal.
3. Anatomical mapping after surgical ligature of the CBD.
4. Impassable stricture of the CBD (benign/malignant).
5. Control of stent positioning in difficult anatomical situations.

REFERENCES

1. Gostout CJ, Bender CE. *Gastroenterology* 1988;95:156–163.
2. Dowsett JF, Vaira D, Hatfield AR, et al. *Gastroenterology* 1989; 96:1180–1186.
3. Tam PC, Lai EC, Hui WM, Chan SC. *Am J Gastroenterol* 1990; 85:207–209.
4. Sommer A, Burlefinger R, Bayersdorffer E, Ottenjann R. *Dtsch Med Wochenschr* 1987;112:747–751.
5. Hagenmüller F, Schwacha H. In: Sackmann M, ed. *Diagnosis and management of biliary stones.* London: Bailliere Tindall, 1992;785–817.
6. Benner KG, Ivancer K, Porayko MK, Rosch J. *Gastrointest Endosc* 1992;38:506–509.
7. Tytgat GNJ, Bartelsmann JFWM, den Hartog Jager FCA, Huibregtse K, Mathus-Vliegen EMH. *Dig Dis Sci* 1986;(suppl):57S.
8. Brambs HJ, Billmann P, Pausch J, Holstege A, Salm R. *Endoscopy* 1986;18:52–54.
9. Reiber A, Brambs HJ, Friedl P. *Fortschr Med* 1990;108:565–567.
10. Tsang TK, Crampton AR, Bernstein JR, Buto S, Cahan IA. *Am J Med* 1990;88:344–348.
11. Huddart RA, Hubbard CS, Dickinson RJ. *Clin Radiol* 1991;43: 103–106.
12. Polydorou AA, Cairns SR, Dowsett JF, et al. *Gut* 1991;32: 685–689.
13. Marsh WH, Cunningham IT. *Am J Gastroenterol* 1992;87: 985–990.
14. Hall RI, Denyer ME, Chapman AH. *Surgery* 1990;107:224–227.
15. Huibregtse K, Carr-Locke DL, Cremer M, et al. *Endoscopy* 1992;24:391–394.
16. Ee H, Laurence BH. *Endoscopy* 1992;24:431–432.

Advanced Therapeutic Endoscopy, 2nd Ed.,
edited by J. S. Barkin and C. A. O'Phelan.
Published by Raven Press, Ltd., New York, 1994.

CHAPTER 37

The Use of Stents in Biliary and Pancreatic Disease

Stephen E. Silvis

Biliary stenting has been done for almost a century (1). Until the last two decades these drains were placed in the biliary tree at surgery. Now they can be placed in the ducts by percutaneous transhepatic (2–6) or endoscopic transpapillary routes (7–18). In well-controlled studies the endoscopic route has been shown to be superior to both the transhepatic and surgical drainage in malignant biliary obstruction (19–22). Without controlled studies, stenting of the bile duct has been felt to be of value in benign strictures (23–26), biliary tract leaks (27–35), and when common bile duct stones cannot be removed (36–39). Over the past decade stenting of the pancreatic duct has been considered to be of value for patients with recurrent (40–42) or chronic (43,44) pancreatic pain, pancreatic fistula (45,46), and in some instances for drainage of a pancreatic pseudocyst (43). Stents probably should be used when pancreatic sphincterotomy is done (47). In this chapter I discuss the most efficient stents, the best methods of inserting the stents, and their role in various diseases.

BILIARY BYPASS FOR MALIGNANCY OF THE BILE DUCT

Malignancy of the bile duct, pancreas, and gallbladder will be covered together. Clinically, following cholangiogram, and after biopsy, it is difficult to tell which disease is present in the patient. The technique of biliary stenting was first described by Soehendra and Reynders-Frederix (9) in 1980. It has been applied throughout the world and is now the standard for treating obstructive jaundice secondary to malignancy in

patients who are not operative candidates. This literature is well reviewed by Naggar et al. (48), who found 856 cases in eight publications in the English language on endoscopic bile duct stenting. There were 702 patients in four open series (49–52), and 154 in four randomized trials (19–22) comparing endoscopic insertion of endoprostheses to percutaneous stents or surgical bypass. The stent diameters were from 7 to 12 Fr. Survival was not affected by the therapy because the natural history of the underlying malignancy has overwhelming precedence. The procedure was successful in nine out of ten patients. The procedure related mortality was 1.3% and 30-day mortality was 12%. Overall complication rates of cholangitis, fever, and hemorrhage were 20% (48).

Speer et al. (19) reported a single controlled trial of endoscopic versus percutaneous stent placement in 75 patients with malignant obstruction. It showed that in the endoscopic group 81% had relief of jaundice with endoscopic stenting and 61% cleared of jaundice with percutaneous treatment. There was a 30-day mortality of 15% in the endoscopic group versus 33% in the percutaneous group. The higher mortality after percutaneous stents was due to complications associated with liver puncture. Bornman et al. (53) pointed out that the complications in this study are much higher than in their earlier experiences (5) and that most of the differences would disappear with a lower complication rate.

Three randomized controlled trials of endoscopic stent versus surgical bypass studied 111 patients (20–22). Fewer complications and shorter hospitalizations are seen in endoscopic stenting with the initial procedure. This difference disappears during follow-up because of clogged endoprostheses causing cholangitis and requiring stent changes. The most important unsolved problem is the tendency for the endoprostheses to clog, producing cholangitis.

S. E. Silvis: Department of Medicine, Gastrointestinal Section, Department of Veterans Affairs, Veterans Administration Medical Center, Minneapolis, Minnesota 55417.

An additional problem is the 10% to 15% of patients in whom endoscopic stenting is extremely difficult or impossible. Three developments have markedly affected the success rate for stenting. They are the development of low friction guidewires, the precut technique of sphincterotomy, and combined techniques. Two low-friction guidewires have been developed [Tracer wire (Wilson-Cook), and Glidewire (Microvasive)]. I have found a slight difference in the two wires, but have found both helpful in entering a tight papilla or passing a small stricture. When the precut technique was first described (54), I was quite concerned about its application. This concern was expressed by others (55). Recently, this technique has been carefully reviewed by Shakoor and Geenen (56), who concluded that this technique was safe and effective when used cautiously. I have found it surprisingly safe and also extremely helpful.

Dowsett et al. (57) reported 74 patients who had a combined endoscopic and percutaneous approach. All of the patients had failed an initial endoscopic procedure and had major contraindications for surgery. The first step was obtaining percutaneous transhepatic access to the biliary tree. This was successful in all but one case. The combined procedure is done by passing a guidewire and the transhepatic catheter down the common bile duct to exit the papilla. It is then grasped by a forceps and retrieved up the endoscopic channel. The guidewire is controlled on both ends and can be useful in stone removal and stenting of malignant obstructions. The bile duct is drained externally for an average of 3.4 days before the combined procedure. One patient died during this period from hemorrhage associated with a liver puncture. This combined procedure was performed on 72 patients and was successful in 60. In 16 patients stent change was necessary after the procedure; 13 (81%) of them were done endoscopically and 3 required another combined procedure. Robertson et al. (58) reported that their success rate of placing stents improved from 67% to 97% when they started performing combined percutaneous and endoscopic procedures. This is a procedure requiring high technical skill. With all of these special techniques (tracer wires, precuts, and combined procedures) the success rate should be greater than 95%.

A number of authors (59–62) have pointed out that lesions at the hilum of the liver represent a severe form of obstruction. Ducreux et al. (63) reported 103 patients with hilar obstruction in their institution. Obstruction was produced by carcinoma of the bile duct, liver metastases or primary hepatocellular carcinoma, and carcinoma of the gallbladder. They were successful in 66 of 92 patients (72%) in placing a 10 or 12 Fr Amsterdam prosthesis. The prosthesis functioned without further procedure in 49 cases (53%). Cholangitis was the main complication and occurred in 25 of the 92 patients. The mortality was 43%. The large mortality was related to incomplete drainage with infectious complications. These authors concluded that endoscopic drainage should be avoided in patients with high-grade biliary hilar obstruction.

Huibregtse et al. (64) and Deviere et al. (65) have a less pessimistic view. In the first report, stent placement was successful in 86% of 64 patients with carcinoma of the gallbladder. Satisfactory drainage occurred in 81% of these patients with normalization of the bilirubin in 37 of 44 patients who survived more than 30 days. Procedure-related mortality was 3.1%; 30-day mortality was 14.5%, and the mean survival was 161 days. They considered stent placement the treatment of choice in these patients who have hilar obstruction.

In Deviere et al.'s (65) study, stent placement was successful in 68 of 70 patients with hilar strictures. In patients with type II and III malignant strictures, they frequently found the need for placing multiple stents. Type I strictures involve only the common hepatic duct, type II involves the right and left hepatic, and type III strictures involve multiple branches. When endoscopic retrograde cholangiopancreatography (ERCP) is performed, stenting should be completed as soon as possible, draining as much of the liver as possible. They put them in by transhepatic route if they could not get multiple stents in endoscopically, and they believe that this should be done before any cholangitis develops.

Dowsett et al. (66) reported the successful treatment of 13 of 16 patients by endoscopic stenting after failure of cholecystojejunostomy. The patients had a mean survival of 3.5 months, and the authors felt that it was valuable palliation.

ENDOSCOPIC TREATMENT OF BILIARY FISTULAS

Biliary fistulas can be produced by abdominal trauma or surgical operations on the biliary tract. They may drain into the peritoneal cavity, other abdominal viscera, or out through the skin. A total of 96 patients have been reported in the literature whose biliary fistulas were treated by endoscopic methods (27–35). These treatments were a combination of endoscopic sphincterotomy, bile duct stenting, and/or stone extraction. In a few instances all three of the techniques have been utilized. Two of these reports [Davids et al. (31) and Ponchon et al. (32)] represent 79 of the 96 patients. It is valuable to address these two studies in some detail. Davids et al. (31) discuss 55 patients. Successful ERCP was performed in 54 of the 55. Thirty-three of their patients had common bile duct obstruction at ERCP (18 strictures, 15 stones). The one failure was a patient with a Billroth II in whom they were unable to find the papilla. Five of the patients had surgical clips on their bile ducts that totally obstructed their bile ducts and were referred to surgery. The remainder of the patients were treated endoscopically, successfully in 48 out of the 49 cases. Forty-three of these patients had excellent results with closure of the fistulas. However, five of the patients had continued sepsis, which resulted in fatal outcomes.

In the other large series, Ponchon et al. (32) reported 24 patients. They were able to demonstrate the site of the fistula in 22 of the 24 patients. Sphincterotomy or biliary stent placement resulted in rapid resolution of the fistula in 16 patients. Twelve of the 16 patients, who were draining from the gallbladder, cystic duct, or the common bile duct, had success with endoscopic stenting. In the eight patients who were draining from intrahepatic bile ducts, only four were helped by endoscopy. Ward et al. (35) report three patients in whom sphincterotomy allowed the healing of biliary fistulas after liver transplantation. Wolfsen et al. (67) report on patients with various problems involving the bile duct after liver transplantation. Therapeutic ERCP was successful in 16 of 17 patients using sphincterotomy, balloon dilatation of strictures, and/or stone extraction.

In these studies, successful endoscopic management of biliary fistulas required demonstration of the fistula at ERCP. Intrahepatic lesions did not do well in Ponchon et al.'s (32) experience, and patients required percutaneous drainage of an associated abscess or biloma. Distal bile duct obstruction had to be relieved to decrease the intrabiliary pressure. In spite of a significant failure rate with endoscopic treatment of biliary fistulas, this condition represents a very difficult problem that can often be managed successfully with endoscopy. It has the advantage of a much lower morbidity than surgical repairs. Even when the endoscopic procedure is not successful it may allow for the surgery to be elective.

ENDOSCOPIC TREATMENT OF BENIGN BILIARY STRICTURES

Until recently strictures of the bile duct were treated exclusively by surgery. There is now a total of four articles (23–26) that report the endoscopic treatment of 130 patients by balloon dilatation with or without plastic stent insertion after the dilatation. In these patients there were good to excellent results in 103 cases (79%). The largest series, consisting of 101 patients, was reported by Davids et al. (24); 35 were treated by surgery and 66 were treated with stenting. Stent placement was successful in 94% of the patients. Nineteen of the 66 patients required dilatation prior to stenting. The plan was to place two 10 Fr plastic endo-

prostheses; the stents were electively changed every three months for one year. With successful stenting of the ducts, all of the patients had relief of the jaundice. After one year the stents were removed. Fifteen of these patients presented with bile leaks and 12 patients had common bile duct stones. Referral to surgery was made in ten patients because of total disconnection of the biliary tree. In a 42-month follow-up period after removal of the stents, 17% of the patients had recurrence of the stricture. The group from Toronto (68) has recently reported that 73% of their patients had good or excellent results from endoscopic treatments when followed 6.5 years. These results, although not controlled, compare favorably to biliary surgery. If the stricture recurs, biliary surgery may be necessary, which then may be planned as an elective procedure (69).

Foerster et al. (70) and Rossi et al. (71) reported the treatment of biliary strictures with self-expanding metal mesh stents. Foerster et al. treated seven patients with wire mesh stents who had failed treatment with plastic stent placement, dilatation, and/or repeated laparotomies for their biliary stricturing. In a follow-up period of eight months there was no stent occlusion, and prosthetic-related complications occurred in only one patient. This patient developed a biliary duodenal fistula of unknown origin, and subsequently a liver abscess that responded to antibiotic therapy.

Rossi et al. (71) implanted the stents percutaneously for relief of biliary strictures. They evaluated 47 patients who did not have sclerosing cholangitis and nine patients with sclerosing cholangitis. Thirty-three of the 47 patients were successful with balloon dilatation alone. The 14 patients who failed dilatation had wire mesh stents inserted. After a follow-up of 23 months the treatment was successful in 45 out of 47 (96%). Only three of nine patients with sclerosing cholangitis were successfully treated. There was one procedure-related death (a patient died of septic shock three days after the stone removal). Other complications included two pleural effusions, and three significant hemorrhages, which required embolization of the hepatic artery branches.

Although the use of wire mesh stents appears to have satisfactory results, they have one very distinct disadvantage. This stent cannot be removed. In my opinion they should only be used in benign strictures when the patient has relapsed after attempted surgical treatment or has a prohibitively high operative risk.

Complications of biliary surgery have been treated by interventional radiology. These procedures have been well reviewed by vanSonnenberg et al. (72) and Zuidema et al. (73). There are no direct comparisons of endoscopic versus transhepatic treatment of biliary complications. However, the data of Speer et al. (7)

on stents in the treatment of malignant obstruction showed that there were fewer complications from endoscopic stent placement in comparison to stent placement transhepatically. It is clear that both approaches can result in a successful outcome. All authors who write about the endoscopic treatment of biliary leaks emphasize that fluid collections or abscesses must be drained either surgically or percutaneously. It is obvious that a high degree of skill in both of these techniques should be available for groups who plan to treat complications of biliary and pancreatic surgery.

Davids et al. (74) report a comparison of surgery and endoscopic treatment for benign strictures. At their institution in Amsterdam they had 35 patients treated with surgery and 66 endoscopically. The immediate complications were higher with surgery than with endoscopy, 26% versus 8%. However, late complications occurred only in the endoscopic group where recurrent cholangitis was a significant problem. The total complication rate was 26% in the surgery group and 35% in the endoscopic group. The recurrence rate was 17% in both groups. Seventy-one percent of the surgery group and 82% of the endoscopic patients had good to excellent results. These authors concluded that complete transection, failure of previous repairs, or failures of endoscopic therapy are indications for surgery. They believe that all other patients are candidates for endoscopic stenting as the initial procedure.

ROLE OF BILIARY STENTS AND THE MANAGEMENT OF COMMON BILE DUCT STONES

Nasobiliary tubes and biliary stents have been useful for patients with bile duct stones who have contraindications for sphincterotomy. A small percentage of our population is anticoagulated for many reasons. When stones and cholangitis are discovered in these patients it is frequently undesirable to reverse the anticoagulation. These problems are well managed by short-term stenting of the bile duct. Cotton et al. (39) report 17 patients who were followed for two to five years. Two of these patients developed complications that required surgery. Five died of other causes. Nordback (37) reports on 104 patients (collected from the literature and his experience) managed with long-term stenting because of overwhelming difficulties in stone removal. They were followed for 3 to 59 months. Seventeen percent of the patients experienced jaundice, and 3% had acute cholangitis. These complications were easily managed with antibiotics and exchange of the stent. In only 2% of the patients was biliary surgery essential. This technique is valid in the occasional patient with a large stone, where one is unable to trap it in a lithotripsy basket.

ROLE OF ENDOSCOPIC STENTING IN PANCREATIC DISEASE

Chronic pancreatitis may entrap and obstruct the bile duct as it passes through the pancreas. Deviere et al. (44) reported 25 patients presenting with biliary stenosis and significant cholestasis due to chronic pancreatitis. They had excellent short-term results from common bile duct (CBD) stenting in these patients. However, their symptoms almost invariably recurred when the stent was removed. Interestingly, 10 of their 25 patients had stent migration. This is much higher than their previous report of 8%. The authors felt that this may be related to the character of the stricture in these patients with chronic pancreatitis and wondered if it could be reduced by placing two stents in the duct at the same time. We (75) have found that stenting of the dilated bile duct in chronic pancreatitis can be useful in the differential diagnosis of the cause of pain in these patients. If the pain disappears following stenting of the bile duct, we have confidence that biliary bypass will relieve the pain; therefore, nothing need be done to the pancreas. We did not have the same difficulty with migration of the stents, possibly because our patients did not have ampullary sphincterotomies.

Stenting of the pancreatic duct has been utilized for pancreatic ductal disruption with peripancreatic fluid collections or pancreaticocutaneous fistulas. Kozarek et al. (45) reported on 18 patients; 16 had complete resolution of the drainage from the disrupted pancreatic duct. All of these patients had undergone previous percutaneous or surgical drainage of the peripancreatic fluid, and had drainage tubes placed in chronic fistula tracts. Complications included mild pancreatitis in two patients, and two patients developed stent inclusion with recurrent pancreatitis. They noticed important duct changes related to the stent in 9 of the 18 patients, thus raising the question of whether this is an ongoing process. These authors concluded that transpapillary treatment of ongoing pancreatic ductal disruption has the potential of cure without surgery and of changing the urgent to elective surgery.

We (46) have reported four patients who had pancreatic duct disruption. Three of these patients had an immediate marked reduction in pancreatic drainage from the fistula, which promptly ceased draining. One patient had recurring obstruction of the pancreatic stent, probably related to thick pancreatic fluid that was infected. It must be emphasized that peripancreatic fluid collections must be drained along with the stent replacement. This technique appears to be of significant benefit in patients with ductal disruption.

Pancreatic stenting has been used in patients with acute relapsing and chronic pancreatitis. Kozarek et al. (42) reported on 17 patients, 9 of whom had acute relapsing pancreatitis, and 8 with chronic pancreatitis.

Two patients had subsequently undergone surgery; six patients had continued long-term stent placement with marked reduction of chronic pain or attacks of recurrent pancreatitis. All six pseudocysts resolved, but one recurred and required surgery.

The largest series of patients with chronic pancreatitis treated endoscopically is reported by Cremer et al. (43) from Brussels. Between 1985 and 1989 they treated 75 patients with severe chronic pancreatitis and distal stricture with upstream dilatation. They stented the main pancreatic duct in 54 patients and the minor papilla in 21 patients with 10 Fr plastic endoprostheses. All patients had had endoscopic pancreatic sphincterotomy, and 84% received extracorporeal shock wave lithotripsy to assist in stone removal. Once the stent was functioning satisfactorily a marked relief of pain occurred in 71 of 75 patients (95%). No explanation for the persisting pain in the other four patients was found. Eleven of these patients underwent pancreaticojejunostomy after confirmation of pain relief following decompression of the main pancreatic duct. The mean length of stent patency was 12 months. Early occlusion was often due to small stones that the authors thought were passing from the secondary ducts into the stent. Disappearance of the stricture was observed in only seven patients. Twenty-two of the patients had 18 Fr metal mesh stents placed in the pancreatic duct. The authors concluded that when stenting of the main pancreatic duct relieves the pain, it indicates that pancreatic duct obstruction is causing the discomfort. In their experience these patients uniformly responded to pancreaticoenteric decompression.

The group from Wisconsin has published two articles (40,41) on their experience with stents in the pancreatic duct. In the initial article (40), 35 patients with relapsing pancreatitis were treated with a stent across the major or minor papilla. Seventeen of the 35 patients had major symptomatic improvement with a decrease in the frequency of severe pain and emergency room visits. The second article (41) is a randomized controlled trial of 19 patients with pancreas divisum who had had at least two documented episodes of severe pancreatitis. They were randomized to either dorsal stent placement (10 patients) or controls (9 patients). The stents were kept in for one year and then permanently removed. Three of the 10 patients had stent migration (two into and one out of the pancreatic duct). The control group had five hospitalizations and two emergency room visits for abdominal pain; there were none in the stent treated group. Pancreatitis was documented with an elevated amylase once in the stent group and seven times in the control group. Nine of ten patients in the stented group reported symptomatic improvement; only one of the nine patients in the control group improved. All of these differences are statistically significant.

Endoscopic treatment of pancreas divisum by sphincterotomy of the minor papilla has been recommended by Lehman et al. (47) who treated 52 patients with pancreas divisum and recurrent pancreatitis. The average follow-up was 1.7 years. They found that patients with acute recurrent pancreatitis benefited from minor papilla sphincterotomy more frequently than those with chronic pancreatitis (76% vs. 27%) or chronic pain (76% vs. 25%). Complications occurred in 15% of the procedures. They were primarily mild pancreatitis; however, one patient died of a pancreatic abscess after a failed cannulation. Stents were left in for a mean of 24.2 days with a range of 7 to 103. They had stent occlusion in 48% of their patients, migration of the stent in 6%, and ductal changes were seen at stent removal in 50%. Thirteen percent of the patients had edema in the stent region; three had the appearance of chronic pancreatitis, and one had diffuse duct dilatation on pancreatograms. Early stent removals were probably related to stent obstruction. The authors recommend the procedure only for patients who have acute relapsing pancreatitis, and not for those with chronic pancreatitis or chronic pancreatic pain.

Harrison and Hamilton (76) report a very interesting patient with pancreatic cancer who had severe pain and elevated amylase. He had a stricture of the main pancreatic duct close to the ampulla. They initially placed a 7 Fr stent in this duct, which promptly relieved the pain. When it clogged, an 8 Fr stent was placed, which remained patent for another month. When it obstructed, the pain recurred and the amylase rose again. A 10 Fr straight stent relieved the pain, which did not return in the remaining two months of the patient's life. Hamilton (*personal communication*) has seen one additional patient with the same response. Both of the patients had markedly elevated serum amylase during acute attacks of pain. Harrison and Hamilton have not tried this in the usual patient with pain from carcinoma pancreatic pain. It may be worthwhile to try stenting the pancreatic duct in patients with chronic pain from pancreatic carcinoma.

We must be cautious in treating the pancreas with endoscopic methods. Complications can be very severe. Approaching the pancreatic duct from either the major or minor papilla is more difficult than from the biliary tree. The margin of error in sphincterotomy or stent placement is very small. It is desirable if most of these patients are treated in a few centers.

MISCELLANEOUS CONDITIONS THAT HAVE BEEN SUCCESSFULLY TREATED WITH ERCP STENTING

Binnie et al. (77) reported a patient who was successfully treated for Mirizzi syndrome by biliary stenting.

This was followed by a laparoscopic cholecystectomy. We have used biliary stents to successfully manage acute cholangitis in two patients with Mirizzi syndrome.

Buse and Edmundowicz (78) reported on a patient who had a dilated bile duct and recurring right upper quadrant pain with evidence of cholestasis. The bile duct appeared to be blocked by a large duodenal diverticulum. With a stent in the duct, her symptoms disappeared. She remained asymptomatic for two months with the stent in place, at which time an elective choledochojejunostomy was performed. The patient remained asymptomatic after the surgical procedure. The authors used the stenting technique to predict the response to surgery.

Tamada et al. (79) reported 14 patients with acute cholecystitis who were treated by placing an endoprosthesis into the cystic duct. The pain improved in 10 of the 14 cases. In the five patients with fever, the temperature promptly returned to normal after stenting; however, they were on antibiotics at the same time. The authors do not define when they anticipate that this technique would be of value. It could be useful in the patient with severe acute cholecystitis who is at extremely high risk for surgery.

Lombard et al. (80) stented six jaundiced patients with primary sclerosing cholangitis. Five showed marked improvement within weeks of stenting. The serum bilirubin fell from 266 μg per liter to 65 μg per liter after one month. This was sustained in a follow-up of 12 to 49 months. This is the preferred technique in patients with primary sclerosing cholangitis because surgery or percutaneous drainage may interfere with a future liver transplant. I have also found that stenting is useful in patients with primary sclerosing cholangitis.

WIRE MESH STENTS

The channels of early endoscopes were only large enough to allow the use of 5 Fr or 7 Fr stents. These small stents plugged quickly and offered little effective treatment. New instruments were designed that allowed an 11.5 Fr stent to be inserted across the ductal obstructions. These larger stents remained patent for a much longer time and provided useful treatment (81). Despite investigations into materials and physical design of the stents, plastic stents invariably obstruct and require replacement in three to six months (82–86). This may be true of any stenting device. The mean survival of these patients is under one year. If the length of stent patency can be significantly prolonged, one stent should be all that a patient would require. This is the ultimate goal.

This problem of stent obstruction has been studied in some detail over the last number of years. Iaccarino et al. (87) placed very large stents in the biliary tree transhepatically. This markedly reduced the incidence of catheter obstruction with sepsis. Most of the stents they used were between 14 and 20 Fr; however, occasionally a 28 Fr catheter was inserted in the biliary tree. For as long as 12 months, there was no catheter obstruction in 173 patients.

Speer et al. (88) showed improved results with 10 Fr when compared to 8 Fr stents. However, the 8 Fr stents were single or double pigtail and the 10 Fr stents were straight stents with side flaps. Therefore, it was hard to determine whether differences were related to form or diameter. In an elegant study, Speer et al. (89) reported light and electron microscopy of blocked and functioning stents. The lumen was blocked by a matrix of bacterial cells and extracellular products, including calcium bilirubin, calcium palmitate, and cholesterol embedded within a matrix. Bacteria were attached to the stent surface by a fibrillar matrix. They believed the first event in stent occlusion is forming this biofilm over the surface of the stent. They suggested that the use of bactericidal agents in the plastics used in the manufacturing of the stents might reduce adhesion and stent clogging. However, Browne et al. (90) did not find improvement in patency when the stents were impregnated with bactericidal agents.

An *in vitro* study by Scheeres et al. (91) compared how the shape of the stent and the diameter affect flow rate. Increasing the diameter from a 7 Fr to a 10 Fr stent tripled the flow rate both in the straight and pigtail design, whereas change from a pigtail to a straight stent increased flow by about 30% in the 10 Fr stent and approximately 50% in the 7 Fr stent. These differences were present both in normal and dilated bile duct diameters. They concluded that large straight stents were the preferable endoprostheses to treat obstructed biliary ducts.

Recently, wire stents have been introduced that are either self-expanding or are expanded by balloon dilatation (92–106). This allows insertion of the stent over a small-diameter endoprosthesis delivery device. The stent expands up to 10 mm (30 Fr). Two randomized controlled studies comparing these wire to plastic stents have been completed (107,108). Davids et al. (107) reported on 105 patients with malignancy of the distal bile duct. They randomized patients with distal bile duct carcinoma to a metal versus a polyethylene (PE) stent. The first wire stent remained patent for 273 days (range 14–363 days) compared to 126 days (range 7–482) for the PE stent. The first stent clogged in 16 (33%) of the patients with metal stents and 30 (54%) of the PE stents. The causes of stent occlusion were very different in the two groups. Four of the metal and 29 of the PE stents occluded with sludge. Tumor ingrowth occurred in 10 of the metal stents and none of the PE stents. Two of the metal stents kinked and one of the PE stents was dislodged. As expected, there was no difference in survival between the two groups. There were 64 ERCPs in the metal stent group and 102 in the plastic group. A total of seven patients had duodenal stenosis, two with the metal stents and five in the PE group. The authors concluded that self-expanding metal stents have a longer patency than plastic stents and offer adequate palliation in patients with unresectable malignant distal bile duct obstruction. The wire stents were much more expensive; however, the decrease in the number of ERCPs more than balances the costs.

In the second report by Carr-Locke et al. (108) they studied 182 patients with biliary cancer from a number of centers. The stent patency was shorter in the PE stents, which were 2.8 times more likely to obstruct than the Wallstents. Sixteen percent of the patients with plastic stents had obstruction compared to 37% with the PE stents. This study from the United States confirms Davids et al.'s (107) from Europe.

We (109) reasoned that by combining the advantages of the metal mesh stents and PE stents we could solve this problem of obstruction of stents. This could be done by coating the wire with plastic. The wires appeared to pass down through the mucosa, frequently beyond the submucosa. This is probably happening when the metal stents plug with tumor ingrowth, i.e., the apparent tumor ingrowth may be the wires being passed through the tumor rather than the tumor growing through the wires. The plastic coat does not interfere with the delivery of the stent; it actually slightly increases its radial expansive forces. We are currently planning a controlled study when coated stents become available.

COMPLICATIONS OF BILIARY AND PANCREATIC STENTING

When done endoscopically, stenting procedures have all the complications of ERCP, plus some unique complications related to inserting the stent. When performed transhepatically they have the problems of transhepatic cholangiography, which are primarily bleeding, sepsis, and bile leaks. The difficulties have been shown to be fewer in patients treated with endoscopic transpapillary stenting than with percutaneous transhepatic stenting (17).

Problems Directly Related to the Stenting

The most common difficulty with stents is sepsis caused by blockage of the stent. All currently available stents have this problem; however, with different stents the mechanism of the obstruction changes. Wire mesh stents rarely obstruct from the sludging of biliary solids within the stents; however, the tumor can grow

between the wire meshes of the stent, or the wire mesh can penetrate the tumor during expansion. Bleeding and clot formation in the biliary tree have produced obstruction in both plastic and wire mesh stents (110). There is a higher incidence of stent migration with plastic stents (107,108). When the top of the wire mesh stent is at the turn in the bile duct, kinking can be produced with recurrence of biliary obstruction. This kinking has been corrected by placing a plastic stent inside the wire mesh stent (107,108).

Occlusion from tumor ingrowth has been treated by coagulating the material within the stent with a bipolar electrode (105), laser (95), or by heater probe (111). The group from Amsterdam has had success by just placing a plastic stent within the wire mesh stent (107). They postulate that movement of the stents relative to each other may produce a sheering action that keeps the material from blocking the stent. Ell et al. (111) report on a metal mesh stent fracturing after they had exposed it three times to an endoscopic heater probe. Treating the tumor ingrowth with a heater probe is a blind procedure; the wire mesh is used as a guide to coagulate back and forth through the narrowed area until the probe is close to the mesh. It is not surprising that stent damage occurs with this technique.

When plastic stents obstruct they are replaced. This is usually done by snaring the obstructed stent with a polyp snare or a Dormia basket. When the occluded stent has been removed, the new stent is replaced in the usual manner by passing a guidewire into the duct, then the dilating catheter, followed by the new stent. This is usually quite easy; however, occasionally it is difficult to get a wire back into the duct. Various techniques have been described to facilitate a stent replacement. Soehendra et al. (112) report a method of replacing the stent by a screw device attaching to the stent that can then be pulled up through the endoscope. This is performed by passing a guidewire up the old stent, passing the screwing device down over the guidewire, then rotating to tighten it. This allows leaving the guidewire in place where it is ready to accept the new stent.

Martin (113) describes a technique of passing the guidewire up the stent to be replaced. He passes a 4-mm biliary dilating balloon over the guidewire into the stent. The balloon is inflated inside the stent, allowing the stent to be pulled out of the duct and up the scope. This leaves the guidewire in place to accept the new stent. Hsu (114) reports a technique of passing a guidewire up through the clogged stent followed by the passage of a biopsy forceps through the stent. This can be done with a standard ERCP biopsy forceps. All of these techniques have a very significant disadvantage. The stent is full of bacterially contaminated material; when a guidewire is passed up the stent, the contaminated material is introduced deeply within the biliary tree. I am concerned about producing biliary sepsis. Therefore, my personal practice is to snare and replace these obstructed stents.

Sepsis is almost invariably related to poor drainage of the biliary tree. This complication is most feared because it has a severe morbidity and mortality. Motte et al. (115) reviewed the experience of their group from Brussels. They reported on 34 patients who experienced septicemia within three days of endoscopic biliary stenting and compared this to a matched group of 71 patients without this complication. The risk factors identified before the procedure were prior cholangitis and leukocytosis. The drainage procedure was considered complete if at least one stent was in place above a common bile duct stricture and two stents above a hilar stricture, and a cholangiogram was obtained showing complete drainage of contrast with aerobilia. Thirty-one of the 34 septic patients had incomplete drainage but only 3 of the 71 uninfected patients had incomplete drainage. Another striking difference was in the percentage of patients with hilar strictures: 19 of 34 septic patients (56%) with hilar strictures compared to 11 of 71 (15%) in the noninfected patients. This confirmed that the primary factor producing biliary sepsis following stenting is inadequate drainage. The authors emphasize that if there is any question of adequate drainage, antibiotics need to be given, including coverage for pseudomonas infection.

Stent migration can be a significant problem. These patients usually present with recurrent obstruction because the stent has migrated below the upper end of the stricture. The stent can impact into the duodenal wall, causing obstruction. I can find only a single case of migration of a metal mesh stent; all others were plastic (116). It was recovered endoscopically. Ruffolo et al. (117) report two cases where stents migrated out of the bile duct and became lodged in the colon. Both stents were removed endoscopically and the patients were treated with antibiotics. They recovered without incidence. There have been stent perforations of the duodenum. Lowe et al. (118) report gastric air as a sign of perforation of one of these stents. Smith et al. (119) report the endoscopic recovery of a stent that had perforated the duodenal wall.

Biliary stents migrate up the bile duct as well. Some of these stents can be captured in either a Dormia-type basket or snare removed from the bile duct. In my experience, when they are difficult or impossible to remove, placing another stent across the papilla has functioned satisfactorily. Zissin et al. (120) and Mallat et al. (121) report the fracturing of biliary stents in three patients. They were able to remove both fragments and the patients recovered without incident. Schuller et al. (122) reported two patients who each had a stent in place for two years and developed a large calculus around their stents. These patients did well with place-

ment of another stent parallel to the calculus. Neither of the patients responded to ursodiol, which is not surprising because these are not cholesterol stones.

I could only find two cases where acute cholecystitis followed stenting of the CBD. This is surprising with the extensive use of stenting (123). One would expect that stents in the CBD would often obstruct the cystic duct. We anticipated that acute cholecystitis would be seen with some frequency. It is unclear to me why this is a rare event.

Unique complications with expandable stents in five patients has been reported by Jowell et al. (124). In their cases the delivery device became caught on the end of the stents. This occurred when the upper end of the stent was impacted in a tight area of stricturing. This restrains the upper end of the expandable metal stent, which must expand slightly to clear the catheter delivery device. The first patient had the plastic delivery catheter cut off in the duodenum with a neodymium:yttrium-aluminum garnet (Nd:YAG) laser. The catheter remained in place and drained bile without a problem. Two patients had the catheters coiled in the stomach. One of these patients passed the delivery catheter in the stool three weeks later. The other patient died after five months without recurrence of obstructive jaundice. In two patients there was delay in release of the delivery device, but steady firm pressure produced a sudden release. This occurred immediately after implantation in one patient and the next day in the other case. Since this report I have had a case of entrapment of the delivery device. The upper end of the delivery device was cut off and a 90 cm, 10 Fr multipurpose guiding catheter (Model #RS210-004A, Schneider, Inc., Plymouth, MN) was passed over the delivery catheter. With a steady forward pressure on the renal angiocath, and pulling back on the delivery catheter, it slid into the renal angiocath. The whole device was then removed without difficulty.

Unique complications of pancreatic duct (PD) stents occur (125–128). Kozarek (125) has reported that 72% of patients with initially normal pancreatograms had duct changes after stenting. Some of the changes appeared to be related to stent occlusion (pseudocyst and diffuse enlargement), or direct stent trauma edema with irregular stenosis with side-branch dilation. Gulliver et al. (127) report that in patients who had a normal pancreatogram prior to stent placement, 80% had diffuse changes in the duct following the stenting. Five patients had focal narrowing at the tip of the stent. There was improvement in 60% of the patients with changes in the PD among those who had repeat ERCP. Nineteen of their patients had an abnormal pancreatogram at the time of stenting. Seven of these showed improvement, eight had no change, and four deteriorated. Barkun et al. (128) report new pancreatic duct changes that were reversible in 73% of their patients.

Immediately after stent removal, 17% of the pancreatograms remained normal, 78% had mild changes, and 5% had severe changes with marked irregularity and clubbing. They repeated the ERCP on 14 of the patients with abnormal pancreatic ducts in 6 to 12 months. At that time 12 of the 13 patients with mild abnormalities had a normal PD. The patients with severe changes had persistent abnormalities.

With these marked changes in the ERCP, pancreatic stents should probably not be used except in controlled clinical trials, in patients with very severe symptoms before stenting, and in patients with pancreatic cutaneous fistulas.

CONCLUSION

The stenting of the biliary and pancreatic ducts is now established in clinical medicine, certainly for the bile duct although perhaps not for the pancreatic duct, where the indications are much fewer and the risks much higher.

Since endoscopic stenting of the common bile duct has become the standard treatment for inoperative biliary malignancies, we place a stent when the diagnosis is made. In our hospitals when there remains a question of whether to treat the patient with a Whipple procedure, we place an 8.5 Fr stent in the duct, which can be removed at the time of surgery. If the patient is not treated surgically the prosthesis can be replaced with a larger plastic (11.5 Fr) or wire mesh (30 Fr) stent at a later time. The choice between a wire mesh and a larger plastic stent remains undecided. The length of patency of the wire stent is about twice as long as for the plastic stent; however, they both tend to occlude, with many patients requiring more than one stent. The wire mesh stents are more expensive and cannot be removed. These factors make this a subjective clinical decision. I place a wire mesh stent in the bile duct of the patient who has a reasonably long life expectancy.

The treatment of bile duct leaks and strictures with endoscopic stents has been remarkably good. They are clearly indicated as the first treatment of these difficult problems. In this era of laparoscopic cholecystectomy (lap-chole) we probably will see more leaks and bile duct injuries. In addition, common bile duct exploration remains difficult during lap-chole. Because of lap-chole, sphincterotomy will be used to remove more CBD stones than we have in the past. The role of stents for retained common bile duct stones remains a valid option for the stone that is extremely difficult to remove. Although stenting of the bile duct is technically somewhat difficult it remains a low-morbidity procedure to establish a biliary drainage.

Endoscopic treatment of the pancreas has proceeded much more slowly, in part because of the difficulties

performing pancreatic sphincterotomy and placing wires and stents in the pancreatic duct. In addition, pancreatitis has been a feared complication of ERCP. We have been reluctant to manipulate the pancreas in the same degree that the bile duct is instrumented. The CBD was vigorously approached, at least in part, because of the long experience with surgery on these very durable structures.

Pancreatic duct stenting in rupture of the duct with percutaneous fistula or localized collection of pancreatic juice appears to be a useful procedure. Remember, peripancreatic collections must be drained surgically or percutaneously. The pancreatic duct stent will not remove large volumes of extrapancreatic fluid.

Treatment of chronic pancreatitis, recurrent pancreatitis, and pancreatic pain by endoscopic methods appears to be effective at a few centers. Whether this should be done by pancreatic sphincterotomy, stenting, or stone removal, or not done at all, remains an unanswered question. Patient selection may be a critical factor. In skilled hands, selected patients appear to benefit at least for the short term. The stent-induced changes in the pancreatic duct raise concern that the treatment could have a long-term harmful effect. We must follow these studies carefully to define the role of endoscopic treatment of pancreatic disease in clinical medicine.

REFERENCES

1. Halsted WS. Contributions to the surgery of the bile passages especially of the common bile duct. *Boston Med Surg J* 1899; 141:645–654.
2. Okuda K, Tanikawa K, Emura T, et al. Nonsurgical percutaneous transhepatic cholangiography—diagnostic significance in medical problems in the liver. *Am J Dig Dis* 1974;19:21–36.
3. Ring EJ, Oleaga JA, Feinman DB, Husted JW, Lunderquist A. Therapeutic application of catheter cholangiography. *Radiology* 1978;128:333–338.
4. Perieras RV Jr, Rheingold OJ, Hutson D, et al. Relief of malignant obstructive jaundice by percutaneous insertion of a permanent prosthesis in the biliary tree. *Ann Intern Med* 1978;89: 589–593.
5. Bornman PC, Harries-Jones EP, Tobias R, Van Stiegmann G, Terblanche J. Prospective controlled trial of transhepatic biliary endoprosthesis versus bypass surgery for incurable carcinoma of head of pancreas. *Lancet* 1986;1:69–71.
6. Denning DA, Ellison EC, Carey LC. Preoperative percutaneous transhepatic decompression lowers operative morbidity in patients with obstructive jaundice. *Am J Surg* 1981;141:61–65.
7. Speer AG, Cotton PB, Russell RCG, et al. Randomised trial of endoscopic versus percutaneous stent insertion in malignant obstructive jaundice. *Lancet* 1987;2:57–62.
8. Siegel JH, Yatto RP. Approach to cholestasis: an update. *Arch Intern Med* 1982;142:1877–1879.
9. Soehendra N, Reynders-Frederix V. Palliative bile duct drainage: a new endoscopic method of introducing a transpapillary drain. *Endoscopy* 1980;12:8–11.
10. Huibregtse K, Tytgat GN. Palliative treatment of obstructive jaundice by transpapillary introduction of large bore bile duct endoprothesis. *Gut* 1982;23:371–375.
11. Kiil J, Kruse A, Rokkjaer M. Endoscopic biliary drainage. *Br J Surg* 1987;74:1087–1090.

12. Ott DJ, Gilliam JH III, Zagoria RJ, Young GP. Interventional endoscopy of the biliary and pancreatic ducts: current indications and methods. *AJR* 1992;158:243–250.

13. Hatfield ARW. Palliation of malignant obstructive jaundice—surgery or stent? *Gut* 1990;31:1339–1340.

14. McLean GK, Burke DR. Role of endoprostheses in the management of malignant biliary obstruction. *Radiology* 1989;170:961–967.

15. Cotton PB. Nonsurgical palliation of jaundice in pancreatic cancer. *Surg Clin North Am* 1989;69:613–627.

16. Lindstrom E, Anderberg B, Olaison G, Ihse I. Endoscopic biliary drainage in malignant bile duct obstruction. *Acta Chir Scand* 1988;154:277–281.

17. Huibregtse K, Katon RM, Coene PP, Tytgat GNJ. Endoscopic palliative treatment in pancreatic cancer. *Gastrointest Endosc* 1986;32:334–338.

18. Cotton PB. Endoscopic biliary stents—trick or treatment? *Gastrointest Endosc* 1986;32:364–365.

19. Speer AG, Cotton PB, Russell RCG, et al. Randomised trial of endoscopic versus percutaneous stent insertion in malignant obstructive jaundice. *Lancet* 1987;2:57–62.

20. Shepherd HA, Royle G, Ross APR, Diba A, Arthur M, Colin-Jones D. Endoscopic biliary endoprosthesis in the palliation of malignant obstruction of the distal common bile duct: a randomized trial. *Br J Surg* 1988;75:1166–1168.

21. Andersen JR, Sorensen SM, Kruse A, Rokkjaw M, Matzen P. Randomized trial of endoscopic endoprosthesis versus operative bypass in malignant obstructive jaundice. *Gut* 1989;30:1132–1135.

22. Dowsett JF, Russell RCG, Hatfield ARW, et al. Malignant obstructive jaundice: a prospective randomized trial by-pass surgery versus endoscopic stenting. *Gastroenterology* 1989;96:A128.

23. Berkelhammer C, Kortan P, Haber GB. Endoscopic biliary prostheses as treatment for benign postoperative bile duct strictures. *Gastrointest Endosc* 1989;35:95–101.

24. Davids PH, Rauws EA, Coene PP, Tytgat GN, Huibregtse K. Endoscopic stenting for post-operative biliary strictures. *Gastrointest Endosc* 1992;38:12–18.

25. Geenen DJ, Geenen JE, Hogan WJ, Schenck J, Venu RP, Johnson GK, Jackson A Jr. Endoscopic therapy for benign bile duct strictures. *Gastrointest Endosc* 1989;35:367–371.

26. Deviere J, Baize M, Vandermeeren A, Buset M, Delhaye M, Cremer M. Endoscopic stenting for biliary strictures. *Acta Gastroenterol Belg* 1992;55:295–305.

27. Kozarek RA, Traverso LW. Endoscopic stent placement for cystic duct leak after laparoscopic cholecystectomy. *Gastrointest Endosc* 1991;37:71–73.

28. Deviere J, van Gansbeke D, Ansay J, de Toeuf J, Cremer M. Endoscopic management of a post-traumatic biliary fistula. *Endoscopy* 1987;19:136–139.

29. Gholson CF, Burton F. Closure of a controlled biliary fistula complicating partial cholecystectomy with endoscopic biliary stenting. *Am J Gastroenterol* 1992;87:248–251.

30. Smith AC, Schapiro RH, Kelsey PB, Warshaw AL. Successful treatment of nonhealing biliary-cutaneous fistulas with biliary stents. *Gastroenterology* 1986;90:764–769.

31. Davids PHP, Rauws EAJ, Tytgat GNJ, Huibregtse K. Postoperative bile leakage: endoscopic management. *Gut* 1992;33:1118–1122.

32. Ponchon T, Gallez JF, Valette PJ, Chavaillon A, Bory R. Endoscopic treatment of biliary tract fistulas. *Gastrointest Endosc* 1989;35:490–498.

33. Sedgwick ML, Denyer ME. Treatment of a postoperative cholecystocutaneous fistula by an endoscopic stent. *Br J Surg* 1989;76:159–160.

34. Musher DR, Gouge T. Cutaneous bile fistula treated with ERCP-placed large diameter stent. *Am Surg* 1989;55:653–655.

35. Ward EM, Wiesner RH, Hughes RW, Krom RAF. Persistent bile leak after liver transplantation: biloma drainage and endoscopic retrograde cholangiopancreatographic sphincterotomy. *Radiology* 1991;179:719–720.

36. Foutch PG, Harlan J, Sanowski RA. Endoscopic placement of

37. Nordback I. Management of unextractable bile duct stones by endoscopic stenting. *Ann Chir Gynaecol* 1989;78:290–292.

38. Dill JE. Endoscopic stenting for biliary stones after Billroth II gastrectomy [Letter]. *Am J Gastroenterol* 1989;84:1591–1592.

39. Cotton PB, Forbes A, Leung JW, Dineen L. Endoscopic stenting for long-term treatment of large bile duct stones: 2 to 5 year follow-up. *Gastrointest Endosc* 1987;33:411–412.

40. McCarthy J, Geenen JE, Hogan WJ. Preliminary experience with endoscopic stent placement in benign pancreatic disease. *Gastrointest Endosc* 1988;34:16–18.

41. Lans JI, Geenen JE, Johanson JF, Hogan WJ. Endoscopic therapy in patients with pancreas divisum and acute pancreatitis: a prospective, randomized, controlled clinical trial. *Gastrointest Endosc* 1992;38:430–434.

42. Kozarek RA, Patterson DJ, Ball TJ, Traverso LW. Endoscopic placement of pancreatic stents and drains in the management of pancreatitis. *Ann Surg* 1989;209:261–266.

43. Cremer M, Deviere J, Delhaye M, Baize M, Vandermeeren A. Stenting in severe chronic pancreatitis: results of medium-term follow-up in seventy-six patients. *Endoscopy* 1991;23:171–176.

44. Deviere J, Devaere S, Baize M, Cremer M. Endoscopic biliary drainage in chronic pancreatitis. *Gastrointest Endosc* 1990;36:96–100.

45. Kozarek RA, Ball TJ, Patterson DJ, Freeny PC, Ryan JA, Traverso LW. Endoscopic transpapillary therapy for disrupted pancreatic duct and peripancreatic fluid collections. *Gastroenterology* 1991;100:1362–1370.

46. Erickson R, Yakshe P, Freeman M, Vennes J, Silvis S. Resolution of pancreatic-cutaneous fistulae by endoscopic transpapillary pancreatic duct stenting: a case series. *Am J Gastroenterol* 1992;87:1283.

47. Lehman GA, Sherman S, Nisi R, Hawes RH. Pancreas divisum: results of minor papilla sphincterotomy. *Gastrointest Endosc* 1993;39:1–8.

48. Naggar E, Krag E, Matzen P. Endoscopically inserted biliary endoprosthesis in malignant obstructive jaundice. A survey of the literature. *Liver* 1990;10:321–324.

49. Leung JWC, Emery R, Cotton PB, Russell RCG, Vallon AG, Mason RR. Management of malignant obstructive jaundice at The Middlesex Hospital. *Br J Surg* 1983;70:584–586.

50. Siegel JH, Snady H. The significance of endoscopically placed prostheses in the management of biliary obstruction due to carcinoma of the pancreas. Results of non-operative decompression in 277 patients. *Am J Gastroenterol* 1986;81:634–640.

51. Huibregtse K, Katon RM, Coene PP, Tytgat GNJ. Endoscopic palliative treatment in pancreatic cancer. *Gastrointest Endosc* 1986;32:334–338.

52. Walta DC, Fausel CS, Brant B. Endoscopic biliary stents and obstructive jaundice. *Am J Surg* 1987;153:444–447.

53. Bornman PC, Terblanche J, Harries-Jones EP, Marks IN. Endoscopic versus percutaneous stents for malignant jaundice [Letter]. *Lancet* 1987;2:689.

54. Huibregtse K, Katon RM, Tytgat GNJ. Precut papillotomy via fine needle knife papillotome: a safe and effective technique. *Gastrointest Endosc* 1986;32:403–405.

55. Cotton PB. Precut papillotomy—a risky technique for experts only [Editorial]. *Gastrointest Endosc* 1989;35:578–579.

56. Shakoor T, Geenen JE. Pre-cut papillotomy. *Gastrointest Endosc* 1992;38:623–627.

57. Dowsett JF, Vaira D, Hatfield ARW, et al. Endoscopic biliary therapy using the combined percutaneous and endoscopic technique. *Gastroenterology* 1989;96:1180–1186.

58. Robertson DA, Ayres R, Hacking CN, Shepherd H, Birch S, Wright R. Experience with a combined percutaneous and endoscopic approach to stent insertion in malignant obstructive jaundice. *Lancet* 1987;2:1449–1452.

59. Beazley RM, Blumgart LH. Malignant stricture at the confluence of the biliary tree: diagnosis and management. *Surg Ann* 1985;17:125–141.

60. Marsh WH, Cunningham JT. Endoscopic stent placement for obstructive jaundice secondary to metastatic malignancy. *Am J Gastroenterol* 1992;87:985–990.

biliary stents for treatment of high risk geriatric patients with common duct stones. *Am J Gastroenterol* 1989;84:527–529.

61. Lameris JS, Stoker J, Dees J, Nix GAJJ, Van Blakenstein M, Jeekel J. Non-surgical palliative treatment of patients with malignant biliary obstruction—the place of endoscopic and percutaneous drainage. *Clin Radiol* 1987;38:603–608.
62. Stanley J, Gobien RP, Cunningham J, Andriole J. Biliary decompression: an institutional comparison of percutaneous and endoscopic methods. *Radiology* 1986;158:195–197.
63. Ducreux M, Liguory CL, Lefebvre JF, et al. Management of malignant hilar biliary obstruction by endoscopy. Results and prognostic factors. *Dig Dis Sci* 1992;37:778–783.
64. Huibregtse K, Schneider B, Coene PP, Tytgat GN. Endoscopic palliation of jaundice in gallbladder cancer. *Surg Endosc* 1987; 1:143–146.
65. Deviere J, Baize M, de Toeuf J, Cremer M. Long-term follow-up of patients with hilar malignant stricture treated by endoscopic internal biliary drainage. *Gastrointest Endosc* 1988;34: 95–101.
66. Dowsett JF, Cairns SR, Vaira D, Polydorou AA, Hatfield ARW, Russell RCG. Endoscopic endoprosthesis insertion following failure of cholecystojejunostomy in pancreatic carcinoma. *Br J Surg* 1989;76:454–456.
67. Wolfsen HC, Porayko MK, Hughes RH, Gostout CJ, Krom RAF, Wiesner RH. Role of endoscopic retrograde cholangiopancreatograpy after orthotopic liver transplantation. *Am J Gastroenterol* 1992;87:955–960.
68. Walden D, Raijman I, Fuchs G, et al. Long term follow-up of endoscopic stenting (ES) for benign postoperative bile duct strictures (BPBDS). *Gastrointest Endosc* 1993;39:335.
69. Branum G, Schmitt C, Baillie J, et al. Management of major biliary complications after laparoscopic cholecystectomy. *Ann Surg* 1993;217:532–541.
70. Foerster EC, Hoepffner N, Domschke W. Bridging of benign choledochal stenoses by endoscopic retrograde implantation of mesh stents. *Endoscopy* 1991;23:133–135.
71. Rossi P, Salvatori FM, Bezzi M, Maccioni F, Porcaro ML, Ricci P. Percutaneous management of benign biliary strictures with balloon dilation and self-expanding metallic stents. *Cardiovasc Intervent Radiol* 1990;13:231–239.
72. vanSonnenberg E, Casola G, Wittich GR, et al. The role of interventional radiology for complications of cholecystectomy. *Surgery* 1990;107:632–638.
73. Zuidema GD, Cameron JL, Sitzmann JV, et al. Percutaneous transhepatic management of complex biliary problems. *Ann Surg* 1983;197:584–593.
74. Davids PHP, Tanka AKF, Rau WS, et al. Benign biliary strictures: surgery or endoscopy? *Ann Surg* 1993;217:237–243.
75. Meier PB, Silvis SE, Daigle-Bjerke A, Vennes JA. Nonoperative biliary drainage differentiates chronic pancreatitis (CP) from biliary pain in CP patients with a benign bile duct strictures. *Gastrointest Endosc* 1991;37:250.
76. Harrison MA, Hamilton JW. Palliation of pancreatic cancer pain by endoscopic stent placement. *Gastrointest Endosc* 1989; 35:443–445.
77. Binnie NR, Nixon SJ, Palmer KR. Mirizzi syndrome managed by endoscopic stenting and laparoscopic cholecystectomy. *Br J Surg* 1992;79:647.
78. Buse PE, Edmundowicz SA. Proximal common bile duct obstruction secondary to a periampullary duodenal diverticulum: successful treatment with endoscopic stenting. *Gastrointest Endosc* 1991;37:635–637.
79. Tamada K, Seki H, Sato K, et al. Efficacy of endoscopic retrograde cholecystoendoprosthesis (ERCCE) for cholecystitis. *Endoscopy* 1991;23:2–3.
80. Lombard M, Farrant M, Karani J, Westaby D, Williams R. Improving biliary-enteric drainage in primary sclerosing cholangitis: experience with endoscopic methods. *Gut* 1991;32: 1364–1368.
81. Siegel JH, Pullano W, Kodsi B, Cooperman A, Ramsey W. Optimal palliation of malignant bile duct obstruction: experience with endoscopic 12 French prostheses. *Endoscopy* 1988; 20:137–141.
82. Leung JWC, del Favero G, Cotton PB. Endoscopic biliary prostheses. A comparison of materials. *Gastrointest Endosc* 1985;31:93–95.
83. Lammer J, Stoffler G, Petek WW, Hofler H. In vitro long-term perfusion of different materials for biliary endoprostheses. *Invest Radiol* 1986;21:329–331.
84. Coene PPLO, Groen AK, Cheng J, Out MMJ, Tytgat GNJ, Huibregtse K. Clogging of biliary endoprostheses: a new perspective. *Gut* 1990;31:913–917.
85. Rey JF, Maupetit P, Greff M. Experimental study of biliary endoprosthesis efficiency. *Endoscopy* 1985;17:145–148.
86. Matsuda Y, Shimakura K, Akamatsu T. Factors affecting the patency of stents in malignant biliary obstructive disease: univariate and multivariate analysis. *Am J Gastroenterol* 1991;86: 843–849.
87. Iaccarino V, Niola R, Porta E. Silicone biliary stents. *AJR* 1987;148:471–473.
88. Speer AG, Cotton PB, MacRae KD. Endoscopic management of malignant biliary obstruction: stents of 10 French gauge are preferable to stents of 8 French gauge. *Gastrointest Endosc* 1988;34:412–417.
89. Speer AG, Cotton PB, Rode J, et al. Biliary stent blockage with bacterial biofilm. A light and electron microscopy study. *Ann Intern Med* 1988;108:546–553.
90. Browne S, Schmalz M, Geenen J, Venu R, Johnson GK. A comparison of biliary and pancreatic stent occlusion in antibiotic-coated vs conventional stents. *Gastrointest Endosc* 1990;36: 206.
91. Scheeres D, O'Brien W, Ponsky L, Ponsky J. Endoscopic stent configuration and bile flow rates in a variable diameter bile duct model. *Surg Endosc* 1990;4:91–93.
92. Huibregtse K, Cheng J, Coene PPLO, Fockens P, Tytgat GNJ. Endoscopic placement of expandable metal stents for biliary strictures—a preliminary report on experience with 33 patients. *Endoscopy* 1989;21:280–282.
93. Domschke W, Foerster E. Endoscopic implantation of large-bore self-expanding biliary mesh stents. *Gastrointest Endosc* 1990;36:55–57.
94. Lammer J, Klein GL, Kleinert R, Hausegger K, Einspieler R. Obstructive jaundice: use of expandable metal endoposthesis for biliary drainage. *Radiology* 1990;177:789–792.
95. Neuhaus H, Hagenmuller F, Griebel M, Classen M. Percutaneous cholangioscopic or transpapillary insertion of self-expanding biliary metal stents. *Gastrointest Endosc* 1991;37:31–37.
96. Salomonowitz EK, Antonucci F, Heer M, Stuckmann G, Egloff B, Zollikofer CL. Biliary obstruction: treatment with self-expanding metal prostheses. *J Vasc Interv Radiol* 1992;3: 365–370.
97. Neuhaus H, Hagenmuller F, Classen M. Self-expanding biliary stents: preliminary clinical experience. *Endoscopy* 1989;21: 225–228.
98. Alvarado R, Palmaz JC, Garcia OJ, Tio FO, Rees CR. Evaluation of polymer-coated balloon-expandable stents in bile ducts. *Radiology* 1989;170:975–978.
99. Carrasco CH, Wallace S, Chamsangavej C, et al. Expandable biliary endoprosthesis: an experimental study. *AJR* 1985;145: 1279–1281.
100. Mueller PR. Metallic endoprosthesis: boon or bust. *Radiology* 1991;179:603–605.
101. Martin EC, Laffey KJ, Bixon R, Getrajdman GI. Gianturco-Rosch biliary stents: preliminary experience. *J Vasc Interv Radiol* 1990;1:101–105.
102. Jackson JE, Roddie ME, Chetty N, Benjamin IS, Adam A. The management of occluded metallic self-expandable biliary endoprostheses. *AJR* 1991;157:291–292.
103. Gillams A, Dick R, Dooley JS, Wallsten H, El-Din A. Self-expandable stainless steel braided endoprosthesis for biliary strictures. *Radiology* 1990;174:137–140.
104. Lameris JS, Stoker J, Nijs HGT, et al. Malignant biliary obstruction: percutaneous use of self-expandable stents. *Radiology* 1991;179:703–707.
105. Cremer M, Deviere J, Sugai B, Baize M. Expandable biliary metal stents for malignancies: endoscopic insertion and diathermic cleaning for tumor ingrowth. *Gastrointest Endosc* 1990;36: 451–457.
106. Hausegger KA, Kleinert R, Lammer J, Klein GE, Fluckiger

F. Malignant biliary obstruction: histologic findings after treatment with self-expandable stents. *Radiology* 1992;185:461–464.

107. Davids PHP, Groen AK, Rauws EAJ, Tytgat GNJ, Huibregtse K. Randomised trial of self-expanding metal stents versus polyethylene stents for distal malignant biliary obstruction. *Lancet* 1992;340:1488–1492.

108. Carr-Locke DL, Ball TJ, Connors PJ, et al. Multicenter randomized trial of Wallstent biliary endoprosthesis versus plastic stents. *Gastrointest Endosc* 1993;39:310.

109. Silvis SE, Sievert CE Jr, Vennes JA, Abeyta B, Brennecke LH. Comparison of covered vs uncovered wire mesh stents in the canine biliary tract. *Gastrointest Endosc* 1994;40:17–21.

110. Vanangunas A, Ehrenpreis E. Endoscopic evacuation of hematobilia induced by large bore self-expanding biliary mesh stent [Letter]. *Gastrointest Endosc* 1991;37:101–103.

111. Ell C, Wolfgang EF, Fleig WE, Hochberger J. Broken biliary metal stent after repeated electrocoagulation for tumor ingrowth. *Gastrointest Endosc* 1992;38:197–198.

112. Soehendra N, Maydeo A, Eckmann B, Bruckner M, Nam V Ch, Grimm H. A new technique for replacing an obstructed biliary endoprosthesis. *Endoscopy* 1990;22:271–272.

113. Martin DF. Wire guided balloon assisted endoscopic biliary stent exchange. *Gut* 1991;32:1562–1564.

114. Hsu D. Recanalization of clogged biliary stent. *Gastrointest Endosc* 1990;36:322–323.

115. Motte S, Deviere J, Dumonceau JM, Serruys E, Thys JP, Cremer M. Risk factors for septicemia following endoscopic biliary stenting. *Gastroenterology* 1991;101:1374–1381.

116. Plotner A, Lewis BS. Duodenal migration and retrieval of metallic biliary stent. *Gastrointest Endosc* 1991;37:496–497.

117. Ruffolo TA, Lehman GA, Sherman S, Aycock R, Hayes A. Biliary stent migration with colonic diverticular impaction. *Gastrointest Endosc* 1992;38:81–83.

118. Lowe GM, Bernfield JB, Smith CS, Matalon TAS. Gastric pneumatosis: sign of biliary stent-related perforation. *Radiology* 1990;174:1037–1038.

119. Smith FCT, O'Connor HJ, Downing R. An endoscopic technique for stent recovery used after duodenal perforation by a biliary stent. *Endoscopy* 1991;23:244–245.

120. Zissin R, Novis B, Rubinstein Z. Case report: broken intracholedochal stent. *Clin Radiol* 1992;45:46–47.

121. Mallat A, Saint-Marc Girardin MF, Meduri B, Liguory C, Dhumeaux D. Fracture of biliary endoprosthesis after endoscopic drainage for malignant biliary obstruction. Report of two cases. *Endoscopy* 1986;18:243–244.

122. Schuller AM, Rezk GJ, Lyon DT. Calculus formation around common bile duct stents: a complication of long-term biliary drainage. *Gastrointest Endosc* 1991;37:581–582.

123. Leung JW, Chung SC, Sung JY, Li MK. Acute cholecystitis after stenting of the common bile duct for obstruction secondary to pancreatic cancer. *Gastrointest Endosc* 1989;35:109–110.

124. Jowell PS, Cotton PB, Huibregtse K, et al. Delivery catheter entrapment during deployment of expandable metal stents. *Gastrointest Endosc* 1993;39:199–202.

125. Kozarek RA. Pancreatic stents can induce ductal changes consistent with chronic pancreatitis. *Gastrointest Endosc* 1990;36:93–95.

126. Derfus GA, Geenen JE, Hogan WJ. Effect of endoscopic pancreatic duct stent placement on pancreatic ductal morphology. *Gastrointest Endosc* 1990;36:206.

127. Gulliver DJ, Edmunds S, Baker ME, et al. Stent placement for benign pancreatic diseases: correlation between ERCP findings and clinical response. *AJR* 1992;159:751–755.

128. Barkun AN, Jones S, Putnam WS, Baillie J, Parker S, Cotton PB. Endoscopic treatment of patients with pancreas divisum and pancreatitis. *Gastrointest Endosc* 1990;36:206.

Advanced Therapeutic Endoscopy, 2nd Ed.,
edited by J. S. Barkin and C. A. O'Phelan.
Raven Press, Ltd., New York © 1994.

CHAPTER 38

Endoscopic Management of Large Bile Duct Stones

Isaac Raijman and Gregory B. Haber

Experience with endoscopic removal of common bile duct stones now spans two decades since the pioneering work of Kawai et al. (1) and Classen and Demling (2). This novel approach was initially viewed with healthy skepticism and rekindled old surgical concerns about the long-term effects of disrupting the normal sphincter mechanisms, particularly in the patient under 40. Today, in the era of laparoscopic cholecystectomy, the endoscopic treatment of bile duct stones is the preferred method for all ages. The challenge of the second decade of endoscopic treatment has been the removal of the large or inaccessible stone.

ENDOSCOPIC SPHINCTEROTOMY

Endoscopic electrocautery to divide the sphincter of Oddi has been shown to be a safe and effective method, little changed since the first cut. The "bowstring" papillotome configuration for standard cuts is universally employed. There are a variety of materials and designs, employed by individual endoscopists according to their preference. There are two types of cutting wire, a single strand of stainless steel and a braided wire, the former better for cutting current and the latter better for distributing coagulation current. A bipolar sphincterotome is currently under investigation (3). The electrical generator supplies a pure cutting or coagulation current, or a choice of blended currents. Theoretically, a pure cut minimizes the risk of thermal damage, possibly a factor in inducing pancreatitis, whereas the

I. Raijman: Gastroenterology and Therapeutic Endoscopy, Rosedale Medical Centre, Toronto, Ontario, Canada

G. B. Haber: Department of Gastroenterology, University of Toronto, The Wellesley Hospital, Toronto, Ontario, Canada.

blended or pure coagulation current should prevent bleeding. The current may be altered according to specific requirements. A stretched-out mucosa with a thinner muscle component, such as in a diverticulum, may be cut too quickly in a "zipper" fashion when a pure cutting current is used. On the other hand, a blended current may cut too slowly through a thickened, chronically inflamed papilla, giving rise to a "blanching" coagulative necrosis without cutting the tissue. In our unit, we use the Meditron UGI 3000. We routinely set the generator on blend 1 or 2 (choice of three blends), which provides for 50% to 75% coagulation current.

Two other important factors in determining the nature of the cut are (a) the length of the wire in contact with the tissue—the shorter the wire in contact with tissue, the greater the energy density of the transmitted current; and (b) the degree of tension of the wire against the tissue, determined by the pulling force on the papillotome catheter and the degree of bowing of the tip of the papillotome. If there is a strong pull of the papillotome or a tight bow of the tip, there will be a tendency for a rapid cut.

Of the various designs available, we prefer a longer 30 to 35 mm cutting wire, which is bowed to 35% to 50% of its original length. Bowing a longer wire creates a deeper bow in the catheter, which serves to stabilize the sphincterotome in the duct and to ensure good wire-tissue contact. In addition, the use of a flat metal plate in the distal end of the sphincterotome catheter allows for a reliable 12 o'clock bending of the sphincterotome tip, as well as allowing preshaping of the tip in various directions, which is sometimes important in achieving cannulation in the presence of distorted anatomy, such as with a periampullary diverticulum.

The most important consideration in performing endoscopic sphincterotomy is to have complete control of all the elements. This starts with adequate patient sedation, and duodenal paralysis and full insufflation of the duodenal loop, which will efface the mucosal folds and delineate the intramural bile duct. This is necessary for determining the permissible length of the sphincterotomy, which must not exceed the upper margin of the roof of the papilla. The endoscopist must accurately assess the length of the cut using the markers on the sphincterotome to establish the depth of insertion and making note of the degree of bowing, which alters the length of exposed wire. The safest approach for the novice is to make short sequential cuts along the roof of the papilla, using the shortest cut sufficient for stone removal.

In the large-stone situation, it is often difficult to assess the adequacy of a cut for stone removal. One reason for this is that the endoscopically visible bulge in the duodenal wall (the roof of the papilla) representing the intramural portion of the bile duct may not represent the total length of the biliary sphincter, which may extend behind the duodenal wall. A balloon may be pulled through the papilla to determine whether all of the sphincter muscle has been cut, but a simpler method is to pull a partially bowed sphincterotome through the papilla and the degree of resistance will aid in establishing the adequacy of the cut. Not uncommonly, a short inflammatory stricture of the distal bile duct, just behind the sphincter where a stone typically impacts, is not fully appreciated after sphincterotomy and may be one of the reasons for failed stone extraction using conventional methods.

In very difficult cannulations it may be necessary to make a small blind cut in the 10 to 12 o'clock direction to allow access into the bile duct. This has been termed a precut or less commonly an infundibulotomy. It is carried out usually with needle cautery, making short strokes from the papillary orifice onto the roof of the papilla or in the reverse direction. The major drawback with this approach is the difficulty determining the appropriate depth and the tendency to create blind submucosal tracks. We prefer a modified bow-string papillotome with the nose cut short, with only 1 to 2 mm of catheter beyond the wire. This permits insertion into the papillary orifice, establishing a foothold prior to cutting in the bile duct direction. Among 394 consecutive sphincterotomies in our unit, this precut technique was necessary in only six patients. For most endoscopists, it may be more prudent to refer the patient to a more experienced endoscopist rather than to overutilize the precut with its inherent risks.

In patients with Billroth II (B-II) anastomosis, we approach the papilla with a side-viewing endoscope. Once deep cannulation of the bile duct is achieved, we perform papillotomy at the 5 to 6 o'clock position over a 7 French straight stent with the needle-knife papillotome. Once an adequate papillotomy has been ob-

tained, the stent is withdrawn through the endoscope and stone extraction is performed. We have had good success and minimal morbidity using this technique (4). Among the commercially available B-II papillotomes, the Soehendra design can be employed with end-viewing endoscopes, while the "shark's fin" or the sigmoid-shaped papillotomes are utilized with the side-viewing endoscopes.

STONE EXTRACTION—STANDARD MODALITIES

Extraction of biliary concretions following endoscopic sphincterotomy with either a Dormia basket or a balloon clears the common bile duct in approximately 90% of the cases, including some cases with large stones impacted in the papilla.

The balloons are available in various sizes, with the size chosen appropriate for the size of the duct. The advantage of a balloon is the ability to deflate and remove it when a stone cannot be pulled out. On the other hand, if forceful extraction is necessary, there are drawbacks to the balloon, which include stretching of the catheter tubing or rupture of the balloon, thereby limiting its usefulness in difficult cases. In a grossly dilated duct, even large balloons tend to slide alongside the stone, preventing extraction.

The dormia baskets are available in several sizes with four, six, or eight wire strands squared or spiral in configuration. Some baskets have a fixed handle, whereas others have detachable components. These devices allow for wire-guided passage of a catheter beyond a stone in a difficult location, e.g., the intrahepatic duct. Once the catheter is positioned beyond the stone, the wire is withdrawn, and a specialized basket is inserted through the catheter and beyond the stone, allowing entrapment.

We prefer a basket for standard removal because of the ability to pull with greater force, as well as to crush soft stones without the need for additional devices. A balloon, however, is useful in clearing small stones and debris that are more difficult to trap in a basket.

When multiple stones are encountered, extraction from the bile duct should start with the most distal stone or fragment in order to avoid stone impaction due to a logjam effect just above the ampulla. Should this occur, a useful maneuver to disengage a basket from a stone when it cannot be pulled out is to open the basket and to advance the catheter beyond the stone, then retract the basket from above the stone. This may have to be repeated but will usually allow for removal of the basket. A stone is most easily captured when there is some space between it and the bile duct wall to allow for some movement and play between the stone and the basket wire. It may be useful, therefore, to push a stone located in the preampullary segment of the duct higher upstream with the basket to facilitate entrapment.

Success of Standard Stone Removal Techniques

We reviewed our experience in 400 consecutive patients referred for bile duct stone removal from June 1989 to July 1991. Successful cannulation was achieved in 397 patients (99.3%) and successful sphincterotomy in 394 patients (98.5%). Among the 394 patients, only 6 required precut technique. Bile duct stone clearance was achieved in 371 patients (93%). The mean number of procedures to achieve ductal clearance was 1.2 (1–5). Nine patients underwent surgery (two failed CBD cannulation and seven after endoscopic therapy) and 18 had endoscopic stents inserted as planned definitive therapy (mean age 86.4 years). Four of these came to eventual surgery, with one postoperative death. A periampullary diverticulum was found in 71 (18%) and a biliary stricture in 18 (4.5%) patients. Among the 372 successful stone clearance patients, nonstandard techniques (see below) were employed in 53 (14.2%). It is evident from this experience that routine methods are highly successful, with only a relatively small group of patients requiring additional therapy, bearing in mind that we are a tertiary referral center and have a disproportionate number of difficult cases. Successful clearance rates of stones from the bile duct are reported in the 85% to 90% range (5,6).

In the presence of large, impacted, or multiple stones, fragmentation may be necessary before extraction. Surgical intervention may be required when endoscopic retrieval of stones has failed. However, it is associated with a high morbidity and mortality in elderly patients, in those with associated systemic illnesses, or in those acutely ill (7). In these circumstances, other options include extracorporeal shock wave lithotripsy in conjunction with endoscopic removal (6–11), insertion of an endoprosthesis (12,13), mechanical lithotripsy (11,14–18), electrohydraulic lithotripsy (11,19–22), laser lithotripsy (23–30), and biliary perfusion with stone-dissolving agents (31–33) when the other approaches are unsuccessful or impractical.

Nonstandard Techniques of Biliary Stone Removal

Dissolution Therapy

Chemical dissolution of biliary stones, mainly cholesterol stones, has been tried with either ether, chloroform, mono-octanoin, glycermono-octanoin, MTBE (methyl-tert-butyl ether), and 1% ethylenediaminetetraacetic acid (EDTA)/bile acid solution. The results are disappointing, with a 50% to 60% success rate in dissolving CBD stones (31–33). MTBE is an aliphatic ether that may, upon contact with stones, dissolve them. Most of these studies have been performed in patients with cholecystolithiasis. However, in patients with common bile duct stones, results have been poor and associated with a high incidence of neurological side effects, elevation of liver enzymes, and duodenitis (33). Better results and fewer side effects may be obtained with infusion of mono-octanoin, and it may even dissolve stones not affected by MTBE (33). In a review of 343 patients, intraductal infusion of mono-octanoin was successful in only 34% with minor and major side effects in 67% and 5%, respectively (34). We have not had any experience with the use of stone dissolution. As stated by others, the "chemical revolution" has not yet taken place in the bile ducts (6).

Mechanical Lithotripsy

The simple mechanistic approach of a "nutcracker" has become a standard for stones too large to be extracted intact either because of the size of the stone, or a relatively small duct size or stricture through which an average size stone cannot be extracted. Of all the endoscopic alternatives for difficult stone extraction, mechanical lithotripsy is the most practical and economical. This method depends entirely on the ability to entrap and crush the stone in a wire basket.

There are two types of mechanical lithotriptors: one is through-the-scope (TTS) (Olympus Corp.) (Fig. 1) and the other is outside-the-scope (OTS) (Soehendra design, Wilson-Cook) (Fig. 2). The latter necessitates withdrawal of the endoscope after removing the basket handle. The basket handle usually has to be cut off with pliers unless it is designed for detachment. The basket wire is left in place with the basket sleeve usually sliding off as the endoscope is withdrawn. Then, a metallic coil-spring sleeve is advanced over the basket wire, with subsequent crushing of the stone. This method is preferred for stones lodged in the distal duct at the level of the papilla. The metal sleeve is not meant to be advanced up the duct as the tension on the basket wire during lithotripsy causes straightening of the sleeve, which may then tear the mucosa at the junction of the duct and the duodenum. It is important to ensure that the basket is closed tightly on the stone prior to withdrawing the endoscope so that the basket does not slip off the stone as the endoscope is being pulled out and during the actual lithotripsy.

The TTS lithotriptor is designed for use within the endoscope with passage of a single unit, comprising a Teflon catheter with the basket and a retractable coil-spring steel sheath through the operating channel. The basket is extended and opened and the stone is trapped by moving the basket in a to-and-fro motion. Once the

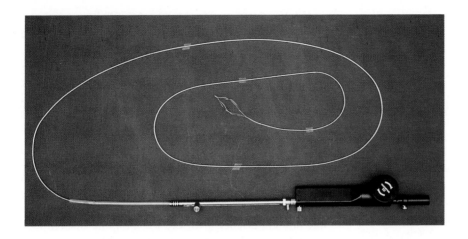

FIG. 1. Through-the-scope (TTS) mechanical lithotriptor.

stone is entrapped, the basket is pulled against the steel sheath. Then, the wheel of the lithotriptor handle is turned clockwise forcing the basket against the steel catheter, fragmenting the stone (Fig. 3). The TTS lithotriptor has a somewhat cumbersome design at present and is expensive. However, it eliminates the need for endoscope removal and does not waste a basket, as occurs with the OTS method.

In our retrospective review of 400 stone removal cases, we successfully used mechanical lithotripsy in 34 instances for common bile duct stones with a mean diameter of 22 mm (range 16–34). In three instances, the lithotriptor failed to entrap the stone, for a success clearance rate of 91%. Binmoeller et al. (11), using the OTS system, treated 33 of 108 patients and cleared the bile duct in all. In 30 patients, Shaw et al. (16) successfully captured and fragmented large CBD stones in 97% of the cases, and cleared the CBD in 93%. Siegel et al. (17) reported a success rate of 94% in 93 patients. More recently, we analyzed our data in 92 patients requiring mechanical lithotripsy: 82 were treated with OTS and 10 with TTS, with successful stone fragmentation and stone clearance in 85 patients (92%) (18). In this group of patients, we encountered

equipment failure in 7.6%, the principal problem being wire breakage of the basket or at soldering points along the cable with the earlier designs of the OTS systems. Problems advancing the coil spring cable over the Teflon catheter have occurred with crimping of the catheter using the TTS device (18).

Overall, mechanical lithotripsy is very useful, effective, and a relatively inexpensive device that is universally successful when the stone can be trapped.

Shock Wave Contact Lithotripsy

The uniquely challenging bile duct stone problem is that of the impacted stone that cannot be entrapped in a basket or dislodged with a balloon. We have employed direct contact shock devices, including pulsed yttrium-aluminum garnet (YAG) laser, pulsed dye laser, and electrohydraulic spark discharge to fracture stones visualized with "mother-daughter" peroral choledochoscopy. "Mother-daughter" endoscopy is a technique employing the dedicated fiberoptic "mother" duodenoscope with a 5.5-mm operating channel that allows passage of a 4.5-mm "daughter" miniscope. The

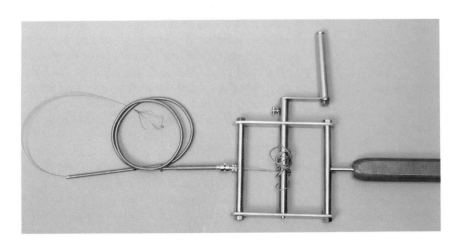

FIG. 2. Outside-the-scope (OTS) mechanical lithotriptor.

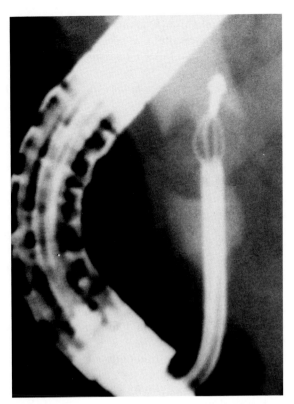

FIG. 3. The stone forced against the steel coil-spring catheter causing fragmentation.

mother duodenoscope elevator has limited mobility and is not useful for routine instrumentation. It is therefore advisable to perform cholangiography and sphincterotomy with a standard duodenoscope prior to insertion of the mother endoscope. Given the limited utility of the mother endoscope, an ample sphincterotomy should be performed to facilitate passage of the daughter endoscope through the papilla.

A prototype 3.4-mm daughter endoscope has been developed with a 1.2-mm operating channel and two-way angulation (30). This can be passed through a standard therapeutic duodenoscope, which allows for use of the same duodenoscope during the entire procedure.

An important aspect of shock wave lithotripsy is the ability to irrigate the bile duct both to provide the appropriate fluid medium (half normal saline) for the shock wave as well as to flush the sediment and debris that limit visibility. In addition, a fluid medium increases by tenfold the fragmentation force of electrohydraulic lithotripsy (25). In our early experience, a previously inserted pigtailed nasobiliary catheter was used for the purpose but it was an added step to the procedure, and the nasobiliary tube was easily dislodged during subsequent insertion of the mother endoscope. We have now adopted a much simpler approach using a Tuohey-Borst valve on the operating channel of the daughter endoscope, which allows for passage of the laser wave-guide or electrohydraulic probe and simultaneous instillation of half normal saline or contrast through a side arm (Fig. 4).

When the larger 3 French electrohydraulic probes are used there is increased resistance to fluid instillation around the fiber in the operating channel and a tendency for fluid backup through the rubber cap on the valve, necessitating the additional occlusion of the valve opening with the endoscopist's finger. The procedure demands the skills of two endoscopists, the more difficult chore being that of the mother endoscope operator. There is a limited range of motion of the tip of the daughter endoscope and its correct positioning is accomplished by alterations in the angle of entry through the papilla. The choledochoscopic image is projected onto a monitor with a camera attachment to magnify the rather small field of vision and to permit

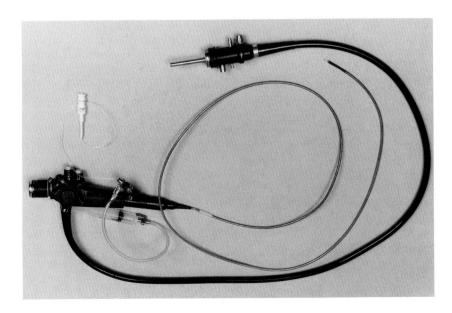

FIG. 4. "Mother" endoscope containing the "daughter" endoscope, which contains the electrohydraulic probe. Note the Tuohey-Borst valve holding the probe in the accessory channel of the "daughter" endoscope.

the mother endoscopist to orchestrate the movement of both endoscopes, as well as the shock-wave probe, and to "fire" when the stone is adequately targeted. All of the probes are particularly difficult to see endoscopically and it is critical to ascertain the position of the probe so as to avoid ductal injury. The probe may deflect outside the field of vision and it is best to retract and re-advance it to bring it into view. Fluoroscopic tracking of the probe is also possible with the metallic electrohydraulic probe and with the laser guides, which have a metallic coating applied. With uncoated laser guides, preloading a 3-Fr metal-tipped catheter, with the laser tip fixed 5 mm beyond the polyethylene catheter tip, facilitates localization of the laser tip both endoscopically and fluoroscopically. Another problem with the preexisting electrohydraulic probes is the lack of stiffness along the length of the probe prohibiting easy passage through the operating channel (Fig. 5). Due to difficulties with kinking, it is necessary to preload the probe into the operating channel of the choledochoscope prior to insertion.

The principle of electrohydraulic lithotripsy (EHL) is the generation of a high-amplitude mechanical shock wave by creating a "spark gap" in a fluid medium. We have found EHL to be highly effective in conjunction with peroral cholangioscopic guidance in 18 of 19 consecutive cases. The single failure was due to inability to target the stone in an angulated duct distorted from prior T-tube insertion. In all 18 patients with successful stone fragmentation, the bile duct was cleared with a dormia basket. In 4 of these, the size of the stone fragments required further mechanical lithotripsy.

Binmoeller et al. (11) successfully fragmented large extrahepatic stones (median 2.6 cm) in 64 of 65 patients using EHL with peroral cholangioscopy. The failure included a patient with a high-grade distal bile duct stricture in whom the daughter scope could not be advanced. Complete fragmentation and stone removal was achieved in one session in 50 patients, two ses-

sions in 13, and three sessions in 1. Bruckner et al. (22) described a case that was successfully treated with EHL in a patient that failed extracorporeal shock wave lithotripsy (ESWL).

Similar success has been achieved with laser modalities. With the flashlamp pulsed neodymium:yttrium-aluminum garnet (Nd:YAG) laser, light is converted into thermal energy. With the Q-switched Nd:YAG laser, light energy is transformed into mechanical energy by producing an optical breakdown with resultant shock waves that can fragment the stones (23–26). The energy of the laser is absorbed by the stone, thus heating its surface, which ionizes the stone material creating mechanical stress waves that fragment the stone (26) (Fig. 6). A problem with continuous wave Nd:YAG laser is that it may simply drill holes in the stone (24). We have had a limited experience with two patients, one with pulsed dye laser and one with Nd:YAG laser, both with peroral cholangioscopy. We were unsuccessful in both patients. One of the failures responded to EHL and mechanical lithotripsy while the other, a patient with intrahepatic stones, was treated with a biliary endoprosthesis. Ponchon et al. (26) used a dye laser in 25 patients with a mean stone size of 18 mm. It was 100% successful when performed under direct visualization (choledochoscope), while it was only 36% successful when fluoroscopic control was used. Overall, ductal clearance was achieved in 88% of the cases. A recent multicenter trial using a Candela flashlamp excited dye laser in 25 patients with large CBD stones, median size 18 mm, reported a success rate in clearing the duct in 80% (20 patients) (29). These authors used a "mother and baby" endoscopic system in 18 of their patients. Recently, new miniscopes of 3.4 and 3.7 mm that can be advanced into the common bile duct via a standard therapeutic duodenoscope were successfully used in four of five patients with large common bile duct stones using a flashlamp excited dye laser (30).

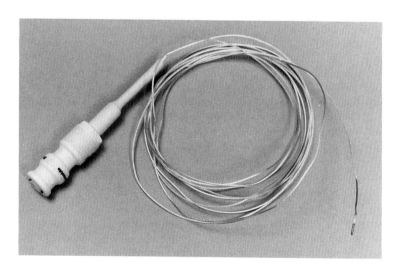

FIG. 5. View of the electrohydraulic probe. Note areas of kinking of the probe shaft.

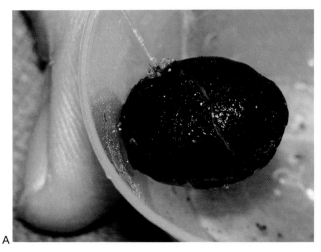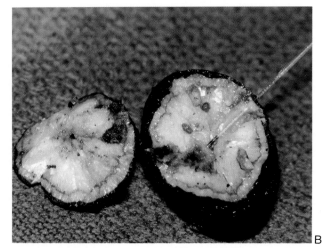

FIG. 6. A,B: *In vitro* laser lithotripsy.

In our experience with laser modalities and EHL, the latter has the advantage of fragmenting stones with fewer shots and in a shorter time, and is inexpensive. The theoretical advantage of laser is that the risk of perforation or bile duct injury may be less. However, this may have little clinical significance when performed under cholangioscopic control.

A recent technological advance has been achieved employing back-scattered laser light in order to differentiate between stone and tissue. This automated stone-tissue recognition system has been integrated into a new flashlamp pumped rhodamine dye laser (Lithognost, Telemit, Germany). The critical advantage of this device is the ability to break stones using fluoroscopic two-dimensional imaging only, passing the fiber through a standard duodenoscope. A malpositioned fiber will automatically shut off within nanoseconds before damage to the duct wall occurs. Using this device, Neuhaus et al. (30) recently reported successful laser lithotripsy and bile duct clearance in 40 of 41 patients with no laser-related complications.

Extracorporeal Lithotripsy

Extracorporeal shock wave lithotripsy (ESWL) has been successfully used in the treatment of common bile duct stones. However, it is expensive, requires repeated ESWL sessions, and several endoscopic procedures for placement of a nasobiliary tube and then for stone fragment removal. ESWL was recently used in 80 patients with "giant" CBD stones, obtaining duct clearance in 90.6% of the cases (8). Complementary mechanical or intracorporeal EHL was used in 23% of the cases. A recent trial showed a 30% failure rate of bile duct clearance with ESWL in conjunction with endoscopic retrograde cholangiopancreatography (ERCP) (9). Others have used ESWL in the treatment of impacted basket and stone in the common bile duct (10). ESWL may be of particular benefit for intrahepatic stones. In a report from Germany it was used in ten patients with intrahepatic stones, with clearing of the bile ducts in seven after a median of eight sessions (11).

Biliary Endoprosthesis for Retained Stones

Biliary endoprostheses have been used as a long-term measure in high-risk patients with unextractable CBD stones. During the study period, we treated 18 high-risk patients with endoscopic stents inserted as definitive therapy (mean age 86.4 years). During follow-up, 8 patients were without biliary symptoms with no further intervention required. Four patients underwent surgery, with stones found and removed in 3. One patient died of postoperative complications. Five patients died of unrelated causes and one patient was lost to follow-up. Dufek et al. (12) treated 15 patients with biliary endoprosthesis, with 13 remaining symptom-free 2 years after insertion. Soomers et al. (13) reported 34 symptomatic elderly patients treated with sphincterotomy and biliary endoprosthesis, with 10 patients surviving 26 months. Stenting of bile duct stones are efficacious probably by preventing stone impaction and allowing bile to flow both through and around the stent.

CONCLUSION

Only uncommonly can stones in the common bile duct be difficult to remove endoscopically, provided endoscopic expertise is available. The initial treatment of large stones should always include an attempt with a basket, as these stones are often soft and can be fragmented. The next option should be mechanical lithotripsy since it is a cheap and readily available instrument with a high success rate in clearing the duct. Electrohydraulic and laser lithotripsy are effective options but can only be employed with direct visual control, either peroral or percutaneous cholangioscopy. The development of smaller choledochoscopes will undoubtedly facilitate these therapies. Endoprostheses as definitive therapy should be reserved for those at high risk for surgery and in whom all endoscopic maneuvers have failed. Extracorporeal shock wave lithotripsy, when available, provides a viable option. We do not recommend the routine use of dissolving agents because of their variable success rate, the associated morbidity, and the time demands. Surgical removal is appropriate in low-risk patients in whom endoscopic efforts have failed.

REFERENCES

1. Kawai K, Akasaka Y, Murakami K, et al. *Gastrointest Endosc* 1974;20:148–151.
2. Classen M, Demling L. *Dtsch Med Wochenschr* 1974;99:496–497.
3. Tucker RD, Sievert CE, Platz CE, Vennes JA, Silvis SE. *Gastrointest Endosc* 1992;38:113–117.
4. Walden D, Raijman I, Fuchs E, Kandel G, Marcon NE, Kortan P, Haber GB. *Gastrointest Endosc* 1993;39:348.
5. Cotton PB. *Gut* 1984;25:587–597.
6. Classen M, Hagenmuller F, Knyrim K, Frimberger E. *Endoscopy* 1988;20:21–26.
7. Vandermeeren A, Delhaye M, Gabbrielli A, Cremer M. *Gastroenterology* 1990;98:A265.
8. Sackmann M, Ippisch E, Sauerbruch T, Holl J, Brendel W, Paumgartner G. *Gastroenterology* 1990;98:392–396.
9. Staritz M, Rambow A, Groose A, et al. *Gut* 1990;31:225–235.
10. Merrett M, Desmond P. *Endoscopy* 1990;22:92.
11. Binmoeller KF, Bruckner M, Thonke F, Soehendra N. *Endoscopy* 1993;25:201–206.
12. Dufek V, Benes J, Chmel J, Kordac V. *Endoscopy* 1990;5:240 [Letter].
13. Soomers AJ, Nagengast FM, Yap SH. *Endoscopy* 1990;22:24–26.
14. Riemann JF, Seuberth K, Demling L. *Endoscopy* 1982;14:226–230.
15. Schneider MU, Matek W, Bauer R, Domschke W. *Endoscopy* 1988;20:248–253.
16. Shaw MJ, Dorsher PJ, Vennes JA. *Am J Gastroenterol* 1990;85:796–798.
17. Siegel JH, Ben-Zvi JS, Pullano WE. *Gastrointest Endosc* 1990;36:351–356.
18. Fuchs E, Kortan P, Raijman I, Walden D, Haber G. *Gastrointest Endosc* 1993;39:266.
19. Silvis SE, Siegel JH, Katon RM, Hughes R, Sievert CE, Sivak MV. *Gastrointest Endosc* 1986;32:155–156.
20. Siegel JH, Ben-Zvi JS, Pullano WE. *Gastrointest Endosc* 1990;36:134–136.
21. Mo LR, Hwang MH, Yeuh SK, Yang JC, Lin C. *Gastrointest Endosc* 1988;34:122–125.
22. Bruckner M, Grimm H, Soehendra N. *Endoscopy* 1990;22:234–235.
23. Ell Ch, Wondrazek F, Frank F, Hockberger J, Lux G, Demling L. *Endoscopy* 1986;18:95–96.
24. Ell Ch, Hochberger J, Muller D, Zirnbigl H, Giedl J, Lux G, Demling L. *Endoscopy* 1986;18:92–94.
25. Teng P, Nishioka NS, Anderson RR, Deutsch TF. *IEEE J Quant Elect* 1987;23:1845–1852.
26. Ponchon T, Gagnon P, Valette PJ, et al. *Gastroenterology* 1991;100:1730–1736.
27. Berci G, Hamlin JA, Daykhovsky L, Paz-Partlow M. *Gastrointest Endosc* 1990;36:137–138.
28. Ell C, Hochberger J, Muller D, Demling L. *Gut* 1988;29:746–751.
29. Cotton PB, Kozarek RA, Schapiro RH, et al. *Gastroenterology* 1990;99:1128–1133.
30. Neuhaus H, Hoffmann W, Classen M. *Endoscopy* 1992;24:208–214.
31. Leuschner U, Baumgartl H, Klempa J. In: Classen M, Geenen J, Kawai K, eds. *Nonsurgical biliary drainage.* Berlin: Springer, 1984;81.
32. Di Padova C, Di Padova F, Montorsi W, Tritapepe R. *Gastroenterology* 1986;91:1296–1300.
33. Jarrett LN, Balfour TW, Bell GD, Knapp DR, Rose DH. *Lancet* 1981;1:68–70.
34. Palmer KR, Hofmann AF. *Gut* 1986;27:196–202.

Advanced Therapeutic Endoscopy, 2nd Ed.,
edited by J. S. Barkin and C. A. O'Phelan.
Raven Press, Ltd., New York © 1994.

CHAPTER 39

Laser Therapy: Role in Biliary Tract Disease

Markus Goldschmiedt

The acronym *laser* (*l*ight *a*mplification and *s*timulated *e*mission of *r*adiation) reflects the process by which a form of energy is converted into light energy. LASER light differs from ordinary light (such as a light from a lamp) because it is *monochromatic* (beam is composed of photons of the same wavelengths or color), *collimated* (the photons travel in the same direction or parallel to each other and do not diverge as they travel outward), and *coherent* (all the waves are in phase and all their peaks move synchronously). LASER is to light as music is to noise.

TYPES OF LASER

Neodymium:yttrium-aluminum garnet (Nd:YAG) and dye lasers have been used in the pancreatobiliary tracts. The physics and specifications of each type of laser are beyond the scope of this chapter, but some practical points are worth mentioning.

The Nd:YAG laser can be delivered by noncontact and contact delivery systems. In the noncontact system the laser can be delivered to the tissue via transmission through a quartz fiber with a silicon and Teflon coating. The fiber is held away from the tissue. Contact delivery systems are made of a neutral synthetic sapphire crystal attachment or shaping of the fiber itself to convert laser energy into thermal energy, creating a laser probe of about 1700°F. Different geometric configurations of laser contact probes are available to shape the laser energy distribution to the desired target area.

Dye lasers have the capacity of varying their output wavelength and are being used for selective destruction of malignant cells, without injury to surrounding cells. The patient is injected with a hematoporphyrin deriva-

tive that is selectively absorbed by malignant cells. The user selects the laser output wavelength that is absorbed by the hematoporphyrin-stained malignant cell and the laser will then destroy primarily these stained cells. Dye lasers are also used for lithotripsy (see below).

APPLICATIONS OF LASER IN THE BILIARY TREE

Endoscopic Sphincterotomy

Endoscopic sphincterotomy (EST) has gained wide acceptance as a therapeutic approach to disorders of the ampulla of Vater and pancreatobiliary tracts. Despite refinements in endoscopes and techniques, selective deep bile duct cannulation, one of the requirements for EST, is unsuccessful in 5% to 19% of cases even in the hands of experienced endoscopists (1–3). In these cases, a precut papillotomy can be used to slit open the roof of the ampulla and expose the common bile duct opening. Precut can be obtained by using a modified traction-type sphincterotome, in which the cutting wire extends to the tip of the catheter, or by using a needle knife catheter. Conventional blended electrosurgical current is used to incise the ampulla with both techniques.

Laser EST has been performed in two patients with "sclerosis" of the ampulla, two cases of impacted stones, and one patient with previous Billroth II partial gastrectomy (4,5). The technique involves the use of a noncontact Nd:YAG laser fiber with a "shooting distance" from the ampulla of 5 mm. No complications were reported in this small series of patients (6,7).

It may also be possible to perform laser EST using contact laser probes, a technique similar to the use of a needle knife.

In summary, laser EST can be performed in selected

M. Goldschmiedt: Parkland Memorial Hospital, Dallas, Texas 75235.

patients in whom selective deep cannulation is not feasible with conventional techniques. It is unknown if precut using a laser is safer than precut with conventional blended electrosurgical current. The high cost of laser equipment will likely preclude its widespread use for EST.

Ampullary Villous Adenomas and Tumors

Ampullary villous adenomas appear to be a premalignant condition with a significant risk for carcinoma in situ (8,9). Standard therapy is surgical resection of the ampulla or pancreaticoduodenectomy (8,9). Endoscopic treatment is used in the treatment of ampullary tumors, primarily for patients unfit for surgery. Endoscopic therapy includes EST, diathermic snare resection of the tumor, and laser photodestruction using Nd:YAG or dye laser (7,10,11). Sander (7) reported six patients with ampullary tumors in whom laser photodestruction was successful in allowing initial bile duct instrumentation. Furthermore, local remission with laser photodestruction was achieved in three (two carcinomas and one adenoma).

Ponchon et al. (10) reported 11 patients with villous adenomas of the ampulla of Vater in whom curative endoscopic treatment was accomplished. Three patients underwent complete resection of tumor with snare alone. In three patients in whom snare resection was not complete, laser photodestruction was used to ablate visible tumor. Only one of the three patients had recurrence of tumor at 24 months. This patient was treated again with additional laser photodestruction. Five patients underwent laser photodestruction without previous snare resection. Repeated biopsies at 14, 15, 51, 52, and 53 months did not reveal residual villous tissue. This study also reported eight patients with adenocarcinoma of the ampulla of Vater who underwent laser photodestruction for palliation. Photodynamic (dye laser) therapy was used in one patient and Nd:YAG laser in seven. Tumor destruction was incomplete in all cases. Complications related to laser therapy were mild pancreatitis in two and ulcerative duodenitis in one.

Abulafi et al. (11) reported ten patients with periampullary carcinoma unsuitable for surgery who were treated with photodynamic dye laser therapy. In the four patients who had tumors confined to the ampulla, biopsy-proven remission was obtained in three. In the three patients with localized extension of the tumor, all had significant reduction in tumor mass. In the three patients with tumor-induced duodenal stenosis, only one had significant reduction in tumor mass. In this series the only complication was moderate skin sensitivity reaction in three patients.

In summary, patients unfit for surgery with ampul-

lary villous adenomas and small carcinomas can be treated with Nd:YAG laser or photodynamic therapy in order to obtain local remission. Although some "curative" cases have been reported, a randomized trial is warranted before it can be recommended as primary therapy. Local debulking may be feasible in advanced tumors.

Common Bile Duct Stones

EST followed by removal of common bile duct stones is successful in 80% to 95% of patients (4,12,13). Large stones are usually approached with mechanical lithotripsy (5) with success rates as high as 90% in experienced centers (14,15). Failure of mechanical lithotripsy is usually due to inability to capture a large stone, poor access to the stone, or tight impaction. In those cases, fragmentation of stones can be attempted using extracorporeal lithotripsy (16,17) or intracorporeal electrohydraulic (18–21) or laser lithotripsy (see below) (Fig. 1).

Laser Lithotripsy with the Continuous Wave Nd:YAG Laser

In 1981 Orii et al. (22) reported two patients in whom transcutaneous transhepatic cholangioscopy was per-

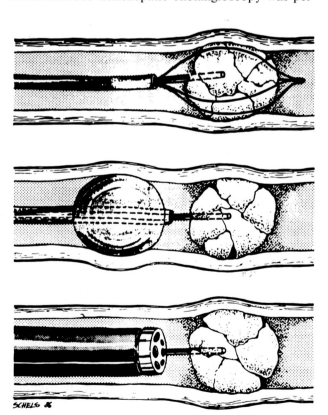

FIG. 1. Variations of endoscopic retrograde lithotripsy; basket or balloon catheter systems with a central bore for the light guide laser system to be used under fluoroscopic control and lithotripsy under direct visualization.

formed, and an Nd:YAG laser fiber was introduced into the common bile duct to disintegrate bilirubinate stones. The authors extended their study and concluded that continuous wave Nd:YAG laser lithotripsy was efficacious for crushing bilirubin stones but inadequate against cholesterol stones (23). Ell et al. (24) demonstrated that continuous wave Nd:YAG laser could fragment stones to an adequate extent in only 10% of cases. In most cases only thermal melting and drilling effects were seen. Thus, the authors concluded that continuous wave Nd:YAG laser should not be used due to its poor efficacy and its high risk of thermal injury to the bile duct.

Laser Lithotripsy with the Pulsed or Q-Switched Nd: YAG Laser

These systems differ from the continuous wave system because the energy is emitted in bursts or pulses. This allows high energy delivery during a very short period of time. The first attempts to disintegrate stones with a flashlamp pulsed Nd:YAG laser were published by Brown et al. (25). However, the authors had disappointing results and abandoned biliary lithotripsy with this technique (26). In 1986, Ell et al. used a flashlamp pulsed Nd:YAG laser and showed that gallstones could be adequately fragmented in vitro, in an animal model (27) and in a patient with giant common bile duct stones (28). The authors also had success in fragmenting gallstones with a Q-switched Nd:YAG laser (29).

Ell et al. (30) extended their studies and reported nine patients with common bile duct stones that could not be removed with conventional methods and underwent laser lithotripsy with a flashlamp pulsed Nd:YAG laser. In eight of the nine patients the stones could be fragmented, and in six patients concrements were removed from the bile duct. Laser lithotripsy was performed under direct visualization using the Olympus mother-daughter dual endoscope system in two patients and under radiological control using a specially developed basket or balloon in the rest. There were no complications due to the laser lithotripsy.

Laser Lithotripsy with the Pulsed Dye Laser

In 1987, Nishioka et al. (31) demonstrated that a flashlamp pulsed dye laser was adequate to fragment gallstones, with cholesterol stones being more difficult to fragment than pigment stones. It appears that the laser pulse is absorbed and heats the stone surface to a temperature sufficient to ionize some of the material and form a plasma (32–36). The plasma is a microscopic cloud of a rapidly expanding cavity of electrons. This rapid expansion creates stress waves that produce damage to the stone. In experimental models the

flashlamp pulsed dye laser proved to be efficacious and safe for fragmentation of biliary stones (37–39). In some studies, there was no evidence of tissue damage to the bile duct wall during experiments in cadavers and resection specimens (38,39), and in one study this laser produced significantly less damage to the gallbladder and bile duct tissue than electrohydraulic lithotripsy (37).

Since Kozarek et al. (38) reported the first successful case of lithotripsy using the dye laser through an Olympus mother-daughter dual endoscope system, several studies have used this laser system for biliary lithotripsy (40–44). Cotton et al. (40) reported 25 patients with large stones who did not respond to standard nonoperative treatment and were treated with a flashlamp dye laser (Candela Laser Corporation, Wayland, MA). Laser lithotripsy was successful in 23 patients with a subsequent clearance of bile duct stones in 20 patients, with an overall success of 80%. Failure of treatment in five patients was due to inability to accurately target the stone to allow laser treatment (one case), unsuccessful fragmentation of a stone (one case), and insufficient fragmentation of the stone to permit duct clearance (three cases). No complications occurred during the study. Nineteen patients were treated through a peroral endoscopic route (Olympus mother-daughter dual endoscope system in 10, experimental minifiberscope through the standard duodenoscope in 2, and in 7 patients laser treatment was aimed under fluoroscopic control). Six patients were approached through a previously established percutaneous drain. This study proved laser lithotripsy with the Candela laser to be effective and safe.

Ponchon et al. (42) used a flashlamp pulsed dye laser (Pulsolith; Technomed International, Lyon, France) to fragment biliary stones in 25 patients. Prior to laser treatment, all patients underwent endoscopic retrograde cholangiopancreatography (ERCP) and EST. Seven patients who had a T-tube from previous surgery underwent laser lithotripsy through a choledochoscope followed by removal of fragments in all patients. Fourteen patients were approached through ERCP and laser lithotripsy was performed under fluoroscopic control. Satisfactory fragmentation of stones and bile duct clearance was accomplished in only 5 out of the 14 patients (36%). Failures were thought to be due to (a) inability to position the balloon catheter against the stone (one case), (b) inability to pass the choledochoduodenal angle with the optic fiber during its insertion through the balloon catheter or basket (five cases), (c) tangential instead of perpendicular positioning of the fiber with respect to the stone (two cases), and (d) fracture of the fiber within its sheath during the introduction maneuvers through the balloon catheter (one case). Ten patients, including six who failed ERCP laser lithotripsy, underwent percutaneous transhepatic choledochoscopy. Satisfactory fragmentation and bile duct clearance was accomplished in all patients. Complications were noted in four patients: bile duct perforation with the percutaneous guidewire (one case) and fevers and chills with negative blood cultures (three cases). No direct complications due to the use of the laser were seen. Overall adequate fragmentation and bile duct clearance was possible in 22 out of 25 patients (88%). However, under direct visualization with the choledochoscope the success rate was 100% and with ERCP and fluoroscopic control the success rate was only 36%.

Hawes et al. (43) treated 14 patients with the pulsed dye laser. Ten patients were approached with a choledochoscope through a preexisting T-tube (five cases) or a percutaneous transhepatic approach (five cases), three patients had peroral cholangioscopy with the mother-daughter dual endoscope system, and one patient with a special basket. Stones were fragmented in 13 out of 14 patients (93%) and duct clearance was accomplished in 12 (86%). No complications were reported in this series. Neuhaus et al. (44) treated 14 patients with dye laser lithotripsy. Seven patients were approached with the mother-daughter dual endoscope system and 7 patients were approached via a percutaneous tract and cholangioscopy. Stone fragmentation and duct clearance was successful in 12 patients (86%). Failure in 2 patients was due to inadequate visualization of the stone. The only complication was cholangitis in one patient.

A rhodamine-6G dye laser with a stone recognition system (Lithognost, Telemit Electronic, GMBH, München, Germany) has been recently described (45–47). This laser has an integrated microprocessor-controlled stone recognition system that checks at the beginning of the emission of every laser pulse whether the fiber tip is in contact with the stone. If there is no stone contact, an ultrafast optical switch will be activated to cut off the further emission of the laser pulse. Only 10% of the total laser pulse energy is emitted, being harmless to the tissue.

Currently, an alexandrite laser is being tested for biliary lithotripsy and appears to be as efficacious as the coumarin and rhodamine-6G dye lasers (48,49).

In summary, laser lithotripsy under direct visualization appears to be safe and effective (Table 1). The efficacy of laser lithotripsy is dependent on proper positioning and good laser-stone contact.

Pancreatic Stones

Although it is unclear if pancreatic calculi are the result of, or a contributing cause of, recurrent or chronic pancreatitis, some reports indicate that removal of pancreatic calculi improve the patient's subsequent pain or pancreatitis course (50–53). Current endoscopic methods to remove pancreatic calculi include EST followed by balloon or basket retrieval (50–52) and extracorporeal lithotripsy (54,55).

Laser fragmentation using a dye laser has been tried on a few occasions (45,56,57). The paucity of reports when compared to bile duct stone lithotripsy is due to the lack of consensus in the medical community that removal of pancreatic calculi is helpful in ameliorating the course of pancreatitis, the relatively smaller number of patients with intraductal pancreatic calculi, and the technical difficulties associated with deep cannulation and instrumentation of the pancreatic duct. Renner (56) treated eight patients with intraductal pancreatic lithiasis and severe symptoms with the Candela dye laser (MDL-2000, Boston, MA). Pancreatic calculi disintegrated easily when good laser fiber–stone contact was achieved. Unfortunately, we do not have complete information in all patients nor long-term follow up to make any conclusions.

WHAT TO EXPECT IN THE FUTURE

The future will probably bring us improved labeling of tumor cells and in wavelength recognition that may allow very accurate destruction of tumor cells sparing the surrounding normal tissue. Introduction of laser fibers into the biliary tree may allow laser photodestruction of intraductal tumors under direct visualization (Nd:YAG) or fluoroscopic control (dye laser). Technological advances in stone recognition systems

TABLE 1. *Laser lithotripsy with the pulsed dye laser*

Authors	No. patients	Success in fragmenting stones	Clearance of bile duct stones	Complications
Cotton et al. (40)	25	92%	80%	None
Berci et al. (41)	1	100%	100%	None
Ponchon et al. (42)	25	88%	88%	n = 4 (16%), none related to the laser
Hawes et al. (43)	14	93%	86%	None
Neuhaus et al. (44)	14	86%	86%	n = 1 (7%), cholangitis
Kozarek et al. (38)	1	100%	100%	None
Total	80	90%	84%	n = 5 (6%), none related to the laser

may allow us to fragment large common bile duct and pancreatic duct stones in a very efficient, safe, and cost-effective fashion.

REFERENCES

1. Siegel JH. Precut papillotomy: a method to improve success of ERCP and papillotomy. *Endoscopy* 1981;12:130–133.
2. Huibregtse K, Katon RM, Tytgat GNJ. Precut papillotomy via fine-needle knife papillotome: a safe and effective technique. *Gastrointest Endosc* 1986;32:403–405.
3. Shakoor T, Geenen JE. Pre-cut papillotomy. *Gastrointest Endosc* 1992;38:623–627.
4. Rauws EAJ, Huibregtse K, Tytgat GNJ. *Endoscopic removal of common bile duct stones. Limits and pitfalls.* In: Tytgat GNJ, Huibregtse K, eds. *Bile and bile duct abnormalities. Pathophysiology, diagnosis and management.* Stuttgart, New York: Georg Thieme Verlag, 1989;39–42.
5. Demling L, Seuberth K, Riemann JF. A mechanical lithotripter. *Endoscopy* 1982;14:100–101.
6. Sander R, Poesl H. Endoscopic papillotomy with Nd:YAG laser. *Endoscopy* 1985;17:115–116.
7. Sander R. Papillotomy. In: Riemman JF, Ell C, eds. *Lasers in gastroenterology. International experiences and trends.* Stuttgart, New York: Georg Thieme Verlag, 1989;53–57.
8. Rosenberg J, Welch JP, Pyrtek LJ, Walker M, Trowbridge P. Benign villous adenomas of the ampulla of Vater. *Cancer* 1986; 58:1563–1568.
9. Ryan DP, Schapiro RH, Warsaw AL. Villous tumors of the duodenum. *Ann Surg* 1986;203:301–306.
10. Ponchon T, Berger F, Chavaillon A, Bory R, Lambert R. *Cancer* 1989;64:161–167.
11. Abulafi AM, Swain CP, Allardyce R, Van Someran RNM, Williams NS, Ainley CC. Photodynamic therapy for malignant tumors of the ampulla of Vater. *Gastrointest Endosc* 1992;38: A263.
12. Heinerman PM, Boeckl O, Pimpol W. Selective ERCP and preoperative stone removal in bile duct surgery. *Ann Surg* 1989; 209:267–272.
13. Geenen JE, Vennes JA, Silvis SE. Resume of a seminar on ERS. *Gastrointest Endosc* 1981;27:31–38.
14. Schneider MU, Matek W, Bauer R, Domschke W. Mechanical lithotripsy of bile duct stones in 209 patients. Effect of technical advances. *Endoscopy* 1988;20:248–253.
15. Siegel JH, Ben-Zvi JS, Pullano WE. Mechanical lithotripsy of common duct stones. *Gastrointest Endosc* 1990;36:351–356.
16. Weber J, Adamek HE, Riemann JF. Extracorporeal piezoelectric lithotripsy for complicated bile duct stones. *Am J Gastroenterol* 1991;86:196–200.
17. Johlin FC, Loening SA, Maher JW, Summers RW. Electrohydraulic shock wave lithotripsy (ESWL) fragmentation of retained common duct stones. *Surgery* 1988;104:592–599.
18. Brückner M, Grimm H, Soehendra N. Electrohydraulic lithotripsy of complicated choledocholithiasis. *Endoscopy* 1990;22: 234–235.
19. Ligoury CL, Bonnel D, Canard JM, Cornud F, Dumont JL. Intracorporeal electrohydraulic shock wave lithotripsy of common bile duct stones: preliminary results in 7 cases. *Endoscopy* 1987; 19:237–240.
20. Siegel JH, Ben-Zvi JS, Pullano WE. Endoscopic electrohydraulic lithotripsy. *Gastrointest Endosc* 1990;36:134–136.
21. Leung JWC, Chung SCS. Electrohydraulic lithotripsy with peroral choledochoscopy. *Br Med J* 1989;299:595–598.
22. Orii K, Nakahara A, Takase Y, Ozaki A, Sakita T, Iwasaki Y. Choledocholithotomy by YAG laser with a choledochofiberscope: case reports of two patients. *Surgery* 1981;90:120–122.
23. Orri K, Ozaki A, Takase Y, Iwasaki Y. Lithotomy of intrahepatic and choledochal stones with YAG laser. *Surg Gynecol Obstet* 1983;156:485–488.
24. Ell C, Hochberger J, Müller D, Giedl J, Lux G, Demling L. Gallensteinlithitripsie mittels Neodym YAG-Dauerstrichlaser. Unpublished data.
25. Bown SG, Mills TN, Watson GN, Swain P, Wickman JE, Salmon PR. Laser fragmentation of biliary calculi. XII International Congress of Gastroenterology, Lisbon, Portugal, September 16–22, 1984.
26. Watson GN, McNichols TA, Wickman JE. The fragmentation of urinary and biliary calculi. Fourth Annual Conference on Lasers in Medicine and Surgery. London, January 22,23, 1986.
27. Ell Ch, Hochberger J, Müller D, Zirngibil H, Giedl J, Lux G, Demling L. Laser lithotripsy of gallstones by means of a pulsed Neodmium-YAG laser. In vitro and animal experiments. *Endoscopy* 1986;18:92–94.
28. Lux G, Ell C, Hochberger J, Müller D, Demling L. The first successful endoscopic retrograde laser lithotripsy of common bile duct stones in man using a pulsed Neodmium-YAG laser. *Endoscopy* 1986;18:144–145.
29. Ell Ch, Wondrazek F, Frank F, Hochberger J, Lux G, Demling L. Laser-induced shockwave lithotripsy of gallstones. *Endoscopy* 1986;18:95–96.
30. Ell Ch, Lux G, Hochberger J, Müller D, Demling L. Laser lithotripsy of common bile duct stones. *Gut* 1988;29:746–751.
31. Nishioka NS, Levins PC, Murray SC, Parrish JA, Anderson RR. Fragmentation of biliary calculi with tunable dye lasers. *Gastroenterology* 1987;93:250–255.
32. Nishioka NS, Teng P, Deutsch TF, Anderson RR. Mechanism of pulsed laser fragmentation of urinary and biliary calculi. *Lasers Life Sci* 1987;1:231–245.
33. Teng P, Nishioka NS, Farinelli WA, Anderson RR, Deutsch TF. Microsecond long flash photography of laser-induced ablation of biliary and urinary calculi. *Lasers Surg Med* 1987;7:394–397.
34. Teng P, Nishioka NS, Anderson RR, Deutsch TF. Acoustic studies of the role of immersion in plasma-mediated laser ablation. *IEEE J Quant Elect* 1987;23:1845–1852.
35. Dretler SP. Laser lithotripsy: a review of 20 years of research and clinical applications. *Lasers Surg Med* 1989;9:454–457.
36. Nishioka NS, Kelsey PB, Kibbi AG, Delmonico F, Parrish JA, Anderson RR. Laser lithotripsy: animal studies of safety and efficacy. *Lasers Surg Med* 1988;8:357–362.
37. Birkett DH, Lamont JS, O'Keane JO, Babayan RK. Comparison of a pulsed dye laser and electrohydraulic lithotripsy on porcine gallbladder and common bile duct in vitro. *Lasers Surg Med* 1992; 12:210–214.
38. Kozarek RA, Low DE, Ball TJ. Tunable dye laser lithotripsy: in vitro studies and in vivo treatment of choledocholithiasis. *Gastrointest Endosc* 1988;34:418–421.
39. Murray A, Basu R, Fairclough PD, Wood RFM. Gallstone lithotripsy with the pulsed dye laser: in vitro studies. *Br J Surg* 1989; 76:457–460.
40. Cotton PB, Kozarek RA, Schapiro RH, Nishioka NS, Kelsey PB, Ball TJ, Putnam WS, Barkun A, Weinerth J. Endoscopic laser lithotripsy of large bile duct stones. *Gastroenterology* 1990; 99:1128.
41. Berci GB, Hamlin JA, Daykhosvsky L, Paz-Partlow M. Common bile duct laser lithotripsy. *Gastrointest Endosc* 1990;36: 137–138.
42. Ponchon T, Gagnon P, Valete PJ, Henry L, Chavaillon A, Thieulin F. Pulsed dye laser lithotripsy of bile duct stones. *Gastroenterology* 1991;100:1730–1736.
43. Hawes RL, Kopecky KK, Lehman GL, Sherman S. Prospective evaluation of the utility and safety of the pulsed dye laser in the management of difficult bile duct stones. *Gastrointest Endosc* 1991;37:A257.
44. Neuhaus H, Hoffman W, Hogrefe A, Classen M. Cholangioscopic dye laser lithotripsy in the nonsurgical treatment of difficult bile duct stones. *Gastrointest Endosc* 1991;37:A254.
45. Neuhaus H, Hoffman W, Classen M. Laser lithotripsy of pancreatic and biliary stones via 3.4mm and 3.7mm miniscopes: first clinical results. *Endoscopy* 1992;24:208–214.
46. Ell C, Hochberger J, May A, Mendez L, Bauer R, Fleig WR, Hahn EG. Laserlithotripsy of difficult bile duct stones by means of a rhodamine-6G dye laser with an integrated automatic stone/tissue detection system (STDS). Abstract form submitted to *Digestive Disease Week*, American Gastroenterological Association, Boston, May 16–19, 1993.
47. Neuhaus H, Hoffman W, Classen M. Endoscopic laser litho-

tripsy with an automatic stone recognition system for basket impaction in the common bile duct. *Endoscopy* 1992;24:596–599.

48. Neuhaus H, Hoffman W, Zillinger C, Classen M. Pulsed dye and alexandrite laser lithotripsy of bile duct stones: clinical results. Abstracts to the *European Digestive Disease Week*. Amsterdam, October 20–26, 1991. *Hepatogastroenterology* 1991;A24.

49. Hochberger J, Bredt M, Mueller G, May A, Eckhard H, Ell C. Laser lithotripsy of gallstones: alexandrite and rhodamine-6G versus cumarin dye laser: fragmentation and fiber burn-off in vitro. Submitted to *Biomedical Optics*, Los Angeles, January 16–22, 1993.

50. Haber G, Sherman S, Miller L, Hawes R, Ponich T, Kortan P, Lehman G. Pancreatic duct stones: frequency of successful removal and improvement in symptoms. *Gastrointest Endosc* 1990;36:202–203.

51. Ponsky JL, Duppler DW. Endoscopic sphincterotomy and removal of pancreatic duct stones. *Am Surg* 1987;53:613–616.

52. Schneider MU, Lux G. Floating pancreatic duct concretions in chronic pancreatitis. Pain relief by endoscopic removal. *Endoscopy* 1985;17:8–10.

53. Hansell DT, Gillespie G, Imrie CW. Operative transampullary extraction of pancreatic calculi. *Surg Gynecol Obstet* 1985;163:17–20.

54. Neuhaus H. Fragmentation of pancreatic stones by extracorporeal shock wave lithotripsy. *Endoscopy* 1991;23:161–165.

55. Delhaye M, Vandermeeren A, Baize M, Cremer M. Extracorporeal shock-wave lithotripsy of pancreatic calculi. *Gastroenterology* 1992;102:610–620.

56. Renner IG. Laser fragmentation of pancreatic stones. *Endoscopy* 1991;23:166–170.

57. Feldman RK, Freeny PC, Kozarek RA. Pancreatic and biliary calculi: percutaneous treatment with tunable dye laser lithotripsy. *Radiology* 1990;174:793–795.

Advanced Therapeutic Endoscopy, 2nd Ed.,
edited by J. S. Barkin and C. A. O'Phelan.
Raven Press, Ltd., New York © 1994.

CHAPTER 40

Ampulla: Motility and Stricture

Rama P. Venu and Joseph E. Geenen

The ampulla of Vater, situated at the confluence of the terminal common bile duct and pancreatic duct, is embedded in the bosom of the major duodenal papilla. Because of this unique anatomical relationship, disorders involving the ampulla can often affect the papilla and vice versa. It is, therefore, not surprising that in day-to-day clinical practice papilla and ampulla are used interchangeably.

Although the major duodenal papilla was first described as early as 1720 by Abraham Vater, the Wittenberg anatomist, this unique structure received little, if any, attention for nearly two centuries. Hypotonic duodenography was one of the earliest techniques utilized for the evaluation of structural disorders of the papilla. Cineradiography following contrast instillation via a surgically placed T-tube provided valuable information regarding the dynamics of the sphincter of Oddi. With the advent of a lateral-viewing endoscope, the ampullary region became accessible for endoscopic inspection, tissue acquisition, radiography, and manometry (1). Significant progress also has been made in our understanding of the physiology and pathophysiology of the sphincter of Oddi (SO) (2).

In recent years, endoscopic ultrasonography (EUS) has added a new dimension in the study of ampullary disorders (3). This innovative technique offers several possibilities. EUS has been shown to be helpful in the diagnosis of certain ampullary disorders such as choledochocele and duodenal duplication cyst (4). Accurate staging of periampullary carcinoma is also possible with EUS (5,6). Limited experience suggests that EUS is particularly useful to assess recurrence of periampullary tumors following local resection (7).

ANATOMY

The ampulla of Vater is formed by the union of the terminal end of the common bile duct and pancreatic duct (Fig. 1). It courses downward through the duodenal wall and the major duodenal papilla before it exits at the summit of the papilla. The ampulla is 5 to 15 mm in length and 1 to 3 mm in diameter. The ampulla is entwined by circular and longitudinal smooth muscle fibers that constitute the sphincter of Oddi. These smooth muscle fibers interdigitate with the duodenal musculature and may extend for a variable length toward the terminal end of the common bile duct and pancreatic duct (8,9). The mucous membrane lining the ampulla of Vater has longitudinal and transverse folds

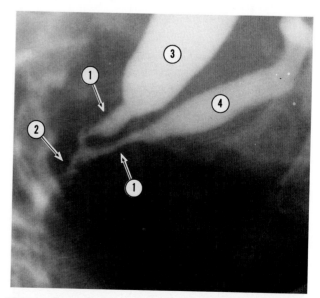

FIG. 1. Radiographic picture of the ampulla of Vater obtained at ERCP. The ampulla *(2)* is formed by the union of the terminal ends *(1)* of the bile duct and pancreatic duct.

R. P. Venu: Department of Medicine, Section of Digestive and Liver Disease, University of Illinois at Chicago, Chicago, Illinois 60612.

J. E. Geenen: Department of Gastroenterology, Medical College of Wisconsin, Milwaukee, Wisconsin 53226.

(8). These smooth mucosal folds, fashioned like Venetian pleats, help to prevent influx of duodenal contents into the bile duct. The vascular supply of the ampulla is derived from the arterial plexus formed by the ventral and dorsal branches of the retroduodenal artery. This vessel is usually located approximately 35 mm away from the papillary orifice (9,10).

The ampullary region is innervated by both the sympathetic and parasympathetic nervous system via the gastroduodenal nerve, which ends in a plexus containing numerous ganglion cells within the sphincter of Oddi zone (11). Adrenergic nerves appear to be more sparse and may innervate the smooth muscle cells indirectly. The intrinsic cholinergic nerve apparatus is richly developed and the ganglion cells of the myenteric plexus and submucosal plexus appear to have a predominance of cholinergic nerves.

Endoscopic and Radiographic Anatomy

The ampulla of Vater per se is less accessible for direct visualization during endoscopic retrograde cholangiopancreatography (ERCP). However, endoscopic evaluation of the papilla might provide valuable information regarding the ampullary region (12). The major duodenal papilla is a pinkish, nipple-like structure situated at the second part of the duodenum in its posteromedial wall (Fig. 2). A vertical fold of mucous membrane located caudad to the papilla is the most useful landmark for localizing the papilla. A transverse mucosal fold is commonly seen at the superior margin of the papilla. On occasion, this fold may form a hood-like covering, hiding the papillary orifice.

The size and shape of the papilla may vary from person to person. Even in the same subject, the configuration of the papilla may change depending upon the contraction or relaxation of the sphincter muscle. The papillary orifice is located at the summit of the papilla. It is a small, irregularly shaped, slit-like orifice surrounded by reticulated mucous membrane. Close endoscopic inspection might reveal the closing and opening of the papillary orifice and the flow of golden yellow bile.

Radiographically the ampulla appears as a smooth, tapering structure extending from the distal end of the common bile duct to the papillary orifice. The confluence of the common bile duct, pancreatic duct, and ampulla assumes three different configurations. The most common configuration is Y-shaped. Less frequently, a V- or U-shaped configuration can be observed. Fluoroscopic monitoring after contrast instillation can demonstrate rhythmic, contractile activity of the sphincter muscle encircling the ampulla. Meticulous observation during these phasic contractions may also reveal contrast drainage from the bile duct into the duodenum through the ampullary segment.

Attention to certain technical details is vital to the radiographic diagnosis of ampullary lesions (13). Thus, early radiographic spot pictures soon after instilling a few milliliters of contrast material into the bile duct can better demonstrate small tumors of the ampulla. After completion of contrast instillation into the bile duct, upright and recumbent spot films of the distal choledochus should be taken. In the upright position, gallstones gravitate to the ampulla enabling us to differentiate them from air bubbles, which migrate upward. A fixed, irregular filling defect at the distal choledochus usually indicates ampullary neoplasm.

Ampulla—Motility

The anatomy of the sphincter muscle as we understand it now is largely based on the painstaking autopsy studies by Boyden (14). The terminal end of the bile duct and the pancreatic duct along with the ampulla are invested with smooth muscle fibers that constitute the SO. The smooth muscle fibers consist of both circular and longitudinal muscles that interdigitate with the duodenal musculature. Boyden identified three distinct bands of smooth muscle fibers surrounding the terminal bile duct, pancreatic duct, and ampulla. This conglomeration of smooth muscle fibers is seen encircling the distal common bile duct, pancreatic duct, and ampulla. Boyden coined the terms *sphincter choledochus*, *sphincter pancreaticus*, and *sphincter papillae* for

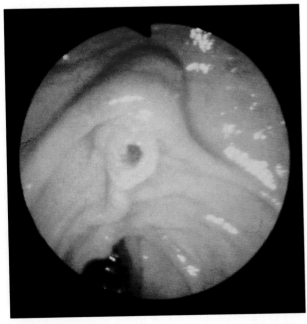

FIG. 2. Endoscopic view of the papilla. Note the vertical fold located caudad and transverse fold located cephalad to the papilla proper.

these so-called minisphincters. However, manometric studies in humans reveal the sphincter of Oddi as a single motor unit.

Recent studies in experimental animals and humans have shown that under normal conditions the SO is in a state of tonic contraction (15). The basal pressure of the SO is about 5 mm above the common bile duct pressure. The bile duct, on the other hand, serves as a passive conduit to facilitate bile flow. Several studies have demonstrated that the SO is a dynamic structure undergoing rhythmic contractions followed by relaxations (15–17). These so-called phasic contractions occur at a rate of 3 to 5 per minute. These contractile activities originate at the proximal end of the sphincter and are propagated in a caudad fashion similar to peristalsis. Cineradiographic studies in conjunction with motility studies in opossum have shown that during the phasic contractions, bile is milked into the duodenum from the ampulla and sphincter zone. At the same time, bile flow from the bile duct to the SO zone practically ceases during phasic contractions.

Following the phasic contractions, the sphincter relaxes allowing bile flow from the bile duct into the sphincter zone. The next contraction wave that follows sweeps the bile into the duodenum again and the cycle is repeated. Thus, the sphincter of Oddi plays a pivotal role in regulating the flow of bile into the duodenum. The sphincter exhibits an occlusive as well as a pumping mechanism. Under fasting conditions, the sphincter offers resistance to the flow of bile into the duodenum, diverting the bile into the gallbladder. Following a meal, the gallbladder contracts and the sphincter relaxes, allowing free flow of bile into the duodenum. Cholecystokinin (CCK)-octapeptide, an enteric peptide, seems to be the mediator of this unique physiolog-

ical phenomenon (18,19). The sphincter also takes part in the migrating motor complexes (MMC).

A number of neural, endocrine, and pharmacological agents influence the sphincter motor function. Several enteric peptides have been shown to modulate the function of SO. Thus, glucagon relaxes the sphincter muscle, and this property of glucagon is utilized to accomplish sphincter and duodenal relaxation during ERCP. In addition, gastrin, secretin, cholinergic agents, morphine, and histamine have also been shown to influence sphincter motor function (20,21).

SPHINCTER OF ODDI MANOMETRY TECHNIQUE

For SO manometry, a highly compliant, constantly perfused manometric catheter is commonly utilized. The catheter is 200 cm long and 1.7 mm in outer diameter. It has three different lumina that open near the tip. These lateral orifices are spaced 2 mm apart, the most distal orifice being located 5 mm away from the catheter tip. The catheter is constantly perfused with bubble-free water using a minimally compliant hydraulic capillary system at a flow rate of 0.25 ml per minute. A second indifferent catheter attached to the external surface of the duodenoscope measures the duodenal pressure continuously.

For manometric study, the catheter is initially advanced well inside the bile duct or pancreatic duct beyond the sphincter zone. After a short period of equilibration, the common bile duct pressure is recorded for 1 to 3 minutes. The catheter is then slowly pulled and stationed at the SO zone to record the pressure at the sphincter zone (Fig. 3). The slow withdrawal of the catheter or "pull-through" is carried out at an incre-

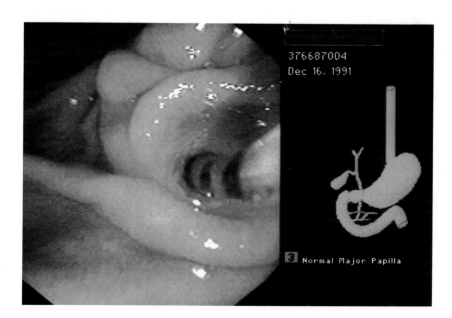

FIG. 3. Endoscopic picture showing the manometric catheter stationed at the SO zone.

SPHINCTER OF ODDI PRESSURE RECORDING
(Station Pull-through Technique)

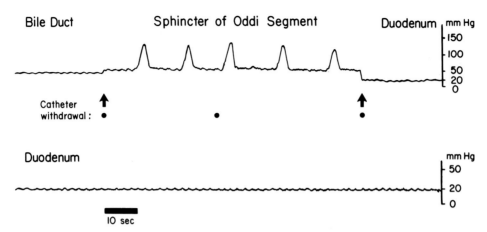

FIG. 4. SO manometry tracing. Note the basal SO pressure is about 5 mm above the common bile duct pressure. Superimposed on the basal SO pressure are seen rhythmic phasic wave contractions.

ment of 1 to 2 mm. Recordings are performed at each station for about 1 to 2 minutes. The pull-throughs are repeated at least three times for reproducibility and accuracy. The mean basal SO pressure is averaged from the basal pressure recorded by all three catheter orifices during a minimum of two sphincteric pull-throughs. We have determined the normal sphincter basal pressure of 15 ± 5 mm Hg based on SO manometry from several normal subjects. Superimposed on the basal tone are high amplitude phasic wave contractions occurring at a mean frequency of 4 ± 0.5 per minute (Fig. 4). Phasic wave contractions usually measure 150 ± 16 mm Hg in amplitude and 4.3 ± 0.5 seconds in duration. The phasic waves are propagated in an antegrade fashion in the majority of subjects. However, 17% of phasic wave contractions in normal subjects can be simultaneous and 10% can be retrograde.

Abnormal Manometric Tracing

Several investigators have identified well-defined abnormalities in the manometric tracing (22). The most commonly observed abnormality consists of an elevated SO basal pressure. A basal pressure ≥40 mm Hg (Fig. 5) is considered to be abnormal in our laboratory. Endoscopic sphincterotomy in these subjects has been shown to be extremely helpful in decreasing the pressure and accomplishing symptomatic improvement (23).

Paradoxical response of the sphincter motility to CCK-octapeptide is another interesting abnormality noted in patients with presumed SO dysfunction (24). In normal subjects, intravenous administration of CCK-octapeptide abolishes the phasic wave activity and decreases the basal pressure. In patients with SO

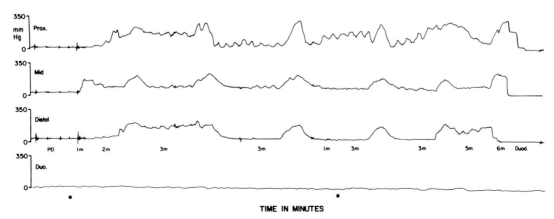

FIG. 5. Manometric tracing for a patient with SO dysfunction showing elevated SO basal pressure.

dysfunction, this enteric peptide causes a paradoxical increase in the basal pressure. This situation is similar to the response of the lower esophageal sphincter in achalasia patients. Increased amplitude of phasic wave contractions has also been reported in patients with SO dysfunction, although rarely. An amplitude >250 mm Hg is considered to be abnormal. Increased frequency of phasic wave contractions >8 per minute, sometimes referred to as tachyoddia, is yet another abnormal manometry finding among patients with SO dysfunction (25). Rapid phasic contractions can prevent the flow of bile into the duodenum and thus can cause functional obstruction. Retrograde sequence of phasic wave contractions is another rare manometric abnormality. The retrograde contractions may prevent bile flow into the duodenum causing functional obstruction and thus SO dysfunction.

Besides these well-defined abnormalities, prolonged phasic wave contractions or low basal tone have also been noted rarely in patients with SO dysfunction. The significance of these rare abnormalities is unclear.

SPHINCTER OF ODDI DYSFUNCTION

Definition

Sphincter of Oddi dysfunction is an ill-defined clinical entity manifested by a group of signs and symptoms resulting from an impedance to biliary pancreatic outflow. SO dysfunction may be caused by a chronic inflammatory process and fibrosis leading to structural narrowing. This condition is often referred to as papillary stenosis. When SO dysfunction results from a motor abnormality of the sphincter, it is commonly referred to as SO dyskinesia.

The pathogenesis of SO dyskinesia is less clear. Denervation or spasm of the sphincter muscle may account for this entity.

Clinical Features

SO dysfunction is commonly seen in middle-aged women. Although most patients may have had prior cholecystectomy, recent reports have shown that SO dysfunction may be seen in patients with intact gallbladder (26). Epigastric or right upper quadrant abdominal pain constitutes the leading symptom in these patients. Pain is characteristically postprandial and may last for several hours. It may be associated with nausea and/or vomiting. The commonly observed symptoms of biliary tract obstruction such as fever, chills, and jaundice are characteristically absent. Some patients may present with acute recurrent pancreatitis.

Laboratory evaluations may reveal transient elevation of liver function tests or amylase. Other investigations such as upper GI examination, ultrasonography, or computed tomography (CT) scan of the abdomen are helpful mainly to rule out such conditions as peptic ulcer disease or neoplasm.

ERCP in SO Dysfunction

ERCP plays an important role in the evaluation of patients presenting with SO dysfunction. A dilated common bile duct and/or pancreatic duct with a smooth narrowing of the ampullary segment is characteristically seen in patients with papillary stenosis. However, the bile duct may be completely normal in many patients with SO dysfunction. Similarly, delayed drainage of contrast material (≥45 minutes) may also be seen in some patients with SO dysfunction. While dilated bile duct and delayed contrast drainage are findings suggestive of SO dysfunction, they are infrequently seen among patients with SO dysfunction and the more common application of ERCP is to rule out other causes of biliary tract obstruction such as common bile duct stone, choledochocele, and bile duct stricture. These entities often present with a clinical picture not unlike that of SO dysfunction.

Other Noninvasive Tests

Since SO manometry is a difficult test to perform, a number of noninvasive tests have recently been designed. The earliest such test is the *morphine/Prostigmin test*. Both of these agents cause spasm of the sphincter leading to biliary colic and elevated liver function tests in patients with suspected sphincter of Oddi dysfunction. The test consists of administering morphine (1 mg) and Prostigmin (10 mg) parenterally followed by laboratory evaluation of the blood for liver function tests and serum amylase. A tenfold increase from the baseline in the transaminase levels or serum amylase is considered to be a positive test (27). However, recent reports indicate that the morphine/Prostigmin test is inaccurate and unreliable (28).

Secretin Ultrasonography

Secretin ultrasonography has been shown to be a useful diagnostic test for papillary stenosis or SO dysfunction. Secretin is a potent secretogogue that causes voluminous outpouring of pancreatic juice. This can result in distention of the pancreatic duct in patients with SO dysfunction. Ultrasonography is utilized for measuring ductal diameter following secretin, and an increase in the diameter of the bile duct ≥2 mm from the baseline is considered to be diagnostic of SO dysfunction (29). Despite the initial enthusiasm, application of this test in clinical practice awaits more elaborate studies.

Fatty Meal Ultrasonography

Ingestion of a fatty meal results in endogenous release of CCK, which enhances biliary flow. In patients with suspected SO dyskinesia, following baseline ultrasonographic measurement of the diameter of the bile duct, Lipomul is given orally. The enhanced biliary flow in the presence of impedance to bile drainage in SO dyskinesia will result in distention of the bile duct, which can be detected by ultrasonography. The bile duct diameter is then determined at 15, 45, and 60 minutes. An increase in the diameter ≥ 2 mm reportedly indicates SO dyskinesia (30). Similar to ultrasonography, fatty meal ultrasound also needs further clinical trial before it can be employed in day-to-day clinical practice.

Quantitative Hepatobiliary Scintigraphy (QHS)

QHS is yet another noninvasive test designed to identify patients with partial biliary tract obstruction including SO dysfunction (31). Following a minimal fast of 4 hours, 5 MCi of diisopropylphenyl carbamoyl methyl aminoacetic acid is administered intravenously. Radioactive counts are then taken over the abdomen for 90 minutes. A positive test is indicated by a clearance rate of <63% in 45 minutes.

While these noninvasive tests are very attractive because of their simple nature, SO manometry seems to be the gold standard for the diagnosis of SO function, at least for the time being.

Ampulla—Stricture

A variety of pathological disorders can result in structural narrowing or stricture of the ampulla. Broadly, ampullary strictures can be classified into benign or malignant stricture. While the clinical presentation of an ampullary stricture is monotonously similar, the management of benign strictures is entirely different from that of malignant strictures. This fact emphasizes the importance of definitive diagnosis of ampullary strictures. Significant advance has been made recently in the preoperative diagnosis of ampullary strictures.

Benign Ampullary Strictures

Benign strictures of the ampulla are sometimes referred to as papillary stenosis. However, the term *papillary stenosis* seems to be more appropriate for stenosis of the ampulla resulting from chronic inflammation and fibrosis. When the ampullary narrowing is a consequence of spasm of the sphincter of Oddi, it is usually referred to as sphincter of Oddi dyskinesia.

The etiology of papillary stenosis includes gallstone migration, instrumental injury, chronic pancreatitis, duodenal Crohn's disease, and sclerosing cholangitis.

Histological findings of papillary stenosis consist of a wide variety of abnormalities from chronic inflammation with infiltration of lymphocytes to chronic inflammatory reaction and severe fibrosis. Sometimes adenomyosis also may be seen.

Of the various causes of papillary stenosis, common bile duct stones constitute the most frequent one. Small gallstones migrating through the ampulla are believed to cause chronic irritation and inflammation leading to cicatrization. Papillary stenosis is often noted in patients with choledochoduodenal fistula, which results from an abnormal migration of the common bile duct stone through the duodenal wall cephalad to the papillary orifice. This observation lends further credence to the etiological association of migrating gallstones to papillary stenosis.

Ampullary Strictures and Tumors of the Ampulla

Benign and malignant tumors can cause structural narrowing of the ampulla. The common benign tumors include adenoma, villous adenoma, leiomyoma, neurofibroma, hemangioma, or hamartoma (32–34). There seems to be an increased incidence of ampullary adenomas in patients with familial polyposis and Gardner's syndrome.

Malignant tumors of the ampulla can be primary or metastatic (35,36). Primary malignancy can originate from the papilla, common bile duct, pancreatic duct, or descending duodenum. Oftentimes it is difficult to determine the exact site of origin of these tumors. Therefore, these tumors are often collectively referred to as periampullary carcinoma. Occasionally, neuroendocrine tumors such as gastrinoma or carcinoid may also originate in the ampulla. Metastatic cancers of the ampulla can arise from carcinoma of the breast, renal cell carcinoma, lymphoma, or malignant melanoma.

ERCP in Ampullary Tumors

Endoscopic inspection during ERCP reveals certain characteristic features in ampullary tumors. The papilla is often enlarged and irregular (Fig. 6). The mucous membranes lining the tumor mass is usually smooth in benign tumors, while ulceration, increased friability, and spontaneous bleeding are characteristic of malignancy. Cholangiography can also demonstrate certain typical findings in ampullary tumors. A fixed,

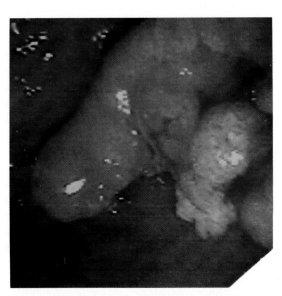

FIG. 6. Endoscopic view of papillary tumor. Note the enlarged papilla, which is irregular and friable.

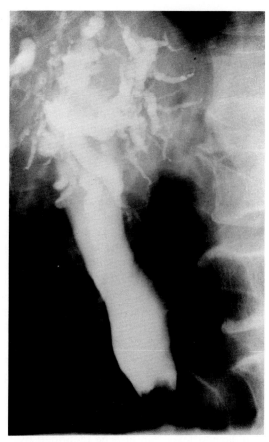

FIG. 7. Cholangiography from a patient with ampullary carcinoma. Note the irregular filling defect at the terminal end of the common bile duct, which is dilated.

irregular filling defect of the terminal common bile duct is the most common finding (Fig. 7). The lower end of the bile duct may be broad, bulbous, and clubbed instead of the normal, tapered appearance of the intramural segment of the bile duct. The bile duct and/or pancreatic duct are usually dilated and the contrast drainage may be prolonged. In some patients with periampullary carcinoma, the terminal end of the common bile duct will be narrow and adynamic. In this situation, differentiation between benign papillary stenosis and malignancy may be difficult if not impossible. While endoscopic and radiographic findings can be helpful in differentiating benign tumors from malignant tumors, an accurate diagnosis rests on tissue acquisition and histological evaluation.

Ampullary Stricture Diagnosis

Clinical Features

Since the ampulla is strategically located at the confluence of the common bile duct and the pancreatic duct, ampullary disorders often cause symptoms resulting from partial or complete obstruction of these vital structures. It is easy, therefore, to understand that many ampullary disorders share a number of common signs and symptoms:

1. Biliary tract obstruction. Nearly one-third of patients with ampullary stricture present with signs and symptoms related to biliary tract obstruction. These symptoms may be intermittent or progres-

sive, especially in those patients with malignant strictures. Biliary colic, jaundice, fever, chills, pruritus, and weight loss are some of the common presenting symptoms.
2. Acute recurrent pancreatitis. Recurrent episodes of acute pancreatitis are another common presentation of ampullary strictures. Impedance to pancreatic flow may be the underlying mechanism leading to pancreatitis. Attacks of pancreatitis are often characterized by severe abdominal pain, nausea, vomiting, fever, leukocytosis, and elevated serum amylase and/or lipase.
3. Occult gastrointestinal bleeding. Chronic gastrointestinal bleeding and iron deficiency anemia are not uncommon among patients with papillary carcinoma. Such bleeding usually results from ulceration of the tumor mass.

There are several physical findings that can be observed in patients with ampullary strictures. The most common findings include jaundice, fever, abdominal tenderness, hepatomegaly, and an enlarged gallbladder.

Laboratory Evaluation

Laboratory studies are quite helpful in the diagnosis of ampullary disorders. The most commonly observed laboratory abnormality includes hypochromic, microcytic anemia, elevated liver function tests (bilirubin, SGOT, SGPT, alkaline phosphatase), and elevated serum amylase or lipase. In patients with papillary carcinoma, the stool may be positive for occult blood.

Other Diagnostic Studies

The commonly employed imaging studies such as upper GI, abdominal ultrasonography, and CT scan are usually normal or nondiagnostic in patients with periampullary disorders. An occasional patient with a relatively large papillary tumor might show a polypoid filling defect in the descending duodenum on an upper GI examination. The most common abnormality noted on CT scan of the abdomen or ultrasonography is a dilated bile duct and/or pancreatic duct. However, these diagnostic modalities rarely demonstrate a tumor mass.

Endoscopic ultrasonography seems to be quite promising in patients with ampullary tumors. The tumor mass can be identified in over 90% of patients with EUS. In malignant tumors, the depth of invasion to the muscular layer can also be identified by EUS. Additionally, metastases to the regional lymph nodes and vascular structures can also be recognized using EUS. Thus, accurate staging of the carcinoma based on TNM specification is possible in this situation, which can be helpful for management decisions.

Tissue Diagnosis

Tissue acquisition using a conventional or regular biopsy forceps constitutes one of the easiest techniques available. Multiple biopsies, especially from the edges and base of the ulcerated lesion, are desirable. The major limitation of this technique is the relatively small size of the specimen, which is often inadequate for accurate histological interpretation. This difficulty can be overcome by using a "jumbo" biopsy forceps. This relatively larger biopsy forceps can be advanced through a large, lateral-viewing endoscope with a 3.7 to 4.2 mm channel size. However, tumors confined to the submucosal plane with a normal mucosal covering might still escape accessibility. In this context, multiple biopsies following endoscopic sphincterotomy have been shown to be extremely helpful for obtaining adequate tissue samples (37). By performing endoscopic sphincterotomy, the ampullary segment is flayed out and thus the tumor is exposed and becomes readily accessible to a biopsy forceps.

Large particle biopsy using a polypectomy snare has also been reported to be successful, especially when other techniques fail (38). However, this technique may be complicated with bleeding. Using these various techniques, an accurate diagnosis of ampullary tumors can be made in about 90% of patients. However, it should be remembered that a negative biopsy by no means can rule out malignancy involving the ampulla.

Ampullary Disorders—Management Guidelines

Endoscopic therapy plays a major role in the management of various ampullary disorders. Endoscopic sphincterotomy (ES), the forerunner of such procedures, constitutes the most commonly employed therapeutic modality. ES is highly successful in the management of papillary stenosis (39–41). The therapeutic principle for the management of SO dyskinesia relies on accomplishing sphincteric relaxation using pharmacological agents or sphincter ablation with ES or surgical intervention. Various pharmacological agents such as nitrate, calcium channel blockers, anticholinergics, bile acid, and hormonal agents have been shown to be useful in relieving symptoms associated with SO dyskinesia (42,43). These agents remain the first-line therapy for SO dyskinesia in most patients. However, lack of compliance and less than optimal symptom relief have prompted the need for more definitive intervention.

Conventionally, surgery offers a favorable outcome that is predictable and permanent. Various operations performed for biliary dyskinesia include sphincteroplasty, sphincterotomy, and septectomy (44). Generally, these are reported to be successful in most patients with biliary dyskinesia.

Many investigators have noted that endoscopic sphincterotomy can offer partial or complete relief of symptoms seen in patients with SO dyskinesia. However, there seems to be an increased frequency of complication rate when endoscopic sphincterotomy is performed in patients with SO dyskinesia.

Patients with ampullary carcinoma and obstructive jaundice who are at high operative risk can be managed by endoprosthesis. An occasional patient with a papillary tumor can also be managed with laser ablation. However, cannulation of the common bile duct can be difficult in the presence of papillary carcinoma. A yellowish speck may be the only clue to identify the papillary orifice in many patients. If cannulation is difficult, a needle-knife sphincterotome can be utilized to incise the tumor and thus to open up the ampulla. However, it should be emphasized that since surgery is the only hope for cure, all patients with periampullary carcinoma should be considered for curative resection.

In conclusion, the ampulla, which is strategically located at the confluence of three anatomic structures, can be affected by motility disorders and strictures. The advent of ERCP, biliary manometry, and endosonography have enhanced the prospect of accurate diagnosis of ampullary disorders. Endoscopic therapy offers an attractive, nonoperative alternative for a number of ampullary disorders.

REFERENCES

1. Blumgart LH. Duodenoscopy and endoscopic retrograde choledochopancreatography: present position in relation to periampullary and pancreatic cancer. *J Surg Oncol* 1975;7:107–119.
2. Geenen JE, Hogan WJ, Dodds WJ, et al. Intraluminal pressure recording from human sphincter of Oddi. *Gastroenterology* 1980;78:317–324.
3. Tio TL, Tytgat GN. Endoscopic ultrasonography in staging local resectability of pancreatic and periampullary malignancy. *Scand J Gastroenterol* 1986;123(suppl):135–142.
4. Tio TL, Rohde P, Sie LH, Tytgat GN. Endosonography in the pre-operative diagnosis of choledochocele. *Gastrointest Endosc* 1992;38:381–383.
5. Tio TL, Tytgat GN, Cikot RJ, Houthoff HJ, Sars PR. Ampullopancreatic carcinoma: preoperative TNM classification with endosonography. *Radiology* 1990;175:455–461.
6. Mukai H, Nakajima M, Yasuda K, et al. Evaluation of endoscopic ultrasonography in the pre-operative staging of carcinoma of the ampulla of Vater and common bile duct. *Gastrointest Endosc* 1992;38:676–683.
7. Tio TL, Mulder CJ, Eggink WF. Endosonography in staging early carcinoma of the ampulla of Vater. *Gastroenterology* 1992;102:1392–1395.
8. Dardinski VJ. The anatomy of the major duodenal papilla, with special reference to its musculature. *J Anat* 1934;69:469.
9. Stolte M. Some aspects of the anatomy and pathology of the papilla of Vater. In: Classen M, Geenen JE, Kawai K, eds. *The papilla of Vater and its diseases.* Baden-Baden, Koln, and New York: Verlag-Gerhard, Witzstrock, 1979;3–13.
10. Sterling JA. Significant factors concerning the papilla of Vater. *Am J Dig Dis* 1953;20:124–128.
11. Burnett W, Gairns FW, Bacsich P. Some observations on the innervation of the extrahepatic biliary system in man. *Ann Surg* 1964;159:8–26.
12. Venu RP, Geenen JE. Diagnosis and treatment of disease of the papilla. In: Classen M, ed. *Clin Gastroenterol* 1986;15:439–456.
13. Moss AA, Goldberg HI, Stewart ET. Endoscopic papillotomy. In: Stewart ET, Vennes JA, Geenen JE, eds. *Atlas of endoscopic retrograde cholangiopancreatography.* St. Louis: CV Mosby, 1977;19–28.
14. Boyden EA. Anatomy of the choledochoduodenal junction in man. *Surg Gynecol Obstet* 1957;106:647–652.
15. Toouli J. Motor function of the opposum sphincter of Oddi. *J Clin Invest* 1983;71:208–220.
16. Carr-Locke DL, Gregg JA. Endoscopic manometry of pancreatic and biliary sphincter zones in man. Basal results in healthy volunteers. *Dig Dis Sci* 1981;87:971–974.
17. Csendes A. Pressure measurements in biliary and pancreatic duct systems in controls and in patients with gallstones, previous cholecystectomy, or common bile duct stones. *Gastroenterology* 1979;77:1203–1210.
18. Behar J, Biancani P. Effect of cholecystokinin and the octapeptide of cholecystokinin on the feline sphincter of Oddi and gallbladder. Mechanisms of action. *J Clin Invest* 1980;66:1231–1239.
19. Toouli J, Hogan WJ, Geenen JE, et al. Action of cholecystokinin-octapeptide on sphincter of Oddi basal pressure and phasic wave activity in humans. *Surgery* 1982;92:497–503.
20. Honda R, Toouli J, Dodds WJ, et al. Effect of enteric hormones on sphincter of Oddi and gastrointestinal myoelectric activity in fasted conscious opossums. *Gastroenterology* 1983;84:1–9.
21. Helm JF, Venu RP, Geenen JE, et al. Effects of morphine on the human sphincter of Oddi. *Gut* 1988;29:1402–1407.
22. Toouli J, et al. Manometric disorders in patients with suspected sphincter of Oddi dysfunction. *Gastroenterology* 1985;88:1243–1250.
23. Geenen JE, Hogan WJ, Dodds WJ, Toouli J, Venu RP. The efficacy of endoscopic sphincterotomy after cholecystectomy in patients with sphincter of Oddi dysfunction. *N Engl J Med* 1989;320;2:82–87.
24. Rolny P, Arleback A, Funch-Jensen P, et al. Paradoxical response of sphincter of Oddi to intravenous injection of cholecystokinin or ceruletide. Manometric findings and results of treatment in biliary dyskinesia. *Gut* 1986;27:1507–1511.
25. Hogan WJ, Geenen JE, Venu RP, et al. Abnormally rapid phasic contractions of the human sphincter of Oddi (tachyodia). *Gastroenterology* 1983;84:1189.
26. Venu RP, Geenen JE, Hogan WJ, Johnson GK, Schmalz MJ. Patients with biliary-type pain and a normal appearing gallbladder: where is the problem? *Gastroenterology* 1992;102:4(2):A336.
27. Nardi GL, Acosta JM. Papillitis as a cause of pancreatitis and abdominal pain: role of evocative test, operative pancreatography and histologic evaluation. *Ann Surg* 1966;164:611–621.
28. LoGiudice JA, Geenen JE, Hogan WJ. Efficacy of the morphine-prostigmin test for evaluating patients with suspected papillary stenosis. *Dig Dis Sci* 1979;24:455–458.
29. Warshaw AL, Simeone J, Schapiro RH, et al. Objective evaluation of ampullary stenosis with ultrasonography and pancreatic stimulation. *Am J Surg* 1985;149:65–72.
30. Darweesh RM, Dodds WJ, Hogan WJ, et al. Roscoe Miller award. Fatty-meal sonography for evaluating patient with suspected partial common duct obstruction. *Am J Roentgenol* 1988;151:63–68.
31. Darweesh R, Dodds WJ, Hogan WJ, et al. Efficacy quantitative hepatobiliary scintigraphy and fatty-meal sonography for detecting partial common duct obstruction. *Gastroenterology* 1987;92(5):1363.
32. Sivak MV. Clinical and endoscopic aspects of tumors of ampulla of Vater. *Endoscopy* 1988;20(suppl 1):211–217.
33. Kahrilas PJ, Hogan WJ, Geenen JE, et al. Chronic recurrent pancreatitis secondary to a submucosal ampullary tumor in a patient with neurofibromatosis. *Dig Dis Sci* 1987;32(1):102–107.
34. Venu RP, Rolny P, Geenen JE, et al. Ampullary hamartoma: endoscopic diagnosis and treatment. *Gastroenterology* 1991;100:795–798.
35. Yamaguchi K, Enjoji M. Carcinoma of ampulla of Vater. A clinicopathologic study and pathologic staging of 109 cases of carcinoma and 5 cases of adenoma. *Cancer* 1987;59:506–515.
36. Venu RP, Rolny P, Geenen JE. Ampullary tumor caused by metastatic renal cell carcinoma. *Dig Dis Sci* 1991;36:376–378.
37. Nakao NL, Siegel JH, Stenger RJ, Gelb AM. Tumors of the ampulla of Vater: early diagnosis by intraampullary biopsy during endoscopic cannulation. Two case presentations and a review of literature. *Gastroenterology* 1982;83:459–464.
38. Safrany L. Duodenoscopy and biopsy in international workshop. Classen M, Geenen J, Kawai K, eds. *The papilla of Vater and its diseases.* Baden-Baden, Koln, New York: Verlag-Gerhard, Witzstrock, 1979;66–71.
39. Lasson A. The postcholecystectomy syndrome: diagnostic and therapeutic strategy. *Scand J Gastroenterol* 1987;22:897–902.
40. Neoptolemos JP, Bailey IS, Carr-Locke DL. Sphincter of Oddi dysfunction: results of treatment by endoscopic sphincterotomy. *Br J Surg* 1988;75:454–459.
41. Roberts-Thomson IC, Toouli J. Is endoscopic sphincterotomy for disabling biliary-type pain after cholecystectomy effective? *Gastrointest Endosc* 1985;31:370–373.
42. Guelrud M, Mendoza S, Rossiter G. Effect of nifedipine on sphincter of Oddi motor function in humans. Studies in healthy volunteers and patients with biliary dyskinesia. *Gastroenterology* 1987;92(5.2):1418.
43. Bar-Meir S, et al. Nitrate therapy in a patient with papillary dysfunction. *Am J Gastroenterol* 1983;78:94–95.
44. Moody FG, Berenson MM, McClosky D. Transampullary septectomy for post-cholecystectomy pain. *Ann Surg* 1977;186:415–423.

Advanced Therapeutic Endoscopy, 2nd Ed.,
edited by J. S. Barkin and C. A. O'Phelan.
Raven Press, Ltd., New York © 1994.

CHAPTER 41

Endoscopic Management of Postoperative Bile Duct Injuries

K. Huibregtse, V. K. Parasher, M. N. Schoeman, and E. A. J. Rauws

Traditionally, patients with postoperative bile duct injuries were seen by the surgeons. More recently, gastroenterologists and radiologists applying nonsurgical treatment modalities have also become involved in the management of these patients. Partly due to a change in referral pattern and partly due to the higher incidence of bile duct injuries in laparoscopic cholecystectomy, the number of patients referred for possible endoscopic therapy has at least tripled in the last 3 years. In this chapter we discuss what endoscopic options are available and for which patients.

BILIARY LEAKAGE

Postoperative bile leakage leading to internal and/or external fistulae is an infrequent but serious complication of biliary tract surgery (1,2). Subclinical bile leaks may occur in 50% of cases, but clinically significant leaks occur in less than 3% of cases (3). Most subclinical leaks heal spontaneously. The incidence of clinical bile leaks after laparoscopic cholecystectomy is reported to be between 1% and 3% (4,5). Postoperative biliary leakage is generally caused by inadvertent injury to the bile duct during surgery. Rupture of the small ducts of Luschka during cholecystectomy may remain undetected during surgery. Inadequate closure of the cystic duct stump due to misplacement or displacement of clips may result in biliary leakage. A distal obstruction caused by biliary stones or strictures may provoke or maintain biliary leakage.

The clinical presentation includes progressive jaundice, persistent shoulder pain, ileus, external biliary fistulae, ascites, fever, peritonitis, and sepsis (6,7). However a more insidious presentation with anorexia, slightly elevated liver function tests, and subfebrile temperature has been reported (8). A sterile bile leak may cause biliary ascites, which manifests as diffuse abdominal pain and ileus. Leukocytosis with elevation of liver functions may be seen. The presence of these findings 4 to 5 days after surgery with a delayed postoperative recovery should alert the physician to the presence of a bile leak.

Computed tomography (CT) scan and ultrasonography may show the presence of free fluid or abscess, but the source of the fluid cannot usually be localized with these techniques. Because the biliary tract is decompressed by the leak, the biliary tree is generally not dilated on CT or ultrasound. Hepatobiliary scanning can also confirm the presence of a leak in almost all patients, but generally is unable to pinpoint the anatomical site of the leak. Endoscopic retrograde cholangiopancreatography (ERCP), on the other hand, is the preferred diagnostic modality since it not only reveals the location of the leak, but simultaneously offers a variety of therapeutic options. ERCP also reveals exacerbating factors such as a retained stone or bile duct stricture (Figs. 1–3). The most common sites of biliary leaks are the cystic duct stump, followed by the hepatic duct and bile duct.

MANAGEMENT

The choice of therapeutic options is large with no definite consensus on optimal management. Repeat laparoscopy offers the advantage of cleaning the peritoneum and visualizing the porta hepatis. However, it is not always possible in the acute phase. Furthermore,

K. Huibregtse, V. K. Parasher, M. N. Schoeman, and E. A. J. Rauws: Department of Gastroenterology and Hepatology, Academic Medical Center, University of Amsterdam, 1105 AZ Amsterdam, The Netherlands.

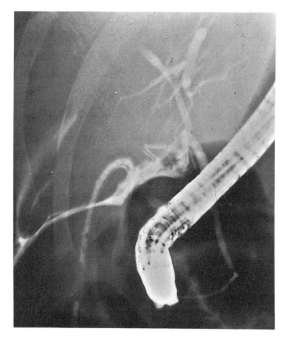

FIG. 1. Cystic duct stump leakage.

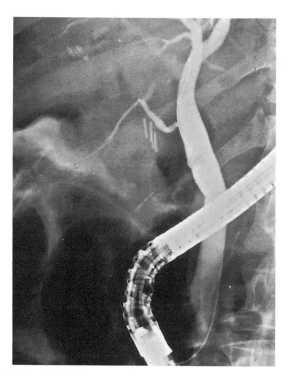

FIG. 3. Bile leakage from small aberrant bile duct.

identification of the site of the leakage is usually not possible. Morbidity and mortality of this approach is about 8% (9). Laparotomy for open surgical repair of bile duct injuries is associated with even higher morbidity (22–37%) and mortality (3–18%) (10). Reoperation for bile duct fistula is complicated by persistent fistula in about 30% and may cause bile duct strictures during further prolonged follow-up (11).

Percutaneous drainage, although suitable for localized collections, carries inherent risks of hemorrhage, sepsis, and perforation (12,13). Percutaneous puncture of the biliary system is more difficult because it is generally not dilated. There is also the risk of the formation of a biliary fistula if the leak is complicated by a resid-

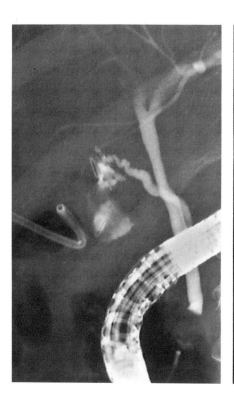

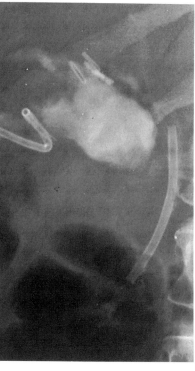

FIG. 2. **Left:** Cystic duct stump leakage. Percutaneous drain in bile collection. **Right:** Endoprosthesis inserted through the sphincter of Oddi. Large bile collection visible, which is drained percutaneously.

ual stone or distal biliary stricture. The risks are also increased in the presence of biliary ascites.

Endoscopic treatment of bile leaks is proven to be safe and effective (8,14–24). The aim of the endoscopic approach is to eliminate or reduce the intraductal pressure gradient maintained by the sphincter of Oddi, residual stones, and strictures, and thereby to allow unhindered bile flow into the duodenum. The advantages of the endoscopic approach are to identify and treat the biliary leak without general anesthesia. Moreover, the postprocedural hospital stay is mostly minimal. Options for endoscopic treatment of postsurgical bile leaks are sphincterotomy, sphincterotomy and stent placement, stent placement without sphincterotomy, or nasobiliary drainage. (Our treatment protocol consists of insertion of a short stent, when bile leakage from the cystic duct stump or from a hepatic radical is present.) In the case where the leak is maintained by a distal obstruction by a stone or stricture, the distal obstruction is treated by endoscopic stone removal or stent insertion. Controversy remains when a leak occurs with no distal obstruction. Sphincterotomy alone, temporary stenting without sphincterotomy, and nasobiliary aspiration all remain viable choices. In the case of a leak from the common duct proper a stent is placed alongside the site of leakage to prevent stricturing of the bile duct during healing process of the bile leak. After endoscopic treatment a prompt therapeutic response is expected within 1 to 5 days. The precise time period necessary for the leak to close is difficult to determine, as early closure may not imply complete healing. Mostly the stent is left in place for several weeks to months, but the optimal duration of stent placement is unknown. Percutaneous drainage of abdominal biloma, already present at the time of endoscopic treatment, may be required.

RESULTS OF ENDOSCOPIC THERAPY FOR POSTOPERATIVE BILE LEAKS

We described our findings in 54 patients (8). Endoscopic therapy was performed in 48 patients and was successful in 90%. The mean interval between surgery and therapy was 37 days. Twenty-seven of the 54 patients had bile leaks after open cholecystectomy, resulting in a biliary cutaneous fistula. Distal bile duct obstruction was present in 60%. An excellent outcome (clinical and radiological) was achieved in 43 patients (90%). Five patients died of ongoing sepsis, notwithstanding surgical and percutaneous abscess drainage procedures.

Foutch et al. (24) recently described 23 patients. Eleven had bile leaks due to laparoscopic cholecystectomy. Eleven of the patients had evidence of distal obstruction, stones were present in seven patients, am-

pullary stenosis in three, and malignant stenosis in one. Endoscopic treatment included sphincterotomy with or without nasobiliary drain or endoprosthesis and was effective in all 23 patients. Five patients required additional percutaneous drainage of bile collections. The only complication was minor bleeding after sphincterotomy controlled endoscopically. In summary, endoscopic therapy in bile duct leaks is effective and relatively safe. Cystic duct stump leaks in particular appear to do well with this therapy. Prospective studies are now needed to determine the most optimal endoscopic treatment and duration of stent placement. It is also clear that close cooperation between the endoscopist and the surgeon is essential in the management of these patients.

Postoperative Biliary Strictures

Postoperative stricturing of the bile duct is nearly always the result of direct surgical trauma during operation. The damage is usually seen after cholecystectomy or bile duct exploration but may follow upper abdominal operations. Postoperative biliary strictures occur in 0.2% to 0.5% of patients undergoing an open surgical procedure (25,26) and in 0.5% to 2.7% of patients undergoing a laparoscopic cholecystectomy (4,5). Ischemia due to vascular insufficiency is also considered another mechanism for postoperative biliary strictures (27). Postsurgical strictures present with jaundice, which may be silent even with complete bile duct transection, fever, and excessive biliary drainage via a T-tube or biliary fistula. Although most patients present early, within weeks after the surgery, some develop symptoms years later. Elevated serum bilirubin and alkaline phosphatase are seen in the majority of patients. Ultrasound and computed tomography are occasionally helpful but biliary dilatation is absent in about 60% of all patients. Direct cholangiography is the diagnostic method of choice and may show a short smooth stricture often located near the cystic duct stump, common hepatic duct, or at the bifurcation.

The management of patients with benign postoperative biliary strictures is a challenge because the majority of patients are young and require a good long-term result. Treatment is aimed at restoring biliary flow, surgically or nonsurgically.

Surgical options are hepaticojejunostomy with Roux-en-Y reconstruction, hepaticoduodenostomy, or end-to-end anastomosis (28–30). Even in skilled hands the surgical mortality ranges from 4% to 14%. Recurrent strictures lead to intrahepatic cholelithiasis and repeated attacks of cholangitis. This complication may develop in 10% to 30% of patients (31,32). With the advent of nonsurgical methods for the treatment of malignant biliary strictures these techniques have also been applied in benign biliary strictures. The nonoperative alternatives include percutaneous transhepatic balloon dilatation and stent placement (33–38) and endoscopic balloon dilatation with or without stent placement (39–45).

Percutaneous Balloon Dilatation

Percutaneous transhepatic balloon dilatation has been employed in several studies with a success rate of 40% to 85%, after a mean follow-up of 16 to 33 months (33,36). Repeated dilatations may be required because of restricturing after a single dilatation. Percutaneous transhepatic dilatation may be associated with complications such as hemorrhage, bile leakage, and sepsis (36–38). This procedure is contraindicated in the presence of ascites, cirrhosis, or coagulopathy.

Endoscopic Balloon Dilatation

Balloon dilatation has also been carried out endoscopically (40,41). Gruntzig-type balloons, made of polyethylene, are used with a diameter of 4 to 10 mm and a length of 2 to 8 cm. The balloons are inserted over a guidewire that has been previously passed through the stricture. The balloons are insufflated to a pressure of 4 to 6 atmospheres. There are no definite data, however, as to how many seconds the stricture must be dilated or how many times during one session the dilatation needs to be carried out. The patient's tolerance of the dilatation and the contour of the waist of the balloon are some of the suggested indicators of the adequacy of the dilatation. Dilatation may be repeated at 3- to 6-month intervals until a 10 mm balloon can be easily inflated at the stricture site. More frequent dilatations may also be clinically indicated.

The largest series of patients with endoscopic balloon dilatation has been reported by Geenen et al. (41). In 16 out of 20 patients dilatation could be successfully performed. In the remaining 4 patients, the passage of the guidewire or the balloon was not possible. During the mean follow up of 22.4 months (range 6–68 months) clinical improvement was observed in all 16, with improvement of the liver functions and resolution of cholangitis, jaundice, and pruritus. Radiographic improvement was found in 14 out of the 20 patients with an increase in the diameter of the stricture in 10 patients. It was concluded that endoscopic dilatation of postoperative bile duct strictures appears to be safe and effective. Temporary stent placement may be required only in a minority of tight strictures.

Endoscopic Stent Placement

The technique of endoscopic stent insertion is well established and described in detail elsewhere (46). The

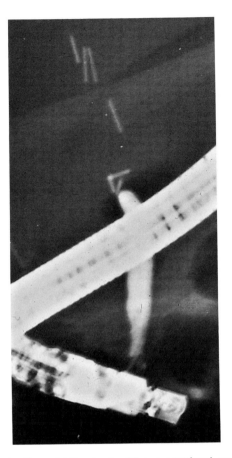

FIG. 4. A clipped bile duct without proximal communication.

optimal number of stents required to dilate the stricture and the duration of stent placement remain unknown.

Between 1981 and 1990 80 patients were referred for endoscopic management of benign postoperative biliary strictures (45). At ERCP, 10 of the patients had a complete obstruction (Fig. 4), 20 had a concomitant bile leak, and 17 had retained or recurrent common bile duct (CBD) stones. Endoscopic treatment was attempted in 70 patients and was successful in 66 patients (94%) (Figs. 5 and 6).

Patients were treated with two 10 Fr endoprostheses left in situ for 1 year. The stents were electively exchanged every 3 months to prevent complications of endoprostheses clogging. Early complications occurred in seven patients and included minor bleeding after the sphincterotomy, procedure-related cholangitis, or ongoing cholangitis. Two patients developed pancreatitis. One of those was operated and eventually died 25 days later due to a cerebral vascular accident. The 30-day mortality was 2.5%.

Most late complications during the period of stenting were due to clogging of the endoprosthesis. Late complications included one episode of cholangitis (4), two or more episodes of cholangitis (10), and recurrent cho-

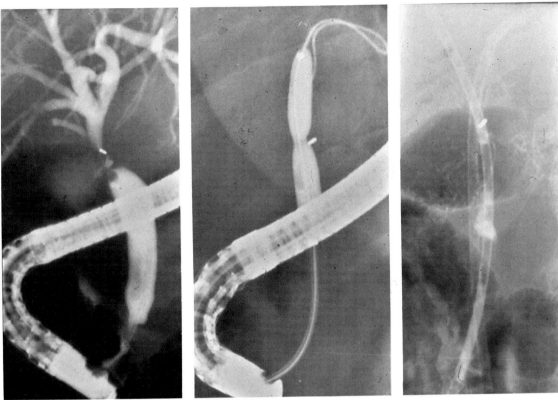

FIG. 5. A firm postoperative stricture *(left)* is dilated by balloon insufflation *(middle)* before the placement of two 10 Fr stents *(right)*.

lestasis (2). Stent exchange relieved the symptoms in most patients. In two patients stent migration into the bile duct occurred. During the period of endoscopic treatment surgery was carried out in six patients because of failed complete drainage in four, stent migration in one, and personal preference in another. Six patients died. The causes of death were all nonbiliary. The endoprostheses were still *in situ* at the time of evaluation in eight patients. In 46 patients the stents were removed and these patients were followed for a median period of 42 months (range 4–99 months) (Table 1). In 38 patients, an excellent (no clinical symptoms, stable liver enzymes) or good result (only one episode of cholangitis) was achieved. Recurrent stricturing occurred in 8 patients (17%) after a median period of 95 days. Of these 8 patients, 6 underwent hepaticojejunostomy. The remaining 2 patients were again treated endoscopically. Extraction of recurrent

CBD stones was necessary in 2 patients. These results showed that 83% of 46 patients were effectively treated after 1 year of endoscopic stenting with a mean follow-up period of 42 months.

Similarly, Geenen et al. (42) reported favorable results after balloon dilatation or stent placement in 88% of 25 patients with a mean follow-up of 46 months. The results of stenting therapy were less satisfactory, however, in a study from Berkelhammer et al. (44), where a good response was found in 74% of 25 patients with a shorter follow-up period of 19 months. This group has recently published the long-term follow-up (6.5 years) in these patients (47): 3 patients died of unrelated causes, 13 of 22 (59%) had an excellent response (no biliary symptoms, normal LFT, and no further intervention), 3 (14%) had good response (no biliary symptoms, stable LFT $\geq 1.5 \times$ normal, no further intervention) and 6 (27%) had poor response (biliary symptoms, cholangitis after stent removal, increasing LFT or surgical/radiological intervention). Patients treated within 3 months after the surgical trauma showed the most favorable results.

SURGICAL OR NONSURGICAL MANAGEMENT?

Comparative studies have not been performed. Pitt et al. (48) compared the results of percutaneous balloon

TABLE 1. *Follow-up of 46 patients after stent removal*

Follow-up (mean/range)	38 (4–96) months
Recurrent stricture	8 (17%)
Endoscopy	3
Surgery	5
Recurrent stones	2 (4%)
Mortality (nonbiliary)	6

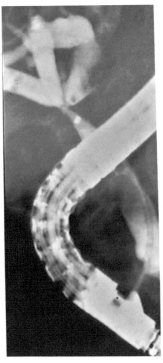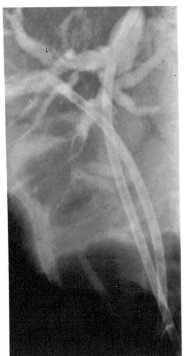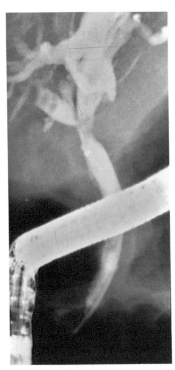

FIG. 6. A benign stricture at the bifurcation *(left)* is treated with two 10 Fr endoprosthesis *(middle).* Control cholangiogram after 3 months showed a good dilatation of the stricture *(right).*

dilatation and surgical repair in the same institution and during the same period of time. They showed superiority of surgery over percutaneous balloon dilatation.

Davids et al. (49) compared the results of surgery and endoscopic stenting in our institution during the same time period (Table 2). Thirty-five patients were treated surgically and 66 by endoscopic stenting. Patient characteristics, initial trauma, previous repair, and level of obstruction were comparable in both groups. Surgical therapy consisted of constructing a biliary digestive anastomosis in normal ductal tissue. Endoscopic therapy consisted in placement of two endoprostheses with trimonthly elective exchange for a 1-year period. Mean length of follow-up was 15 months (range 10–85 months) and 42 months (range 4–99 months) for surgery and endoscopy, respectively.

Early complications occurred more frequently in the surgically treated group ($p <.03$). Late complications during therapy occurred only in the endoscopically treated group. In 46 patients the endoprosthesis was subsequently removed; 17% in both groups had restricturing. The long-term success rate in both groups was similar.

CONCLUSION

Endoscopic treatment of postoperative bile duct injuries is safe and effective in the majority of patients. In the early postoperative phase it has a reduced morbidity and mortality compared to reoperation and usually provides a satisfactory long-term result. Drainage of the biliary tree via the percutaneous transhepatic approach has also been reported to be effective, but the incidence of complications is higher than that of endoscopic drainage. In addition, puncture of a nondilated biliary tree can be difficult and dangerous. Endoscopic therapy also allows treatment of the primary problem as well as any exacerbating factor, such as retained CBD stones or biliary stricture.

The choice between the available therapeutic options is essentially determined by local expertise and preference. There are no controlled trials to support one over the other. We generally recommend endoscopic treatment initially with or without the aid of a rendezvous procedure. This appears to be the safest and most effective first step. If endoscopic therapy fails or the long-term result is unsatisfactory, then reoperation is still feasible. The reverse approach is usually

TABLE 2. *Comparison between surgical and endoscopic treatment*

	Surgery	Endoscopy
Patients (no.)	35	66
Early complications (%)	26	8
30-day mortality	0	1
1-yr complications (%)	0	27
Outcome for no. of patients	35	46
Excellent	25	33
Good	4	5
Poor	6 (17%)	8 (17%)

impossible unless an access loop is fashioned at the time of surgery for subsequent endoscopic therapy.

REFERENCES

1. Hills ThM, Westbrook KC, Caldwell FT, Read RC. Surgical injury of the common bile duct. *Am J Surg* 1977;134:712–716.
2. Hadjis NS, Blumgart LH. Injury to segmental bile ducts. *Arch Surg* 1988;123:351–353.
3. Raute M, Schaup W. Iatrogenic damage of the bile ducts caused by cholecystectomy. *Langenbecks Arch Chir* 1998;373:345–354.
4. The Southern Surgeons Club. A prospective analysis of 1518 laparoscopic cholecystectomies. *N Engl J Med* 1991;324:1073–1078.
5. Deziel DJ, Millikan KW, Economou SG, Doolas A, Ko ST, Airan MC. Complications of laparoscopic cholecystectomy: a national survey of 4,292 hospitals and an analysis of 77,604 cases. *Am J Surg* 1992;165:9–14.
6. Collins PG, Gorey TF. Iatrogenic biliary stricture: presentation and management. *Am J Surg* 1984;71:900–902.
7. Andrén-Sandberg AA, Johansson S, Bengmark S. Accidental lesions of the common bile duct at cholecystectomy. *Am J Surg* 1985;201:452–455.
8. Davids PHP, Rauws EAJ, Coene PPLO, Tytgat GNJ, Huibregtse K. Postoperative bile leakage: the endoscopic management. *Gut* 1992;33:1118–1122.
9. Brooks DC, Becker JM, Connors PL, Carr-Locke DL. Management of bile leaks following laparoscopic cholecystectomy. *Surg Endosc* 1993;7:292–295.
10. Browden IW, Dowling JB, Koontz KK, Litwin MS. Early management of postoperative injuries of the extrahepatic biliary tract. *Ann Surg* 1987;205:649–658.
11. Czerniak A, Thompson JN, Soreide O, Benjamin IS, Blumgart LH. The management of fistulae of the biliary tract after injury to the bile duct during cholecystectomy. *Surg Gynecol Obstet* 1988;167:33–38.
12. van Sonnenberg E, Giovanna C, Wittich GR, et al. The role of interventional radiology for complications of cholecystectomy. *Surgery* 1990;107:632–638.
13. Zuidema GD, Cameron JL, Sitzman JV, et al. Percutaneous transhepatic management of complex biliary problems. *Ann Surg* 1983;197:584–593.
14. Kozarek R, Ganna R, Baerg R, Wagonfeld J, Ball TK. Bile leak after laparoscopic cholecystectomy. Diagnostic and therapeutic application of endoscopic retrograde cholangiopancreatography. *Arch Intern Med* 1993;152:1040–1043.
15. Sauerbruch T, Wienzierl M, Holl J, Pratschke E. Treatment of postoperative bile fistulas by internal endoscopic drainage. *Gastroenterology* 1986;90:1998–2003.
16. van Steenbergen W, Haemers A, Pelemans et al. Postoperative biliocutaneous fistula: successful treatment by insertion of an endoprosthesis. *Endoscopy* 1987;19:34–36.
17. Deviere J, van Gansbeke D, Ansay J, du Toeuf J, Cremer M. Endoscopic management of post-traumatic biliary fistula. *Endoscopy* 1987;19:136–139.
18. Del Olmo L, Meroño E, Moreira VF, Garcia T, Garcia-Plaza A. Successful treatment of postoperative external biliary fistulas by endoscopic sphincterotomy. *Gastrointest Endosc* 1988;34:307–309.
19. Ponchon T, Gallez JF, Valette PJ, Chavaillon A, Bory R. Endoscopic treatment of biliary tract fistula. *Gastrointest Endosc* 1989;35:490–498.
20. Binmoeller KF, Katon RM, Sheidman. Endoscopic management of postoperative biliary leaks: review of 77 cases and report of two cases with biloma formation. *Am J Gastroenterol* 1991;86:227–231.
21. Liguory C, Vitale GC, Lefebre JF, Bonnel D, Cornud F. Endoscopic treatment of postoperative biliary fistula. *Surgery* 1991;100:779–784.
22. Kozarek RA, Traverso LW. Endoscopic stent placement for cystic duct leak after laparoscopic cholecystectomy. *Gastrointest Endosc* 1991;37:71–73.
23. Kozarek RA. Endoscopic management of bile duct injury. *Gastrointest Clin North Am* 1993;3:261–269.
24. Foutch PG, Harlan JRE, Hoefer M. Endoscopic therapy for patients with a postoperative biliary leak. *Gastrointest Endosc* 1993;39:416–421.
25. Glenn F. Iatrogenic injuries to the biliary ductal system. *Surg Gynecol Obstet* 1978;146:430–434.
26. Way LW, Barnhoft RA, Thomas MJ. Biliary stricture. *Surg Clin North Am* 1981;61:963–972.
27. TerBlanche J, Allison HF, Northover JMA. An ischemic basis for biliary strictures. *Surgery* 1983;94:52–57.
28. Ganst JF, Nano SE, Grundfast-Bromatouski S, Vogt D, Hermann RE. Benign biliary strictures: an analytic review (1970–1989). *Surgery* 1986;99:409–413.
29. Barker FM, Winkler M. Permanent access hepaticojejunostomy. *Br J Surg* 1984;71:1988–1991.
30. Moosa AR, Meyer AD, Stabile B. Iatrogenic injury to the bile duct: who, how, where? *Arch Surg* 1990;125:1028–1031.
31. Pitt HA, Miyamato T, Parapatis KS. Factors influencing outcome in patients with post-operative biliary stricture. *Am J Surg* 1982;144:14–21.
32. Pellegrini CA, Thomas MJ, Way LW. Recurrent biliary stricture: pattern of recurrence and outcome of surgical therapy. *Am J Surg* 1984;147:175–180.
33. Salomonowitz E, Castandeda-Zuniger WR, Lund G, et al. Balloon dilatation of benign biliary strictures. *Radiology* 1984;151:613–616.
34. Vogel SB, Howard RJ, Coridi J, Hawkins IF. Evaluation of percutaneous transhepatic balloon dilatation of benign biliary strictures in high risk patients. *Am J Surg* 1985;149:73–79.
35. Gallacher DJ, Kadir S, Kaufman SL, et al. Nonoperative management of benign postoperative biliary strictures. *Radiology* 1985;156:625–629.
36. Mueller PR, van Sonnenberg E, Ferrucci JT, et al. Biliary stricture dilatation: multicenter review of clinical management in 73 patients. *Radiology* 1986;160:17–22.
37. Trambert JJ, Bon KM, Zajko AB, Starzi TE, Inatsuki S. Percutaneous transhepatic balloon dilatation of benign biliary strictures. *AJR* 1987;149:945–948.
38. Williams HJ Jr, Bender CE, May GR. Benign postoperative biliary strictures: dilatation with fluoroscopic guidance. *Radiology* 1987;163:629–634.
39. Vallon SB, Mason RR, Laurance BH, et al. Endoscopic retrograde cholangiography in post-operative bile duct strictures. *Br J Radiol* 1982;55:32–35.
40. Foutch PG, Sivak MV Jr. Therapeutic endoscopic balloon dilatation of the extrahepatic biliary ducts. *Am J Gastroenterol* 1985;80:575–580.
41. Geenen JE, Derfus D, Welch JM. Biliary balloon dilatation. *Endosc Rev* 1985;2(1):10–16.
42. Geenen DJ, Geenen JE, Hogan WJ, et al. Endoscopic therapy for benign bile duct strictures. *Gastrointest Endosc* 1989;35:267–271.
43. Huibregtse K, Katon RM, Tytgat GNJ. Endoscopic treatment of postoperative biliary strictures. *Endoscopy* 1986;18:133–137.
44. Berkelhammer L, Kortan P, Haber GD. Endoscopic biliary prosthesis as treatment for benign postoperative bile duct strictures. *Gastrointest Endosc* 1989;35:95–101.
45. Davids PHP, Rauws EAJ, Coene PPLO, Tytgat GNJ, Huibregtse K. Endoscopic stenting for postoperative biliary strictures. *Gastrointest Endosc* 1992;38:12–18.
46. Huibregtse K. *Endoscopic biliary and pancreatic drainage.* Stuttgart: Georg Thieme Verlag, 1988.
47. Walden D, Raijman I, Fuchs, Kandel G, Marcon N, Kortan P, Haber G. Long term follow up of endoscopic stenting (ES) for benign post-operative bile duct strictures (BPBDS). *Gastrointest Endosc* 1993;39:335(abst 349).
48. Pitt HA, Kaufman SOL, Coleman JL. Benign postoperative biliary strictures: operate or dilate? *Ann Surg* 1989;218:417–425.
49. Davids PHP, Tanka AK, Rauws EAJ, van Gulik ThM, van Leeuwen DJ, de Wit LTh, Verbeek PLM, Huibregtse K, van der Heyde MN, Tytgat GNJ. Benign biliary strictures: surgery or endoscopy. *Ann Surg* 1993;217:237–243.

Advanced Therapeutic Endoscopy, 2nd Ed.,
edited by J. S. Barkin and C. A. O'Phelan.
Raven Press, Ltd., New York © 1994.

CHAPTER 42

The Role of ERCP in Laparoscopic Cholecystectomy

Lee McHenry, Jr. and Alvin M. Zfass

In just 5 years, laparoscopic cholecystectomy has revolutionized the approach to the patient with symptomatic gallstones. Since its introduction in 1989 by the European surgeons, Dubois and Perissat, and in the United States by Reddick, Olsen, and Phillips, laparoscopic cholecystectomy has captured the forefront in the management of gallstone disease (1–3). Laparoscopic cholecystectomy has been embraced by the general public and by general surgeons and their medical colleagues as the procedure of choice, replacing open cholecystectomy. The shortened postoperative recovery time and a more desirable cosmetic result are obvious benefits of the procedure. The evolution in laparoscopic cholecystectomy has been swift, and with this rapid evolution it has become necessary for gastroenterologists to stay abreast of new developments regarding the advantages and shortcomings of this therapeutic option. For example, the gastroenterologist's approach to patients with suspected choledocholithiasis in the preoperative setting, as well as the investigation of jaundice and bile leaks in the postoperative setting, present new, critical decision options.

The initial enthusiasm of the laparoscopic surgeon and the gastroenterologist to obtain a preoperative endoscopic retrograde cholangiopancreatography (ERCP) in patients with symptomatic gallstones has changed remarkably over the past 5 years (Fig. 1). Early in the laparoscopic cholecystectomy era, the surgeon was less experienced in obtaining an intraoperative cholangiogram and not enthusiastic about attempting laparoscopic retrieval of common bile duct stones. During this early period, the gastroenterologist was called upon to perform preoperative ERCP when patients were suspected of having common bile duct stones. Some clinical algorithms considered preoperative ERCP as "routine" prior to laparoscopic cholecystectomy to define the biliary anatomy, to remove unsuspected common bile duct (CBD) stones, and to decrease intraoperative complications. This routine use of preoperative ERCP prior to laparoscopic cholecystectomy was quickly viewed as endoscopic "overkill" as only 5% to 10% of patients had unsuspected CBD stones. Additionally, preoperative definition of the biliary anatomy by ERCP had a low yield (4). As experience with laparoscopic surgery grew, the confidence of the laparoscopic surgeon in obtaining an intraoperative cholangiogram (IOC) grew. Intraoperative cholangiography can be performed by many laparoscopic surgeons in over 90% of cases. The performance of IOC adds only 10 minutes of operative time to the laparoscopic cholecystectomy and has few complications. The technique of IOC can be expected to improve in the future as newer cholangiographic catheters and techniques are introduced (5,6).

Each year in the United States alone an estimated half a million patients undergo cholecystectomy, of which 85% to 90% are performed by the laparoscopic method. In this cost-driven medical environment, gastroenterologists and surgeons are required to choose from superb endoscopic and laparoscopic techniques in order to optimize outcomes. This approach maximizes investment and enables patients to receive the most cost-effective care with, it is hoped, fewer complications. These objectives can be obtained with cur-

L. McHenry, Jr. and A. M. Zfass: Division of Gastroenterology, Department of Medicine, Medical College of Virginia, Richmond, Virginia 23292.

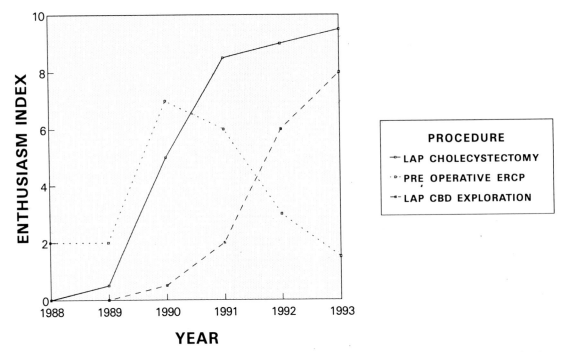

FIG. 1. Evolution of laparoscopic cholecystectomy and ERCP from 1988 to 1993. A rise in the enthusiasm for laparoscopic cholecystectomy and laparoscopic extraction of common duct stones resulted in a fall in the enthusiasm for preoperative ERCP.

rent knowledge of treatment algorithms and a realistic consideration of the expertise of the surgeon and the gastroenterologist. For example, the gastroenterologist must consider where the operators are on the so-called learning curve of laparoscopic cholecystectomy and endoscopic extraction of CBD stones. This steep curve has impact on any proposed algorithm. Unfortunately, no controlled studies have addressed this issue.

Approximately 500,000 patients will undergo cholecystectomy this year. The following are three algorithms useful in planning cholecystectomy:

Algorithm 1: Laparoscopic cholecystectomy and intraoperative cholangiography with attempt at laparoscopic retrieval of common duct stones. Postoperative ERCP and endoscopic sphincterotomy (ES) for retained common duct stones.

Algorithm 2: Preoperative ERCP ± ES in patients with suspected CBD stones followed by laparoscopic cholecystectomy.

TABLE 1. *Professional costs in 500,000 laparoscopic cholecystectomies*

	Algorithm		
	1	2	3
Lap. chole.	945,750,000	945,750,000	945,750,000
ERCP	6,075,000	50,625,000	442,500,000
Total	$951,825,000	$996,375,000	$1,388,250,000

Algorithm 3: Routine preoperative ERCP ± ES in all patients followed by laparoscopic cholecystectomy.

The potential cost differentials of the algorithms are shown in Table 1. The potential cost savings for professional costs is minimal (4.6%) when algorithm 1 is compared with algorithm 2. However, algorithm 3 is 45% more expensive when compared with algorithm 1, yet has no proven benefit in patient outcome. Whether the gastroenterologist advocates preoperative ERCP ± ES in patients at high risk for harboring CBD stones or laparoscopic cholecystectomy with attempted transcystic retrieval of CBD stones depends on the expertise of the operating surgeon and endoscopist.

CAN THE PRESENCE OF COMMON BILE DUCT STONES BE PREDICTED?

The presence of CBD stones may be suspected on the basis of abnormal liver function tests. In a retrospective review of patients who underwent open cholecystectomy and operative cholangiography, Del Santo et al. (7) evaluated the preoperative serum levels of lactic dehydrogenase, aspartate aminotransferase, total bilirubin and alkaline phosphatase in 195 consecutive patients with symptomatic cholelithiasis. When all four of these biochemical tests were normal, no patient had a CBD stone visualized by intraoperative cholangiography. However, as the number of abnormal biochemical tests increased from one to four, the frequency of CBD stones increased from 17% to 50%. This study suggests that abnormal preoperative liver function tests will predict the presence or absence of CBD stones. Lacaine et al. (8) noted that in patients with no previous jaundice, normal alkaline phosphatase, and a CBD diameter <12 mm, common bile duct stones were identified in less than 5% of patients.

Neoptolemos et al. (9) evaluated the laboratory biochemical criteria in patients who presented with suspected acute gallstone pancreatitis. The discriminating variables that were helpful in detecting CBD stones at time of ERCP included alkaline phosphatase >220 IU/L, total bilirubin >3.2 mg/dl, γ-glutamyl transpeptidase (GGT) >225 IU/L, and age >70 years. The single best predictor of the presence of a CBD stone was a serum bilirubin >3.2 mg/dl (sensitivity of 80%, specificity of 80%). If all four criteria were present, the specificity for detecting CBD stones increased to 93%.

In conclusion, patients with no abnormalities of liver chemistries and a normal size CBD have choledocholithiasis <5% of the time. The greater the number of liver biochemical abnormalities (alkaline phosphatase, total bilirubin, aspartate aminotransferase, GGT, lactate dehydrogenase), the greater the likelihood of CBD stones with an incidence ranging from 15% to 50%. Advanced age (>70 years) increases the likelihood of CBD stones in patients undergoing cholecystectomy for symptomatic cholelithiasis.

The sensitivity of preoperative extracorporeal ultrasonography in detecting CBD stones is low (13% to 55%) (10). In addition, the specificity of this test is poor (<70%) when compared with endoscopic or intraoperative cholangiography.

In an effort to improve the sensitivity and specificity of ultrasound, attempts have been made to maneuver the ultrasound closer to the CBD. A technique reported by Mosnier et al. (11) using a 7.5-mHz ultrasound probe inserted through a small incision at the time of open cholecystectomy to evaluate the CBD was evaluated in 131 patients with normal liver chemistries. The CBD was visualized by intraoperative ultrasound in 98% of patients and CBD stones were visualized in ten patients with a sensitivity of 95% and specificity of 100%. This diagnostic test required on average only 7 minutes of additional intraoperative time and compares favorably with intraoperative cholangiography (sensitivity of 95%, specificity of 92%). Studies of intraoperative ultrasonography during laparoscopic cholecystectomy are warranted.

Intravenous cholangiography, a relatively insensitive test for detecting CBD stones, was originally introduced in 1953 but fell out of favor over the ensuing 20 years because of a significant incidence (10%) of contrast reactions and, rarely (0.5%), anaphylactic shock. Recently in the British literature (12), intravenous cholangiography has resurfaced using a lower os-

molarity contrast agent, meglumine iotroxate, in the preoperative evaluation of patients suspected of CBD stones. This technique requires tomography for adequate visualization of the CBD, has a >10% false-negative rate for detection of CBD stones, and is associated with a high (2–5%) contrast reaction. In this era of diagnostic ERCP, intravenous cholangiography is not likely to be a useful technique.

MANAGEMENT OF CBD STONES IN THE LAPAROSCOPIC ERA

Although the natural history of choledocholithiasis has not been well studied, observations by previous authors have established a high complication rate of CBD stones that were not removed at cholecystectomy. In 1941, Millbourn noted his experience of following 38 patients, with documented CBD stones at the time of cholecystectomy, for 6 months to 13 years (13). Twenty-one of 38 patients (55%) became symptomatic with biliary colic, jaundice, or cholangitis over this time period. Johnson and Hosking (14) reported similar results with over 50% of patients with retained CBD stones developing symptoms with resultant serious complications in nearly 25% of patients. From this experience, it can be recommended that retained CBD stones should be removed to prevent both short- and long-term complications.

Over the past 5 years, laparoscopic surgeons have developed successful techniques of imaging the CBD during laparoscopic cholecystectomy. With refined laparoscopic equipment (catheters, choledochoscopes) for accessing the CBD via the transcystic route or through a laparoscopic choledochotomy, CBD stones can be removed in over 70% (50–90%) of cases. Carroll and Phillips (15) reported their impressive results in 78 patients with CBD stones detected at the time of laparoscopic cholecystectomy. Common bile duct stones were removed in 62 patients (79%), with the majority (90%) being removed via the transcystic route. Laparoscopic choledochotomy is technically feasible for stones that are too large to be removed through the cystic duct. However, laparoscopic choledochotomy is a technique that requires microscissors and choledochoscopy, and it tethers the patient to a T-tube for weeks, eliminating the simplicity of the "no tubes" notion. Postoperative ERCP with endoscopic sphincterotomy remains the most appropriate alternative when CBD stones cannot be removed via the transcystic route.

Endoscopic sphincterotomy (ES), first developed over 15 years ago, has allowed the biliary endoscopist the opportunity to extract CBD stones without resorting to surgical intervention. The technique of ES is well described and the short-term complications of pancreatitis, bleeding, and perforation occur in <6% of patients. In the laparoscopic cholecystectomy era, ERCP and ES are being increasingly performed in young patients and patients with small (<7 mm) bile ducts with suspected or documented CBD stones. In patients with CBD stones, one series noted a higher complication rate of ES in patients with small (<10 mm) diameter bile ducts (10.4%) than in patients with large (>10 mm) diameter bile ducts (2.6%) (16). Other methods besides endoscopic sphincterotomy, such as sphincter dilation (medical or mechanical), may obviate complications of sphincterotomy in patients with a small (<7 mm) bile duct and small CBD stones. Staritz et al. (17) reported their success in 21 patients using nitroglycerin at the time of endoscopic stone removal. Thirty of 32 stones were removed successfully (size 6–12 mm) with this technique with no noted complications. Another series reported the efficacy of balloon sphincteroplasty in 26 patients with small (<1.5 cm) CBD stones. A 6- to 8-mm balloon was inflated to 10 psi for 60 seconds × 2 and stones were extracted with a retrieval balloon or Dormia basket. The success rate in stone removal was 70% with one reported complication of mild pancreatitis (18). Papillotomy was successful in the remaining eight patients with no complications. Further trials are ongoing to evaluate medical and mechanical sphincter dilation in the overall management of bile duct stones.

ENDOSCOPIC MANAGEMENT OF LAPAROSCOPIC BILE DUCT INJURY

The overall complication rate of laparoscopic cholecystectomy appears to be reduced when compared with conventional open cholecystectomy (19,20). However, this lower overall complication rate includes a higher bile duct injury rate (laparoscopic cholecystectomy, 0.5–2.7%; open cholecystectomy, 0.2–0.5%). There is no question that the incidence of bile duct injury during laparoscopic cholecystectomy is indirectly proportional to the laparoscopic experience of the surgeon, with the highest rates (2.3%) in the first 15 laparoscopic cholecystectomies as compared with 0.1% for subsequent laparoscopic cholecystectomies (19). Other reasons have been cited for the increased rate of bile duct injuries with laparoscopic cholecystectomy, such as limited visual field, inadequate exposure, variant anatomy, and injudicious use of laser or cautery (20). With this background, it can be expected that the rate of bile duct injury will gradually decrease over the next several years as experience increases.

The most dreaded bile duct injury with laparoscopic cholecystectomy is the common bile or hepatic duct transection with resultant biliary stricture. The duct injury, if recognized at the time of surgery, may be addressed with primary duct anastomosis or with hepaticojejunostomy. The natural history of bile duct injury and surgical repair during laparoscopic cholecystectomy is not yet known.

Endoscopic therapy of postoperative bile duct strictures is now considered to be routine (21). The endoscopic approach to postoperative strictures has included an initial stricture dilation and placement of a 7 or 10 Fr biliary endoprosthesis with a trade-out of stents every 3 months for at least 1 year. The stricture is dilated on subsequent exchanges to accommodate two 10 Fr biliary endoprostheses in order to bridge the stricture to the widest diameter possible. In one series, biliary endoprosthesis placement was successful in 94% of patients (66 of 70 patients) with postoperative strictures. The endoprostheses were removed in 46 patients at 1 year with a long-term success (asymptomatic) in 83% at a mean follow-up of 42 months. Similar techniques and results have been described by others with a long-term success in 66% to 84% after stent removal (22–25). Endoscopic management of postoperative biliary strictures compares favorably with surgical intervention.

Bile duct leaks after laparoscopic cholecystectomy may present in the first several postoperative days with pain, jaundice, bile leak from the trocar wounds, biloma, or bile ascites. The leak is usually from the cystic duct stump, although occasionally it may occur from an anomalous branch of the right hepatic duct. The principle in treating this complication is to decrease the transphincteric pressure gradient from the bile duct to the duodenum to allow free flow of bile with resultant closure of the bile duct leak. Closure of the leak may be accomplished endoscopically by various techniques including biliary sphincterotomy, bile duct stents, and/or nasobiliary drains (25–28).

The most common approach to bile duct leaks is placement of a 10 Fr biliary endoprosthesis across the leak for 1 month. The bile duct leak can be successfully treated in 75% to 100% of cases using this technique (25–28). If a fluid collection, or biloma, coexists with the leak, percutaneous aspiration with ultrasound guidance is required the following day. Sphincterotomy alone is successful in closing biliary fistula in 28 of 37 patients (76%) with an average time to closure of the leak of 2.4 ± 1.6 days (28). In three patients with bile ascites complicating a laparoscopic bile duct injury, nasobiliary drainage was successful in resolving the large volume of the bile ascites rapidly (3–5 days) (26,27).

CONCLUSIONS

Laparoscopic cholecystectomy has rapidly supplanted conventional open cholecystectomy for the treatment of symptomatic cholelithiasis over the past

5 years. With further refinement in laparoscopic instrumentation and techniques, it can be expected that the laparoscopic surgeon will, in time, effectively manage patients with coexistent choledocholithiasis. Until that time comes, however, it is important for the therapeutic endoscopist to be able to diagnose and treat CBD stones, in both the pre- and postoperative setting. The gastroenterologist must also be cognizant of the methods, success rates, and potential pitfalls of endoscopic interventional techniques such as sphincterotomy, sphincter dilation, and stone extraction. Lastly, the gastroenterologist must be able to understand, diagnose, and endoscopically treat the complications of bile duct leak and/or stricture in this new era of laparoscopic cholecystectomy.

REFERENCES

1. Dubois F, Icard P, Berthelot G, Levard H. Coelioscopic cholecystectomy. *Ann Surg* 1991;211:61–62.
2. Perissat J, Collet DR, Belliard R. Gallstones, laparoscopic treatment, intracorporeal lithotripsy followed by cholecystostomy or cholecystectomy: a personal technique. *Endoscopy* 1989;21:373–374.
3. Reddick EJ, Olsen DO. Laparoscopic laser cholecystectomy. A comparison with mini laparotomy cholecystectomy. *Surg Endosc* 1989;3:131–133.
4. Neuhaus H, Feussner H, Ungeheuer A, Hoffmann W, Siewert JR, Classen M. Prospective evaluation of the use of ERC prior to laparoscopic cholecystectomy. *Endoscopy* 1992;24:745–749.
5. Spaw AT, Reddick EJ, Olsen DO. Laparoscopic laser cholecystectomy: analysis of 500 procedures. *Surg Laparosc Endosc* 1991;1:2–7.
6. Flowers JL, Zucker KA, Graham SM, Scovill WA, Imembo AL, Bailey RW. Laparoscopic cholangiography: results and indications. *Ann Surg* 1992;215(3):209–216.
7. Del Santo P, Kazarian KK, Rogers JF, Bevins PA, Hall JR. Prediction of operative cholangiography in patients undergoing elective cholecystectomy with routine liver function chemistries. *Surgery* 1985;98(1):7–11.
8. Lacaine F, Corlette MB, Bismuth H. Preoperative evaluation of the risk of common bile duct stones. *Arch Surg* 1980;115:1114–1116.
9. Neoptolemos JP, London NJ, Bailey I, Carr-Locke DL. The role of clinical and biochemical criteria and endoscopic retrograde cholangiopancreatography in the urgent diagnosis of common bile duct stones in acute pancreatitis. *Surgery* 1986;100(4):732–742.
10. Cronan JJ. Ultrasound diagnosis of choledocholithiasis: a reappraisal. *Radiology* 1986;161:133–134.
11. Mosnier H, Audy J-DR, Boche O, Guivarc'h M. et al. Intraoperative sonography during cholecystectomy for gallstones. *Surg Gynecol Obstet* 1992;174:469–473.
12. Joyce WP, Keane R, et al. Intravenous cholangiography: identification of bile duct stones in patients undergoing laparoscopic cholecystectomy. *Br J Surg* 1991;78:1174–1176.
13. Millbourn E. On reoperation for choledocholithiasis. *Acta Chir Scand* 1941;86(suppl):65.
14. Johnson A, Hosking S. Appraisal of the management of bile duct stones. *Br J Surg* 1987;74:555–560.
15. Carroll B, Phillips E. Laparoscopic removal of common duct stones. Laparoscopic cholecystectomy and surgical endoscopy. *Gastrointest Endosc Clin North Am* 1993;3(2):239–248.
16. Sherman S, Ruffolo T, Hawes R, Lehman G. Complications of endoscopic sphincterotomy. *Gastroenterology* 1991;101:1068–1075.
17. Staritz M, Poralla T, Dormeyer H, Buschenfelde K. Endoscopic removal of common bile duct stones through the intact papilla after medical sphincter dilation. *Gastroenterology* 1985;88:1807–1811.
18. Mac Mathuna P, White P, Lennon J, Crowe J. Balloon sphincteroplasty for removal of bile duct stones: an alternative to papillotomy? *Gastroenterology* 1993;104(4):A369.
19. Southern Surgeons Club. A prospective analysis of 1518 laparoscopic cholecystectomies. *N Engl J Med* 1991;324:1073–1078.
20. Deziel DJ, Millikan KW, Economou SG, Doolas A, Ko S, Airan MC. Complications of laparoscopic cholecystectomy: a national survey of 4,292 hospitals and an analysis of 77,604 cases. *Am J Surg* 1993;165:9–14.
21. Davids PHP, Rauws EAJ, Coene PPLO, Tytgat GNJ, Huibregtse K. Endoscopic stenting for postoperative biliary strictures. *Gastrointest Endosc* 1992;38:12–18.
22. Berkelhammer C, Kortan P, Haber GB. Endoscopic biliary prostheses as treatment for benign postoperative biliary strictures. *Gastrointest Endosc* 1989;35:95–101.
23. Geenen DJ, Geenen JE, Hogan WJ, et al. Endoscopic therapy for benign bile duct strictures. *Gastrointest Endosc* 1989;35:367–371.
24. Ponchon T, Galez J-F, Vallette PJ, Chavaillon A, Bory R. Endoscopic treatment of biliary tract fistulae. *Gastrointest Endosc* 1989;35:490–498.
25. Manoukian AV, Schmalz MJ, Geenen JE, Hogan WJ, Venu RP, Johnson K. Endoscopic treatment of problems encountered after cholecystectomy. *Gastrointest Endosc* 1993;39(1):9–14.
26. Foutch PG, Harlan JR, Hoefer M. Endoscopic therapy for patients with a post-operative biliary leak. *Gastrointest Endosc* 1993;39:416–421.
27. Howell DA, Bosco JJ, Sampson LN, Bula V. Endoscopic management of cystic duct fistulas after laparoscopic cholecystectomy. *Endoscopy* 1992;24:796–798.
28. Liguory C, Vitale GC, Lefebre JF, Bonnel D, Cornud F. Endoscopic treatment of postoperative biliary fistulae. *Surgery* 1991;110:779–784.

Advanced Therapeutic Endoscopy, 2nd Ed.,
edited by J. S. Barkin and C. A. O'Phelan.
Raven Press, Ltd., New York © 1994.

CHAPTER 43

Laparoscopic Cholecystectomy: An Underutilized or Overutilized Technique?

Stephen Wise Unger

Since its first published report in 1989 (1) and its dramatic development in the United States and Europe, laparoscopic cholecystectomy has gone from a technical tour de force to a standard of surgical practice with a rapidity unprecedented in modern surgery. This rise in popularity has been fueled by physician interest, industry promotion, and patient demand. The extraordinary postgraduate training program undertaken to satisfy the demand for surgeons in the United States has been a topic of discussion among surgical societies, academic institutions, lay press, government regulatory agencies, third-party carriers, and the legal profession. Clearly, as the furor surrounding the procedure settles down, the medical community will be able to more clearly decide whether this represents an over- or underutilized technique.

This chapter reviews the history, technique, instrumentation, indications, and results of laparoscopic cholecystectomy, and discusses the legitimacy of the utilization of the technique.

HISTORY

While Kelling is usually given credit for originating laparoscopy in 1901, placing a cystoscope in an air-filled abdominal cavity of a dog, the first major series of human laparoscopies, and also thoracoscopies, is credited to H. C. Jacobeus and was reported in 1911 (2). Reports of laparoscopy appeared, detailing small clinical series, well into the 1920s; however, aside from describing changes in position and questioning the insufflating gas choice, none advanced the procedure be-

yond what was originally described. John C. Ruddock (3) described a large, clinical experience of some 500 cases, including laparoscopic biopsies performed in the United States in the 1930s. Janos Veress, in 1938, described the spring-loaded needle that bears his name for use in instituting pneumoperitoneum. Most consider the gynecologist Kurt Semm to be the father of modern laparoscopic surgery. He developed many of the techniques of modern pelviscopy, pioneered hand instrumentation especially modified for those procedures, and developed machines for controlled automatic gas insufflation. As introduction of the Hopkins rod lens system greatly improved the optical portion of the procedure with its adoption in the 1960s (4), the adaptation of video imaging to the procedure in the late 1980s relieved the surgeon of the obligation of holding the scope and allowed him to use both hands, stand up straight, and operate. While Mouret, a French gynecologist, is universally credited with performing the first laparoscopic cholecystectomy (5), the technique was simultaneously developed by several workers in North America and France, including Reddick and Olsen (6), Saye and McKernon (7), Dubois et al. (5), and Perisatt et al. (8).

INSTRUMENTATION

Instrumentation for laparoscopic cholecystectomy has developed rapidly from the crude pelviscopy instrumentation available at the end of the 1980s. At that time, almost all insufflators were low flow, almost all hand instruments were single action with few configurations of tip, and almost all trocars and insufflating needles were nondisposable, having changed very little from the instrumentation used in the 1940s. Light sources were primarily designed for direct viewing and

S. W. Unger: Department of Surgical Endoscopy and Laparoscopy, Mount Sinai Medical Center of Greater Miami, Miami Beach, Florida 33140.

the articulated arms available for teaching or assistance. In describing the instrumentation for present-day cholecystectomy, all modern innovations will be included.

Needles and Trocars

Insufflating needles are used for the initiating step in introducing the pneumoperitoneum. The principle of function is that of a spring-loaded needle with a blunt stylet. As the needle is pressed against the fascia or peritoneum, the needle is exposed, but as the needle pierces and perceives the loss of resistance associated with entrance into the abdominal cavity, the blunt stylet appears. This needle has been modified in disposable form to incorporate the spring-loaded blunt stylet feature, but also to offer a few advantages of guaranteed sharpness and sterility (in particular, precluding the chance of clogging with solid debris and/or dried body fluids). In addition, the spring mechanism is usually encased in plastic and is thus not interfered with by the operator's hand. Finally, there usually is a visual marker demonstrating the presence or absence of the exposed needle tip.

Trocars, disposable and nondisposable, share many characteristics, including a sharp stylet and gas-tight valve and gasket mechanism to allow scope and instrument insertion without loss of insufflating medium. Most have an insufflating port. Newer, disposable trocars incorporate features that make their use safer in laparoscopic surgery and facilitate manipulations. These include safety devices that protect the underlying viscera from the sharp stylet of the trocar; variations include spring-loaded shields that lock over the sharp tip on introduction into the abdominal cavity or trocar tips that actually retract on insertion. In addition, newer devices may include internal balloons or struts to keep the trocar from falling out or a skin adhesive mechanism or screw type shaft to hold the trocar in place. To date there are no data to prove that disposable trocars are safer or even more efficacious. However, there is significant enough surgeon preference, because of the sum of the benefits, to justify the use in spite of their increased cost. Trocars and needles of both disposable and nondisposible varieties are pictured in Fig. 1.

Staplers

A great amount of research and development has gone into the making of automatic stapling devices. In the early 1980s, devices were single-fire staplers that had to be loaded for each use. Present-day staplers feature multiple reloadable fires and do not have to be removed between each firing. This greatly facilitates usage, and in emergency situations where multiple bleeding sites or multiple structures might have to be clipped, offers significant safety advantage (Fig. 2.)

Instrumentation

Initially hand instrumentation was confined to simple straight or curved scissors, single-action ratcheted and nonratcheted clamps for grasping and dissecting, flat spatulas for cautery, and large graspers for extracting tissue or morselating specimens. Intense research and development engendered new features, such as particular variations of tip-gripping surface, rotational ability of shafts, adaptation of monopolar and bipolar

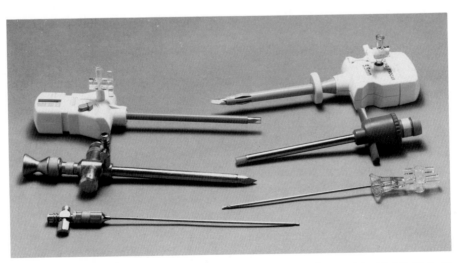

FIG. 1. Two insertion needles *(foreground)*: reusable *(left)* and disposable *(right)*. Note the inclusion of the spring mechanism in the plastic housing on the disposable. There are also two disposable trocars *(background)*, both of which have different safety devices to shield the tip on insertion. The reusable ones *(center)* don't have these safety devices.

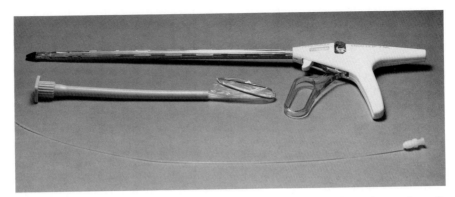

FIG. 2. *(top to bottom)*: An automatic endoscopic stapler that fires 20 staples; an insertion device with a partially exposed plastic retrieving bag; and a cholangiogram catheter, which is the type used for cystic duct cholangiography.

cautery and incorporation of suction irrigation systems into the hand instrumentation. In addition, a host of ancillary devices (Figs. 2 and 3) have been designed to include a variety of collecting bags, tissue graspers, and hand instruments with a variety of unique tips (for example, Babbock, Allis, and Kelly tips), tissue retractors, tissue and stone morselators, and multiple cholangiography devices. Finally, as attention has been directed to the common bile duct, more emphasis has been placed on flexible choledochoscopy instrumentation, including stone baskets, dilating balloons, Fogerty balloons, and crushing instruments including electrical and laser stone fragmenting instrumentation.

Mechanical Equipment

As laparoscopic cholecystectomy has become more sophisticated the actual machine support has also be-

come more sophisticated. Almost essential is a good high-flow insufflator, which allows the surgeon to monitor intraabdominal pressure and CO_2 flow rate and is able to provide high-flow (up to 10 L per minute) insufflation. These high flows obviate the chronic problem of gas leak and loss of pneumoperitoneum with multiple trocars and multiple instruments.

Most operating room configurations include two monitors, one at each of the patient's shoulders, thus allowing the surgeon and assistant to look straight across the table during the procedure. Depending on surgeon and medical center preference, a VCR or still-photography device may be interposed into the system, allowing documentation and archiving of these procedures. The archiving of the visual record, for obvious reasons, is being looked at carefully by both risk management agencies and the legal profession and may be a source of potential liability or protection. No national

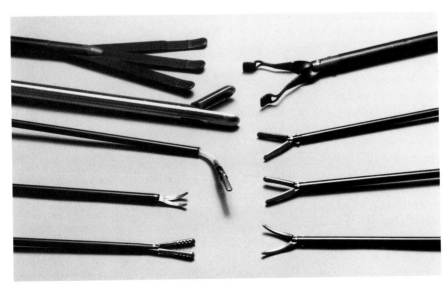

FIG. 3. The variety of tips of hand instruments, and a retractor device *(upper left hand corner)*. These are but some of the many varieties of hand instruments now available on both the reusable and disposable market.

standard for visual documentation has been reached as yet. The camera is a further instrumental variation, and quality of the image is directly related to the sophistication of both the monitor and the camera. The ability of the camera system to process changes in light exposure and to zoom or focus with varying depth of field greatly affects the eventual image.

Suction irrigation systems are also an important part of the hardware armamentarium. These vary from devices as simple as hanging IV bags to complex mechanical devices with pressure jet flow for hydrodissection. The configuration of the suction irrigation probe may vary from devices as simple as a cannula with a single hole on the end to screened tip probes with detachable or inserted hand instrumentation and cauterizing devices.

TECHNIQUE

The vast majority of centers performing laparoscopic cholecystectomies are using variations of the methods of Reddick and Olsen (6). This is a four-trocar technique. In short, after nasogastric and bladder intubation and drainage, the procedure is started by placing a Veress needle in the umbilicus, and a pneumoperitoneum is created. A 10- or 11-mm trocar is then inserted in the umbilicus, pointing toward the pelvis, and, if the patient has had prior surgery in the lower abdomen, an alternate upper abdominal puncture technique is used and a 5-mm trocar may be inserted. This allows visualization of the umbilical area to look for adhesions before placing the larger trocar. Alternatively, the procedure may be a semi-open variation of the Hassan technique (9), and this has been popularized as the primary method of insertion by some authors (10).

Once the abdomen has been accessed, a systematic exploration is accomplished, which should include changes in table position to maximize exposure with reverse Trendelenburg and left side down tilt as the eventual position for the laparoscopic cholecystectomy. Three operating trocars are placed, two 5-mm trocars in the right subcostal anterior axillary line and midclavicular line and a 10- or 11-mm trocar in the epigastrium.

The operation proceeds with elevation of the gallbladder cephalad with grasping forceps placed through the two lateral trocars and operating through the epigastric trocar. The cystic duct is identified and clipped. There is intense controversy (11–15) with respect to whether the cystic duct cholangiogram should be performed or not, but if it is used to delineate anatomy, it is performed by placing a catheter into the cystic duct and either clipping it in place or clamping it to the cystic duct. Once anatomy is defined, the duct and artery are clipped and transected, and the gallbladder

is dissected away from the liver bed. The majority of surgeons are using monopolar cautery, but a minority still use laser and some centers are working with bipolar cautery instrumentation. Finally, the gallbladder is separated from the liver, the laparoscope is transferred to the epigastrium, and the gallbladder is brought out through the umbilicus. The field is irrigated and aspirated, and the wounds are closed. Some centers use fascial sutures for the umbilical closure and some do subcuticular, while others do staple or suture closure of the wounds. A drain may be placed in the right upper quadrant, and this is easily performed laparoscopically.

INDICATIONS

Initial indications for laparoscopic cholecystectomy were very restrictive. In Reddick and Olsen's (6) first series and in the early large series prior to surgery, obesity, old age, and acute cholecystitis were contraindications (5,7,8). As surgical expertise has improved, series devoted to these indications have been published.

Adhesions from prior surgery handled by alternate puncture technique and/or open insertion and adhesiolysis have been dismissed as a potential contraindication (10,16).

Obesity (17–20), initially thought to be a contraindication, can be handled well laparoscopically. The avoidance of short- and long-term wound problems and the early mobilization, decreasing the possibility of pulmonary emboli and pulmonary complications, makes laparoscopy the procedure of choice for obesity. Technical modifications, including cephalad placement of the viewing trocar and occasional use of extra-long trocars and instruments, simplify the procedure.

Elderly patients usually have either a small, contracted gallbladder secondary to multiple attacks over many years or have remarkably floppy, long gallbladders. The scarred, fibrotic, frozen triangle of Calot seen in the contracted gallbladder mandates cholangiography to avoid common bile duct injury (12,13), while floppy, long gallbladders require walking down the fundus with the upper grasper and placing the redundant gallbladder over the liver, thus making the case routine.

Acute cholecystitis (16,21–25) has been described at length by several authors. While not for novices, several technical modifications make these cases manageable. These include rapid needle decompression of the gallbladder, blunt and hydrodissection in the triangle of Calot, aggressive graspers for holding the friable fundus, mandatory cholangiography, and specimen bags for extraction.

Pregnancy may remain as a contraindication (26–28) and portal hypertension may greatly complicate the procedure, although cases have been described in both of these settings.

RESULTS

Initial results by the few centers that began laparoscopic cholecystectomy early were surprisingly free of significant complications. Conversion rates range from 5% to 12%, common bile duct injury rates from 0% to 2%, and in Airan and Ko's (29) review of some 36,000 cases, injuries were very rare, although these studies have been criticized somewhat because of their reliability: an individual's morbidity may be underreported. As larger series appeared documenting multiple inexperienced, but properly trained, surgeons' results, alarming morbidity was identified, especially with respect to cystic duct leaks, common duct injuries, and even death. Estimates from the New York State Health Department (30,31) suggested a technical error rate of 2% in patients undergoing laparoscopic cholecystectomy and the department issued an edict defining criteria to allow surgeons to perform the procedure, including a 15- to 20-case preceptorship. In our series of some 500 patients, common bile duct injury rate is 0%, conversion rate for elective cases is 0%, conversion rate for acute cholecystitis is approximately 5%, and mortality is 0.2%. Not surprisingly, in our center where rigid training and proctorship criteria have been adhered to, our overall morbidity, regardless of the surgeon performing the procedure, with respect to common bile duct and other serious complications has been extraordinarily low.

DISCUSSION

It is estimated that half a million cholecystectomies are performed annually in the United States. Transiently, this number may be even higher since there is a latent population that had avoided open surgery and may be much more willing to undergo laparoscopic surgery. As 50,000 surgeons in the United States have been trained in laparoscopic surgery, laparoscopic cholecystectomy has been developed as a standard of care. Intense study, applying the principles of laparoscopic surgery to almost every manifestation of gallstone disease, has allowed laparoscopic cholecystectomy to be performed electively, in patients regardless of body habitus, in pediatric patients (32,33), in obese and morbidly obese patients, in patients with a significant prior surgery, in patients who have had pancreatitis, in patients with portal hypertension, and in patients with markedly altered anatomy, including situs inversus (34–37).

In short, there are now few contraindications to laparoscopic cholecystectomy, being limited to those patients who are unable to undergo general anesthesia, those patients with refractory and retractable bleeding disorders, those patients with advanced pregnancy, and possibly those patients with carcinoma. More frequently, management of the common bile duct is being addressed by preoperative endoscopic stone removal (38–40) or intraoperative transcystic common duct exploration (41,42) and even laparoscopic common bile duct exploration (43).

Laparoscopic cholecystectomy, for all intents and purposes, has replaced open cholecystectomy in the United States as the primary way of handling gallbladder disease surgically. In that setting it is hard to see it in the long-term as being an over- or underutilized technique. Rather, it is a technique that is being applied to a disease when there is a surgical indication. The unique application of this technology to a specific disease in which the laparoscopic procedure is identical to that done with open surgery, and the operative procedure is simple enough that it can be learned by almost all surgeons with reasonable hand-eye coordination, has made this acceptance almost universal in less than 3 years. The morbidity and mortality rates are still being accumulated, and until the learning curves are completely erased the gold standard for those numbers has not been determined yet. However, one could estimate that, with increasing expertise of the general surgical population, the morbidity of the laparoscopic cholecystectomy should equal or even fall below that of open cholecystectomy.

REFERENCES

1. Reddick EJ, Olsen DO, Daniell JF, Saye WB, McKernon B, Muller W, Hoback M. Laparoscopic laser cholecystectomy. *Laser Med Surg News* 1989;7:38–40.
2. Stellato TA. History of laparoscopic surgery. *Surg Clin North Am* 1992;72:997–1002.
3. Ruddock JC. Peritoneoscopy. *Surg Gynecol Obstet* 1937;65:623.
4. Berci G, Kont LA. A new optical system in endoscopy—with special reference to cystoscopy. *Br J Urol* 1969;41:564.
5. Dubois F, Icard P, Berthelot G, Levard H. Coelioscopic cholecystectomy—preliminary report of 36 cases. *Ann Surg* 1990;211: 60–62.
6. Reddick EJ, Olsen DO. Laparoscopic laser cholecystectomy—a comparison with minilap cholecystectomy. *Surg Endosc* 1989; 3:131–133.
7. McKernon JB. Laparoscopic cholecystectomy. *Am Surg* 1991; 57:309–312.
8. Perisatt J, Collet D, Belliard R. Gallstones: laparoscopic treatment—cholecystectomy, cholecystostomy and lithotripsy. Our own technique. *Surg Endosc* 1990;4:1–5.
9. Hassan HM. A modified instrument and method for laparoscopy. *Am J Obstet Gynecol* 1971;110:886–887.
10. Fitzgibbons RJ, Salerno GM, Filipi CJ. Open laparoscopy. In: Zucker KA, Baily RW, Reddick EJ, eds. *Surgical laparoscopy.* St. Louis: Quality Medical Publishing, 1991;87–97.
11. Blatner ME, Wittgen CM, Andries CH, Kaminski DL. Cystic duct cholangiography during laparoscopic cholecystectomy. *Arch Surg* 1991;126:646–649.

12. Sackier JM, Berci G, Phillips E, Carroll B, Shapiro S, Paz Partlow M. The role of cholangiography in laparoscopic cholecystectomy. *Arch Surg* 1991;126:1021–1026.
13. Corbitt JD, Cantwell DV. Laparoscopic cholecystectomy with operative cholangiogram. *Surg Laparosc Endosc* 1991;1:229–232.
14. Flowers JL, Zucker KA, Graham SM, Scovill WA, Imbembo AL, Baily RW. Laparoscopic cholangiography—results and indications. *Ann Surg* 1992;215:209–216.
15. Lillemoe KD, Yeo CJ, Talamini MA, Wang BH, Pitt HA, Gadacz TR. Selective cholangiography—current role in laparoscopic cholecystectomy. *Ann Surg* 1992;215:669–676.
16. Reddick EJ, Olsen DO, Spaw A, Baird D, Asbun H, O'Reilly M, Fisher K, Saye W. Safe performance of difficult laparoscopic cholecystectomy. *Am J Surg* 1992;161:377–381.
17. Collet D, Edye M, Mague E, Perissat J. Laparoscopic cholecystectomy in the obese patient. *Surg Endosc* 1992;6:186–188.
18. Schirmer BD, Dix J, Edge S, Hyser MJ, Hanks J, Aguilar M. Laparoscopic cholecystectomy in the obese patient. *Ann Surg* 1992;216:146–152.
19. Unger SW, Scott JS, Unger HM, Edelman DS. Laparoscopic approach to gallstones in the morbidly obese patient. *Surg Endosc* 1991;5:116–117.
20. Unger SW, Unger HM, Edelman DS, Scott JS, Rosenbaum G. Obesity: an indication rather than a contraindication to laparoscopic cholecystectomy. *Obesity Surg* 1992;2:29–31.
21. Unger SW, Edelman DS, Scott JS, Unger HM. Laparoscopic treatment of acute cholecystitis. *Surg Laparosc Endosc* 1991;1:14–16.
22. Phillips EH, Carrol B, Bello JM, Fallas MJ, Daykhovsky L. Laparoscopic cholecystectomy in acute cholecystitis. *Am Surg* 1992;58:273–276.
23. Fletcher DR, O'Riordon B, Hardy KJ. Laparoscopic cholecystectomy for complicated gallstone disease. *Surg Endosc* 1992;6:179–182.
24. Wilson RG, MacIntyre IM, Nixon SJ, Sanders JH, Varma JS, King PM. Laparoscopic cholecystectomy as a safe and effective treatment for severe acute cholecystitis. *Br Med J* 1992;305:394–396.
25. Zucker KA, Bailey RW, Flowers J. Laparoscopic management of acute and chronic cholecystitis. *Surg Clin North Am* 1992;72:1045–1068.
26. Arvidsson D, Gerdin E. Laparoscopic cholecystectomy during pregnancy. *Surg Laparosc Endosc* 1991;1:193–194.
27. Schribe JH. Laparoscopic appendectomy in pregnancy. *Surg Endosc* 1990;4:100–102.
28. Soper NJ, Hunter JG, Petrie RH. Laparoscopic cholecystectomy during pregnancy. *Surg Endosc* 1992;6:115–117.
29. Airan MC, Ko ST. Assessment of quality of care in laparoscopic cholecystectomy. *Am Coll Med Qual News* 1992;7:85–87.
30. Newner RP, Imperato PJ, Alcorn CM. Serious complications of laparoscopic cholecystectomy in New York State. *NYS J Med* 1992;92:179–181.
31. Altman LK. *New York Times* June 14, 1992;141:1.
32. Davidoff AM, Branum GD, Murray EA, Chong WK, Ware RE, Kinney TR, Pappas TN, Meyers WC. The technique of laparoscopic cholecystectomy in children. *Ann Surg* 1992;215:186–192.
33. Ware RE, Kinney TR, Casey JR, Pappas TN, Meyers WC. Laparoscopic cholecystectomy in young patients with sickle hemoglobulinopathies. *J Pediatr* 1992;120:58–61.
34. Scott-Connor CE, Hall TJ. Variant arterial anatomy in laparoscopic cholecystectomy. *Am J Surg* 1992;163:590–592.
35. Hugh TB, Kelly MD, Li B. Laparoscopic anatomy of the cystic artery. *Am J Surg* 1992;163:593–595.
36. Campos L, Sipes E. Laparoscopic cholecystectomy in a 39 year old woman with situs inversus. *J Laparosc Surg* 1991;1:123–125.
37. Drover JW, Nguyen KT, Pace RF. Laparoscopic cholecystectomy in a patient with situs inversus viscerum—a case report. *Can J Surg* 1992;35:65–66.
38. Hunter JG, Soper NJ. Laparoscopic management of bile duct stones. *Surg Clin North Am* 1992;72:1077–1097.
39. Arregui ME, Davis CJ, Arkush AM, Nagan RF. Laparoscopic cholecystectomy combined with endoscopic sphincterotomy and stone extraction or laparoscopic choledochoscopy and electrohydraulic lithotripsy for management of cholelithiasis with choledocholiasis. *Surg Endosc* 1992;6:10–15.
40. Vitale GC, Larsen GM, Wieman TJ, Cheadle WG, Miller FB. The use of ERCP in the management of common bile duct stones in patients undergoing laparoscopic cholecystectomy. *Surg Endosc* 1993;7:9–11.
41. Baily RW, Zucker KA. Laparoscopic cholangiography in management of choledocholithiasis. In: Zucker KA, Baily RW, Reddick EJ, eds. *Surgical laparoscopy*. St. Louis: Quality Medical Publishing, 1991;201–225.
42. Appel S, Krebs H, Fern D. Techniques for laparoscopic cholangiography and removal of common duct stones. *Surg Endosc* 1992;6:134–137.
43. Petelin JB. Laparoscopic approach to common duct pathology. *Surg Laparosc Endosc* 1991;1:33–41.

Advanced Therapeutic Endoscopy, 2nd Ed.,
edited by J. S. Barkin and C. A. O'Phelan.
Raven Press, Ltd., New York © 1994.

CHAPTER 44

Advances in Diagnostic Laparoscopy

Anthony Albanese and Lennox J. Jeffers

In the past 5 years, there has been a tremendous resurgence of laparoscopy in the United States and around the world. While gynecologists have been performing, adhesion lysis, cyst drainage, and tubal ligation laparoscopically for many years, more complex procedures to restore fertility and remove diseased ovaries and/or fallopian tubes are now commonly performed (1). Laparoscopic cholecystectomy, appendectomy, herniorrhaphy, hemicolectomy, hiatal hernia repair, and vagotomy are now performed (2–7) and taught to general surgical residents throughout the country. The explosion of articles describing new techniques and equipment has resulted in the birth of two new journals—*The Journal of Laparoendoscopic Surgery* and *Surgical Laparoscopy and Endoscopy*. The use of laparoscopy for diagnosis by gastroenterologists and hepatologists, while less common, has benefited from the new equipment and technology.

NEW EQUIPMENT

There are many reasons for the recent growth in laparoscopic procedures, but the greatest is the enhanced optics provided by video chip technology. Video systems allow an operator to perform laparoscopy from a comfortable position, while assistants, instructors, or colleagues view the procedure on monitors in real time, or later on videocassette. This facilitates performing complex tasks laparoscopically, which would be too difficult for a single operator. Depending on his needs, the laparoscopist can choose from any number of instruments ranging in design from well-known, reliable rigid systems, to new semiflexible

systems with endoscope-like controls (8). With the various rigid systems available, operators may choose forward or oblique viewing optical systems, with either wide angle or distortion-free "flat" lenses. The flexible system is forward viewing and relies on its deflectable tip to allow the laparoscopist to see around corners and view structures at the desired angle (Fig. 1). With either system, video recording and still video photography can be performed at the touch of a button. Mavagraphs can produce high-quality color pictures up to a size of 5" by 7" in less than 1 minute. Some instruments utilize "super image technology," enabling them to produce clear video images that are larger than life-size.

Another recent technological advancement has been the creation of small sonographic probes. These probes range in size from 3 to 20 mm, and several can be passed through a "second puncture" site to scan the gallbladder or common bile duct for stone (9). The design of these probes varies greatly; some use single-element transducers that are mechanically moved, and others use multiple elements to form a sector or linear array scanning device. These high-frequency probes (5 to 20 mHz) give very good resolution of thin structures, but penetration into solid organs has characteristically been poor. Prototype instruments have been used in Italy, Germany, and The Netherlands since 1980, examining solid organs with varying degrees of success. Instruments producing frequencies at the lower end of the spectrum provide better solid organ penetration, but lose fine structural details. In the past few years, instruments have become available that utilize an adjustable multiple focus transducer to provide good resolution and adequate penetration to thoroughly examine the liver and spleen (Aloka, Tokyo) (Fig. 2). The 7.5-mHz electronic linear array sonographic probe can be inserted through a 10-mm trocar and used for any number of indications from staging malignancy to iden-

A. Albanese and L. J. Jeffers: Divisions of Gastroenterology and Hepatology, University of Miami school of Medicine, and Veterans Administration Medical Center, Miami, Florida 33101.

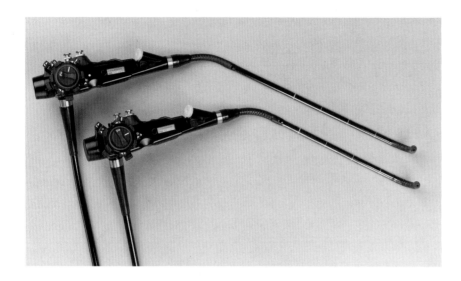

FIG. 1. Flexible laparoscope. 380 mm long *(top)* and length 350 mm *(bottom)*.

tifying biliary stones to determining the vascularity of intraperitoneal structures. Studies are currently under way to determine whether or not this tool can be used to reliably detect masses in the liver, aid in their identification, and guide biopsies.

NEW INDICATIONS

As the indications for surgical laparoscopy have expanded, so have the indications for diagnostic laparoscopy. An excellent, well-referenced review of the role of laparoscopy in staging cancer can be found in the first edition of this book (10). The chapter outlines the use of laparoscopy in patients with esophageal, gastric, pancreatic, gallbladder, biliary, hepatocellular, colonic, and ovarian carcinoma. Also reviewed is the use of laparoscopy for staging lymphoma (Hodgkin's), and diagnosing liver and peritoneal metastatic disease,

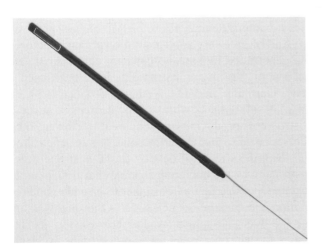

FIG. 2. A 7.5-mHz electronic linear array ultrasound laparoscopic probe with cable attachment.

which may not be detectable by computed tomography (CT) scan. Other recent publications have confirmed the use of laparoscopy in combination with CT in the staging of pancreatic and biliary tract malignancies (11) and early identification of hepatocellular carcinoma (12).

A second area where laparoscopy has proven to be useful is in the diagnosis and treatment of chronic active hepatitis, particularly hepatitis C. Before the FDA approval of second-generation tests for the diagnosis, and α-interferon for the treatment of hepatitis C, the presence or absence of early cirrhosis in a patient with chronic active hepatitis was only of academic interest. Now, a body of literature is evolving that suggests that patients with early cirrhosis do not respond well to standard treatment regimens of interferon therapy (13). These patients should be referred to hepatology centers to possibly undergo new treatment protocols, and should undergo evaluation with the highest degree of sensitivity (that is reasonably possible) to determine the presence or absence of early cirrhosis. Laparoscopic visualization combined with liver biopsy has been shown in multiple studies to be more sensitive at detecting early cirrhosis than liver biopsy alone (14,15). Right and left lobe liver biopsy at the time of laparoscopy is currently the most sensitive technique for determining the presence of early cirrhosis (16).

The third area in which laparoscopy has made new inroads is in the evaluation of abdominal pain. In their recent article on the utility of diagnostic laparoscopy for abdominal pain, Easter et al. (17) found laparoscopy "positive" in 37 of 70 patients (53%) with chronic abdominal pain and 4 of 7 (57%) with acute pain. While 53% positive examinations might not seem like a high yield in the patients with chronic abdominal pain, the strict inclusion criteria (undiagnosed pain for greater than 12 years despite medical evaluation) validate the importance of the test.

The fourth area in which laparoscopy has proven useful is the diagnosis of peritoneal infection. The epidemics of AIDS and drug-resistant tuberculosis have made it necessary to obtain material for culture to accurately diagnose and treat previously unusual peritoneal infections (18–22).

Laparoscopy should be considered in patients with unexplained ascites when fluid analysis and CT of the abdomen and pelvis do not reveal a definitive etiology.

NEW TECHNIQUES

The techniques used to perform diagnostic laparoscopy have changed in more subtle ways than those for surgical laparoscopy. Recent literature has confirmed the safety of performing this procedure in the GI station, revealing no significant difference in wound infections or anesthetic complications when compared to cases performed in the operating room (23,24). Good reviews of the standard diagnostic technique can be found in several textbooks (10,25–27). After giving informed consent for the procedure, the patient may be premedicated with intramuscular injections of 25 to 100 mg of meperidine, 25 to 50 mg of promethazine (to reduce nausea), and 0.6 mg of atropine (to dry secretions, slow bowel motility, and reduce the incidence of vagal-mediated bradycardia). Sedation can be maintained during the procedure with small intravenous aliquots of meperidine and midazolam (or diazepam). The abdomen is prepped and draped in sterile fashion and suitable area for trocar placement (usually 2 cm to the left and 2 cm cephalad of the umbilicus) is anesthetized with 1% lidocaine. In many surgical procedures, the first trocar is placed through the umbilicus. Portal hypertension is suspected in many medical/diagnostic cases, and the immediate periumbilical area is avoided because of its proximity to the falciform ligament and the ligamentum teres. History of major abdominal surgery was previously thought to be a relative contraindication to diagnostic laparoscopy. Several groups have recently demonstrated that it can be performed safely and effectively by placing the initial Veress needle and trocar 5 cm away from the surgical scar, and using direct visual guidance if other trocars are necessary (28,29).

Our surgical colleagues often place the trocar into the peritoneal cavity directly using the Hassan technique. With the patient under general anesthesia, the abdominal wall is dissected down to the parietal peritoneum. The peritoneum is elevated, and incised to permit trocar placement. Pneumoperitoneum is accomplished by instilling CO_2 gas through the trocar. With their patients awake, most gastroenterologists create the pneumoperitoneum by instilling N_2O gas through a Veress needle before inserting the trocar. Because the interaction between CO_2 and H_2O forms irritating carbonic acid on the peritoneal surfaces, N_2O is the preferred gas when the procedure is performed under conscious sedation. Nitrous oxide (N_2O) is not explosive, but unlike CO_2, it will sustain combustion. Heater probe and bipolar electrocoagulation (BICAP) can be performed safely in N_2O (30), but there is a theoretical risk of combustion with spark-producing monopolar electrosurgical instruments. Some gastroenterologists prefer to use air (which also supports combustion and is absorbed less readily than N_2O) for the pneumoperitoneum.

During insufflation, the patient and equipment are continually monitored to ensure that the gas is actually filling the peritoneal cavity and is not creating an artificial cavity or escaping into the subcutaneous tissue. Once the abdomen is tense and tympanic (usually at a pressure of around 20mm Hg), the Veress needle is withdrawn. Pneumoperitoneum is rechecked and the peritoneum is further anesthetized by aspirating peritoneal gas into a syringe filled with 1% lidocaine and injecting the lidocaine when the needle is withdrawn from the cavity. The incision is lengthened horizontally, and the subcutaneous tissue and muscles are bluntly separated with a hemostat before the trocar is inserted. The disposable trocars made by several companies (Ethicon, U.S. Surgical) are a marked improvement over the sterilizable type. Their sharp tips, whether conical or pyramidal, ensure quick passage through the layers of the abdominal wall. Once the tip passes the resistance of the abdominal wall, it is instantly covered by a spring-loaded retractable sheath, which prevents any further cutting. A characteristic popping sound announces the trocars entry into the peritoneal cavity, and then all pushing and twisting should be stopped. The size of the trocars' sleeve may vary from 5 to 15 mm in diameter, depending on the size of the laparoscope. We have found that the 5- and 7-mm instruments provide adequate illumination for direct examination through the scope, but the 10-mm scope is necessary for good quality video laparoscopy and image reproduction.

After the laparoscope is introduced through the sleeve, the area below the insertion site is examined first to determine if any complication (bleeding or perforation) has occurred. The abdominal cavity is then examined in a sequential, orderly fashion, changing patient position and table height as necessary. Most diagnostic examinations require a second puncture, with a 3- or 5-mm trocar, for either biopsy equipment, suction, or a palpating probe. We have long been able to examine, palpate, brush, aspirate, or biopsy intraperitoneal organs, but some laparoscopists in Japan and Europe have been able to examine and biopsy the pancreas (31,32). Examination of parts of the body and tail of the pancreas can be performed via a supragastric approach by elevating the left liver lobe and looking through the usually transparent lesser omentum. The lesser omentum can be grasped, incised, and passed through with a laparoscope to directly examine, or biopsy the pancreas (31). An infragastric approach has also been described, in which the gastrocolic ligament is incised to permit laparoscopic examination of the pancreas (32). Neither of these techniques allows good visualization of the head or uncinate process of the pancreas.

THE FUTURE

The recent trends toward more types of laparoscopic or minimally invasive surgery will continue. Driven by publicity (patients requesting laparoscopic surgery) and economics (shorter recovery periods, and hospital stays), creative surgeons will continue to expand the current boundaries. The indications for diagnostic laparoscopy are also expanding, and the demand for it will also increase. Diagnostic laparoscopy will, in many areas, probably merge with therapeutic laparoscopy, and be taught in surgical residency programs throughout the country.

Video and endosonographic technology will continue to improve. Several centers in the United States, Japan, and Europe are experimenting with computer-assisted videoendoscopy to determine whether neoplasms reflect unique wavelengths of light. If differences too subtle to be noticed with the human eye could be detected by a computer, the impact on endoscopy and laparoscopy would be profound.

REFERENCES

1. Bruhat MA, Mage G, Chapron C, Pouly JL, Canis M, Wattiez A. Present day endoscopic surgery in gynecology. *Eur J Obstet Gynecol Reprod Biol* 1991;41(1):4–13.
2. *New applications of laparoscopy,* 1st ed. Austin: R.G. Landes Company, 1992.
3. Jacobs M, Verdeja JC, Goldstein HS. Minimally invasive colon resection (laparoscopic colectomy). *Surg Laparosc Endosc* 1991;1:8–13.
4. Pier A, Gotz F, Bacher C. Laparoscopic appendectomy in 625 cases; from innovative to routine. *Surg Laparosc Endosc* 1991; 1:144–150.
5. Baird DR, Wilson JP, Manson EM, et al. An early review of 800 laparoscopic cholecystectomies at a university-affiliated community teaching hospital. *Am Surg* 1992;58:206–210.
6. Cuschieri A, Shimi S, Nathanson LK. Laparoscopic reduction, crural repair, and fundoplication of large hiatal hernia. *Am J Surg* 1992;163:425–430.
7. Schirmer BD, Edge SB, Dix J, Miller AD. Incorporation of laparoscopy into a surgical endoscopy training program. *Am J Surg* 1992;163:46–51.
8. Albanese A, Parker T, Vargas C, et al. Safety and efficacy of a new flexible video laparoscope in diagnostic laparoscopy. *Gastrointest Endosc* 1992;38:271.
9. Ascher SM, Evans SR, Goldberg JA, et al. Intraoperative bile duct sonography during laparoscopic cholecystectomy. *Radiology* 1992;185:493–496.
10. Calmet F, Phillips RS, Jeffers LJ. Laparoscopy, role in staging cancer. In: Barkin J, O'Phelan CA, eds. *Advanced therapeutic endoscopy,* 1st ed. New York: Raven Press, 1990;169–182.
11. Kodali V, Reddy R, Parker T, et al. Role of laparoscopy in pancreatico-biliary malignancy. *Gastrointest Endosc* 1992;38:271.
12. Jeffers LJ, Speigelman G, Reddy KR, et al. Laparoscopically guided fine needle aspiration for the diagnosis of hepatocellular carcinoma: a safe and accurate technique. *Gastrointest Endosc* 1988;34(3):235–237.
13. Camma C, Craxi A, Tine F, et al. Predictors of response to alpha-interferon (IFN) in chronic hepatitis C: a multivariate analysis on 361 treated patients. *Hepatology* 1992;16(2):131A.
14. Nord JH. Biopsy diagnosis of cirrhosis: blind percutaneous versus guided under direct vision techniques—a review. *Gastrointest Endosc* 1982;28:102–104.
15. Pagliaro L, et al. Percutaneous blind biopsy versus laparoscopy with guided biopsy in diagnosis of cirrhosis. *Dig Dis Sci* 1983; 28:39–43.
16. Jeffers LJ, Findor A, Thung SN, Reddy KR, Silva M, Schiff ER. Minimizing sampling error with laparoscopic guided liver biopsy of right and left lobes. *Gastrointest Endosc* 1991;37(2): 266.
17. Easter D, Cuschieri A, Nathanson L, Lavelle-Jones M. The utility of diagnostic laparoscopy for abdominal disorders. *Arch Surg* 1992;127:379–383.
18. Phillips EH, Carroll BJ, Chandra M, et al. Laparoscopic guided biopsy for diagnosis of hepatic candidiasis. *J Laparoendosc Surg* 1992;2:33–38.
19. Jamidar PA, Campell DR, Fishback JL, Klotz SA. Peritoneal coccidioidomycosis associated with human immunodeficiency virus infection. *Gastroenterology* 1992;102:1054–1058.
20. Bhargave DK, Shriniwas, Chopra P, Nihjawan S, Dasarathy S, Kushwaba AKS. Peritoneal tuberculosis: laparoscopic patterns and its diagnostic accuracy. *Am J Gastroenterol* 1992;87: 109–112.
21. Jeffers LJ, Alzate I, Reddy KR, et al. Laparoscopic findings in AIDS and ARC patients. *Gastrointest Endosc* 1991;37(2):267.
22. Mimica M. Usefulness and limitations of laparoscopy in the diagnosis of tuberculous peritonitis. *Endoscopy* 1992;24:588–591.
23. Puccio JE, Kulesza MD, Gordon SC. Should gastroenterologists perform diagnostic laparoscopy in the operating room? *Am J Gastroenterol* 1992;87:1303.
24. Reddy R, Findor A, Jeffers L, et al. Are operating room and anesthesiologist necessary for the performance of diagnostic laparoscopy? *Gastrointest Endosc* 1991;37(2):235.
25. Dagnini G. *Laparoscopy and imaging techniques.* New York: Springer-Verlag, 1990.
26. Boyce W. Laparoscopy. In: Schiff L, Schiff E, eds. *Diseases of the liver,* 6th ed. Philadelphia: JB Lippincott, 1987;444–456.
27. Nord HJ. Technique of laparoscopy. In: Sivak MV, ed. *Gastroenterologic endoscopy,* 1st ed. Philadelphia: WB Saunders, 1987;994–1029.
28. Molina E, Reddy R, Albanese A, et al. Diagnostic laparoscopy in patients with previous extensive abdominal surgery. *Gastrointest Endosc* 1992;38:271.
29. Marti-Vicente A, et al. Peritoneoscopy examination following abdominal operations. *Gastrointest Endosc* 1979;25:144–145.
30. Jeffers LJ, McDonald TJ, Hyder S, et al. The use of two new coagulation probes for control of hemorrhage in laparoscopic liver biopsy. *Gastrointest Endosc* 1989;35:398–402.
31. Ishida H. Peritoneoscopy and pancreas biopsy in the diagnosis of pancreatic disease. *Gastrointest Endosc* 1983;3:211–218.
32. Strauch M, Lux G, Ottenjan R. Infragastric pancreoscopy. *Endoscopy* 1973;5:30–32.

Advanced Therapeutic Endoscopy, 2nd Ed.,
edited by J. S. Barkin and C. A. O'Phelan.
Raven Press, Ltd., New York © 1994.

CHAPTER 45

Role of Diagnostic Laparoscopy in the Staging of All Patients with Gastrointestinal Malignancies

H. Juergen Nord

Diagnostic laparoscopy is one of the oldest gastrointestinal endoscopic procedures, dating back to the turn of the century. Newer noninvasive imaging studies like ultrasonography (US) and computed tomography (CT) have emerged in the 1980s as preferred methods to evaluate the abdomen. They permit image-directed biopsy of abnormal lesions and have led to an overall decline of laparoscopy.

The 1990s, however, have seen a resurgence of new interest in laparoscopy. This is especially true in the rediscovery of laparoscopy by surgeons and a plethora of new data on laparoscopic cholecystectomy and other endoscopic surgical procedures. As the surgical utilization of laparoscopy increases, a new emphasis has been placed on the diagnostic potential of laparoscopy, especially for the evaluation of patients with chronic liver disease, focal liver disease, ascites of unknown cause, diseases of the peritoneum, and the staging of malignancies, especially those involving the gastrointestinal tract. Likewise, well-controlled studies have emerged attesting to the superiority of diagnostic laparoscopy over other imaging studies, especially in the accurate staging of patients with metastatic lesions less than 1 cm in diameter.

CANCER STAGING

As medical and surgical therapy of malignancies has made substantial progress, accurate tumor staging has a major impact on patient management. If a tumor is

found to be limited to the primary site, a curative resection is possible. If the patient undergoes surgery and the tumor is found to have spread beyond its original boundaries, the patient does not benefit from laparotomy, faces the added risk of surgical morbidity and mortality, and is in most cases more appropriately managed with palliative measures.

The TNM method of tumor staging involves the prospective evaluation of patients prior to any therapy in an attempt to determine if the tumor is confined to its original site, has extended to adjacent organs [tumor (T)], involves regional lymph nodes (N), or has spread to distant sites [metastasis (M)]. Tumor staging has a major impact on selection of therapy as well as patient prognosis.

Patients with suspected focal liver disease are a common problem facing the clinician while staging intraabdominal malignancies. This problem may present itself in three different clinical settings. The patient has a primary carcinoma and liver metastases are suspected on clinical grounds (hepatomegaly) or because of abnormal liver function studies. The patient may undergo hepatic US or CT scanning for other reasons and unsuspected focal defects are noted. The question arises: Are the nodules benign or are they malignant lesions? In a patient with known primary carcinoma, hepatic imaging studies may be normal, but metastases are suspected for other reasons. It is important that the true nature of a proven or suspected focal liver defect be determined with the most reliable test, which must include histologic confirmation. Laparoscopy is ideally suited for this purpose.

Surgical and autopsy series have demonstrated that in patients with metastatic liver disease, the hepatic

H. J. Nord: Department of Medicine, Division of Digestive Diseases and Nutrition, University of South Florida, College of Medicine, Tampa, Florida 33606.

surface is involved in 90% (1,2). With proper technique about two-thirds of the hepatic surface can be inspected and biopsied at laparoscopy (3). The left lobe is easily evaluated, an area that is difficult and risky to biopsy percutaneously. Only the most superior region of the right lobe and posterior aspects of both lobes cannot be seen at laparoscopy. Large intrahepatic lesions frequently present with a surface bulge and deep biopsies are usually positive. Small intrahepatic lesions are usually missed. New laparoscopic US probes may increase the diagnostic yield in these situations. One of the main values of laparoscopy lies in the fact that lesions only millimeters in size on the liver, omentum, or peritoneum can be identified and biopsied (4). These foci are usually below the resolution of even newer generation scanners. In situations where a forceps or needle biopsy is technically difficult or risky, cytology by aspiration or abrasion yields excellent results (5,6). In patients with a vascular tumor, like hepatocellular carcinoma, the bleeding risk with needle or forceps biopsy may be substantial. Fine needle aspiration cytology is safe and can have an accuracy of 100% (7).

LAPAROSCOPY VERSUS OTHER IMAGING STUDIES

Ultrasound and/or CT of the abdomen are accepted steps in the initial staging of patients with gastrointestinal malignancy. They have a high degree of sensitivity but differentiation of cirrhosis from focal lesions and false-positive and, more importantly, false-negative results remains a problem (8). If a focal defect is identified with imaging, image-guided biopsy and laparoscopic direct vision biopsy yield comparable results (9). The problem remains for a negative scan or when hepatic or omental/peritoneal lesions are suspected. The superiority of laparoscopy in this clinical setting has been confirmed by several studies (4,9,10). In a study by Brady et al. (10), 47% of negative scan patients had either benign (26%) or malignant (21%) hepatic lesions. The predictive value of a negative CT scan was only 50%; it was 89% for laparoscopy. It would have been 100% if technically unsatisfactory examinations in two patients due to adhesions were excluded. In a follow-up study of 25 patients with suspected metastatic disease but negative CT scan, laparoscopy documented malignancy in 48%. Of those with exudative ascites, 75% had peritoneal metastases (10). In 40 patients with pancreatic cancer and no evidence of peritoneal or hepatic spread by CT scan, 35% were found to have metastases at laparoscopy (4). In three a false-negative laparoscopy had to be considered technically incomplete since a palpating probe was not used in all cases

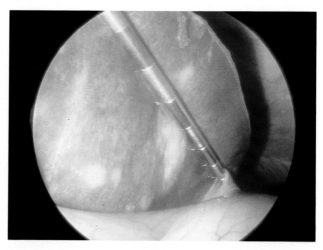

FIG. 1. Adenocarcinoma of the pancreas, metastatic to the undersurface of the left hepatic lobe. This lesion would have been missed without use of the palpating probe. (Reprinted with permission from ref. 28.)

(Fig. 1). Furthermore, it was stated that some of the lesions noted at laparoscopy were so small that they would have easily escaped surgical detection. There is little question that a negative US/CT scan in patients with suspected intraabdominal malignancy is not an appropriate end point of investigation. Laparoscopy is indicated in these patients and will have a significant diagnostic yield.

GASTROINTESTINAL CANCERS

The most common tumors that metastasize to the liver are those of the colon, pancreas, breast, and lung. Laparoscopy therefore will at times detect intraabdominal malignancy that does not have its origin in the abdominal cavity. In some cancers associated with alcohol abuse, like cancer of the esophagus and pancreas, it is often difficult to determine if abnormal liver function tests, hepatomegaly, and abnormal imaging studies are due to chronic liver disease, e.g., cirrhosis or metastatic disease, or if a hepatocellular carcinoma is complicating chronic liver disease. Laparoscopy can settle this dilemma reliably in most cases.

Then should all patients with gastrointestinal malignancies undergo laparoscopic tumor staging prior to surgery? It is difficult to make categorical rules for all cases since these decisions depend on many individual patient factors, the philosophy of the surgeon and oncological team, as well as local availability and endoscopic skill. Ideally, most but not necessarily all patients will benefit. However, before an attempt of curative surgical resection is made, all diagnostic modalities should be exhausted, which includes laparoscopy in many cases to assure that the patient's tumor is correctly and accurately staged.

Hepatocellular Carcinoma

Hepatocellular carcinoma (HCC) is one of the most common malignant tumors in the world. However, in the United States and Western Europe the tumor is relatively rare, with only 1 to 5 cases per 100,000 population. At the time of diagnosis the tumor is usually far advanced, with a poor outlook and short survival time—in North America less than 18 weeks (11). Laparoscopy is suited for confirmation of the diagnosis of HCC by direct vision biopsy and cytology, for detection of peritoneal spread, usually missed by other imaging studies, and for assessment of extent and severity of associated cirrhosis, which frequently determines prognosis and resectability in otherwise localized disease (12). Ultrasonography is the best screening and initial imaging study (together with alpha-fetoprotein). It is especially useful in the detection of vascular invasion, which makes the patient unresectable. However, it diagnosed cirrhosis in only 25 of 54 patients, while laparoscopy found cirrhosis in 42 patients and small peritoneal lesions in 5, all missed with US (13). In selected cases where curative resection seems possible, forceps biopsies should be avoided because of the risk of spreading tumor cells. In one study of 27 consecutive patients fine needle aspiration had an accuracy of 100%, all were found to be unresectable (7). In a French study multifocal disease was noted in 28 of 43 patients (14).

Lightdale (15) reported 11 of 14 patients to be unresectable because of various endoscopic criteria. Of three operated patients one had peritoneal metastases missed at laparoscopy, one had vascular involvement, and one is a long-term survivor. In small lesions it can be difficult to differentiate HCC from regenerating nodules. Clues that can aid the endoscopist and suggest the need for biopsy or cytology include irregular nodules of variable size and color. These lesions are usually lighter in color and often whitish yellow. Even in these difficult cases, the overall diagnosis can be confirmed laparoscopically in 93% of cases (16). In certain select cases of HCC, especially the fibrolamellar cell type, hepatic transplantation has been considered if no extrahepatic spread is present. Metastases on the peritoneum, including the diaphragm and omentum, which preclude successful transplant are usually not detected by US or CT scans but can be clearly recognized at laparoscopy. Ascites, a contraindication to percutaneous liver biopsy, does not preclude laparoscopy and biopsy (12).

In the staging of HCC, US and laparoscopy both have their value and should be considered complementary because the highest diagnostic accuracy is achieved when both procedures are combined (15,17,18).

Carcinoma of the Gallbladder

Gallbladder carcinoma rarely presents with signs, symptoms, or laboratory and x-ray findings that allow a preoperative diagnosis. In the largest series of patients studied laparoscopically, only 10% were suspected clinically. Evidence of metastases to liver and omentum were found in 89 of 98 patients and only 9 were considered resectable. It is of interest that the tumor was partially obscured in 21 of the patients and completely in another 29. In only half could the gallbladder be fully examined. However, because of widespread metastases the diagnosis could be confirmed in almost all patients (19). Similar results were found in another study (20) that confirmed metastatic disease in 81% of 48 patients. The combination of US and laparoscopy confirmed the diagnosis in 100% of cases.

With the increased utilization of laparoscopic cholecystectomy, this aggressive cancer may be diagnosed more frequently and, it is hoped, at an earlier stage.

Pancreatic Cancer

Pancreatic carcinoma carries a poor prognosis and even after "curative" resection tumor recurrence is high. About 35% to 40% of patients considered to have localized disease by imaging studies will have metastatic disease at the time of surgery. Warshaw et al. (4,21) have demonstrated the value of staging laparoscopy in two studies (the first has been previously mentioned). In 35% of 40 patients considered resectable by preoperative studies, laparoscopy demonstrated tumor spread. In all cases the laparoscopic findings changed the management plan. In 88 patients with pancreatic and ampullary carcinoma, using a multifaceted approach of CT, magnetic resonance imaging (MRI), angiography, and laparoscopy plus biopsy, 90% of unresectable tumors were correctly identified. Laparoscopy detected 96% of patients with peritoneal and liver implants (21).

Similar results were obtained in a third study where 42 of 51 patients with preoperative laparoscopy were correctly staged as inoperable. Of the remaining nine patients judged to be resectable, only four were found to be operable. While the majority of hepatic lesions were correctly found with preoperative imaging, omental and peritoneal implants were only noted at laparoscopy (22).

With the ability to adequately palliate patients with cancer of the head of the pancreas and obstructive jaundice with endoscopic or percutaneous stents, surgery has little room in the management of these patients except if intestinal obstruction is imminent (Fig.

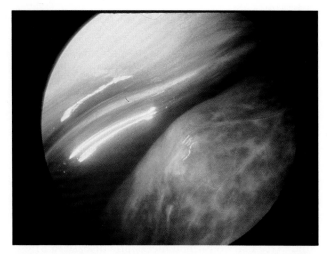

FIG. 2. Adenocarcinoma of the pancreas with obstructive jaundice and ascites, metastatic to the right hepatic lobe. This patient is best palliated with an endoscopically placed biliary stent.

2). The goals of therapy are surgical resection for cure in the small group of patients with truly limited disease, and palliation by nonsurgical means for those unfortunate ones with extensive disease, in an effort to avoid the morbidity and mortality of needless surgery.

Esophageal Carcinoma

Squamous cell carcinoma of the esophagus and adenocarcinoma of the gastroesophageal junction, which has been increasing in recent years, are usually diagnosed at an advanced stage and patients present as poor operative risks. Surgery for these lesions carries one of the highest mortalities for any elective surgical procedure. With a multitude of palliative options available, like radiation therapy, dilation, laser therapy, prosthesis, and photodynamic therapy, adequate palliation and relief of obstruction can be achieved at a low risk. Surgery should be reserved for candidates with a chance for cure after extensive staging, which should also include endoscopic ultrasonography and laparoscopy.

Dagnini et al. (23) demonstrated in a large series distant metastases in one out of four patients. In 369 patients single or multiple metastases were found in 23.7%. Of 250 patients who went to surgery, false-negative findings were found in only 4.4%. This compares favorably to the false-negative rate of 29% for US. It is not surprising that cirrhosis was found in 14.3% of patients, since heavy alcohol consumption is considered a risk factor for esophageal cancer. In 6.7% surgery was rejected because of cirrhosis and severe portal hypertension with otherwise limited disease. Others have confirmed liver metastases in 16% with a false-positive rate for CT scan of 19% in esophageal cancer

(24). A Dutch study, however, found that CT, with no false-negative results and only one false-positive test in 49 patients, was sufficiently sensitive, and laparoscopy was therefore no longer warranted in the routine staging of esophageal cancer (25).

Gastric Cancer

Gastric adenocarcinoma generally has a poor outlook. Palliative surgery has a place in distal gastric cancer with outlet obstruction as well as patients with bleeding when palliative measures like laser therapy fail. Otherwise, surgery should be reserved for those patients with a true chance for curative resection. In a large series of 360 patients, the accuracy of laparoscopy for detecting metastases was 96.5%, clearly superior to other imaging studies (26). In 40 patients considered resectable by US and CT and studied preoperatively by laparoscopy, 40% were found to be unresectable. Of 23 patients who subsequently went to surgery, the tumor could be resected in 20 (27) (Fig. 3).

Patients with gastric carcinoma will greatly benefit from presurgical laparoscopy. In a significant number of patients the subsequent course of therapy will be affected by the endoscopic findings.

Colon Carcinoma

There is little information on the role of laparoscopy in the evaluation of patients with colorectal cancer. The indications for surgery are usually obstruction and bleeding. Preoperative staging is important from a standpoint of prognosis and the decision for adjuvant

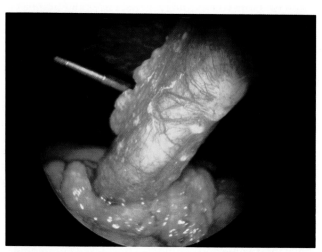

FIG. 3. Adenocarcinoma of the stomach, metastatic to the round ligament. These flat lesions are usually missed with US and CT but easily identified and biopsied at laparoscopy. Note the marked tumor neovascularity.

therapy. The decision for surgery is rarely affected. In patients with rising carcinoembryonic antigen (CEA) levels after surgery, the cause is often liver metastases. A ''second look'' surgery is a frequent next step. When surgical resection of isolated liver metastases is considered, especially if they are late metastases, laparoscopy would offer a reasonable alternative to surgical explorations in these patients to assure that one is indeed dealing with a solitary lesion, provided the liver is not obscured by postoperative adhesions. However, this concept has not been subjected to study.

CONCLUSION

Laparoscopy for staging of intraabdominal malignancies has a high sensitivity and specificity. It is especially useful in cases where metastatic disease is suspected and imaging studies are negative. Laparoscopy is highly accurate and clearly superior to US and CT in this subset of patients. If the decision for surgery is not affected by the presence or absence of metastases, as in patients with obstruction or bleeding, or if surgery provides significant palliation compared to other modalities in patients who are good surgical risks, laparoscopy is not indicated. The greatest value of laparoscopy lies in the fact that it can significantly affect the decision for a curative resection in patients with cancer of the esophagus, stomach, pancreas, and hepatocellular carcinoma, who will not benefit from surgery and are thus not subject to the insult of a needless operation under the guise of palliation if metastases are found (Fig. 4). With many alternatives to palliative surgery available, these patients are best served by nonoperative means. In the staging for patients with gastrointestinal malignancies, laparoscopy is best used selectively, as outlined above.

Laparoscopy is technically easy and safe, it can be performed with conscious sedation only, and it is comparable in cost to image-guided biopsy and significantly less expensive than surgical exploration (28,29).

REFERENCES

1. Foster JH, Berman MM. *Solid liver tumors.* Philadelphia: WB Saunders, 1977.
2. Hogg L, Pack GT. Diagnostic accuracy of hepatic metastases at laparotomy. *Arch Surg* 1956;72:251.
3. Whitcomb FF, Gibbs SP, Boyce HW. Peritoneoscopy for the diagnosis of left lobe lesions of the liver. *Arch Intern Med* 1978;138:126.
4. Warshaw AL, Tepper JE, Shipley WU. Laparoscopy in the staging and planning of therapy for pancreatic cancer. *Am J Surg* 1986;151:76.
5. Cusso X, Marti-Vincente A, Mon'es-Xiol J, Vilardell F. Laparoscopic cytology, an evaluation. *Endoscopy* 1988;20:102.
6. Hajdu SI, E'Ambrosio FG, Fields V, et al. Aspiration and brush cytology of liver. *Semin Diagn Pathol* 1986;3:227.
7. Jeffers L, Speiglman G, Reddy R, et al. Laparoscopically directed fine needle aspiration for the diagnosis of hepatocellular carcinoma: a safe and accurate technique. *Gastrointest Endosc* 1988;34:335.
8. Leuschner M, Leuschner U. Diagnostic laparoscopy in focal parenchymal disease of the liver. *Endoscopy* 1992;24:698.
9. Brady PG, Goldschmid, Chappel G, et al. A comparison of biopsy techniques in suspected focal liver disease. *Gastrointest Endosc* 1987;33:289.
10. Brady PG, Peebles M, Goldschmid S. Role of laparoscopy in the evaluation of patients with suspected hepatic or peritoneal malignancies. *Gastrointest Endosc* 1991;37:27.
11. Kassianides C, Kew MC. The clinical manifestation and natural history of hepatocellular carcinoma. *Gastroenterol Clin North Am* 1987;16:553.
12. Nord HJ, Brady PG. Endoscopic diagnosis and therapy of hepatocellular carcinoma. *Endoscopy* 1993;25:126.
13. Gandolfi L, Muratori R, Solmi L, et al. Laparoscopy compared with ultrasonography in the diagnosis of hepatocellular carcinoma. *Gastrointest Endosc* 1989;35:508.
14. Etienne JP, Chaput JC. La laparoscopie dans le cancer primitif du foie de l'adulte. *Ann Gastroenterol Hepatol (Paris)* 1973;49.
15. Lightdale CJ. Laparoscopy and biopsy in malignant liver disease. *Cancer* 1982;50:2672.
16. Kameda Y, Shinji Y, Nishiuchi M, et al. Detection of minute hepatocellular carcinoma with fatty metamorphosis by laparoscopy. *Endoscopy* 1988;20(suppl):A29.

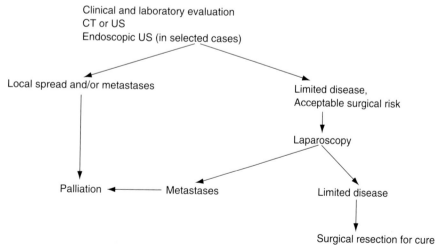

FIG. 4. Staging of gastrointestinal malignancies.

17. Fornari F, Rappaccini GL, Cavanna L, et al: Diagnosis of hepatic lesions: ultrasonically guided fine needle biopsy or laparoscopy. *Gastrointest Endosc* 1988;34:231.

18. Brady PG. Laparoscopy and ultrasonography in the diagnosis of hepatocellular carcinoma [Editorial]. *Gastrointest Endosc* 1989; 35:577.

19. Dagnini G, Marin G, Patella M, et al. Laparoscopy in the diagnosis of primary carcinoma of the gallbladder. *Gastrointest Endosc* 1984;30:289.

20. Kriplani A, Jayant S, Kapur B. Laparoscopy in primary carcinoma of the gallbladder. *Gastrointest Endosc* 1992;38:326.

21. Warshaw AL, Gu Z, Wittenberg J, et al. Preoperative staging and assessment of resectability of pancreatic cancer. *Arch Surg* 1990;125:230.

22. Cuschieri A. Laparoscopy for pancreatic cancer: does it benefit the patient? *Eur J Surg Oncol* 1988;14:41.

23. Dagnini G, Caldironi MW, Marin G, et al. Laparoscopy in abdominal staging of esophageal carcinoma. *Gastrointest Endosc* 1986;32:400.

24. Lightdale CJ, Kelsen DP, Kurtz RC, et al. Staging of the liver in patients with carcinoma of the esophagus with CT and laparoscopy. *Gastrointest Endosc* 1984;30:(A)147.

25. Den Hartog Jager FC, Gortzak E. Peritoneoscopy in the diagnosis of liver metastases. *Dev Oncol* 1984;24:132.

26. Possik RA, Franco EL, Pires DR, et al. Sensitivity, specificity, and predictive value of laparoscopy for the staging of gastric cancer and for the detection of liver metastases. *Cancer* 1986;58:1.

27. Kriplani AK, Kapur ML. Laparoscopy for pre-operative staging and assessment of operability in gastric carcinoma. *Gastrointest Endosc* 1991;37:441.

28. Nord HJ. Technique of laparoscopy. In: Sivak M, ed. *Gastroenterologic endoscopy*. Philadelphia: WB Saunders, 1987;994.

29. Boyce HW, Nord HJ. Laparoscopy. In: Yamada T, ed. *Textbook of gastroenterology*. Philadelphia: JB Lippincott, 1991; 2465.

Advanced Therapeutic Endoscopy, 2nd Ed.,
edited by J. S. Barkin and C. A. O'Phelan.
Raven Press, Ltd., New York © 1994.

CHAPTER 46

Endoscopic Management of Acute Gallstone Pancreatitis

David L. Carr-Locke

Over the last decade, as the technique of, and competency with, therapeutic endoscopic retrograde cholangiopancreatography (ERCP) have evolved, its application to pancreatic disorders has gained increasing attention. The procedures, previously applied to the biliary tract, include pancreatic sphincterotomy of both the major and minor papilla, pancreatic endoprosthesis placement, nasopancreatic drainage, extraction and lithotripsy of pancreatic stones, and balloon or catheter dilatation of pancreatic duct strictures or its orifice. Current nonendoscopic pancreatic treatment modalities are often unsatisfactory in terms of efficacy, morbidity, or inapplicability, such that endoscopic treatment is an attractive alternative. The aims of therapy in pancreatitis are to alleviate acute pain and prevent recurrent attacks.

Early identification of those patients presenting with acute pancreatitis due to gallstone disease is important, as emergency intervention may prevent the development of local and systemic complications. Urgent biliary surgery carries an unacceptably high morbidity and mortality, but ERCP in experienced hands appears to be safe and is the optimal method for the diagnosis of bile duct stones. Two randomized controlled prospective trials have shown an advantage for endoscopic sphincterotomy and bile duct clearance compared with supportive therapy when performed within 24 to 72 hours of admission in those patients considered severe on prognostic scoring systems.

D. L. Carr-Locke: Department of Endoscopy, Brigham and Women's Hospital, and Department of Medicine, Harvard Medical School, Boston, Massachusetts 02115.

ETIOLOGY

Gallstones and alcohol represent the commonest etiologic factors associated with over 80% of the cases of acute pancreatitis. There is an extensive list of other associated conditions (1) with approximately 10% of cases remaining unexplained (2,3). Gallstones are the most common single cause of acute pancreatitis in the Western world and parts of Asia (2–4). The clinical course of acute pancreatitis is variable and there are several established criteria to predict prognosis.

PATHOGENESIS

In 1901, Opie (5) reported a patient who died of fatal pancreatitis with an autopsy demonstrating a small stone impacted at the ampulla of Vater (Fig. 1). He reasoned that this allowed reflux of bile into the pancreatic duct. The "obstructive" theory has been supported by appearances at operative cholangiography and in animal studies, but the importance of bile reflux has been questioned (6). Gallstones are recovered in the feces of 85% to 95% of the cases of acute pancreatitis compared with a 10% recovery in patients with symptomatic cholelithiasis without pancreatitis (7). In patients with acute pancreatitis undergoing urgent operative intervention, an incidence of common bile duct (CBD) stones as high as 63% to 78% has been reported compared with patients undergoing delayed operative procedures with a 3% to 33% incidence of CBD stones (7,8). An alternative hypothesis of an incompetent sphincter of Oddi facilitating reflux of activating duodenal contents containing lysolecithin, bacterial toxin, and enterokinase into the pancreatic duct has been proposed and may be explained by previous gallstone pas-

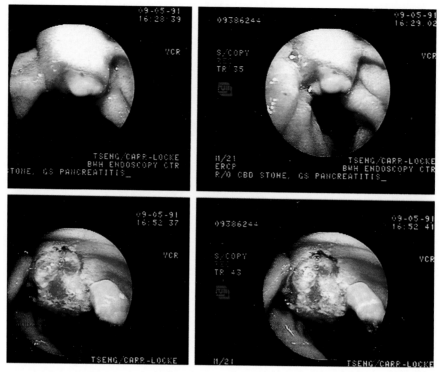

FIG. 1. Endoscopic appearances of impacted stone at the time of ERCP performed during an episode of acute pancreatitis.

sage. Elements of both obstructive and reflux theories seem plausible and may conceivably occur in concert.

MICROLITHIASIS

Up to 30% of patients with acute pancreatitis are considered idiopathic after a careful search for an etiology is unrevealing. This should include a detailed history, laboratory evaluation, and imaging studies with ERCP to exclude alcoholism, hereditary factors, abdominal trauma, pregnancy, medications, infections, hypertriglyceridemia, hypercalcemia, gallstones, tumors of the ampulla or pancreas, sphincter of Oddi dysfunction, vasculitis, penetrating ulcer disease, or congenital anomalies (9). The concept that stones, too small to be visualized on conventional imaging, might cause pancreatitis was proposed more than 50 years ago (10), and recent studies (11,12) have confirmed these previous suggestions that there is an association between microlithiasis and recurrent pancreatitis.

Lee et al. (13) found a 36% incidence of idiopathic pancreatitis in 86 consecutive patients after a conventional workup failed to identify an etiology. These 31 patients were evaluated for the presence of microlithiasis (calcium bilirubinate granules or cholesterol monohydrate crystals) by microscopic examination of centrifuged bile obtained at ERCP or by duodenal

drainage following cholecystokinin (CCK) stimulation. Twenty-three (74%) of those initially classified as idiopathic were found to have evidence of biliary microlithiasis. Serial ultrasonographic examination was positive in only 52% of those patients with microlithiasis, indicating the complementary role of these two diagnostic modalities. Two of the 23 patients with microlithiasis were excluded from the study due to the detection of dilated bile ducts at ERCP. Of the remaining 21 patients, 6 underwent cholecystectomy (microlithiasis in all six pathologic specimens and stones in four), 4 underwent endoscopic papillotomy, and 11 received no definitive therapy. The patients who underwent treatment with papillotomy or cholecystectomy experienced fewer recurrences of acute pancreatitis during follow-up compared with untreated patients (10% vs. 73%). Furthermore, the one treated patient who experienced subsequent pancreatitis and all 9 of the 11 untreated patients who had follow-up bile analysis were found to have persistent microlithiasis on microscopic examination, suggesting but not proving a cause-and-effect relationship between microlithiasis and recurrent pancreatitis. The clinical course of biliary sludge–associated pancreatitis was similar to that of gallstone pancreatitis with a high risk of recurrence for both when left untreated. Pancreatitis should no longer be considered idiopathic until biliary microlithiasis has been excluded.

These findings are remarkably similar to those previously reported by Ros et al. (14). They found a 67% prevalence of microlithiasis in patients with idiopathic pancreatitis, and uncontrolled treatment with cholecystectomy or dissolution therapy (ursodeoxycholic acid) prevented recurrence of pancreatitis in 30 of 31 patients.

Buscail et al. (15) reported the results of endoscopic collection of bile during ERCP in 72 consecutive patients, 50 with proven cholelithiasis (group I) and 22 with clinically suspected stones not demonstrated on ultrasonography or cholangiography (group II). Among the 22 group II patients, 11 had idiopathic pancreatitis and 11 biliary colic associated with transient increase in liver function studies. Microlithiasis was demonstrated in the bile of 41 of the 50 (82%) group I patients. Among the group II patients, all seven with a positive bile examination were subsequently found to have biliary calculi, five at the time of endoscopic sphincterotomy and two in cholecystectomy specimens. None of these seven individuals experienced recurrent biliary or pancreatic symptoms during a mean follow-up of 13 months. In the 15 group II patients without microlithiasis, only one was subsequently shown to have a CBD stone. Based on these results, microscopic examination of bile obtained at ERCP had a sensitivity, specificity, positive predictive value, and negative predictive value of 83%, 100%, 88%, and 93%, respectively, for the presence of occult biliary calculi. This confirms the belief that many such patients have very small gallstones not demonstrable on conventional imaging studies. The possibility that pancreatitis itself might predispose to sludge formation, thereby only serving as a marker for pancreatitis and acting as an innocent bystander, cannot be refuted by these studies. While this may be true in some instances, microlithiasis has a significant association with what was previously termed "idiopathic" pancreatitis. Prospective randomized studies are required to define the clinical spectrum of sludge-associated pancreatitis. The current logical recommendation would seem to be cholecystectomy, reserving dissolution therapy or sphincterotomy for the poor operative risk patient.

PREDICTION OF SEVERITY AND OUTCOME

The majority of patients with acute pancreatitis fully recover within a week or so of the attack with conservative management alone. A mortality of about 10% is reported in unselected clinical series (1). Stratifying patients into mild and severe categories is helpful in directing appropriate management. This stratification also allows direct comparison between groups studied at different institutions and comparison between different treatment modalities. Ranson (3) developed an 11-

TABLE 1. Ranson's criteria to predict severity in acute pancreatitis

On admission	
Age	>55 years
WCC	>16,000/mm^3
Glucose	>200 mg/dl
LDH	>350 U/l
AST	>250 U/l
At 48 hours	
Hct fall	>10%
BUN rise	>5 mg/dl
Ca	<8 mg/dl
PaO$_2$	<60 mm Hg
Base deficit	>4
Sequestration	>6 liters

Severe = 3 or more of the above criteria

From ref. 3.

TABLE 2. Imrie's criteria (modified) to predict severity in acute pancreatitis

Age	>55 years
WCC	>15,000/mm^3
BUN	>45 mg/dl
Glucose	>180 mg/dl
Albumin	<3.2 g/dl
Ca	<8 mg/dl
PaO$_2$	<60 mm Hg
LDH	>500 IU/l

Severe = 3 or more of the above criteria

From ref. 17.

TABLE 3. Apache II scoring system

1. Physiological points
   Temperature
   Mean arterial BP
   Heart rate
   Respiratory rate
   PaO$_2$
   Arterial pH
   Serum sodium
   Serum potassium
   Serum creatinine
   Hematocrit
   White cell count
   Glasgow coma score
2. Age points
3. Long-term health points
   Liver
   Cardiovascular system
   Respiratory system
   Renal system
   Immune system

Total Apache Score = 1 + 2 + 3

TABLE 4. *Balthazar CT grading*

A	Normal
B	Pancreatic enlargement
C	Peripancreatic infiltrate
D	One extrapancreatic fluid collection
E	Two or more extrapancreatic fluid collections

From ref. 18.

factor system to predict severity (Table 1) and Imrie's group (16) proposed a more simplified eight-factor system. A modified Imrie system is now widely used in Europe (17) (Table 2). The validity of these systems is now accepted and they are widely applied to stratify patients. Additional methods of predicting severity such as Apache II scores (Table 3), C-reactive protein concentrations, computed tomography (CT) grading (Table 4), trypsinogen activation peptide (TAP), leukocyte elastase, peritoneal lavage, and others are increasingly being used (18,19).

URGENT TREATMENT

Surgical

Early surgical intervention to prevent progression of the current attack to one of greater severity and to reduce the chance of recurrence has been challenged due to the high risk of surgical morbidity and mortality. The majority of cases of acute pancreatitis fall into the mild category and respond to conservative management alone. Those cases predicted severe by either Ranson or Glasgow criteria cause the greatest controversy. Common bile duct stones are found in 30% to 60% of the patients who die from gallstone-associated pancreatitis, but these stones are not always impacted in the ampulla. Evaluation of the surgical literature on the treatment of gallstone-associated pancreatitis remains difficult because patients have not usually been stratified into mild or severe cases and historical controls are often used to compare results. Acosta et al. (4) reported only 1 death in 46 patients (2.2%) in the group treated by urgent surgical intervention as compared with 14 deaths in 86 patients (16%) of the historical control group, and Stone et al. (8) undertook a randomized prospective study with 1 death in 36 patients (2.8%) for urgent surgery and 2 deaths in 29 patients (6.9%) for early or delayed surgery, but in neither study was there any differentiation between mild and severe cases. Ranson (3) urged nonoperative intervention after experiencing a high mortality for surgery during the acute phase of gallstone pancreatitis. In the most recent prospective randomized surgical study Kelly and Wagner (20) demonstrated a mortality rate of 48% in patients with predicted severe attacks operated upon

early compared with a still unacceptable 11% mortality rate for those operated upon later. Thus, surgical opinion would point toward avoidance of biliary surgery during the acute phase of pancreatitis, especially when classified as severe.

Endoscopic

The initial application of ERCP and endoscopic sphincterotomy (ES) in acute gallstone-associated pancreatitis began as sporadic case reports from various centers around the world (1). The feared complications of endoscopic sphincterotomy, including exacerbation of pancreatitis, cholangitis, hemorrhage, and perforation, were not realized. All authors commented on how rapidly some patients improved with establishment of effective drainage and normalization of laboratory values.

The Leicester group published the first prospective randomized controlled trial of urgent ERCP for acute pancreatitis due to gallstones (21). They randomized 121 patients with gallstone pancreatitis to receive either conventional conservative treatment or to undergo urgent ERCP (within 72 hours), accompanied by ES and stone extraction only in those whose ERCP showed stones in the CBD (Fig. 2). Patient stratification was based on modified Glasgow criteria. Sixty-two patients were randomized to conventional treatment and 59 patients were randomized to ERCP. Common bile duct stones were found in 63% of the predicted severe group but only 26% of those with predicted mild attacks. All bile duct stones were removed endoscopically without complication. This study had four important findings (Table 5): (a) ERCP could be safely performed in acute pancreatitis by an experienced endoscopist; (b) there was a significant reduction in major complications of severe acute pancreatitis secondary to gallstones following ERCP, ES, and stone extraction (12% morbidity compared with 61% morbidity in the conventional group); (c) this reduction was also observed for mortality in those with predicted severe attacks; (d) urgent sphincterotomy nearly halved the hospital stay for those with severe attacks (median 9.5 days versus 17 days). A statistical difference in mortality was not demonstrated. This study provided a rational basis for the application of ERCP/ES and stone extraction in cases of acute pancreatitis associated with gallstones.

A second prospective study from Hong Kong (22), randomized 195 patients with acute pancreatitis of whom 127 had stone disease at ERCP. Sixty-four were randomized to ERCP within 24 hours and ES performed in 37 (58%) as stones were present. In the 63 treated conventionally, 22 subsequently underwent ERCP because of deterioration and 10 each were found

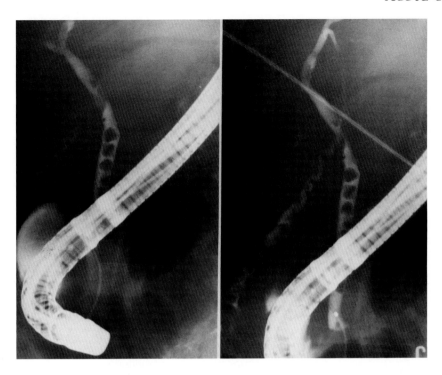

FIG. 2. Radiograph during ERCP for severe acute pancreatitis with several small bile duct stones prior to endoscopic removal.

TABLE 5. *Acute biliary pancreatitis prospective trial ERCP/ES, 1983–87, Leicester*

| | Number of cases | Complications | | Death | Morbidity |
		Pancreas/biliary	Systemic		
Mild	68				
ERCP	34	3	1	0	4 (12%)
Conventional	34	4	0	0	4 (12%)
Severe	53				
ERCP	25	3	3	1 (4%)	6 (24%)
Conventional	28	8	12	5 (18%)	17 (61%) ($p = .007$)

From ref. 21.

to have bile duct stones and gallbladder stones. As in the British study, there was no difference in outcome in the conventionally treated and ERCP groups for those patients with "mild" prognostic scores, but for those with "severe" scores the morbidity was 54% compared with 13% and the mortality 18% compared with 3%, respectively (Table 6). This report from Hong Kong provides important information for those concerned with the management of acute gallstone-associated pancreatitis. It should, however, be considered in conjunction with the only other published prospective randomized controlled trial of ERCP and endoscopic sphincterotomy (ES) in this condition from the United Kingdom (21), which concluded that ES was of significant benefit only in patients with severe acute pancreatitis in whom there was also an increased incidence

TABLE 6. *Acute biliary pancreatitis prospective trial ERCP/ES, 1988–91, Hong Kong*

| | Number of cases | Complications | | Death | Morbidity |
		Pancreas/biliary	Systemic		
Mild	114				
ERCP	56	6	2	0	8 (14%)
Conventional	58	5	1	0	6 (10%)
Severe	81				
ERCP	41	4	5	5 (12%)	9 (22%)
Conventional	40	10	13	9 (23%)	23 (58%) ($p = .003$)

From ref. 22.

of bile duct stones compared with mild cases. While the mechanism for this effect is not fully understood and may be complex, the eradication of concomitant biliary sepsis might play an important role in reducing morbidity and mortality in this subgroup. Thus, the principal findings of the Hong Kong study that ERCP and ES performed within 24 hours of admission reduced biliary sepsis in patients with mild and severe pancreatitis is supportive of the same contention.

The conclusion that all patients with acute pancreatitis should therefore undergo emergency ERCP cannot, however, be extrapolated to other parts of the world for the following reasons: choledocholithiasis is the predominant cause of acute pancreatitis in Hong Kong and it is not uncommon for there to be no coexistent cholelithiasis [21 of 64 (33%) in this report]; there was no attempt at preselection of patients with stone disease compared with other etiologies that would not be appropriate in other geographical areas, as was the case with the previous series; ERCP was used both for diagnosis and therapy, without other imaging modalities; the prognostic scoring system employed probably overpredicted the number of patients with severe pancreatitis, which may have had a significant impact on the incidence of bile duct stones between mild and severe groups and the interpretation of outcome; although there was no statistical difference in morbidity (18% vs. 29%) and mortality (5% vs. 9%) between the ERCP and conservatively treated groups, comparison of outcome in patients with a "severe" score reveals an overall complication rate of 22% versus 57.5%, a local complication rate of 10% versus 28%, and a systemic complication rate of 20% versus 32.5%, respectively. Analysis for those patients with bile duct stones and severe pancreatitis accentuates these differences further.

It should be concluded that the findings from Hong Kong add support for expert endoscopic intervention in acute gallstone-associated pancreatitis at an early stage, but that only patients with severe disease are likely to derive benefit.

ACKNOWLEDGMENT

The author would like to acknowledge the assistance of Dr. Angelo Ferrari in the preparation of the illustrations.

REFERENCES

1. Carr-Locke DL. Endoscopic treatment of biliary acute pancreatitis. In: Beger, Buchler, Malfertheiner, eds. *Standards in pancreatic surgery.* Berlin, Heidelberg: Springer-Verlag, 1993;127–134.
2. Goodman AJ, Neoptolemos JP, Carr-Locke DL, Finlay DB, Fossard DP. Detection of gallstones after acute pancreatitis. *Gut* 1985;26:125–132.
3. Ranson JHC. Etiologic and prognostic factors in human acute pancreatitis: a review. *Am J Gastroenterol* 1982;77:633–638.
4. Acosta JM, Peligrini CA, Skinner DB. Etiology and pathogenesis of acute biliary pancreatitis. *Surgery* 1980;88:118–125.
5. Opie EL. The etiology of acute hemorrhagic pancreatitis. *Johns Hopkins Hosp Bull* 1901;121:182–188.
6. Lerch MM, Saluja AK, Runzi M, Dawra R, Saluja M, Steer ML. Pancreatic duct obstruction triggers acute necrotizing pancreatitis in the opossum. *Gastroenterology* 1993;104:853–861.
7. Acosta JM, Ledesma CL. Gallstone migration as a cause of acute pancreatitis. *N Engl J Med* 1974;290:484–487.
8. Stone HH, Fabian TC, Dunlop WE. Gallstone pancreatitis: biliary tract pathology in relation to time of operation. *Ann Surg* 1981;194:305–310.
9. Steinberg WM. Acute pancreatitis—never leave a stone unturned. *N Engl J Med* 1992;326:635–637.
10. Bockus HL, Sahy H, Willard JH, Pessel JF. Comparison of biliary drainage and cholecystography in gallstone diagnosis with special reference to bile microscopy. *JAMA* 1931;96:311–317.
11. Block MA, Priest RJ. Acute pancreatitis related to minute stones in a radiographically normal gallbladder. *Am J Dig Dis* 1967;12:934–938.
12. Neoptolemos JPN, Davidson BR, Winder AF, Vallance D. Role of duodenal bile crystal analysis in the investigation of "idiopathic" pancreatitis. *Br J Surg* 1988;75:450–453.
13. Lee SP, Nicholls JF, Park HZ. Biliary sludge as a cause of acute pancreatitis. *N Engl J Med* 1992;326:589–593.
14. Ros E, Navarro S, Bru C, Garcia-Puges A, Valderrama R. Occult microlithiasis in 'idiopathic' acute pancreatitis: prevention of relapses by cholecystectomy or ursodeoxycholic acid therapy. *Gastroenterology* 1991;101:1701–1709.
15. Buscail L, Escourrou J, Delvaux M, Guimbaud R, Nicolet T, Frexinos J, Ribet A. Microscopic examination of bile directly collected during endoscopic cannulation of the papilla. Utility in patients with suspected microlithiasis. *Dig Dis Sci* 1992;37:116–120.
16. Osborne DH, Imrie CW, Carter DC. Biliary surgery in the same admission for gallstone-associated pancreatitis. *Br J Surg* 1981;68:758–761.
17. Leese T, Shaw D. Comparison of three Glasgow multifactor prognostic scoring systems in acute pancreatitis. *Br J Surg* 1988;75:460–462.
18. Banks PA. Predictors of severity in acute pancreatitis. *Pancreas* 1991;S7–12.
19. Karimgani I, Porter KA, Langenvin RE, Banks PA. Prognostic factors in sterile pancreatic necrosis. *Gastroenterology* 1993;104:1636–1640.
20. Kelly TR, Wagner DS. Gallstone pancreatitis: a prospective randomized trial of the timing of surgery. *Surgery* 1988;104:600–605.
21. Neoptolemos JP, Carr-Locke DL, London NJ. Controlled trial of urgent endoscopic retrograde cholangiopancreatography and endoscopic sphincterotomy versus conservative treatment for acute pancreatitis due to gallstones. *Lancet* 1988;2:979–983.
22. Fan ST, Lai ECS, Mok FPT, Lo CM, Zheng SS, Wong J. Early treatment of acute biliary pancreatitis by endoscopic papillotomy. *N Engl J Med* 1993;328:228–232.

Advanced Therapeutic Endoscopy, 2nd Ed.,
edited by J. S. Barkin and C. A. O'Phelan.
Raven Press, Ltd., New York © 1994.

CHAPTER 47

Endoscopic Management of Chronic Pancreatitis

Kenneth F. Binmoeller and Nib Soehendra

Chronic pancreatitis is a morphologically multifaceted disease that may present with ductal strictures, stones, and pseudocysts. Encouraged by the successes of therapeutic biliary endoscopy, endoscopists have begun to apply techniques commonly utilized in the biliary tree to the treatment of pancreatic disorders. The techniques described in this chapter, which include pancreatic sphincterotomy, stone extraction, stenting of strictures, and drainage of pseudocysts and abscesses, are still considered largely investigational. However, there is accumulating evidence that these techniques are beneficial when used for the proper indication.

GOAL OF ENDOSCOPIC TREATMENT

Ductal obstruction leading to increased ductal and tissue fluid pressures is thought to be a major factor in the pathogenesis for pancreatic pain and recurrent attacks of pancreatitis (1,2). Surgical procedures to improve ductal drainage have been shown to result in striking relief of pancreatitis pain in a high percentage of cases (3,4). The aim of endoscopic treatment is to accomplish the same result as surgical decompression, but with lower mortality and morbidity.

Currently, the principal indication for surgical or endoscopic decompressive treatment is intractable pain. According to traditional teaching, ductal decompression will not impact upon the natural history of chronic pancreatitis. There is, however, experimental evidence that pancreatic blood flow and exocrine function improve after decompression (5–8). A prospective clinical study by Nealon et al. (9) demonstrated a delay in

K. F. Binmoeller and N. Soehendra: Department of Endoscopic Surgery, University Hospital Eppendorf, Hamburg, Germany.

functional impairment following early surgical drainage. Only 16% of patients who had drainage developed progressive disease, as compared to 71% who did not. A report by Amman et al. (10) revealed regression of calcification in a third of patients with chronic pancreatitis, the majority of whom had ductal drainage. These studies raise the question of whether relief of pancreatic hypertension early in the course of chronic pancreatitis can arrest progression and possibly even lead to regression of disease.

PANCREATIC SPHINCTEROTOMY

Endoscopic incision of the pancreatic sphincter is commonly a preliminary step to access the pancreatic duct for interventional procedures. Pancreatic sphincterotomy may be indicated when papillary stenosis is suspected to be the underlying cause of chronic pancreatitis. Pancreatic sphincterotomy is performed in an analogous manner to biliary sphincterotomy using a standard Erlangen sphincterotome. Because the intramural segment of the pancreatic duct is shorter than that of the bile duct, the risk of sphincterotomy is inherently greater. To minimize complications, no more than 0.5 cm of the cutting wire should be in contact with tissue when performing the sphincterotomy. We use a papillotome with a short (15-mm) wire. Bowing of the wire should be avoided since this may result in a sudden "zipper" incision. The wire is oriented in the one o'clock position and the incision is made in millimeter increments for a length of about 0.5 cm. Either pure cutting or blended current can be used. The power setting will vary according to the type of diathermy unit employed.

In experienced hands, success rates for pancreatic sphincterotomy approach 90%. Complication rates appear to be similar to those of biliary sphincterotomy (11,12). Huibregtse et al. (13) reported two cases of mild pancreatitis and one perforation in their series of 22 pancreatic sphincterotomies. Cremer et al. reported three cases of cholangitis and one case of hemobilia following pancreatic sphincterotomy in their series of 76 patients (12); they advocated performing a biliary sphincterotomy prior to pancreatic sphincterotomy to avoid biliary complications. In contrast, we have not observed biliary complications associated with selective pancreatic sphincterotomy.

Stenting for Ductal Strictures

The most common finding on endoscopic retrograde pancreatography (ERP) in chronic pancreatitis is a stricture of the main pancreatic duct with upstream dilatation. A stricture may be dominant or multifocal, the latter giving the pancreatogram a typical "chain of lakes" appearance. Ductal strictures can be dilated with catheters or balloons. However, the dilating effect is short-lived, and most endoscopists will follow dilatation by stent placement.

Technique

Following a diagnostic ERP, a sphincterotomy of the pancreatic orifice is usually performed in the manner described previously. A guidewire is passed through the stricture and a Teflon dilating catheter inserted over the guidewire (Fig. 1A). Contrast medium may be injected through the catheter at this point to define the ductal anatomy proximal to the stenosis. The dilating catheter is exchanged for a stent, which is then inserted over the guidewire using a pusher tube (Fig. 1B).

In general, strictures of the pancreas are more difficult to negotiate than biliary strictures. The recent availability of hydrophilic guidewires (Terumo Glidewire, Tokyo, Japan; Tracer wire, Wilson-Cook Medical, Inc., Winston-Salem, NC) has made the passage of tight strictures much easier and safer. Hydrophilic guidewires have a special polymer coating that becomes extremely slippery following immersion in water. The core is made of a titanium/nickel alloy that is steerable and does not kink. Wires with straight and curved tips are available; the 0.032-inch angulated wire is most commonly used. The stricture is negotiated by combining to-and-fro movements with torque. Hydrophlic guidewires are not well suited for over-the-wire stent placement and therefore should be exchanged for a conventional Teflon-coated stainless steel guidewire for this purpose.

Standard pancreatic stents are tubes made of Teflon, polyethylene, or polyurethane with multiple side holes for drainage of side branches. Ductal anchorage is afforded either by pigtails or flaps. We use a stent with a slightly curved tip at the proximal end and flaps at the distal end (Wilson-Cook Medical, Inc). The choice of stent diameter (usually 5, 7, or 10 French) and length depends upon the severity and location of the stricture. The largest stent size should be placed to provide maximal drainage. If a stricture is very tight, a 5-Fr stent can be initially placed and exchanged several weeks later for a larger stent as the stricture dilates.

Results

Preliminary results of stent placement for pancreatic duct strictures have been encouraging. The procedure was technically successful in 72% to 100% of cases reported in published series (12–16). Failure occurred primarily in patients with pancreas divisum (see section below). Improvement of pain has been reported in 75% to 94% of cases, although follow-up was variable (2–69 months). We have treated 93 patients with dominant strictures of the pancreatic duct by stent drainage (5–10 Fr); 69% reported significant improvement of symptoms (amelioration of pain and weight gain) over a mean follow-up of 3.5 years (17).

Pancreatitis following placement of pancreatic stents has been reported by several authors (13–15). This was usually mild and subsided spontaneously. It is unclear whether stent placement increases the risk of pancreatitis above that associated with pancreatography and pancreatic sphincterotomy. McCarthy et al. (18) found that stent insertion alone did not increase the incidence of post-ERCP pancreatitis.

As encountered with biliary stents, pancreatic stents may occlude over time. The exact mechanism is not well understood, but is probably triggered by bacterial colonization (19). Patients may remain asymptomatic if there is adequate drainage alongside the stent, but most patients will experience a relapse of symptoms. Stent patency rates have been found to be extremely variable, with some stents remaining patent for several years. Cremer et al. (12) found the mean stent patency to be 12 months, whereas Geenen and Rolny (20) reported frequent clogging at 4 to 6 months. It is generally recommended that stents be exchanged periodically, usually every 6 months. We perform stent exchanges on an outpatient basis.

Self-expandable metallic stents, which are capable of expanding to a size severalfold greater than standard plastic prostheses, may improve stent patency rates (12). To date, there are no randomized studies evaluating their application in the pancreatic duct. The major problem with currently available expandable stents is that they cannot be removed once having been implanted. Concern about long-term safety has discouraged the application of expandable stents for benign disease.

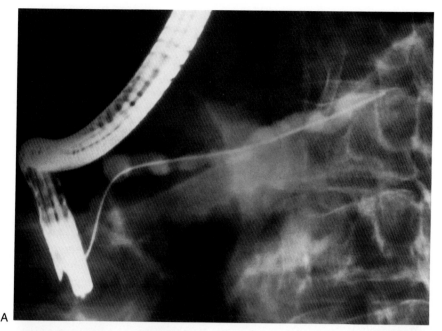

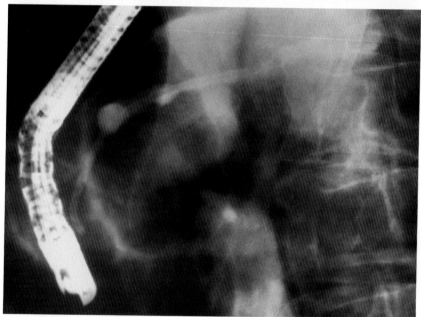

FIG. 1. Pancreatograms showing **A:** guidewire introduced through a dominant stricture in the head portion of the pancreas into a dilated pancreatic duct, and **B:** 7-Fr pancreatic stent inserted into the pancreatic duct.

Stent migration may cause a variety of complications. Duodenal migration may cause injury to the visceral wall. Proximal migration into the duct is usually harmless, but perforation leading to abscess formation has been reported (21). Removal of a proximally migrated stent may be difficult (see chapter "Technique for Retrieval of Migrated Biliary and Pancreatic Stents," by Binmoeller and Soehendra). Various instruments including the mini-snare, basket, and forceps have been used. A special stent removal device (Soehendra stent retriever, Wilson-Cook Medical, Inc.) may be used to remove and replace plastic stents over an indwelling guidewire (22,23). If the above mea-

sures fail, placement of a second stent alongside the original stent can be attempted.

Stents have been reported to induce pancreatic ductal changes of chronic pancreatitis such as ductal dilation and pseudocyst formation. In a retrospective study by Kozarek (24) new ductal changes were observed in six of nine patients with occluded stents, and 3 of 29 patients with nonoccluded stents. These changes normalized or improved after stent removal in the majority of patients. The preliminary results in a study by Derfus et al. (25) confirmed these findings. In their series of 36 patients, 83% had mild to marked pancreatic ductal changes at the time of stent removal;

most changes resolved over time. These studies raise concerns about the long-term consequences of pancreatic stent placement but should not discourage further studies evaluating pancreatic stents. In particular, different stent designs and mechanisms to delay stent clogging warrant investigation.

PANCREAS DIVISUM

Pancreas divisum occurs in approximately 6% of the general population. Because the minor papilla is much smaller than the major papilla, a modified technical approach to sphincterotomy is necessary. The minor papilla is first cannulated with a fine guidewire. We prefer to use a hydrophilic guidewire (0.028-inch with an angulated tip) since it is less prone to cause papillary trauma than a conventional guidewire. A tapered tip catheter (Universal Catheter, Wilson-Cook Medical, Inc.) is used to position the guidewire at the orifice of the minor papilla; with the guidewire slightly extended from the catheter tip, the orifice is gently probed to enter the duct of Santorini. Following cannulation, the wire is advanced under fluoroscopic control into the dorsal duct. The catheter is then pushed over the wire and the hydrophilic guidewire exchanged for a conventional 0.035-inch Teflon-coated wire (26).

Sphincterotomy of the minor papilla can be performed by one of two approaches. A mini-papillotome can be inserted over the guidewire and a 2- to 3-mm incision made (26). Alternatively, a 5 or 7 Fr stent can be inserted across the minor papilla and the sphinctero-

tomy performed over the stent using the needle knife (Fig. 2). The prosthesis serves as a guide rail for the incision. The latter approach is the more popular and is represented in most published studies.

Results of endoscopic therapy in patients with pancreas divisum have been generally favorable (14,16,27–29). In a randomized controlled study of 19 patients with pancreas divisum and acute recurrent pancreatitis, dorsal duct stenting was found to result in significant objective and subjective clinical improvement (28). Lehman et al. (29) evaluated minor sphincterotomy in 52 patients with pancreas divisum and pancreatitis pain and found a significant benefit in patients with acute recurrent pancreatitis, but not in patients with chronic pancreatitis or chronic pain. We have placed stents (3–10 Fr) in 14 symptomatic patients with pancreas divisum accompanied by a dominant dorsal duct stricture of chronic pancreatitis; a significant improvement of symptoms occurred in 71% of patients (mean follow-up of 58 months).

REMOVAL OF PANCREATIC DUCT STONES

Following an adequate pancreatic sphincterotomy, ductal stones can be extracted in the same manner as biliary duct stones using a small Dormia basket or balloon catheter (Fig. 3). Small stones may pass spontaneously.

Although there is some controversy as to whether stones contribute to pancreatic pain, several series have reported pain relief and clinical improvement fol-

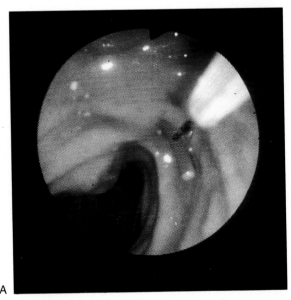
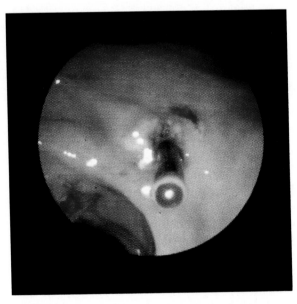

A   B

FIG. 2. Endoscopic views showing minor papilla sphincterotomy over an indwelling stent. **A:** A 7-Fr stent has been inserted into the minor papilla. The needle knife is positioned for minor papilla sphincterotomy. **B:** A small incision has been made.

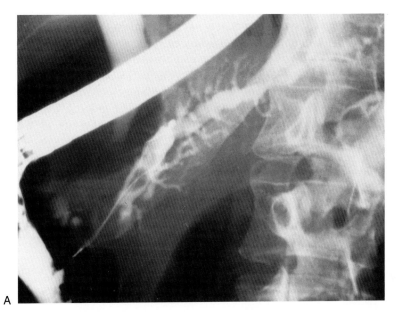
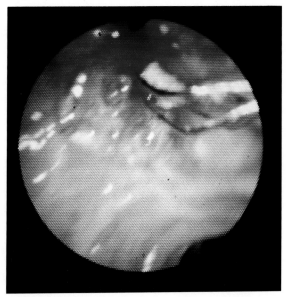

A   B

FIG. 3. Pancreatic stone extraction with the Dormia basket. **A:** Pancreatogram showing stone entrapment with the opened basket. **B:** Endoscopic view of a whitish stone extracted through a pancreatic sphincterotomy.

lowing endoscopic stone extraction (11,13,30). In a study comprising 32 patients with main pancreatic duct stones located primarily in the head, endoscopic extraction was successful in 72% of patients, and 69% improved after endoscopic therapy (30). In patients who failed stone extraction, 50% had partial symptomatic improvement from the pancreatic sphincterotomy alone.

In contrast to biliary stones, pancreatic duct stones are more commonly associated with proximal strictures, making them more difficult to extract. In our experience basket extraction after sphincterotomy was successful in only one-fifth of patients with pancreatic duct stones. To facilitate stone extraction in these difficult cases, several investigators have applied extracorporeal shock wave lithotripsy (ESWL) to fragment stones (31–33). Results have shown high success rates for fragmentation and subsequent ductal clearance, resulting in pain relief in the majority of patients. No significant complications related to ESWL treatment have been reported.

As an alternative to ESWL, pancreatic duct stones can be fragmented intraductally using laser lithotripsy. Experience is currently limited, but preliminary results using the pulsed dye laser have shown this modality to be effective and safe (34,35). An advantage over ESWL is the ability to perform the sphincterotomy, laser procedure, and extraction of fragments at a single session. The pulsed dye laser can be applied under fluoroscopic control or direct vision using an ultrathin miniscope that can be passed via the working channel of the duodenoscope into the pancreatic duct (Fig. 4).

Since there is a risk of ductal wall injury, the latter would seem to be the preferred approach (26).

DRAINAGE OF PSEUDOCYSTS

Depending on the anatomical conditions, pseudocysts can be endoscopically drained by two ap-

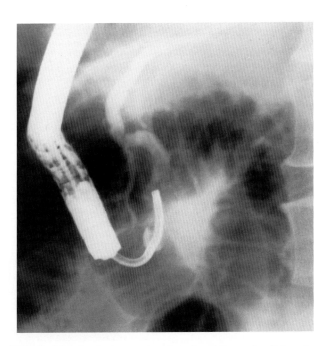

FIG. 4. Pancreatogram showing insertion of a "daughter" miniscope through a "mother" duodenoscope to access the pancreatic duct for intraductal electrohydraulic shock wave lithotripsy.

proaches. Pseudocysts communicating with the pancreatic duct can be drained via the transpapillary route by stent or nasopancreatic catheter placement. Pseudocysts impinging directly upon the stomach or duodenal wall can be drained transmurally by endoscopic cystgastrostomy or endoscopic cystduodenostomy.

Technique

Transpapillary pseudocyst drainage (Fig. 5) is an extension of ductal stenting. Ideally, the stent or nasopancreatic catheter should be inserted directly into the cyst. However, passing a stent across the pancreatic duct leak is often adequate (36).

To appropriately select patients for transmural drainage, the proximity of the cyst to the stomach or duodenum should be established by computed tomography or ultrasonography. At endoscopy, there should be prominent bulging of the stomach or duodenal wall at the site of cyst impingement. The mucosa will typically have a mosaic-type pattern at the site of wall compression.

A diagnostic cyst puncture is initially performed to identify the optimal site of endoscopic drainage. A cystoenterotostomy is then performed to establish a conduit through the wall. This can be accomplished with a variety of endoscopic instruments including the needle knife, papillotome, and laser (36–39). To maintain

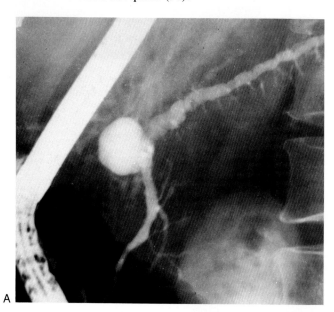
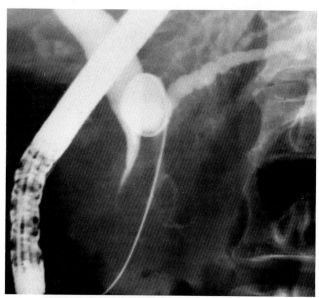
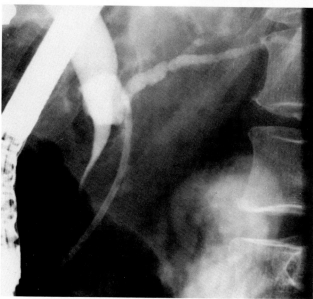

FIG. 5. Pancreatograms showing transpapillary pseudocyst drainage. **A:** A 2 × 2 cm pseudocyst in the head of the pancreas communicating with the pancreatic duct. **B:** Guidewire inserted into the pseudocyst. The biliary tree has been opacified and shows a long, tapered distal common bile duct stricture. **C:** A 7-Fr stent inserted into the draining the pseudocyst.

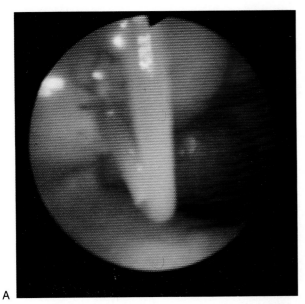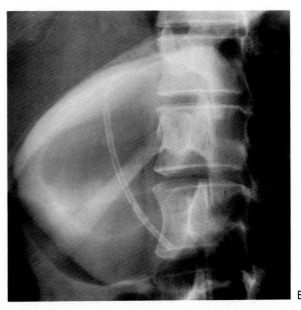

A   B

FIG. 6. Transgastric drainage of a pseudocyst with a 10-Fr stent. **A:** Endoscopic view immediately after stent insertion. A stream of fluid is shown flowing from the distal stent opening. **B:** Abdominal plainfilm showing the 10-Fr stent in the pseudocyst cavity filled with contrast.

drainage, a 10 Fr pigtail stent or nasocystic catheter is inserted over a conventional Teflon-coated guidewire (Fig. 6). Alternatively, Sahel (38) prefers to perform a large (8–20 mm) cystoenterostomy using the papillotome.

To simplify cystoenterotostomy, we devised an instrument that allows for a diagnostic puncture and immediate guidewire placement as a one-step procedure (40). The instrument consists of a retractable injection catheter containing a diathermic wire and an outer 7 Fr Teflon sheath (Fig. 7). Cyst puncture with the injection catheter is facilitated by the application of cautery. Contrast medium is injected through the injection catheter to confirm cyst puncture. The outer sheath is then

Diathermic
Wire

20 G Needle

7 Fr Outer Sheath

|← 15 mm →|

FIG. 7. Instrument for transmural pseudocyst puncture consisting of a retractable inner injection catheter contained in an outer 7-Fr Teflon sheath. Current is applied to the injection needle via a diathermic wire that runs through the inner catheter. Following cyst puncture, the outer sheath is advanced into the cyst and the injection catheter exchanged for a guidewire (40).

advanced into the cyst cavity and the injection catheter exchanged for a guidewire. Cremer et al. (41) have described a similar instrument for cystoenterotostomy consisting of a 10 Fr diathermic sleeve that can be passed over a diathermic needle catheter. Knecht and Kozarek (42) have described a double-channel fistulotome that allows for simultaneous puncture and guidewire placement. A unique advantage of this instrument is the ability to place a stent and nasocystic catheter or two stents over separate guidewires.

Cyst resolution can be monitored by transabdominal ultrasonography (Fig. 8). Most pseudocysts will regress within 10 to 14 days, thereby extruding the stent into the visceral lumen. The stent should be retrieved after documentation of cyst decompression.

Role of Endosonography

Endosonography is an ideal tool to delineate the relationship of the pseudocyst to the bowel wall. In addition to allowing a precise measurement of the distance between the pseudocyst and visceral lumen, endosonography demonstrates the presence of interposed vessels (Fig. 9). Patients demonstrating interposed vessels should be excluded from endoscopic drainage owing to an increased risk of bleeding.

Pseudocyst puncture under endosonographic guidance is a novel application of endosonography. We recently used an echoendoscope equipped with a curved array transducer (Pentax FG-32UA) to perform a guided puncture (43). The transducer emits an image in the axis of the instrumentation plane (Fig. 10). Endo-

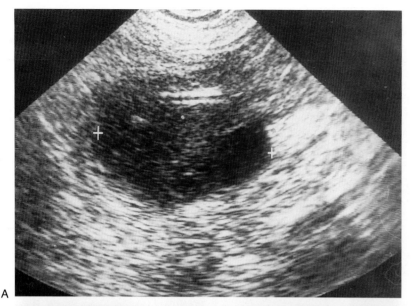

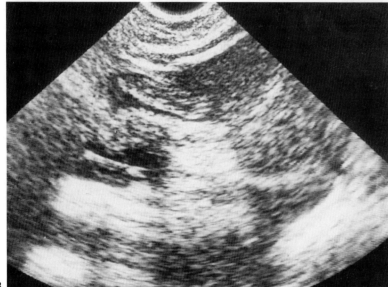

FIG. 8. Transabdominal ultrasonography. **A:** Cyst *(crossbars)* after endoscopic placement of a 10 Fr stent. **B:** The cyst has disappeared after 2 weeks of drainage.

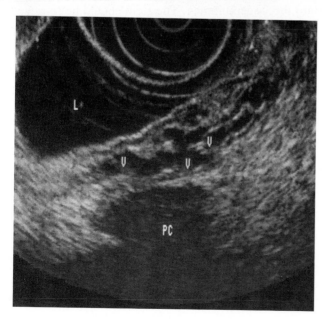

FIG. 9. Endosonography showing interposed vessels (V) between the bowel wall and pseudocyst (PC) in a patient with portal hypertension. L, lumen.

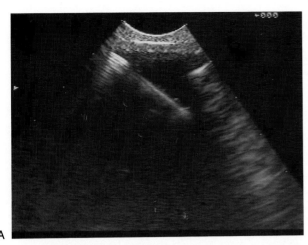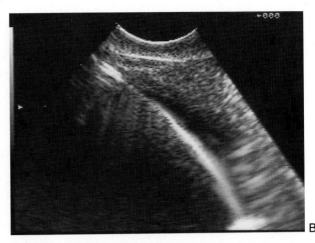

FIG. 10. Pseudocyst puncture and guidewire placement under endosonographic guidance using a curved array instrument. **A:** Needle visualized lengthwise within the pseudocyst immediately following puncture. **B:** A guidewire has replaced the needle. The echoendoscope was subsequently exchanged for a duodenoscope and a 10 Fr stent inserted over the guidewire.

sonographically guided puncture is attractive since it could improve the safety of the procedure and potentially expand the number of cases eligible for endoscopic drainage, in particular, patients who did not have endoscopic evidence of extramural bulging.

Results

Most series have shown high technical success rates resulting in cyst resolution in over 90% of patients (35–37). Bleeding has been the most common and severe complication reported. In our series of 53 patients, drainage was technically successful in 53 of 57 proce-dures followed by cyst resolution in 94% of patients (44). Over a mean follow-up of 22 months, 23% of patients had recurrences, the majority of whom were retreated endoscopically. Procedure-related complications included bleeding, pancreatitis, and gallbladder puncture in 7.5% of patients; there was no mortality. Stent clogging necessitated stent exchanges in 28% of patients and was complicated by abscess formation in two cases.

MANAGEMENT OF PANCREATIC ABSCESSES

The same technique for draining pseudocysts can be applied to the drainage of pancreatic abscesses. In ad-

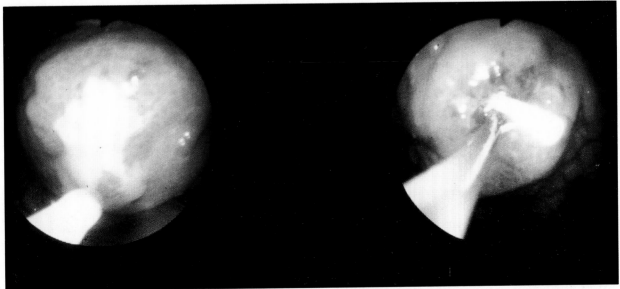

FIG. 11. Endosonographic images showing puncture of a pancreatic abscess through the duodenal wall. **A:** Pus emerging from the abscess cavity after endoscopic puncture. **B:** Placement of a nasocystic catheter (gray) alongside a 10 Fr stent (white).

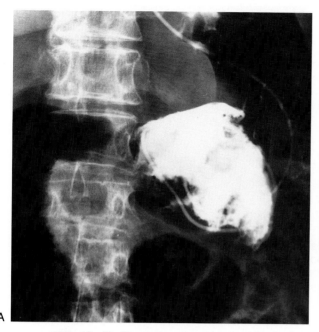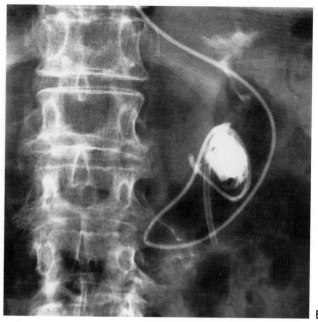

FIG. 12. Radiographs showing transgastric drainage of a pancreatic abscess. **A:** Contrast medium filling of the large abscess cavity immediately following endoscopic insertion of a nasocystic catheter and 10-Fr stent. **B:** Marked reduction in the size of the abscess cavity after 1 week of irrigation and drainage. Stent and nasocystic catheter in position.

dition to a 10 Fr stent, a 7 Fr nasocystic catheter is inserted into the abscess cavity for periodic saline irrigation and antibiotic instillation (Figs. 11 and 12). The nasocystic catheter is withdrawn after 5 to 7 days. We have treated ten patients with pancreatic abscesses (mean size 8.8 cm, range 5–20) by endoscopic drainage; abscesses completely resolved after a mean of 33 days in eight patients (43).

Sealants for Pancreatic Ductal Disruptions

We have been using fibrin glue (Tissucol, Immuno, Heidelberg, Germany; Behriplast, Behringwerke AG, Marburg, Germany) and the cyanoacrylate tissue adhesive Histoacryl (Histoacryl Blau, Braun, Melsungen, Germany) to seal pancreatic ductal disruptions and fistulas refractory to standard drainage procedures (44). The sealant is retrogradely instilled through a catheter whose tip is positioned at the site of the leak or fistulous opening. A theoretical advantage of using Histoacryl is that the fistula is immediately and permanently occluded with a single treatment, whereas fibrin glue application may take several sessions to achieve an effective seal. We have not observed any adverse reactions associated with Histoacryl application for this indication.

CONCLUSION

The novel endoscopic treatments for chronic pancreatitis are technically feasible, appear to be reasonably

safe, and provide substantial relief of pain in the majority of patients. Hence, endoscopic pancreatic drainage may be an acceptable alternative to surgery, particularly in patients who are at higher operative risk. Some patients may prefer this alternative, with the option of surgery if treatment fails. Further, endoscopic management may help select those patients most likely to benefit from surgical management. The ideal patient for endoscopic treatment has yet to be defined. Future endeavors should include prospective trials using objective criteria for treatment benefit (including long-term) and randomized trials comparing endoscopic and surgical treatment.

REFERENCES

1. Ebbehj N, Borly L, Matzen P, Svendsen LB. Pancreatic tissue pressure and pain in chronic pancreatitis. *Pancreas* 1986;1:556–558.
2. Okazaki K, Yamamoto Y, Kagiyama S, Tamura S, Sakamoto Y, Nakazama, et al. Pressure of papillary sphincter zone and pancreatic main duct in patients with chronic pancreatitis in the early stage.
3. Frey CF, Suzuki M, Isaji S, Zhu Y. Pancreatic resection for chronic pancreatitis. *Surg Clin North Am* 1989;69:499.
4. Prinz RA, Greenlee H. Pancreatic duct drainage in 100 patients with chronic pancreatitis. *Ann Surg* 1981;194:313–320.
5. Tiscorna OM, Dreiling DA. Recovery of pancreatic exocrine secretory capacity following prolonged ductal obstruction: bicarbonate and amylase response to hormonal stimulation. *Ann Surg* 1966;164:267.
6. White TT, Magee DF. Recovery of pancreatic exocrine function after controlled duct obstruction. *Surg Gynecol Obstet* 1962;144:463.

7. Karanjia ND, Widdison AL, Leung FW, Lutrin FJ, Reber HA. The effect of decompression of the main pancreatic duct on pancreatic blood flow in chronic pancreatitis. *Pancreas* 1990;3:713.
8. Widdison AL, Alvariz C, Karanjia ND, Reber A. Experimental evidence of beneficial effects of ductal decompression in chronic pancreatitis. *Endoscopy* 1991;23:151–154.
9. Nealson WH, Townsend CM, Thompson JC. Operative drainage of the pancreatic duct delays functional impairment in patients with chronic pancreatitis: a prospective analysis. *Ann Surg* 1988; 208:321–329.
10. Amman RW, Muench R, Otto R, Buehler H, Freiburghaus AU, Siegenthaler W. Evolution and regression of pancreatic calcification in chronic pancreatitis. *Gastroenterology* 1988;95: 1018–1028.
11. Fuji T, Amano H, Ohmura R, Akiyama T, Aibe T, Takemoto T. Endoscopic pancreatic sphincterotomy-technique and evaluation. *Endoscopy* 1989;21:27–30.
12. Cremer M, Deviere J, Delhaye M, Baize M, Vandermeeren A. Stenting in severe chronic pancreatitis: results of medium-term follow-up in 76 patients. *Endoscopy* 1991;23:171–176.
13. Huibregtse K, Schneider B, Vrij AA, Tytgat GNJ. Endoscopic pancreatic drainage in chronic pancreatitis. *Gastrointest Endosc* 1988;34:9–15.
14. McCarthy J, Geenen JE, Hogan WJ. Preliminary experience with endoscopic stent placement in benign pancreatic diseases. *Gastrointest Endosc* 1988;34:16–18.
15. Kozarek RA, Patterson DJ, Ball TJ, Traverso LW. Endoscopic placement of pancreatic stents and drains in the management of pancreatitis. *Ann Surg* 1989;209:261–266.
16. Grimm H, Meyer WH, Nam V Ch, Soehendra N. New modalities for treating chronic pancreatitis. *Endoscopy* 1989;21:70–74.
17. Binmoeller KF, Jue P, Seifert H, Soehendra N. Endoscopic stent drainage for chronic pain in patients with chronic pancreatitis and a dominant stricture: long term results. *Gastrointest Endosc* 1994;40:A100.
18. McCarthy JH, Geenan JE. Pancreatic stents and post ERCP pancreatitis. *Gastrointest Endosc* 1990;36:A201.
19. Provansal-Cheylan M, Bernard JP, Mariani A, et al. Occluded pancreatic endoprostheses-analysis of the clogging material. *Endoscopy* 1989;21:63.
20. Geenen JE, Rolny P. Endoscopic therapy of acute and chronic pancreatitis. *Gastrointest Endosc* 1991;37:377–382.
21. Siegel J, Veerappan A. Endoscopic management of pancreatic disorders: potential risks of pancreatic prostheses. *Endoscopy* 1991;23:77–80.
22. Soehendra N, Maydeo A, Eckmann B, Brückner M, Nam V Ch, Grimm H. A new technique for replacing an obstructed biliary endoprosthesis. *Endoscopy* 1990;22:271–272.
23. Waxman I, Fockens P, Huibregtse K, Tytgat GNJ. Removal of a broken pancreatic stent using a new stent retrieval device. *Gastrointest Endosc* 1991;37:631–632.
24. Kozarek RA. Pancreatic stents can induce ductal changes consistent with chronic pancreatitis. *Gastrointest Endosc* 1990;36: 93–95.
25. Derfus GA, Geenen JE, Hogan WJ. Effect of endoscope pancreatic duct stent placement on pancreatic ductal morphology. *Gastrointest Endosc* 1990;36:206A.
26. Soehendra N, Kempeneers I, Nam V Ch, Grimm H. Endoscopic drainage and papillotomy of the accessory papilla and internal drainage in pancreas divisum. *Endoscopy* 1986;18:129–132.
27. Siegel JH, Ben-Zvi JS, Pullano W, Cooperman A. Effectiveness of endoscopic drainage for pancreas divisum: endoscopic and surgical results in 31 patients. *Endoscopy* 1990;22:129–133.
28. Lans JI, Geenen JE, Johanson JF, Hogan WJ. Endoscopic therapy in patients with pancreas divisum and acute pancreatitis: a prospective, randomized, controlled clinical trial. *Gastrointest Endosc* 1992;38:430–434.
29. Lehman GA, Sherman S, Nisi R, Hawes RH. Pancreas divisum: results of minor papilla sphincterotomy. *Gastrointest Endosc* 1993;39:1–8.
30. Sherman S, Lehman GA, Hawes RH, Ponich T, Miller LS, Cohen LB, Kortan P, Haber GB. Pancreatic ductal stones: frequency of successful endoscopic removal and improvement in symptoms. *Gastrointest Endosc* 1991;37:511–516.
31. Delhaye M, Vandermeeren A, Gabbrielli A, Cremer MP. Lithotripsy and endoscopy for pancreatic calculi: the first 104 patients. *Gastroenterology* 1990;98:A216.
32. Neuhaus H. Fragmentation of pancreatic stones by extracorporeal shock wave lithotripsy. *Endoscopy* 1991;23:161–165.
33. Sauerbruch T, Holl J, Sackmann M, Paumgartner G. Extracorporeal lithotripsy of pancreatic stones in patients with chronic pancreatitis and pain: a prospective follow up study. *Gut* 1992; 33:969–972.
34. Renner IG. Laser fragmentation of pancreatic stones. *Endoscopy* 1991;23:166–170.
35. Neuhaus H, Hoffmann W, Classen M. Laser lithotripsy of pancreatic and biliary stones via 3.4 mm and 3.7 mm miniscopes: first clinical results. *Endoscopy* 1992;24:208–214.
36. Kozarek RA, Brayko CM, Harlan J, Sanowski RA, Cintora I, Kovac I. Endoscopic drainage of pancreatic pseudocysts. *Gastrointest Endosc* 1985;31:322–328.
37. Cremer M, Deviere J, Engelholm L. Endoscopic management of cysts and pseudocysts in chronic pancreatitis: long-term follow-up after 7 years of experience. *Gastrointest Endosc* 1989; 35:1–9.
38. Sahel J. Endoscopic drainage of pancreatic cysts. *Endoscopy* 1991;23:181–184.
39. Buchi KN, Bowers JH, Dixon JA. Endoscopic pancreatic cystogastrostomy using Nd:Yag laser. *Gastrointest Endosc* 1986; 32:112.
40. Binmoeller KF, Seifert H, Soehendra N. Endoscopic pseudocyst drainage: a new instrument for simplified cystenterostomy. *Gastrointest Endosc* 1994;40:112.
41. Cremer M, Deviere J, Baize M, Matos C. New device for endoscopic cystoenterostomy. *Endoscopy* 1990;22:76–77.
42. Knecht GL, Kozarek RA. Double-channel fistulotome for endoscopic drainage of pancreatic pseudocyst. *Gastrointest Endosc* 1991;37:356–357.
43. Grimm H, Binmoeller KF, Soehendra N. Endosonography-guided drainage of a pancreatic pseudocyst. *Gastrointest Endosc* 1992;38:170–171.
44. Binmoeller KF, Walter A, Seifert H, Soehendra N. Endoscopic stenting for pancreatic pseudocyts in 53 patients. *Gastrointest Endosc* 1993;39:A308.
45. Binmoeller KF, Walter A, Seifert H, Soehendra N. Endoscopic therapy for pancreatic abscesses. *Gastrointest Endosc* 1993;39: A308.
46. Brückner M, Grimmn H, Nam VC, Soehendra N. Endoscopic treatment of a pancreatic abscess originating from biliary pancreatitis. *Surg Endosc* 1990;4:227–229.

Advanced Therapeutic Endoscopy, 2nd Ed.,
edited by J. S. Barkin and C. A. O'Phelan.
Raven Press, Ltd., New York © 1994.

CHAPTER 48

Endoscopic Drainage of Pancreatic Pseudocysts

Richard Kozarek

Pancreatic pseudocysts are formed as a consequence of pancreatic ductal disruption with or without subsequent enzyme activation (1,2). Widespread application of abdominal ultrasound and computed tomography (CT) have demonstrated the development and variable resolution of most pancreatic fluid collections (3,4). Nonresolving cysts 6 cm or larger, enlarging pseudocysts, symptomatic pseudocysts, or those that develop the complications of bleeding, perforation, infection, or concomitant organ obstruction (stomach or bile duct) have traditionally undergone surgical intervention (5,6). The latter include internal drainage (cystgastrostomy, cystenterostomy), external drainage, or resective therapy. More recently, interventional radiologists have approached pseudocysts with percutaneous drainage in conjunction with chronic catheter placement (3,6). Results of surgical or radiologic drainage are in part institutionally defined and also dependent on whether the pseudocyst develops in the setting of acute or chronic pancreatitis and whether proximal duct obstruction or discontinuity is present.

In general, multiple series suggest that the majority of pseudocysts can be handled with either of these techniques, that operative and tube related complications approximate 30%, and that 10% to 30% of these cysts will recur (3–9). These are the data that must be considered when reviewing series reporting the endoscopic drainage of pseudocysts.

FISTULIZATION

Technique

Pancreatic pseudocysts can be drained either by creating a fistula through the gut wall (10) or by placing

R. Kozarek: Department of Medicine, University of Washington, and Department of Gastroenterology, Virginia Mason Clinic, Seattle, Washington 98111.

a drain or stent through the papilla (11), but either technique should be preceded by a diagnostic endoscopic retrograde cholangiopancreatography (ERCP) and antibiotic coverage. The former procedure requires an amenable anatomy with an extrinsic bulge on the posterior gastric wall or medial wall of the duodenum. Moreover, less than 1 cm of intervening tissue to incise through and the absence of gastric varices at the incision site have been previous prerequisites in my practice. This has been traditionally defined by CT imaging, although endoscopic ultrasonography is probably a more sensitive diagnostic tool.

The incision itself is undertaken utilizing a needle-knife sphincterotome placed through a therapeutic duodenoscope. I currently utilize a sphincterotome that allows placement of two guidewires through auxiliary channels in the sphincterotome sheath, thereby assuring continued cyst access (12). Cauterization is done with a blended current approximating 40 W and is associated with a sudden "give" and gush of fluid upon cyst entry. At this point, I remove the needle from the sphincterotome, inject contrast, and pass guidewires into the now defined cyst cavity. In the past, most practitioners would extend the poke hole by using a conventional sphincterotome to enlarge either the cystgastrostomy or cystduodenostomy. I would discourage this practice as both bleeding and perforation are possible. Instead, I currently place one or two 10-Fr, 3-cm double-pigtail endoprostheses across the gut wall to maintain chronic drainage and usually place a nasocyst drainage catheter to allow aspiration of cyst fluid for Gram stain, amylase measurements, and culture and sensitivity. The latter catheter, usually removed in 24 to 48 hours, also allows access for contrast studies and assurance of cyst decompression (Fig. 1). I currently retrieve the transgastric or duodenal prostheses after 6 to 8 weeks and invariably the only remaining cavity approximates the diameter of the stent's pigtail.

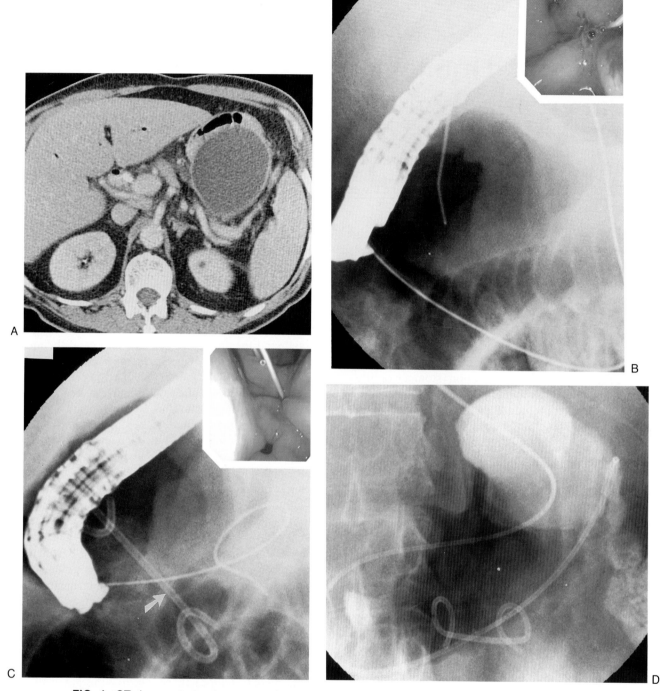

FIG. 1. CT demonstrates large pseudocyst compressing gastric wall **(A)**. Guidewire placement **(B)** into pseudocyst cavity following transgastric fistulization. A 10-Fr double-pigtail stent *(arrow)* placed through gastric wall to drain pseudocyst **(C)** followed by insertion of nasocyst drain into retroperitoneum **(D)**. Latter is usually retrieved after 24 to 48 hours.

Results

In the largest series reported to date, Sahel (13) utilized transduodenal or transgastric fistulization to drain 52 pseudocysts in 46 patients. Two patients had obstructing tumors, 9 acute pancreatitis, and 35 had pseudocysts in conjunction with chronic pancreatitis. He was successful in diverting cyst contents into the upper gastrointestinal tract in 88.5% (46/52) of patients. Complications occurred in 13% (6/46) of the patients and included retroperitoneal perforations early in the author's experience. Other complications included one instance of pseudocyst infection and two cases of bleeding, one of which resulted in the patient's death.

Sahel (14) has subsequently updated his experience utilizing this technique in pseudocysts associated with chronic pancreatitis. Complete cyst resolution was effected in 27 of 36 patients acutely and 4 had partial resolution. In patients followed up for 6 months or longer, 19 of 22 had not recurred while 2 continued to have small pseudocysts. Two patients died in this series, including 1 who developed acute mesenteric infarction.

Two other large series of endoscopic pseudocyst drainage have been reported using this technique. Fröschle et al. (8) undertook endoscopic drainage in 35 patients, reporting a 0% mortality. Cremer et al. (15), in turn, described 33 patients who underwent successful fistulization through the duodenal wall (21 of 22) or stomach (11 of 11). Three complications occurred and included 1 case of pseudocyst infection, 1 instance of bleeding, and 1 case of retroperitonitis. All responded to conservative measures. A 9% recurrence rate was noted following cystduodenostomy and a 19% rate after cystgastrostomy, suggesting either ongoing ductal disruption or early fistula closure.

Additional case reports or small series have been reported by Knecht and Kozarek (12), Kozarek et al. (10), Grimm et al. (16,17), Grewal et al. (18), and Huibregtse et al. (19), as well as additional authors.

TRANSPAPILLARY DRAINS

Technique

In addition to fistulization through the stomach or duodenal wall, pseudocysts can also be drained utilizing transpapillary drains or stents (11,19,20). The latter technique requires diagnostic ERCP to delineate the site of ductal disruption, and with smaller pseudocysts, transpapillary passage of a nasocyst drain directly into the fluid collection (Fig. 2). Alternatively, ductal disruptions can be directly bridged with endoprostheses. Currently, I undertake diagnostic ERCP after antibiotic precoverage and utilize an 0.035-inch nitinol wire (Tracer, Wilson-Cook, Inc., Winston-Salem, NC) to access either the cyst or distal pancreatic duct (Fig. 3). Large cysts are initially decompressed with a 6- to 7-Fr drain for 2 to 3 days after which the ductal disruption is bridged with 5 to 10 Fr endoprostheses. The diameter of the latter is contingent upon pancreatic ductal diameter and care should be taken not to select a stent that occludes multiple ductal side branches (Fig. 4). The latter has been associated with induction of pancreatic ductal changes that radiographically resemble chronic pancreatitis (21). Such changes, while usually reversible several months post-stent retrieval, can at times be permanent. Indwelling endoprostheses should

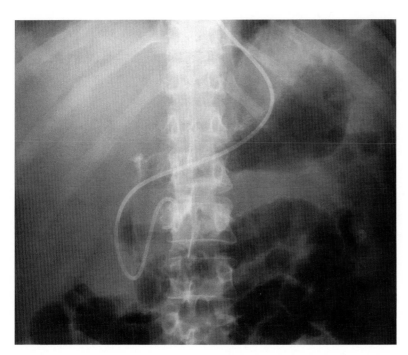

FIG. 2. Transduodenal nasocyst drain inserted into pseudocyst cavity compressing medial duodenal wall.

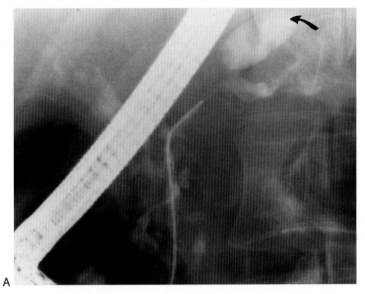 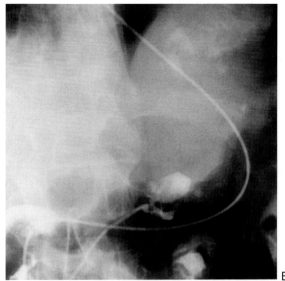

A

B

FIG. 3. A: Guidewire in disrupted pancreatic duct in patient who presented with pancreatitis/splenic flexure ischemia. Note small pseudocyst *(arrow)* **B:** Transpapillary nasocyst drain in patient depicted in A. Patient had dramatic resolution of clinical symptoms/ultimate distal pancreatectomy.

therefore be used with caution in patients with otherwise normal ductal systems, particularly with disruptions in the tail of the gland. Nor should small caliber endoprostheses be placed directly in large cysts with phlegmonous changes, as early occlusion and subsequent abscess formation have been reported (19).

Once a stent has been utilized to bridge a ductal disruption, I currently assure cyst decompression with ultrasound or abdominal CT in several weeks, retrieving the endoprosthesis at 4 to 6 weeks. A repeat diagnostic ERCP is done at this time to assure that residual ductal disruption is not present, which may potentially require surgery.

Results

Although there have been small series reported by Grimm et al. (16) and Huibregtse et al. (19), the largest

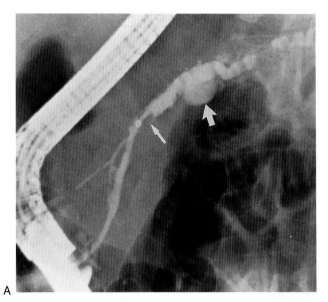 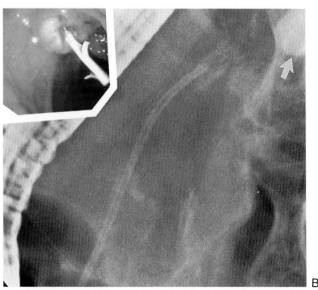

A

B

FIG. 4. A: Small pseudocyst *(large arrow)* in patient with chronic pancreatitis Patient has undergone pancreatic duct (PD) sphincterotomy and stone retrieval. **B:** Note balloon *(small arrow)* at genu. PD stent placement in patient depicted in A. Pseudocyst resolution by 4 weeks despite failure to pass stent beyond cyst *(arrow).*

experience to date has been reported by our group (11). In the latter series, 17 cases of ductal disruption, including 9 patients with severe acute and 8 patients with chronic pancreatitis, underwent transpapillary drain or stent placement. Technically, all procedures were successful and 12 of 14 fluid collections resolved completely. Complications included pseudocyst infection in one patient and stent occlusion with recurrent cyst formation in another. Both complications resolved with stent exchange. Two-thirds of patients ultimately avoided surgery following endoprostheses placement and an additional one-third exchanged urgent surgical intervention for an elective procedure.

PERSPECTIVE

While endoscopic drainage of pancreatic pseudocysts is technically feasible both by fistulization through the gut wall and by transpapillary drain or stent placement, utilization of these techniques must be placed in the perspective of the clinical situation as well as local technical expertise. For instance, small transgastric or transduodenal stents may be inadequate to drain large compartmentalized pseudocysts or fluid collections that contain copious debris. Nor is it possible to safely fistulize through several centimeters of intervening tissue or drain fluid collections through the papilla if no ductal communication persists. In such instances, percutaneous drainage with the advantage of external catheter access or even surgery may be required. Given the foregoing, the endoscopic approach to pancreatic fluid collections is applicable in a subset of patients only. These techniques are currently utilized in approximately one-third of all cysts drained at our institution.

REFERENCES

1. Bank S. Clinical pancreatitis: clinical features and medical management. *Am J Gastroenterol* 1986;81:153–167.
2. Kolars JC, O'Connor-Allen AM, Ansel H, et al. Pancreatic pseudocysts: clinical and endoscopic experience. *Am J Gastroenterol* 1989;84:259–264.
3. Gumaste UV, Dave PB. Pancreatic pseudocyst drainage—the needle or the scalpel? [Editorial]. *J Clin Gastroenterol* 1991;13:500–505.
4. Walt AJ, Bowman DL, Weaver DW, Sachs RJ. The impact of technology on the management of pancreatic pseudocyst. *Arch Surg* 1990;125:759–763.
5. Williams KJ, Fabian TC. Pancreatic pseudocyst: recommendations for operative and nonoperative management. *Am Surg* 1992;58:199–205.
6. Adams DB, Anderson MC. Changing concepts in the surgical management of pancreatic pseudocysts. *Am Surg* 1992;58:173–180.
7. Köhler H, Schafmayer A, Lüdtke FE, et al. Surgical treatment of pancreatic pseudocysts. *Br J Surg* 1987;74:813–815.
8. Fröschle G, Henne-Bruns D, Kremer B, Grimm H. Pancreatic pseudocysts and their interdisciplinary therapy. *Zentralbl Chir* 1991;116:359–368.
9. Duclos B, Loeb C, Jung-Chaigneau E, et al. Non-surgical treatment of cysts and pseudocysts of the pancreas. A study of a series of 33 cases. *Ann Gastroenterol Hepatol* 1991;27:1–5.
10. Kozarek RA, Brayko CM, Harlan J, et al. Endoscopic drainage of pancreatic pseudocysts. *Gastrointest Endosc* 1985;31:322–328.
11. Kozarek RA, Ball TJ, Patterson DJ, et al. Endoscopic transpapillary therapy for disrupted pancreatic duct and peripancreatic fluid collections. *Gastroenterology* 1991;100:1362–1370.
12. Knecht GL, Kozarek RA. Double-channel fistulotome for endoscopic drainage of pancreatic pseudocyst. *Gastrointest Endosc* 1991;37:356–357.
13. Sahel J. Endoscopic cyst gastrostomy and cyst duodenostomy of pancreatic cysts and pseudocysts. *Dig Endosc* 1990;2:218–223.
14. Sahel J. Endoscopic drainage of pancreatic cysts. *Endoscopy* 1991;23:181–184.
15. Cremer M, Devière J, Engelholm L. Endoscopic management of cysts and pseudocysts in chronic pancreatitis: long-term follow-up after 7 years of experience. *Gastrointest Endosc* 1989;35:1–9.
16. Grimm H, Meyer W-H, Nam V Ch, Soehendra N. New modalities for treating chronic pancreatitis. *Endoscopy* 1989;21:70–74.
17. Grimm H, Binmoeller KF, Soehendra N. Endosonography-guided drainage of a pancreatic pseudocyst. *Gastrointest Endosc* 1992;38:170–171.
18. Grewal HP, London NJ, Carr-Locke D, Wood KF. Endoscopic drainage of a recurrent pancreatic pseudocyst. *Postgrad Med J* 1990;66:1081–1083.
19. Huibregtse K, Schneider B, Vrij AA, et al. Endoscopic pancreatic drainage in chronic pancreatitis. *Gastrointest Endosc* 1988;34:9–15.
20. Kozarek RA, Patterson DJ, Ball TJ, Traverso LW. Endoscopic placement of pancreatic drains and stents in the management of pancreatitis. *Ann Surg* 1989;209:261–266.
21. Kozarek RA. Pancreatic stents can induce ductal changes consistent with chronic pancreatitis. *Gastrointest Endosc* 1990;36:93–95.

Subject Index